CLINICAL MANIFESTATIONS
& ASSESSMENT OF
RESPIRATORY DISEASE

Clinical Manifestations & Assessment of Respiratory Disease

TERRY DES JARDINS, M.Ed., R.R.T.

Director
Department of Respiratory Care
Parkland College
Champaign, Illinois

GEORGE G. BURTON, M.D., FACP, FCCP

Medical Director, Respiratory Services
Kettering Medical Center, Kettering, Ohio
Clinical Professor of Medicine and Anesthesiology
Wright State University School of Medicine
Dayton, Ohio

MEDICAL ILLUSTRATIONS BY

TIMOTHY H. PHELPS, M.S., FAMI, CMI

Associate Professor
Johns Hopkins University School of Medicine
Baltimore, Maryland

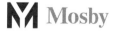 Mosby

St. Louis Baltimore Boston Carlsbad Chicago Naples New York Philadelphia Portland
London Madrid Mexico City Singapore Sydney Tokyo Toronto Wiesbaden

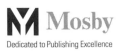

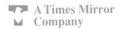

A Times Mirror
Company

Editor: James F. Shanahan
Developmental Editors: Anne Gleason/Jennifer Roche
Project Manager: Mark Spann
Senior Production Editor: Jerry Schwartz
Designer: David Zielinski
Manufacturing Supervisor: Theresa Fuchs

Printed in the United States of America
Composition by Clarinda Company
Printing/binding by Maple-Vail

Mosby–Year Book, Inc.
11830 Westline Industrial Drive
St. Louis, Missouri 63146

ISBN 0-8016-7988-5

95 96 97 98 99 / 9 8 7 6 5 4 3 2 1

To Jane, Jennifer and Michelle,
and to Uncle Jim and Janelle
and
To all the past, present and future
students of respiratory care

To cease smoking is the easiest thing I ever did.
I ought to know because I've done it a thousand times.
Mark Twain

PREFACE

The use of *therapist-driven protocols* (TDPs) is mounting and will soon be an integral part of respiratory health services. TDPs provide much-needed flexibility to respiratory care practitioners and increase the quality of health care, as therapy can be more easily and efficiently modified according to the needs of the patient. Core to the success of TDPs is the quality of the respiratory therapist's *assessment skills* at the bedside and the ability to transfer findings into a plan of treatment that follows agreed-upon guidelines. The respiratory care practitioner must be able to recognize when physician and patient-specific severity indicators have been reached or exceeded and must be able to communicate such concerns to those physicians and other health care workers who appropriately need to hear them.

This textbook is designed to provide the student with the basic knowledge and understanding essential to assess and treat patients with repiratory disease. To meet this objective, the reader is provided with (1) a detailed illustration (both in color and in black and white) of the major *anatomic alterations* of the lungs (or related anatomic structures) caused by the respiratory disorder, (2) the *pathophysiologic mechanisms* that are most commonly activated as a result of the anatomic alterations, (3) an overview of the cardiopulmonary *clinical manifestations* caused by the pathophysiologic mechanics, and (4) the various *treatment modalities* used to offset the clinical manifestations caused by the anatomic alterations and pathophysiologic mechanisms.

Additionally, the student is provided with the basic knowledge and helpful clinical tools to (1) *systematically* gather clinical data, (2) formulate an *assessment* (i.e., the cause of the clinical data), (3) select an appropriate *treatment plan,* and (4) *document* these three essential steps in a clear, precise manner. In writing this textbook, care has been taken to present a realistic balance between the esoteric language of pathophysiology and the simple, straight-to-the-point approach generally preferred by busy students. We have added new features to this edition, including a set of **full-color plates** that allow the reader to see another view of each pathophysiologic state included in the text, and a complete set of brand-new **case studies** that will aid both students *and* instructors in applying the fundamental information covered in this text to the assessment and treatment of respiratory patients. This skill will be more valuable to future respiratory practitioners than ever before.

Terry Des Jardins
George G. Burton

ACKNOWLEDGMENTS

A number of people provided important contributions to the development of the third edition of this textbook. Initially, it is with great pleasure that I welcome George G. Burton, M.D., as a coauthor. Dr. Burton's contributions have been invaluable—especially in regard to (1) the importance of "assessment skills" in the implementation of therapist-driven respiratory care protocols (criteria-based respiratory care), and (2) the demonstration (in the case studies) of how the clinical manifestations presented by the patient suffering from the respiratory disorder under discussion can be systemically collected, organized, assessed, and documented to justify the respiratory care protocols activated.

For his excellent work and extensive amount of time in the (1) initial development of the case study scenarios, (2) reading and editing the assessment portions of the case studies, and (3) reading and editing the respiratory disease chapters, a sincere thank you goes to Dr. Thomas DeKornfeld.

For help in obtaining information regarding various clinical laboratory tests and normal laboratory value ranges, a sincere thank you goes to Marc Des Jardins, M.T., A.S.C.P., and Patricia McKenzie, M.T., A.S.C.P., Chelsea Hospital, Michigan. A special thank you also goes to Judy Tietsort, R.N., R.R.T., Lutheran Medical Center, and Lucy Kester, M.B.A., R.R.T., The Cleveland Clinic Foundation, for their helpful suggestions regarding the (1) respiratory assessment flow chart, and (2) respiratory assessment guide (card) presented in Chapter 3. These assessment tools will, undoubtedly, enhance the respiratory care practitioners' systematic collection, assessment, and documentation of clinical data—the foundation of respiratory care protocols.

Finally, but certainly by no means least, a very special thank you goes to Tim Phelps, Johns Hopkins Hospital, for his wonderful artwork. Tim's renderings of each disease entity presented in the textbook—both in color and black and white—are outstanding.

Terry Des Jardins

HOW TO USE THIS BOOK

Part I, entitled *Assessment Skills As Core To Practitioner Success,* consists of chapters 1, 2, and 3. Collectively, these chapters provide the reader with

1. *the basic skills involved in the patient interview,*
2. *the pathophysiologic basis for the common clinical manifestations associated with respiratory disease,*
3. *the essentials of radiography,*
4. *the fundamentals for collecting and recording the assessment data essential for critical thinking skills.*

In subsequent chapters on the various respiratory diseases, the student is often referred back to Chapter 1 to supplement the discussion on the clinical manifestations commonly associated with each specific disease. For example, Chapter 1 describes the known pathophysiologic mechanisms responsible for the following clinical manifestations associated with respiratory diseases:

- Abnormal chest assessment findings
- Abnormal ventilatory pattern findings
- Abnormal pulmonary function study findings
- Pursed-lip breathing
- Increased anteroposterior chest diameter (barrel chest)
- Use of accessory muscles of inspiration
- Use of accessory muscles of expiration
- Abnormal arterial blood gas findings
- Cyanosis
- Abnormal oxygenation indices
- Abnormal cardiovascular system findings
- Increased central venous pressure/decreased systemic blood pressure
- Polycythemia, cor pulmonale
- Digital clubbing
- Cough, sputum production, and hemoptysis
- Substernal/intercostal retraction
- Chest pain/decreased expansion
- Abnormal hematology, blood chemistry, and electrolyte findings
- Abnormal bronchoscopy findings

Chapters 4 through 31 provide the reader with the essential information regarding common respiratory diseases. Basically, each chapter on a specific respiratory disorder adheres to the following format: anatomic alterations of the lungs, etiology of the disease process, overview of the cardiopulmonary clinical manifestations associated with the disorder, general management of the disorder, case study, and a set of self-assessment questions.

Anatomic Alterations of the Lungs

Each chapter on respiratory disease begins with a detailed illustration showing the anatomic alterations of the lungs caused by the disease. While serious efforts have been made to illustrate each disorder accurately at the beginning of each chapter, artistic license has been taken to emphasize certain anatomic points and pathologic processes.

The subsequent material in each chapter discusses the disease in terms of (1) the *anatomic alterations of the lungs* caused by the disease, (2) the *pathophysiologic mechanisms* activated throughout the respiratory system as a result of the anatomic alterations, (3) the *clinical manifestations* that develop as a result of the pathophysiologic mechanisms, and (4) the basic *respiratory therapy modalities* used to improve the anatomic alterations and pathophysiologic mechanisms caused by the disease. When the anatomic alterations and pathophysiologic mechanisms caused by the disorder are improved, the clinical manifestations should also improve.

Etiology

A discussion of the etiology of the disease follows the presentation of anatomic alterations of the lungs.

Overview of the Cardiopulmonary Clinical Manifestations Associated with the Disorder

The section represents the central theme of the text. The reader is provided with the *clinical manifestations* commonly associated with the disease under discussion. In essence, the student is given a general "baseline" of the *signs* and *symptoms* commonly demonstrated by the patient.

By having a working knowledge—and predetermined expectation—of the clinical manifestations associated with a specific respiratory disorder, the practitioner is in a better position to (1) gather clinical data that is relevant to the patient's respiratory status, (2) formulate an objective—and measurable—assessment, and (3) select an effective and safe treatment plan that is based on a valid assessment. If the appropriate clinical data is not gathered and assessed correctly, the ability to effectively treat the patient is lost.

Many of the clinical manifestations listed refer the reader back to specific pages in Chapter 1 for a broader discussion of the pathophysiologic mechanisms usually responsible for the identified sign or symptom. When a particular clinical manifestation is unique to the respiratory disorder, however, a discussion of the pathophysiologic mechanisms responsible for the sign or symptom is presented in this section.

Because of the dynamic nature of many respiratory disorders, the reader should note the following regarding this section:

1. Because the severity of the disease is influenced by a number of factors (e.g., magnitude of the diseases, age, or general health of the patient), the clinical manifestations may vary remarkably from one patient to another. In fact, the clinical manifestations may vary in the same patient from one time to another. Thus, it should be understood that the patient may demonstrate *all* the clinical manifestations presented, or just a *few*. In addition, many of the clinical manifestations that are associated with a respiratory disorder may never appear in some patients (e.g., digital clubbing, cor pulmonale, or an increased hemoglobin level). As a general rule, however, the patient usually demonstrates most of the clinical manifestations presented during the advanced stages of the disease.
2. Some of the clinical manifestations presented in this section may not actually be measured in the clinical setting for a variety of practical reasons (e.g., age, mental status, or severity of the disorder). They are, nevertheless, considered important and, thus, are presented through extrapolation. For example, the newborn with severe

infant respiratory distress syndrome, who obviously has a restrictive lung disorder as a result of the anatomic alterations associated with the disease, cannot actually perform the necessary maneuvers necessary for a pulmonary function study.

3. It should also be noted that the clinical manifestations presented in this text are only based on the respiratory disorder under discussion. In the clinical setting, the patient often has a combination of respiratory problems, e.g., emphysema compromised by pneumonia. When such a condition exists, the patient will likely present with clinical manifestations related to both pulmonary disorders.

Finally, this section does not attempt to present the "absolute" pathophysiologic bases for the development of a particular clinical manifestation. Again, because of the dynamic nature of many respiratory diseases, the precise cause of some of the clinical manifestations presented by the patient is not always clear. In most cases, however, the pathophysiologic mechanisms responsible for the various signs and symptoms associated with a specific respiratory disorder are known and understood.

General Management or Treatment of the Disease

Each chapter provides an overview of the general management or treatment of the disease. It is not the intent of this text to provide a comprehensive section concerning the management of respiratory disorders. Several excellent textbooks dealing with the subject matter already exist. A general overview of the more common therapeutic modalities used to offset the anatomic alterations and pathophysiologic mechanisms activated by a particular disorder are presented.

It should be stressed that while several respiratory therapy modalities may be safe and effective in treating a respiratory disorder, the respiratory care practitioner must have a clear conception of the following:

1. *How the therapies work to offset the anatomic alterations of the lung caused by the disease*
2. *How the correction of the anatomic alterations of the lung work to offset the pathophysiologic mechanisms*
3. *How the correction of the pathophysiologic mechanisms work to offset the clinical manifestations demonstrated by the patient*

Without the above understanding, the respiratory therapist merely goes through the motions of administering the therapeutic tasks—with no anticipated outcomes that can be measured.

Case Study

The case study provides the reader with a realistic example of (1) the manner in which the patient may present in the hospital with the disorder under discussion, (2) the various clinical manifestations commonly associated with the disease, (3) how the clinical manifestations can be gathered and organized, (4) how an assessment of the patient's respiratory status is formulated from the clinical manifestations, and (5) how the treatment plan is developed from the assessment.

In essence, the case study provides the reader with an example of how the respiratory care practitioner would likely *assess and treat* a patient with the disorder under discussion. In addition, many of the case studies presented in the text *assess and treat* the patient several times, demonstrating (1) the importance of assessment skills, and (2) how therapy is often *up-regulated* or *down-regulated* on a moment-to-moment basis in the clinical setting.

Self-Assessment Questions

Each respiratory disease chapter concludes with a set of self-assessment questions. The student may be asked questions from (1) the disease chapter under discussion, or (2) the appendixes which often provide a broader discussion of the various treatment modalities commonly used to manage the disease under discussion.

Glossary and Appendixes

Finally, a glossary and appendixes are provided at the end of the text. The appendixes include the following:

- A table of symbols and abbreviations commonly used in respiratory physiology
- Medications commonly used in the treatment of cardiopulmonary disorders, including:
  - Sympathomimetic agents
  - Parasympatholytic (anticholinergic) agents
  - Xanthine bronchodilators
  - Corticosteroids
  - Mucolytic agents
  - Expectorants
  - Antibiotic agents
  - Positive inotropic agents
  - Diuretics
- Therapeutic procedures used to mobilize bronchial secretions
- Hyperinflation therapy procedures
- The ideal alveolar gas equation
- Physiologic dead space calculation
- Units of measurement
- Poiseuille's law for flow and pressure
- $P_{CO_2}/HCO_3^-/pH$ Nomogram
- Calculated hemodynamic measurements
- DuBois body surface chart
- Cardiopulmonary profile (representative example)
- Answers to the self-assessment questions

CONTENTS

PART III
INFECTIOUS PULMONARY DISEASES

10. Pneumonia, 231

11. Acquired Immunodeficiency Syndrome, 247

12. Lung Abcess, 257

13. Tuberculosis, 267

14. Fungal Diseases of the Lungs, 277

PART IV
PULMONARY VASCULAR DISEASES

15. Pulmonary Edema, 289

Anatomic Alterations of the Lungs, 289
Etiology, 289
Overview of the Cardiopulmonary Clinical Manifestations Associated with Pulmonary Edema, 291
General Management of Pulmonary Edema, 294
Case Study, 296
Self-Assessment Questions, 298

16. Pulmonary Embolism and Infarction, 301

Anatomic Alterations of the Lungs, 301
Etiology, 301
Overview of the Cardiopulmonary Clinical Manifestations Associated with Pulmonary Embolism, 302
General Management of Pulmonary Embolism, 310
Case Study, 311
Self-Assessment Questions, 313

PART V
CHEST AND PLEURAL TRAUMA

17. Flail Chest, 317

Anatomic Alterations of the Lungs, 317
Etiology, 317
Overview of the Cardiopulmonary Clinical Manifestations Associated with Flail Chest, 318
General Management of Flail Chest, 321
Case Study, 321
Self-Assessment Questions, 324

18. Pneumothorax, 327

Anatomic Alterations of the Lungs, 327
Etiology, 327
Overview of the Cardiopulmonary Clinical Manifestations Associated with Pneumothorax, 330
General Management of Pneumothorax, 335
Case Study, 336
Self-Assessment Questions, 338

PART VI
DISORDERS OF THE PLEURA AND OF THE CHEST WALL

19. Pleural Diseases, 343

Anatomic Alterations of the Lungs, 343
Etiology, 343

PART VII
ENVIRONMENTAL LUNG DISEASE

PART VIII
NEOPLASTIC DISEASE

PART IX
DIFFUSE ALVEOLAR DISEASES

PART XII
OTHER IMPORTANT TOPICS

ASSESSMENT SKILLS AS CORE TO PRACTITIONER SUCCESS

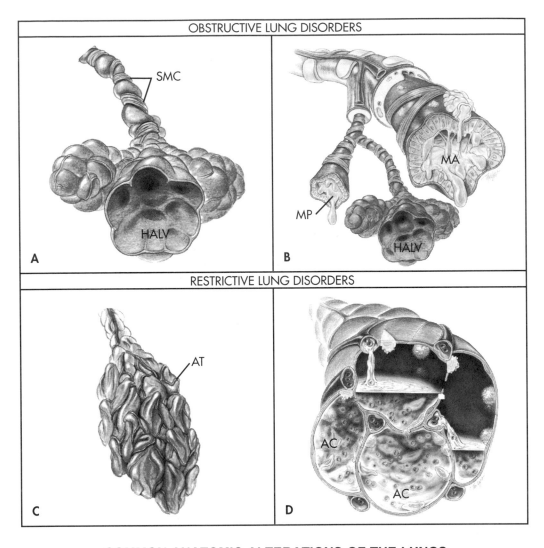

COMMON ANATOMIC ALTERATIONS OF THE LUNGS

FIG 1-1

OBSTRUCTIVE LUNG DISORDERS. **A,** bronchial smooth muscle constriction accompanied by air trapping. **B,** tracheobronchial inflammation accompanied by mucus accumulation, partial airway obstruction, and air trapping (note: when mucus accumulation causes total airway obstruction, alveolar atelectasis ensues). RESTRICTIVE LUNG DISORDERS. **C,** alveolar collapse or atelectasis. **D,** alveolar consolidation. *SMC* = smooth muscle constriction; *HALV* = hyperinflated alveoli; *MA* = mucus accumulation; *MP* = mucus plug; *AT* = atelectasis; *AC* = alveolar consolidation.

CHAPTER 1

PATIENT ASSESSMENT

When the lungs are affected by disease or trauma, they are anatomically altered to some degree, depending on the severity of the process. In general, the anatomic alterations caused by an injury or disease process can be classified as resulting in an **obstructive lung disorder,** a **restrictive lung disorder,** or a **combination of both.** Figure 1-1 illustrates common anatomic alterations that present as either obstructive or restrictive lung disorders. Table 1-1 lists the common respiratory diseases and their general classifications.

When the **normal anatomy of the lungs is altered,** certain **pathophysiologic mechanisms** throughout the cardiopulmonary system are activated. These pathophysiologic mechanisms, in turn, cause a variety of **clinical manifestations** to develop that can be readily identified in the clinical setting (e.g., increased heart rate, depressed diaphragm, or an increased functional residual capacity). To effectively collect clinical data, assess the data (i.e., identify the cause(s) of the data), and treat a specific respiratory disorder, one must first have a basic knowledge and understanding of (1) *the anatomic alterations of the lungs caused by the disease process or trauma;* (2) *the possible pathophysiologic mechanisms activated by the anatomic alterations of the lungs;* and (3) *the various clinical manifestations associated with the disorder.* Without this basic knowledge and understanding, the respiratory care practitioner merely goes through the motions of performing assigned therapeutic tasks with no short- or long-term anticipated outcome that can be measured. In such an environment, the practitioner works in a **task-oriented,** rather than a **goal-oriented,** manner.

That goal-oriented (patient-oriented) respiratory care may become the hallmark of future practice is suggested by analyzing the work performance of our colleague physical therapists. Orders that routinely empower their practice are infinitely more generic than those with which we customarily deal. For example, physical therapists are instructed to "improve back range of motion" or "strengthen quadricep muscle groups," rather than "warm fomentations to low back," or "quadriceps setting exercises with 10-lb ankle weights." Such therapists can up- or down-regulate the intensity of physical therapy on the basis of the patient's needs and capabilities at the point in time when the patient is seen, not on the basis of a two-hour, two-day, or two-week-old physician assessment. **Goal achievement,** not **task completion,** is the way the success of the work is measured.

In today's "sicker in, quicker out" environment, a change is coming to respiratory care. Under fixed-reimbursement programs, shorter lengths of stay have required hospital administrators and medical staff to examine allocation of health care resources. Fully one third of hospitalized patients receive respiratory care services and, thus, such services have come under close scrutiny. Recent clinical practice guidelines such as those developed by the American Association of Respiratory Care (AARC) have come to serve as the basis for **therapist-**

Table 1-1 General Respiratory Disease Classifications			
Respiratory Disorder	Obstructive	Restrictive	Combination
Chronic bronchitis	X		
Emphysema	X		
Asthma	X		
Bronchiectasis*			X
Cystic fibrosis*			X
Pneumoconiosis			X
Pneumonia		X	
Pulmonary edema		X	
Near-drowning		X	
Adult respiratory distress syndrome		X	
Chronic interstitial lung disease		X	
Flail chest		X	
Pneumothorax		X	
Pleural diseases		X	
Kyphoscoliosis		X	
Tuberculosis		X	
Fungal diseases		X	
Idiopathic (infant) respiratory distress syndrome		X	

*Most commonly seen primarily as an obstructive lung disorder.

driven respiratory care protocols (TDP). TDP are also known as **criterion-based respiratory care protocols and treat protocols, or respiratory consult services.**

Protocols are defined as ". . . *patient care plans which are initiated and implemented by credentialed respiratory care workers. These plans are designed and developed with input from physicians, and are approved for use by the medical staff and the governing body of the hospitals in which they are used. They share in common extreme reliance on assessment and evaluation skills. Protocols are by their nature dynamic and flexible, allowing up- or down-regulation of intensity of respiratory services. Protocols allow the respiratory care practitioner authority to evaluate the patient, initiate care, and to adjust, discontinue, or restart respiratory care procedures on a shift-by-shift, or hour-to-hour basis once the protocol is ordered by the physician. They must contain clear strategies for various therapeutic interventions, while avoiding any misconception that they infringe on the practice of medicine.*"

When appropriate guidelines are followed, allocation of respiratory care services has been seen to improve. Indeed, there is hope that under this paradigm, the respiratory care that is inappropriately ordered will be either withheld or modified, whichever is appropriate, and the patients who deserve respiratory care services (but who have not had such ordered) will now be able to receive needed care.

From these observations, it should be understood that the respiratory care worker of today is being asked to actively participate in the now-vital appropriate allocation of respiratory care services. Future respiratory care practitioners must have the basic *knowledge, skills,* and *personal attributes* to effectively collect clinical data, assess the clinical data, and treat their patients. Under the protocol paradigm, specific indications (clinical manifestations) for a particular respiratory care procedure must first be identified. In other words, a specific treatment plan cannot be started, up-regulated, down-regulated, or discontinued without (1) the presence and collection of specific clinical data, and (2) the assessment made from the clinical data (i.e., the cause of the clinical data) to justify a treatment order, or change. In addition, once a particular treatment has been administered to the patient, all outcomes of the

Table 1-2 Comparison of Closed and Open-Ended Questions

Open-Ended	Direct, Closed
Used for narrative information	Used for specific information
Calls for long answers	Calls for short one- or two-word answers
Elicits feeling, options, ideas	Elicits "cold facts"
Builds and enhances rapport	Limits rapport and leaves interaction neutral

treatment must be measurable. *Clearly, the success or failure of protocol work depends on accurate and timely patient assessment!*

Respiratory care assessment in this new construct should include (1) a patient interview, (2) the identification of all cardiopulmonary clinical manifestations demonstrated by the patient, including pertinent laboratory data, pulmonary function studies, and chest radiographic data, (3) an understanding of the pathophysiologic basis for the cardiopulmonary clinical manifestations presented by the patient, and (4) a systematic recording method that can be used to effectively gather clinical data, formulate an assessment, and develop an appropriate treatment plan.

THE PATIENT INTERVIEW

The interview is a meeting between the respiratory care practitioner and the patient. During the interview, data is collected about the patient's feelings regarding his or her condition. During a successful interview, the practitioner (1) gathers complete and accurate data about the patient's impressions about their health, including their description and chronology of any symptoms; (2) establishes rapport and trust so that the patient feels accepted and comfortable to share all relevant information; (3) develops and shows an understanding about the patient's health state, which in turn enhances the patient's participation in identifying problems; and (4) builds rapport to secure a continuing working relationship, which facilitates future assessments, evaluations, and treatment plans.

Interview skills are an art form that takes time and experience to develop. The most important components of a successful interview are communication and understanding. Understanding the various signals of communication is the most difficult part. When understanding—the conveying of meaning—breaks down between the practitioner and the patient, there is no communication. It cannot be assumed that communication happens just because two people can speak and listen.

Although the complete subject of the patient interview is beyond the scope of this textbook, there are a number of important techniques that should be studied and used by the respiratory care practitioner to facilitate the interview process. Such techniques include nonverbal messages, open-ended questions (e.g., "What brings you to the hospital today?"), closed or direct questions (e.g., "Have you ever had this chest pain before?"), and examiner responses. Table 1-2 provides a general comparison of closed and open-ended questions. Table 1-3 presents a general overview of positive and negative nonverbal messages of the interview. Finally, as the patient answers open-ended questions, the examiner's role (or response) is to encourage free expression, but not to let the patient wander off the subject. Again, there are a number of helpful techniques that can be studied and used to enhance this process. For example, the examiner may facilitate the patient's response by showing a genuine concern for the patient, empathy, and the ability to listen, while at the same time preventing the patient from getting off the subject by reflecting, summarizing, or asking for clarification on specific topics previously mentioned by the patient.

Table 1-3 Nonverbal Messages of the Interview

Positive	Negative
Professional appearance	Nonprofessional appearance
Sitting next to patient	Sitting behind a desk
Close proximity to patient	Far away from patient
Turned toward patient	Turned away from patient
Relaxed open posture	Tense closed posture
Leaning toward patient	Slouched away from patient
Facilitating gestures	Nonfacilitating gestures
• Nodding of head	• Looking at watch
Positive facial expressions	Negative facial expressions
• Appropriate smiling	• Frowning
• Interest	• Yawning
Good eye contact	Poor eye contact
Moderate tone of voice	Strident, high-pitched voice
Moderate rate of speech	Speech too fast or too slow
Appropriate touch	Too frequent or inappropriate touch

THE PATHOPHYSIOLOGIC BASIS FOR COMMON CLINICAL MANIFESTATIONS ASSOCIATED WITH RESPIRATORY DISEASES

In addition to the important information that can be gathered during the patient interview, there are a variety of clinical manifestations commonly demonstrated by the patient suffering from a respiratory disorder. Such clinical manifestations can be noted through direct observation (e.g., during the interview process) or from review of the patient's chart, which documents the results of various laboratory tests.

Table 1-4 provides an overview of the knowledge/database necessary for the successful clinical assessment of patients with respiratory disease. A more in-depth discussion of the items presented in Table 1-4 follows.

ABNORMAL CHEST ASSESSMENT FINDINGS

The physical examination of the chest and lungs should be performed in an orderly and consistent fashion. The typical sequence is as follows:

- Inspection
- Palpation
- Percussion
- Auscultation

Inspection

The examiner may obtain a large amount of important information by inspecting the chest and by confirming the presence or absence of certain clinical features. A significant amount of information that has gone unrecognized by the patient can be gathered. During inspection, the examiner should particularly note the following:

- Is the patient short of breath while talking? Does the patient stop to breathe after speaking only a few words?

Table 1-4 Overview of the Knowledge Base Necessary for the Successful Clinical Assessment of Patients with Respiratory Disease

Abnormal Chest Assessment Findings, including:
Inspection   Palpation
Percussion   Auscultation

Abnormal Ventilatory Pattern Findings, including:
Common abnormal ventilatory patterns
  Apnea
  Biot's respiration
  Cheyne-Stokes respiration
  Dyspnea
  Hyperpnea
  Hyperventilation
  Hypoventilation
  Kussmaul's respiration
  Orthopnea
  Tachypnea
Lung compliance and its effect on the ventilatory pattern
Airway resistance and its effect on the ventilatory pattern
The peripheral chemoreceptors and their effect on the ventilatory pattern
The central chemoreceptors and their effects on the ventilatory pattern
The pulmonary reflex(es) and its effect on the ventilatory pattern

Abnormal Pulmonary Function Study Findings, including:
Expiratory maneuver findings characteristic of restrictive lung diseases

Lung volume and capacity findings characteristic of restrictive lung diseases
Expiratory maneuver findings characteristic of obstructive lung diseases
Lung volume and capacity findings characteristic of obstructive lung diseases
Diffusion capacity findings characteristic of pulmonary diseases

Pursed-Lip Breathing

Increased Anteroposterior Chest Diameter (barrel chest)

Use of Accessory Muscles of Inspiration

Use of Accessory Muscles of Expiration

Abnormal Arterial Blood Gas Findings, including:
Acute alveolar hyperventilation with hypoxemia
Acute ventilatory failure with hypoxemia
Chronic ventilatory failure with hypoxemia
Acute alveolar hyperventilation superimposed on chronic ventilatory failure
Acute ventilatory failure superimposed on chronic ventilatory failure
Metabolic acidosis
Metabolic alkalosis
Hypoxemic state

Cyanosis

Abnormal Oxygenation Indices, including:
Arterial oxygen tension
Alveolar-arterial oxygen tension difference

Total oxygen delivery
Arterial-venous oxygen content difference
Oxygen consumption
Oxygen extraction ratio
Mixed venous oxygen saturation
Pulmonary shunting

Abnormal Cardiovascular System Findings, including:
Normal and abnormal heart sounds, murmurs
Common cardiac arrhythmias
  Sinus bradycardia
  Sinus tachycardia
  Sinus arrhythmia
  Atrial flutter
  Atrial fibrillation
  Premature ventricular contractions
  Ventricular tachycardia
  Ventricle flutter
  Ventricular fibrillation
  Asystole
Noninvasive hemodynamic monitoring results
  Increased heart rate (pulse)
  Increased cardiac output
  Increased blood pressure
  Decreased perfusion state
  Pitting edema
Invasive hemodynamic monitoring results
  Central venous pressure
  Right atrial pressure
  Mean pulmonary artery pressure

Pulmonary capillary wedge pressure
Cardiac output
Stroke volume
Stroke volume index
Cardiac index
Right ventricular stroke work index
Left ventricular stroke work index
Pulmonary vascular resistance
Systemic vascular resistance

Increased central venous pressure/decreased systemic blood pressure
(e.g., diseases that affect the major vessels of the chest)

Polycythemia, Cor Pulmonale
Elevated hemoglobin concentration and hematocrit
Distended neck veins
Enlarged and tender liver
Peripheral edema
Pitting edema

Digital Clubbing

Cough, Sputum Production, and Hemoptysis

Substernal/Intercostal Retraction

Chest Pain/Decreased Expansion

Abnormal Hematology, Blood Chemistry, and Electrolyte Findings

Abnormal Bronchoscopy Findings

Abnormal Radiology Findings
(see Chapter 2)

- Are accessory muscles of respiration used during inspiration or expiration?
- The patient's posture while sitting. Individuals in respiratory distress often lean forward when seated, hold on to a stationary object, and hunch their shoulders forward.
- The patient's ventilatory pattern (rate and depth of breathing).
- The patient's inspiratory-to-expiratory ratio (I:E ratio).
- Retractions of the intercostal spaces during inspiration.
- Nasal flaring.
- Pursed-lip breathing.
- Symmetry of the chest.
- Are the scapulae symmetric and the spine straight?
- Is the excursion of the chest wall symmetric? Does the diaphragm move downward and the thoracic cage move upward and outward during each inspiration?
- Is the patient splinting in an attempt to control chest pain by decreasing chest excursion? Splinting suggests the presence of pneumonia, rib fractures, pleural effusion, pneumothorax, or postoperative pain.
- The presence or absence of paradoxical movement of the lower costal margins. During the advanced stages of chronic obstructive pulmonary disease the costal margins first expand on inspiration and then contract.
- The patient's skin condition and color. Is the patient dehydrated? Is the skin cyanotic?
- Are the patient's hands and nail beds cyanotic and is there digital clubbing?
- Does the patient cough and is the cough productive?
- The presence of audible wheezing or rhonchi.
- Are the neck and face veins distended and is there edema of the extremities (indications of congestive heart failure)?
- Surgical scars.
- The presence of a "barrel chest."

External Landmarks

In an examination of the chest and lungs, various anatomic landmarks and imaginary vertical lines drawn on the chest are useful in pinpointing abnormal findings.

Anteriorly, the first rib and its cartilage are fastened to the manubrium directly beneath the clavicle. The second rib and its cartilage are adjacent to the sternal angle. The ribs can be easily numbered once the second rib is identified. The sixth rib and its cartilage are located on the sternum just above the xiphoid process. Anteriorly, the lungs normally extend to about the level of the xiphoid process (Fig 1-2).

Posteriorly, the ribs can be numbered by identifying the inferior angle of the scapulae. The eighth rib usually lies near this point. The examiner may also trace the location of a rib from the front of the chest to the back. In the back the lungs normally extend inferiorly to the level of the ninth or the tenth rib (see Fig 1-2).

As shown in Fig 1-3, a good method for localizing certain findings is to use a reference grid of the following imaginary vertical lines drawn on the chest:

- Midsternal line
- Midclavicular line
- Anterior axillary line
- Midaxillary line
- Posterior axillary line
- Midscapular line
- Vertebral line

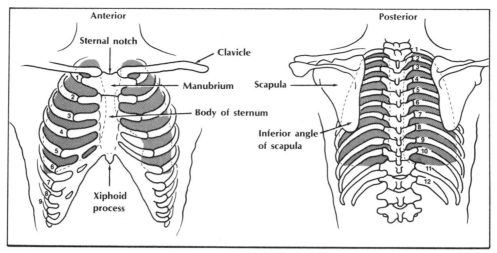

FIG 1-2
Anatomic landmarks of the chest.

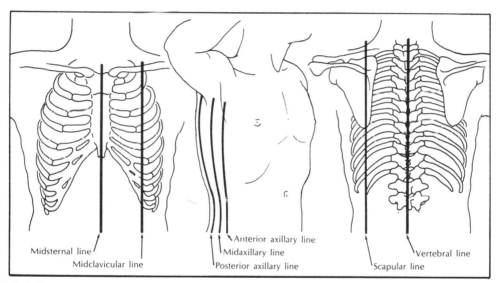

FIG 1-3
Imaginary vertical lines of the chest.

Palpation

Palpation is the process of touching the patient in an effort to evaluate areas of tenderness, tone of the respiratory muscles, any chest wall abnormalities that may or may not be visibly evident, and fremitus.

When palpating the patient's chest for tenderness, muscle tone, and abnormalities, the examiner may use the heel of the hand, the ulnar surface of the hand, or the fingertips. The position of the patient's trachea, for example, can be determined by placing the index finger into the sternal notch. Care should be taken when palpating areas of chest wall tenderness, e.g., over fractured ribs.

Tactile and Vocal Fremitus

Vibration felt over the chest—produced by gas flowing through partially obstructed tracheo-bronchial segments—is known as *tactile fremitus*. The vibration caused by phonation and transmitted through the chest is called *vocal fremitus*. Vocal fremitus is commonly produced by the patient repeating the number "ninety-nine." Palpation should be performed from the top of the chest down and should be done anteriorly and posteriorly (Fig 1-4).

Tactile and vocal fremitus may increase or decrease when additional pulmonary complications are present. *Decreased tactile and vocal fremitus* are caused by respiratory disorders that interfere with the transmission of sounds. Such respiratory problems include (1) chronic obstructive pulmonary disease accompanied by an increased functional residual capacity, (2) tumors of the pleural cavity, and (3) pleural effusion.

When the pulmonary disorder produces consolidation within the lungs, tactile and vocal fremitus increase because liquid and solid materials transmit vibrations more readily than air-filled spaces. Some causes of *increased vocal fremitus* are pneumonia, alveolar collapse or atelectasis, pulmonary edema, lung masses, and pulmonary fibrosis.

Percussion

Percussion of the chest wall is performed to obtain information concerning the presence of air or consolidation within the chest cavity. When percussing the chest, the examiner firmly presses the distal portion of the middle finger of the nondominant hand onto the surface to be examined. No other part of the hand should touch the patient. Using the tip of the middle finger of the dominant hand, the examiner quickly strikes the distal joining of the positioned finger and then immediately withdraws the tapping finger (Fig 1-5). The sounds normally produced by percussion are referred to as resonant sounds. The examiner should percuss from the top down, between the ribs, and compare the sounds generated on the two sides of the chest. Both the anterior and posterior aspects of the chest should be percussed (Fig 1-6).

In a normal lung, the sound created by percussion is transmitted throughout the air-filled lung and is typically described as loud, low in pitch, and long in duration. The sounds elicited by the examiner vibrate freely throughout the large surface area of the lungs and create a sound like that elicited by knocking on a watermelon (Fig 1-7).

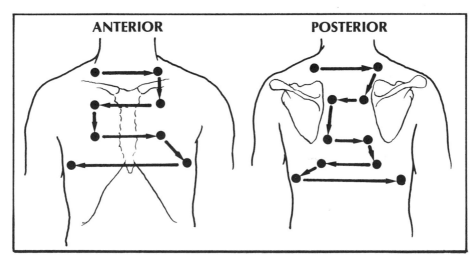

FIG 1-4
Path of palpation for vocal or tactile fremitus.

Abnormal Percussion Notes

- Dull percussion note
- Hyperresonant percussion note

In persons with chest disorders such as pleural thickening, pleural effusion, atelectasis, or consolidation, the sound elicited on percussion does not resonate throughout the lungs. The sounds produced are typically described as dull, flat, or soft, high in pitch, short in duration, and suggestive of those produced by knocking on a full barrel (Fig 1-8).

When the chest is percussed over areas of trapped gas, a hyperresonant note is produced. These sounds are typically described as very loud, low in pitch, long in duration, and reminiscent of those produced by knocking on an empty barrel (Fig 1-9). Such sounds are com-

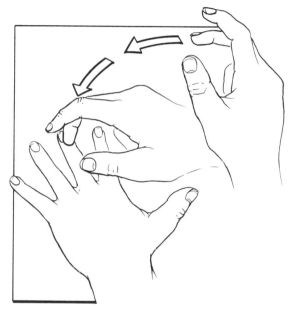

FIG 1-5
Chest percussion technique.

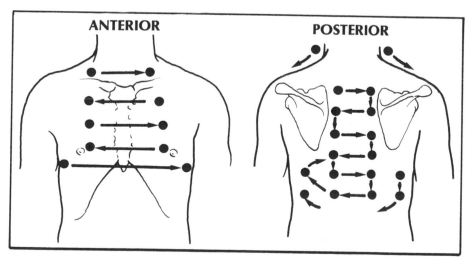

FIG 1-6
Path of percussion.

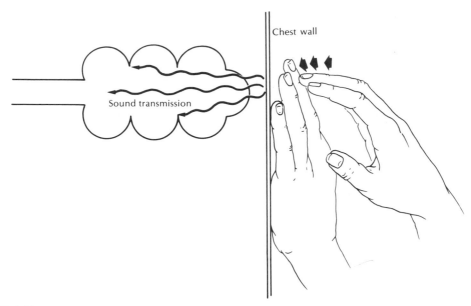

FIG 1-7
Chest percussion of a normal lung.

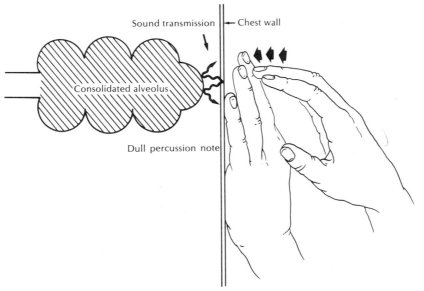

FIG 1-8
A short, dull percussion note is typically produced over areas of alveolar consolidation.

monly elicited in patients with chronic obstructive pulmonary disease and in patients with pneumothorax.

Auscultation

Auscultation of the lungs yields information about the flow of gas through the tracheobronchial tree and the presence of alveolar consolidation, secretions, or bronchial obstruction. The examiner should auscultate the chest from one side to the other and from top to bottom (Fig 1-10). Each area should be listened to while the patient inhales and exhales at a slightly in-

ALVEOLI AFFECTED BY ASTHMA

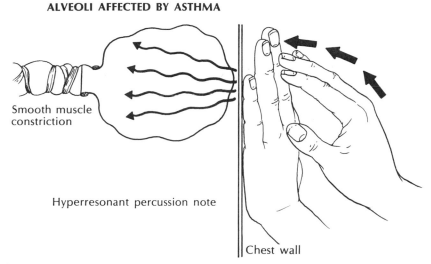

Smooth muscle constriction

Hyperresonant percussion note

Chest wall

FIG 1-9

Percussion becomes more hyperresonant with alveolar hyperinflation.

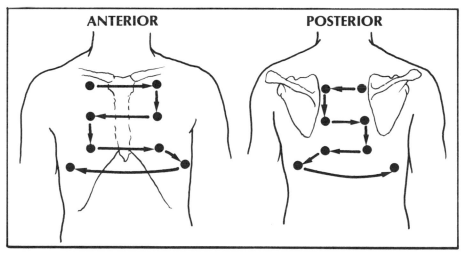

FIG 1-10

Path of auscultation.

creased depth. The examiner should listen to the quality and intensity of the breath sounds and for the presence or absence of adventitious sounds.

Normal Breath Sounds

In the normal lung, the sounds heard on auscultation are the sounds of air rushing through the tubelike structures of the tracheobronchial tree. Since the rate of flow changes very markedly between the trachea and the alveoli, the nature and pitch of the breath sounds change also.

Over the trachea and larger bronchi, the sound is loud and high-pitched and has a so-called tubular or bronchial quality. Such sounds are commonly referred to as normal bronchial breath sounds. Bronchial breath sounds may be louder during expiration, and there is generally a pause between the inspiratory phase and the expiratory phase.

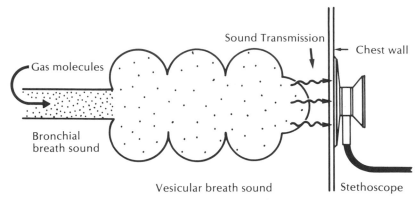

FIG 1-11
Auscultation of vesicular breath sounds over a normal lung unit.

Over the parenchymal areas of normal lungs, the breath sounds are much softer, have a lower pitch, and are much more evident during inspiration. This softer, lower-pitched sound over the parenchymal areas is due largely to the fact that the gas molecules entering the alveoli spread out over a larger surface area and therefore create less gas turbulence. As gas turbulence decreases, breath sounds decrease. The sounds are referred to as *bronchovesicular* or *vesicular sounds* (Fig 1-11).

Abnormal (Adventitious) Breath Sounds

- Bronchial breath sounds
- Diminished breath sounds
- Crackles and rhonchi
- Wheezing
- Pleural friction rubs
- Whispered pectoriloquy

Bronchial Breath Sounds.—If gas molecules are not permitted to dissipate throughout the parenchymal areas (because of alveolar consolidation or atelectasis, for example) the gas molecules have no opportunity to spread out over a larger surface area and therefore to become less turbulent. Consequently, the sounds produced in this area will be louder, since the gas sounds are coming mainly from the tracheobronchial tree and not the lung parenchyma. These sounds are called *bronchial sounds.*

It is commonly believed that the breath sounds in patients with alveolar consolidation should be diminished, since the consolidation acts as a sound barrier. While it may be true that alveolar collapse or consolidation does act as a sound barrier and so reduces bronchial breath sounds, the reduction is not as great as it would be if the gas molecules were allowed to dissipate throughout the lung parenchyma. In addition, liquid and solid materials transmit sounds more readily than air-filled spaces do and therefore may further contribute to the bronchial quality of the breath sound. Thus, when disease causes alveolar collapse or consolidation, there will be harsher, bronchial-type sounds over the affected areas rather than the normal vesicular sounds (Fig 1-12).

Diminished Breath Sounds.—Breath sounds are diminished or distant when auscultated in respiratory disorders that lead to alveolar hypoventilation, regardless of the cause. For example, patients with chronic obstructive pulmonary disease commonly have diminished breath sounds. These patients hypoventilate because of air trapping and increased functional residual

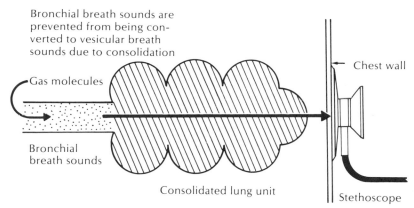

Bronchial breath sounds are prevented from being con- verted to vesicular breath sounds due to consolidation

Chest wall

Gas molecules

Bronchial breath sounds

Consolidated lung unit

Stethoscope

FIG 1-12

Auscultation of bronchial breath sounds over a consolidated lung unit.

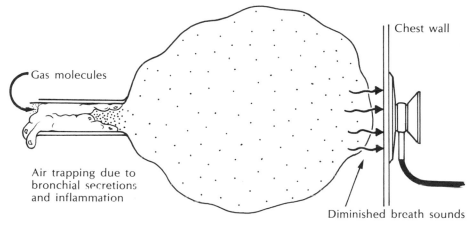

Chest wall

Gas molecules

Air trapping due to bronchial secretions and inflammation

Diminished breath sounds

FIG 1-13

As air trapping and alveolar hyperinflation develop in obstructive lung diseases, breath sounds progressively diminish.

capacity. In addition, when the functional residual capacity is increased, the gas that enters the enlarged alveoli during each breath spreads out over a greater-than-normal surface area, thereby resulting in less gas turbulence and a softer sound (Fig 1-13). Heart sounds may also be diminished in patients with increased functional residual capacity.

Diminished breath sounds are also found in respiratory disorders that cause hypoventilation by compressing the lung. Such disorders include flail chest, pleural effusion, and pneumothorax. Diminished breath sounds are also characteristic of neuromuscular diseases that cause hypoventilation. Such disorders include the Guillain-Barré syndrome and myasthenia gravis.

Crackles and Rhonchi.—Adjectives used in the older literature to describe crackles and rhonchi (moist, wet, dry, crackling, sibilant, coarse, fine, crepitant) depend largely on the auditory acuity and experience of the examiner. They have little value because it is only the presence or absence of crackles or rhonchi that is important. When fluid accumulation is present in a respiratory disorder, there are almost always some crackles or rhonchi, i.e., "bubbly" or "slurpy" sounds accompanying the breath sounds.

Crackles (rales) are usually fine or medium crackling wet sounds and are typically heard during inspiration. Crackles are formed in the small and medium-sized airways and generally do not change in nature after a strong, vigorous cough.

Rhonchi, on the other hand, usually have a coarse, "bubbly" quality and are typically heard during expiration. Rhonchi are formed in the larger airways and often change in nature or disappear after a strong, vigorous cough.

Wheezing.—Wheezing is the characteristic sound produced by airway obstruction. It is found in all bronchospastic disorders and is one of the cardinal findings in bronchial asthma. The sounds are high-pitched and whistling and generally last throughout the expiratory phase. The mechanism of a wheeze is similar to a vibrating reed of a woodwind instrument. The reed, which partially occludes the mouthpiece of the instrument, vibrates and produces a sound when air is forced through it (Fig 1-14).

Pleural friction rubs.—If pleuritis accompanies a respiratory disorder, the inflamed pleural membranes resist movement during breathing and create a peculiar and characteristic sound known as a pleural friction rub. The sound is reminiscent of the sound made by a creaking shoe and is usually heard in the area where the patient complains of pain.

Whispering pectoriloquy.—*Whispered pectoriloquy* is the term used to describe the unusually clear transmission of the whispered voice of a patient as heard through the stethoscope.

When the patient whispers "one, two, three," the sounds produced by the vocal cords are transmitted not only toward the mouth and nose but throughout the lungs as well. As the whispered sounds travel down the tracheobronchial tree, they remain relatively unchanged, but as the sound disperses throughout the large surface areas of the alveoli, it diminishes sharply. Consequently, when one listens with a stethoscope over a normal lung while a patient whispers the "one, two, three," the sounds are diminished, distant, muffled, and unintelligible (Fig 1-15).

When a patient who has atelectasis or consolidated lung areas whispers "one, two, three," the sounds produced are prevented from spreading out over a large alveolar surface area. Even though the consolidated area may act as a sound barrier and diminishes the sounds somewhat, the reduction in sounds is not as great as if the sounds were allowed to dissipate throughout a normal lung. Consequently, the whispered sounds will be much louder and more intelligible over the affected lung areas (Fig 1-16).

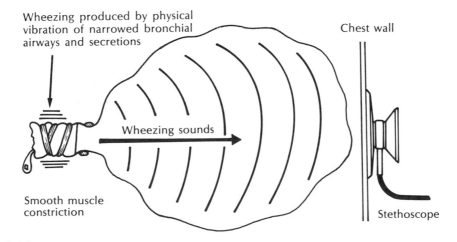

FIG 1-14
Wheezing and rhonchi often develop during an asthmatic episode because of smooth muscle constriction, wall edema, and mucus accumulation.

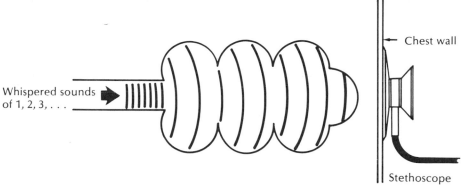

FIG 1-15

Whispered voice sounds auscultated over a normal lung are usually faint and unintelligible.

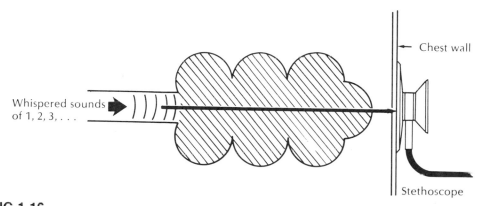

FIG 1-16

Whispered voice sounds heard over a consolidated lung are usually louder and more intelligible in comparison to a normal lung.

ABNORMAL VENTILATORY PATTERN FINDINGS

An individual's ventilatory pattern is composed of a *tidal volume* (V_T), a *ventilatory rate,* and an *inspiratory-to-expiratory ratio* (I:E ratio). In normal adults, the V_T is about 500 ml (7 to 9 ml/kg), the ventilatory rate is about 15 (12 to 18) times per minute, and the normal I:E ratio is approximately 1:2 (i.e., exhalation is usually twice as long as inspiration). In patients with respiratory disorders, however, an abnormal ventilatory pattern is often present. Table 1-5 lists abnormal ventilatory patterns commonly seen in respiratory diseases.

Although the precise etiology may not always be known, the basic cause of an abnormal ventilatory pattern is frequently related to (1) the anatomic alterations of the lungs associated with a specific disorder, and (2) the pathophysiologic mechanisms that develop because of the anatomic alterations. Thus, to fully evaluate and assess the various abnormal ventilatory patterns (rate and volume relationship) seen in the clinical setting, the following pathophysiologic mechanisms that can alter the ventilatory pattern must first be understood:

- Lung compliance
- Airway resistance
- Peripheral chemoreceptors
- Central chemoreceptors

Table 1-5 Common Abnormal Ventilatory Patterns

Apnea	Complete absence of spontaneous ventilation.
Biot's respiration	Characterized by episodes of rapid, uniformly deep inspirations, followed by long periods (10 to 30 seconds) of apnea. Commonly seen in patients suffering from meningitis or increased intracranial pressure.
Cheyne-Stokes respiration	Characterized by apnea lasting 10 to 30 seconds followed by gradually increasing depth and frequency of respirations. Cheyne-Stokes respiration is associated with cerebral disorders and with congestive heart failure.
Dyspnea	A shortness of breath or a difficulty in breathing, of which the individual is aware.
Hyperpnea	An increased depth (volume) of breathing with or without an increased frequency. A certain degree of hyperpnea is normal immediately after exercise. Hyperpnea is associated with respiratory disease, infection, cardiac disease, certain drugs, hysteria, or with the hypoxemia experienced at high altitude.
Hyperventilation	An increased alveolar ventilation caused by an increased ventilatory rate, an increased depth of breathing, or a combination of both that causes the PA_{CO_2} and Pa_{CO_2} to decrease.
Hypoventilation (Hypopnea)	A decreased alveolar ventilation caused by a decreased ventilatory rate, a decreased depth of breathing, or a combination of both that causes the PA_{CO_2} and Pa_{CO_2} to increase.
Kussmaul's respiration	Both an increased depth (hyperpnea) and rate of breathing (tachypnea). Kussmaul's respiration is commonly associated with diabetic acidosis (ketoacidosis).
Orthopnea	A condition in which an individual is able to breathe comfortably only in the upright position.
Tachypnea	A rapid rate of breathing.

- Pulmonary reflex(es)
  - Hering-Breuer reflex
  - Deflation reflex
  - Irritant reflex
  - Juxtapulmonary-capillary receptor (J receptors) reflexes
  - Reflexes from the aortic and carotid sinus baroreceptors
  - Pain/anxiety

Lung Compliance and Its Effect on the Ventilatory Pattern

The ease with which the elastic forces of the lungs accept a volume of inspired air is known as *lung compliance* (C_L). C_L is measured in terms of *unit volume change* per *unit pressure change*. Mathematically, it is written as liters per centimeter of water pressure. In other words, compliance determines how much air, in liters, the lungs will accommodate for each centimeter of water pressure change in distending pressure.

For example, when the normal individual generates a negative intrapleural pressure change of 2 cm H_2O during inspiration, the lungs accept a new volume of about 0.2 L gas. Thus, the C_L of the lungs would be expressed as 0.1 L/cm H_2O:

$$C_L = \frac{\Delta V \ (L)}{\Delta P \ (cm \ H_2O)}$$

$$= \frac{0.2 \ L \ gas}{2 \ cm \ H_2O}$$

$$= 0.1 \ L/cm \ H_2O$$

The normal compliance of the lungs is graphically illustrated by the *volume-pressure curve* (Fig 1-17). When C_L increases, the lungs accept a greater volume of gas per unit pressure change. When C_L decreases, the lungs accept a smaller volume of gas per unit pressure change (Fig 1-18).

Although the precise mechanism is not clear, it is well documented that certain ventilatory patterns occur when lung compliance is altered. For example, when C_L decreases, the patient's breathing rate generally increases while, at the same time, the tidal volume decreases (Fig 1-19). This type of breathing pattern is commonly seen in restrictive lung disorders such as pneumonia, pulmonary edema, and adult respiratory distress syndrome. This breathing pattern is also commonly seen during the early stages of an acute asthmatic attack when the alveoli are hyperinflated—C_L progressively decreases as the alveolar volume increases (see Fig 1-17) at high lung volumes.

Airway Resistance and Its Effect on the Ventilatory Pattern

Airway resistance (R_{aw}) is defined as the pressure difference between the mouth and the alveoli (transairway pressure) divided by flow rate. Thus, the rate at which a certain volume of gas flows through the airways is a function of the pressure gradient and the resistance created by the airways to the flow of gas. Mathematically, R_{aw} is written as follows:

$$R_{aw} = \frac{\Delta P \ (cm \ H_2O)}{\dot{V} \ (L/sec)}$$

For example, if a patient produces a flow rate of 6 L/sec during inspiration by generating a transairway pressure of 12 cm H_2O, R_{aw} would be 2 cm H_2O/L/sec:

$$R_{aw} = \frac{\Delta P}{\dot{V}}$$

$$= \frac{12 \ cm \ H_2O}{6 \ L/sec}$$

$$= 2 \ cm \ H_2O/L/sec$$

Under normal conditions, the R_{aw} in the tracheobronchial tree is about 1.0 to 2.0 cm H_2O/L/sec. However, in obstructive pulmonary diseases (e.g., bronchitis, emphysema, or asthma), the R_{aw} may be very high. An increased R_{aw} has a profound effect on the patient's ventilatory pattern.

When airway resistance increases significantly, the patient's ventilatory rate usually decreases while, at the same time, the tidal volume increases (see Fig 1-19). This type of breathing pattern is commonly seen in obstructive lung diseases (e.g., chronic bronchitis, emphysema, bronchiectasis, asthma, and cystic fibrosis) during the advanced stages.

The ventilatory pattern adopted by the patient in either a restrictive or obstructive lung disorder is thought to be based on minimum work requirements rather than gas exchange efficiency. In physics, work is defined as the force multiplied by the distance moved (work = force × distance). In respiratory physiology, the change in pulmonary pressure (force) mul-

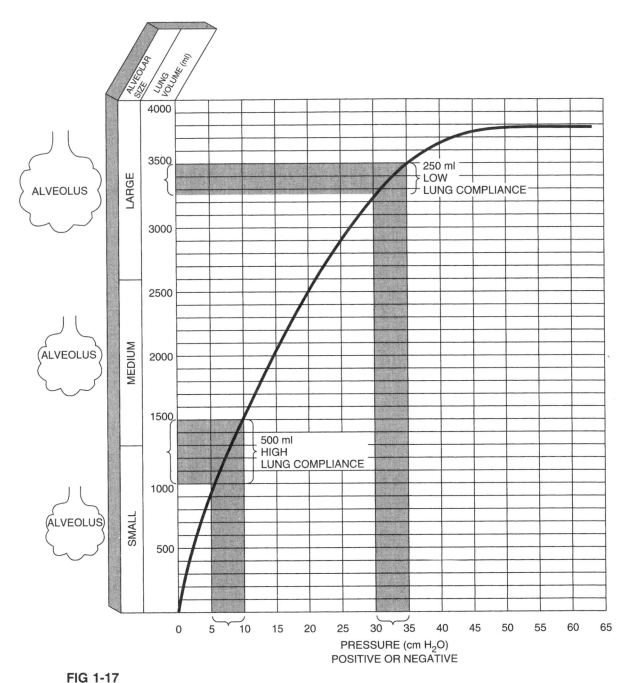

FIG 1-17

Normal volume-pressure curve. The curve shows that lung compliance progressively de-creases as the lungs expand in response to more volume. For example, note the greater vol-ume change between 5 and 10 cm H_2O (small/medium alveoli) than between 30 and 35 cm H_2O (large alveoli). (From Des Jardins T: *Cardiopulmonary Anatomy and Physiology: Essentials for Respiratory Care,* 2nd ed, Albany, NY, Delmar Publishers Inc, 1993. Used by permission.)

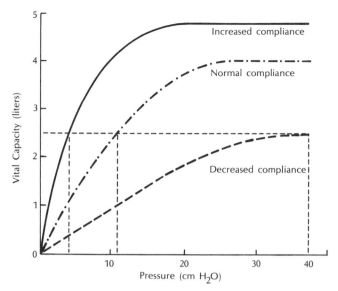

FIG 1-18

The effects of increased and decreased compliance on the volume-pressure curve. Note that as the lung compliance decreases, it takes a greater pressure change to obtain the same volume of 2.5 L (dotted lines).

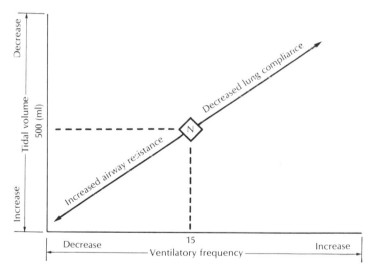

FIG 1-19

The effects of increased airway resistance and decreased lung compliance on ventilatory frequency and tidal volume. N = normal resting tidal volume and ventilatory frequency.

tiplied by the change in lung volume (distance) may be used to quantitate the amount of work required to breathe (work = pressure × volume).

It should be noted that the patient's usual adopted ventilatory pattern may not be seen in the clinical setting because of secondary heart or lung problems. For example, a patient with chronic emphysema who has adopted a decreased ventilatory rate and an increased tidal volume because of the increased airway resistance associated with the disorder will demonstrate an increased ventilatory rate and decreased tidal volume in response to a secondary pneumonia (a restrictive lung disorder superimposed on a chronic obstructive lung disorder).

Thus, it is important to note that because the patient may adopt a ventilatory pattern based on the expenditure of energy rather than on the efficiency of ventilation, it cannot be assumed that the ventilatory pattern acquired by the patient in response to a certain respiratory disorder is the most efficient one in terms of physiologic gas exchange.

The Peripheral Chemoreceptors and Their Effect on the Ventilatory Pattern

The *peripheral chemoreceptors* (also called carotid and aortic bodies) are oxygen-sensitive cells that react to a reduction of oxygen in the arterial blood (Pa_{O_2}). The peripheral chemoreceptors are located at the bifurcation of the internal and external carotid arteries (Fig 1-20) and on the aortic arch (Fig 1-21). Although the peripheral chemoreceptors are stimulated whenever the Pa_{O_2} is less than normal, they are generally most active when the Pa_{O_2} falls below 60 mm Hg (Sa_{O_2} of about 90%). Suppression of these chemoreceptors, however, is seen when the Pa_{O_2} falls below 30 mm Hg.

When the peripheral chemoreceptors are activated, an afferent (sensory) signal is sent to the respiratory centers of the medulla by way of the glossopharyngeal nerve (cranial nerve IX) from the carotid bodies and by way of the vagus nerve (cranial nerve X) from the aortic bodies. Efferent (motor) signals are then sent to the respiratory muscles, and this results in an increased rate of breathing.

In patients who have a chronically low Pa_{O_2} and a high Pa_{CO_2} (e.g., the advanced stages of emphysema), the peripheral chemoreceptors may be totally responsible for the control of ventilation. This is because a chronically high CO_2 concentration in the CSF inactivates the H^+ sensitivity of the central chemoreceptors.

Causes of Hypoxemia

In respiratory disease, a decreased arterial oxygen level (hypoxemia) is the result of decreased ventilation perfusion ratios, pulmonary shunting, and venous admixture.

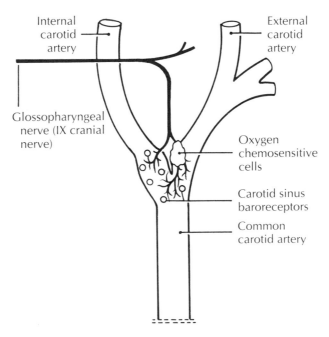

FIG 1-20
Oxygen-chemosensitive cells and the carotid sinus baroreceptors are located on the carotid artery.

Ventilation-Perfusion Ratios

Ideally, each alveolus should receive the same ratio of ventilation and pulmonary capillary blood flow. In reality, however, this is not the case. Alveolar ventilation is normally about 4 L/min and the pulmonary capillary blood flow is about 5 L/min, which makes the overall ratio of ventilation to blood flow 4:5, or 0.8. This relationship is referred to as the *ventilation-perfusion ($\dot{V}/\dot{Q}$) ratio* (Fig 1-22).

In a normal individual in the upright position, the alveoli in the upper portions of the lungs (apices) receive moderate amounts of ventilation and little blood flow. Consequently, the $\dot{V}/\dot{Q}$ ratio throughout this region is higher than 0.8. In the lower regions of the lung, alveolar ventilation is moderately increased, and the blood flow is greatly increased since blood flow is *gravity dependent*. As a result, the $\dot{V}/\dot{Q}$ ratio is lower than 0.8 in this area. In short, the $\dot{V}/\dot{Q}$ ratio progressively decreases from the top to the bottom of the lungs in an individual in the upright position, and the overall average $\dot{V}/\dot{Q}$ ratio is about 0.8. In respiratory disorders, the $\dot{V}/\dot{Q}$ ratio is usually altered.

Increased Ventilation-Perfusion Ratio.—In some disorders such as pulmonary embolic disease, the lungs receive less blood flow in relation to ventilation. When this condition develops, the $\dot{V}/\dot{Q}$ ratio increases. As a result, a larger portion of the alveolar ventilation will not be physiologically effective and is said to be "wasted" or *dead-space ventilation* (Fig 1-23).

Decreased Ventilation-Perfusion Ratio.—In lung disorders such as asthma or pneumonia, the lungs receive less ventilation in relation to blood flow. When this condition develops, the $\dot{V}/\dot{Q}$ ratio decreases. As a result, a larger portion of the pulmonary blood flow will not be

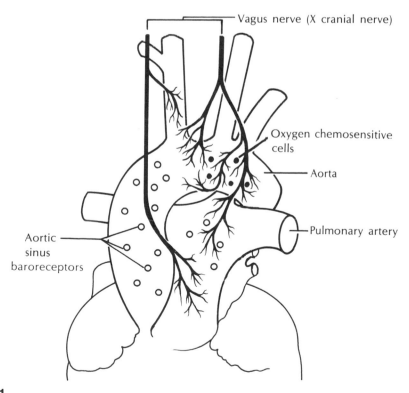

FIG 1-21

Oxygen-chemosensitive cells and the aortic sinus baroreceptors are located on the aorta and pulmonary artery.

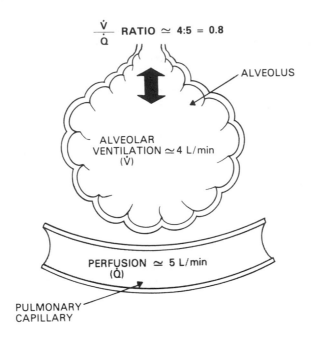

FIG 1-22

The normal overall pulmonary ventilation-perfusion ratio $(\dot{V}/\dot{Q})$ is about 0.8. (From Des Jardins TR: *Cardiopulmonary Anatomy and Physiology: Essentials for Respiratory Care,* 2nd ed, Albany, NY, Delmar Publishers Inc, 1993. Used by permission.)

physiologically effective in terms of molecular gas exchange and is said to be "shunted" blood (see the section on pulmonary shunting below). Generally, when the $\dot{V}/\dot{Q}$ ratio decreases, the Pa_{O_2} decreases and the Pa_{CO_2} increases.

Pulmonary Shunting

There are three forms of pulmonary shunting: the anatomic shunt, the capillary shunt, and the shuntlike effect.

Anatomic Shunt.—An anatomic shunt exists when blood flows from the right side of the heart to the left side without going through the pulmonary capillaries (Fig 1-24, B). Normally, this is about 2% to 5% of the cardiac output. This normal shunted blood comes from the bronchial, pleural, and thebesian veins, which drain into the left atrium. Such shunting can also be caused by congenital heart diseases, intrapulmonary arteriovenous fistulas, and pulmonary vascular abnormalities such as hemangiomas.

Capillary Shunt.—A capillary shunt is commonly caused by alveolar collapse or atelectasis, alveolar fluid accumulation, or alveolar consolidation (see Fig 1-24, C). The sum of the anatomic and capillary shunts is referred to as a *true* or *absolute shunt*. Patients with respiratory disorders causing capillary shunting will be refractory to oxygen therapy since the alveoli are unable to provide any O_2/CO_2 exchange function.

Shuntlike Effect.—When pulmonary capillary perfusion is in excess of alveolar ventilation, a shuntlike effect can develop. Common causes of this form of shunting are hypoventilation, uneven distribution of ventilation (e.g., bronchospasm or excessive mucus accumulation in the tracheobronchial tree), and alveolar-capillary diffusion defects (even though the alveolus may be ventilated in this condition, the blood passing by the alveolus does not have enough

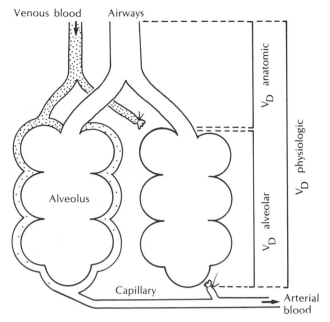

FIG 1-23

Dead-space ventilation (V_D).

Only the inspired air that reaches the alveoli is physiologically effective. This portion of the inspired gas is referred to as alveolar ventilation. The volume of inspired air that does not reach the alveoli is not physiologically effective. This portion of gas is referred to as dead-space ventilation. There are three types of dead spaces: anatomic, alveolar, and physiologic.

Anatomic dead space. Anatomic dead space refers to the volume of gas in the conducting airways: the nose, mouth, pharynx, larynx, and lower portions of the airways down to but not including the respiratory bronchioles. The volume of the anatomic dead space is approximately equal to 1 ml/lb (2.2 ml/kg) of normal body weight.

Alveolar dead space. When an alveolus is ventilated but not perfused with blood, the volume of air in the alveolus is dead space, that is, the air within the alveolus is not physiologically effective in terms of gas exchange. The amount of alveolar dead space is unpredictable.

Physiologic dead space. The physiologic dead space is the sum of the anatomic dead space and the alveolar dead space. Since neither of these two forms of dead space is physiologically effective in terms of gas exchange, the two forms are combined and are referred to as physiologic dead space. (See Physiologic Dead Space Calculation, Appendix XIV.)

time to equilibrate with the alveolar oxygen tension) (see Fig 1-24, D). Pulmonary shunting due to these conditions can generally be corrected by oxygen therapy.

Table 1-6 lists some respiratory disorders associated with capillary shunting and shunt-like effects.

Venous Admixture

The end result of pulmonary shunting is venous admixture, which is the mixing of shunted nonreoxygenated blood with reoxygenated blood distal to the alveoli (i.e., downstream in the pulmonary circulatory system) (Fig 1-25). When venous admixture occurs, the shunted non-reoxygenated blood gains oxygen molecules while, at the same time, the reoxygenated blood loses oxygen molecules. The end result is a blood mixture that has (1) higher Po_2 and Cao_2 values than the nonoxygenated blood, and (2) lower Po_2 and Cao_2 values than the reoxygenated blood—in other words, a blood mixture with Pao_2 and Cao_2 values somewhere between

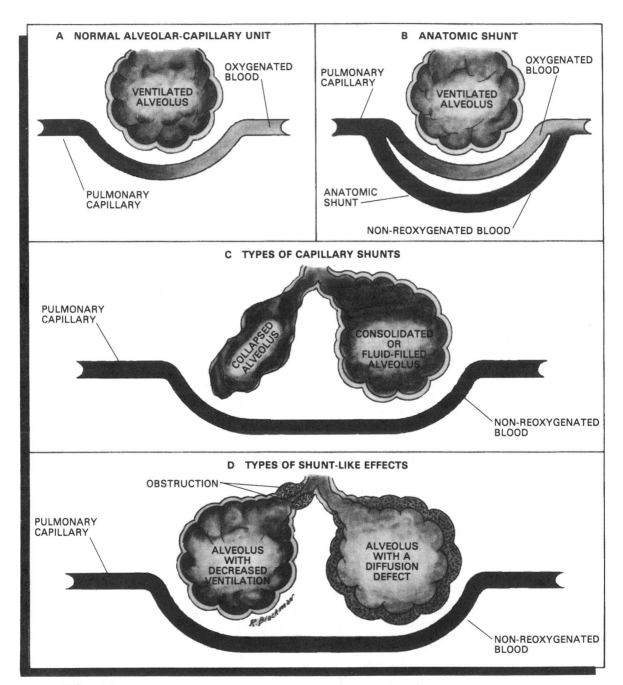

FIG 1-24

Pulmonary shunting. *A*) Normal alveolar-capillary unit; *B*) anatomic shunt; *C*) types of capillary shunts; *D*) types of shuntlike effects. (From Des Jardins T: *Cardiopulmonary Anatomy and Physiology: Essentials for Respiratory Care,* 2nd ed., Albany, NY, Delmar Publishers Inc, 1993. Used by permission.)

Table 1-6 Type of Pulmonary Shunting Associated With Common Respiratory Diseases

Respiratory Disease	Capillary Shunt	Shuntlike Effect
Chronic bronchitis		X
Emphysema		X
Asthma		X
Croup/epiglottitis		X
Bronchiectasis*	X	X
Cystic fibrosis*	X	X
Pneumoconiosis*	X	X
Pneumonia	X	
Lung abscess	X	
Pulmonary edema	X	
Near-drowning	X	
Adult respiratory distress syndrome	X	
Chronic interstitial lung disease	X	
Flail chest	X	
Pneumothorax	X	
Pleural diseases	X	
Kyphoscoliosis	X	
Tuberculosis	X	
Fungal diseases	X	
Idiopathic (infant) respiratory distress syndrome	X	
Smoke inhalation	X	

*Shuntlike effect is most common.

the original values of the reoxygenated and nonreoxygenated blood. Clinically, it is this mixed blood that is sampled downstream (e.g., from the radial artery) to assess the patient's arterial blood gases.

To summarize, the peripheral chemoreceptors are frequently stimulated in respiratory disease because they respond to hypoxemia caused by decreased $\dot{V}/\dot{Q}$ ratio, capillary shunting (or a shuntlike effect), and venous admixture. The decreased arterial oxygen tension, in turn, stimulates the peripheral chemoreceptors to send a signal to the medulla to increase ventilation (Fig 1-26).

Other Factors That Stimulate the Peripheral Chemoreceptors

While the peripheral chemoreceptors are primarily activated by a decreased arterial oxygen level, they are also simulated by a decreased pH (increased H^+ concentration). For example, the accumulation of lactic acid (from anaerobic metabolism) or ketoacids (diabetic acidosis) in the blood increases ventilatory rate almost entirely through the peripheral chemoreceptors. The peripheral chemoreceptors are also activated by hypoperfusion, increased temperature, nicotine, and the direct effect of $Paco_2$. The response of the peripheral chemoreceptors to $Paco_2$ stimulation, however, is relatively small compared to the response generated by the central chemoreceptors.

The Central Chemoreceptors and Their Effect on the Ventilatory Pattern

Although the mechanism is not fully understood, it is now believed that two special respiratory components in the medulla, called the *dorsal respiratory group* (DRG) and the *ventral*

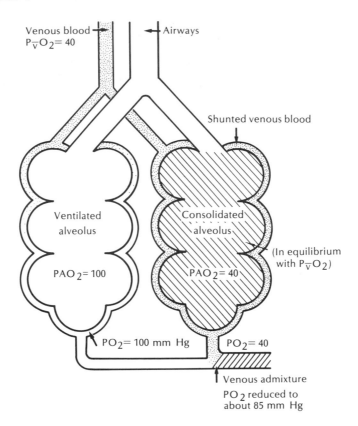

FIG 1-25
Venous admixture occurs when reoxygenated blood mixes with nonreoxygenated blood distal to the alveoli. Technically, the P_{O_2} in the pulmonary capillary system will not equilibrate completely because of the normal $P(A-a)_{O_2}$. The P_{O_2} in the pulmonary capillary system is normally a few mm Hg less than the P_{O_2} in the alveoli.

respiratory group (VRG), are responsible for coordinating respiration (Fig 1-27). Both the DRG and the VRG are stimulated by an increased concentration of hydrogen ions [H^+] in the cerebrospinal fluid (CSF). The H^+ concentration of the CSF is monitored by the central chemoreceptors, which are located bilaterally and ventrally in the substance of the medulla. A portion of the central chemoreceptor region is actually in direct contact with the CSF. It is believed that the central chemoreceptors transmit signals to the respiratory neurons by the following mechanism:

1. When the CO_2 level increases in the blood (e.g., during periods of hypoventilation), CO_2 molecules readily diffuse across the blood-brain barrier and enter the CSF. The blood-brain barrier is a semipermeable membrane that separates circulating blood from the CSF. The blood-brain barrier is relatively impermeable to ions like H^+ and HCO_3^- but is very permeable to CO_2.
2. Once CO_2 crosses the blood-brain barrier and enters the CSF, it forms carbonic acid:

$$CO_2 + H_2O \leftrightarrows H_2CO_3 \leftrightarrows H^+ + HCO_3^-$$

3. Because the CSF has an inefficient buffering system, the H^+ produced from the above reaction rapidly increases and causes the pH in the CSF to decrease.
4. The central chemoreceptors react to the liberated H^+ by sending signals to the respiratory components of the medulla, which in turn increase the ventilatory rate.

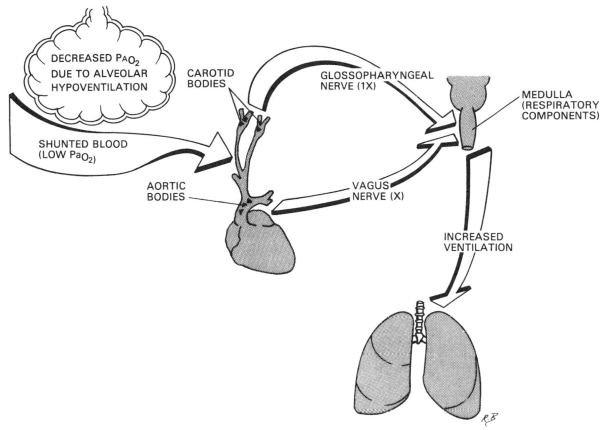

FIG 1-26

Schematic illustration showing how a low Pa_{O_2} stimulates the respiratory components of the medulla to increase alveolar ventilation. As shown, alveolar hypoventilation (decreased $\dot{V}/\dot{Q}$ ratio) leads to shunting and venous admixture. This process causes the Pa_{O_2} to fall. The low Pa_{O_2} stimulates the carotid and aortic bodies to send signals to the medulla. The medulla, in turn, sends out signals to increase ventilation. (From Des Jardins T: *Cardiopulmonary Anatomy and Physiology: Essentials for Respiratory Care,* 2 ed., Albany, NY, Delmar Publishers Inc, 1993. Used by permission.)

    5. The increased ventilatory rate causes the Pa_{CO_2} and, subsequently, the P_{CO_2} in the CSF to decrease. Thus, the CO_2 level in the blood regulates ventilation by its indirect effect on the pH of the CSF (Fig 1-28).

The Pulmonary Reflexes and Their Effect on the Ventilatory Pattern

There are several reflexes that may be activated in certain respiratory diseases, and these influence the patient's ventilatory rate:

Deflation reflex.—When the lungs are compressed or deflated (e.g., atelectasis), an increased rate of breathing is seen. The precise mechanism responsible for this reflex is not known. Some investigators suggest that the increased rate of breathing may simply be due to reduced stimulation of the receptors serving the Hering-Breuer reflex rather than the stimulation of specific deflation receptors. Receptors for the Hering-Breuer reflex are located in the walls of the bronchi and bronchioles. When these receptors are stretched (e.g., during a deep inspiration), a reflex response is triggered to decrease the ventilatory rate. Other investigators, however, feel that the deflation reflex is not due to the absence of receptor stimulation of the

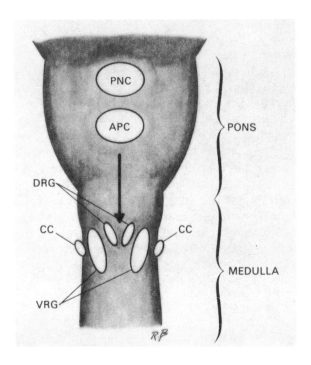

FIG 1-27
Schematic illustration of the respiratory components of the lower brain stem (pons and medulla). *PNC* = pneumotaxic center; *APC* = apneustic center; *DRG* = dorsal respiratory group; *VRG* = ventral respiratory group; *CC* = central chemoreceptors. (From Des Jardins T: *Cardiopulmonary Anatomy and Physiology: Essentials for Respiratory Care,* 2nd ed, Albany NY, Delmar Publishers Inc, 1993. Used by permission.)

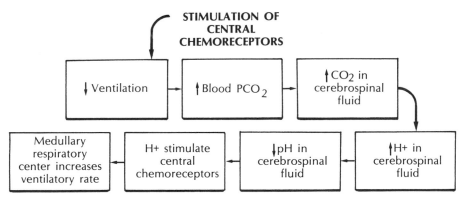

FIG 1-28
The central chemoreceptors are stimulated by hydrogen ions *(H⁺),* which increase in concentration as CO_2 moves into the CSF.

Hering-Breuer reflex, since the reflex is still seen when the bronchi and bronchioles are below a temperature of 8° C. The Hering-Breuer reflex is not seen when the bronchi and bronchioles are below this temperature.

Irritant reflex.—When the lungs are compressed, deflated, or exposed to noxious gases, the irritant receptors are stimulated. The irritant receptors are subepithelial mechanoreceptors located in the trachea, bronchi, and bronchioles. When the receptors are activated, a reflex response causes the ventilatory rate to increase. Stimulation of the irritant reflex may also produce a cough and bronchoconstriction.

Juxtapulmonary capillary receptors (J receptors).—The juxtapulmonary capillary receptors, or J receptors, are located in the interstitial tissues between the pulmonary capillaries and the alveoli. The precise mechanism of this action is not known. When the J receptors are stimulated, a reflex response triggers rapid, shallow breathing. It is believed that the J receptors are activated by:

- Pulmonary capillary congestion
- Capillary hypertension
- Edema of the alveolar walls
- Humoral agents (serotonin)
- Lung deflation
- Emboli in the microcirculation

Reflexes from the aortic and carotid sinus baroreceptors.—The normal function of the aortic and carotid sinus baroreceptors, located near the aortic and carotid peripheral chemoreceptors, is to activate reflexes that cause (1) decreased heart rate and ventilatory rate in response to an increased systemic blood pressure and (2) increased heart rate and ventilatory rate in response to a decreased systemic blood pressure.

Pain/Anxiety

An increased respiratory rate may simply be due to the chest pain or fear and anxiety associated with the patient's inability to breathe. For example, it is not unusual for chest pain and fear to occur in a number of cardiopulmonary diseases such as pleurisy, rib fractures, pulmonary hypertension, and angina. An increased respiratory rate may also be caused by fever. Fever is commonly associated with infectious lung disorders such as pneumonia, lung abscess, tuberculosis, and fungal disease.

ABNORMAL PULMONARY FUNCTION STUDY FINDINGS

Pulmonary function studies play a major role in the assessment of pulmonary disease. The results from pulmonary function studies are used to (1) evaluate pulmonary causes of dyspnea, (2) differentiate between obstructive and restrictive pulmonary disorders, (3) assess severity of the pathophysiologic impairment, (4) follow the course of a particular disease, (5) evaluate the effectiveness of bronchodilator therapy, and (6) assess the patient's preoperative status.

NORMAL LUNG VOLUMES AND CAPACITIES

As shown in Figure 1-29, gas in the lungs is divided into four separate volumes. The four lung "capacities" represent different combinations of lung volumes.

Lung Volumes

- *Tidal volume* (V_T): The volume of gas that normally moves into and out of the lungs in one quiet breath.
- *Inspiratory reserve volume* (IRV): The volume of air that can be forcefully inspired after a normal tidal volume inhalation.

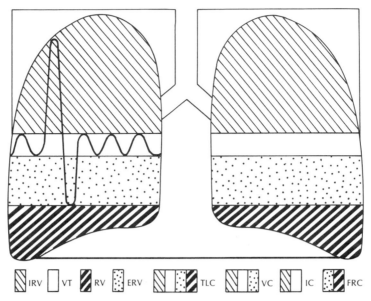

FIG 1-29

Normal lung volumes and capacities. *IRV* = inspiratory reserve volume; V_T = tidal volume; *RV* = residual volume; *ERV* = expiratory reserve volume; *TLC* = total lung capacity; *VC* = vital capacity; *IC* = inspiratory capacity; *FRC* = functional residual capacity.

Table 1-7 Lung Volumes and Capacities (in Milliliters) of Normal Recumbent Subject Between 20 and 30 Years of Age

Measurement	Male	Female
Tidal volume (V_T)	500	400 to 500
Inspiratory reserve volume (IRV)	3,100	1,900
Expiratory reserve volume (ERV)	1,200	800
Residual volume (RV)	1,200	1,000
Vital capacity (VC)	4,800	3,200
Inspiratory capacity (IC)	3,600	2,400
Functional residual capacity (FRC)	2,400	1,800
Total lung capacity (TLC)	6,000	4,200

- *Expiratory reserve volume* (ERV): The volume of air that can be forcefully exhaled after a normal tidal volume exhalation.
- *Residual volume* (RV): The amount of air remaining in the lungs after a forced exhalation.

Lung Capacities

- *Vital capacity* (VC): VC = IRV + V_T + ERV. The volume of air that can be exhaled after a maximal inspiration. There are two major VC measurements: *slow vital capacity* (SVC), or a vital capacity in which exhalation is performed slowly to offset air trapping, and forced vital capacity (FVC), or a vital capacity in which a maximal effort is made to exhale as rapidly as possible to assess the degree of air flow obstruction.

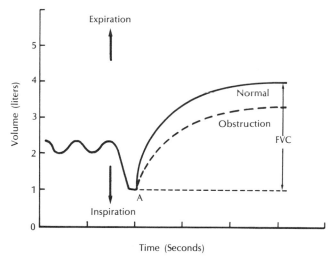

FIG 1-30

Forced vital capacity *(FVC)*. *A* is the point of maximal inspiration and the starting point of an FVC.

- *Inspiratory capacity* (IC): IC = V_T + IRV. The volume of air that can be inhaled after a normal exhalation.
- *Functional residual capacity* (FRC): FRC = ERV + RV. The lung volume at rest after a normal tidal volume exhalation.
- *Total lung capacity* (TLC): TLC = IC + FRC. The maximal amount of air that the lungs can accommodate.

The amount of air the lungs can accommodate varies with age, weight, height, and the sex of the individual. Table 1-7 lists the normal lung volumes and capacities of the average man and woman aged 20 to 30 years.

EXPIRATORY FLOW RATE MEASUREMENTS

In addition to the volumes and capacities that can be measured by pulmonary function testing, it is possible to measure the rate at which gas flows out of the lungs. Such measurements provide data on the patency of the airways, the severity of the airway impairment, and whether the patient has a large-airway or a small-airway problem, and include the following.

Forced Vital Capacity (FVC).—The volume of gas that can be exhaled as forcefully and rapidly as possible after a maximal inspiration. Normally FVC = VC. In obstructive lung disease, however, FVC is reduced when compared to the *slow vital capacity* (Fig 1-30), indicating air trapping with forced exhalation.

Forced Expiratory Volume, Timed (FEV_T).—The maximum volume of gas that can be exhaled over a specific period. This measurement is obtained from an FVC measurement. Commonly used time periods are 0.5, 1.0, 2.0, and 3.0 seconds. Normally, the percentages of the total volume exhaled during these time periods are as follows: $FEV_{0.5}$, 60%; $FEV_{1.0}$, 83%; $FEV_{2.0}$, 94%; and $FEV_{3.0}$, 97%. $FEV_{1.0}$ is the most commonly used measurement. In obstructive disease, the time necessary to forcefully exhale a certain volume is increased (Fig 1-31).

Forced Expiratory Flow $_{200-1,200}$ ($FEF_{200-1,200}$).—The $FEF_{200-1,200}$ (formerly called maximum expiratory flow rate [MEFR]) measures the average rate of airflow between 200 and

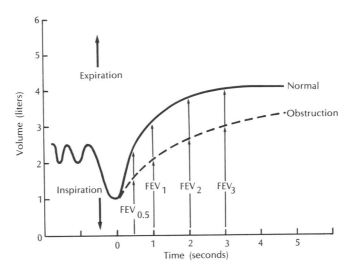

FIG 1-31
Forced expiratory volume timed *(FEV_T)*. In obstructive pulmonary disease, more time is needed to exhale a specific volume.

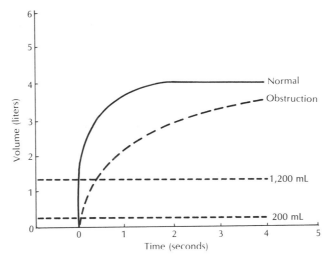

FIG 1-32
Forced expiratory flow 200-1,200 *(FEF_{200-1,200})*. This test measures the average rate of flow between 200 ml and 1,200 ml of an FVC. The flow rate is measured when 200 ml have been exhaled and again when 1,200 ml have been exhaled. The average rate of flow is derived by dividing the combined flow rates by 2.

1,200 ml of an FVC (Fig 1-32). The first 200 ml of the FVC is usually exhaled more slowly than at the average flow rate because of (1) the inertia involved in the respiratory maneuver and (2) the slow initial response of the spirometer.

Because the $FEF_{200-1,200}$ measures expiratory flows at high lung volumes (i.e., the initial part of the forced vital capacity), it is a good index of the patency of large airways. The normal $FEF_{200-1,200}$ for the average healthy male between 20 and 30 years of age is about 8 L/sec (480 L/min). The normal $FEF_{200-1,200}$ in the average healthy female between 20 and 30 years of age is about 5.5 L/sec (330 L/min). In obstructive lung disease, however, flow rates as low as 1 L/sec (60 L/min) have been reported. The $FEF_{200-1,200}$ is a responsive test to determine the patient's response to bronchodilator therapy.

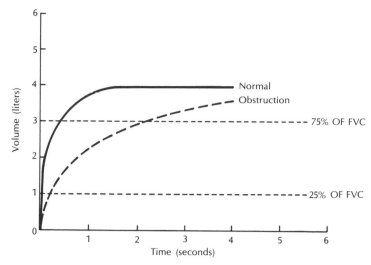

FIG 1-33

Forced expiratory flow 25% to 75% *(FEF₂₅%₋₇₅%)*. This test measures the average rate of flow between 25% and 75% of an FVC. The flow rate is measured when 25% of the FVC has been exhaled and again when 75% of the FVC has been exhaled. The average rate of flow is derived by dividing the combined flow rates by 2.

Forced Expiratory Flow ₂₅%₋₇₅% (FEF₂₅%₋₇₅%).—The $FEF_{25\%-75\%}$ (also known as the maximum midexpiratory flow rate [MMRF]) is the average flow rate during the middle 50% of an FVC measurement (Fig 1-33). This expiratory maneuver is commonly used to assess the status of medium-sized airways in obstructive lung diseases. The normal $FEF_{25\%-75\%}$ in the average healthy male between 20 and 30 years of age is about 4.5 L/sec (270 L/min). The normal $FEF_{25\%-75\%}$ in the average healthy female between 20 and 30 years of age is about 3.5 L/sec (210 L/min). The $FEF_{25\%-75\%}$ progressively decreases in obstructive diseases and with age.

Peak Expiratory Flow Rate (PEFR).—The PEFR (also known as the peak flow rate [PFR]) is the maximum flow rate that can be achieved. This measurement can be obtained from an FVC (Fig 1-34). The normal PEFR in the average healthy male between 20 and 30 years of age is about 10 L/sec (600 L/min). The normal PEFR in the average healthy female between 20 and 30 years of age is about 7.5 L/sec (450 L/min). The PEFR progressively decreases in obstructive diseases and with age.

It should be noted that the PEFR can easily be measured at the patient's bedside with a hand-held *peak flowmeter* (e.g., Wright peak flowmeter). The hand-held peak flowmeter is used to monitor the degree of airway obstruction on a moment-to-moment basis and is relatively small, inexpensive, accurate, reproducible, and easy for the patient to use. In addition, the mouthpieces are disposable, thus allowing the safe use of the same peak flowmeter from one patient to another. PEFR measurements should routinely be performed at the patient's bedside to assess the degree of bronchospasm, effect of bronchodilators, and day-to-day progress. The fact that the PEFR results generated by the patient before and after bronchodilator therapy can serve as excellent, objective data regarding the effectiveness of the therapy. Thus, this device is finding a great use in modern asthma programs.

Maximum Voluntary Ventilation (MVV).—The MVV (formerly called the maximum breathing capacity [MBC]) is the largest volume of gas that can be breathed voluntarily in and out of the lungs in one minute (Fig 1-35). The normal MVV in the average healthy male between 20 and 30 years of age is about 170 L/min. The normal MVV in the average healthy

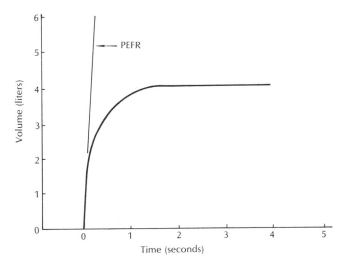

FIG 1-34
Peak expiratory flow rate *(PEFR)*. The steepest *slope* of the $\Delta V/\Delta T$ line is the PEFR ($\dot{V}$).

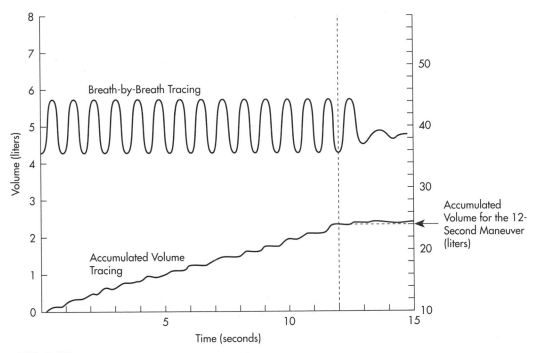

FIG 1-35
Volume/time tracing for a maximum voluntary ventilation (MVV) maneuver

female between 20 and 30 years of age is about 110 L/min. The MVV progressively decreases in obstructive and restrictive pulmonary diseases.

Forced Expiratory Volume in 1 Second/Forced Vital Capacity Ratio (FEV_1/FVC Ratio).—The FEV_1/FVC ratio is used as a broad indicator of airway obstruction. Although a decreased ratio is a reliable measurement of airway obstruction, the absence of a decreased ratio does not exclude the presence of airway (particularly small airway) obstruction.

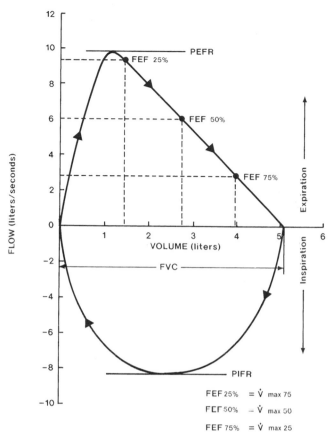

FIG 1-36
Flow-volume loop.

Flow-Volume Loop.—The *flow-volume loop* analysis is helpful in determining the site of airway obstruction. It requires use of a flowmeter (called a pneumotachograph), a spirometer, and a recorder with X-Y graphic capability. As shown in Figure 1-36, the upper half of the flow-volume loop (above the zero flow axis) represents the maximum expiratory flow generated during a forced vital capacity (FVC) maneuver, plotted against volume change. This portion of the curve shows the flow generated between the TLC to RV.

The lower half of the flow-volume loop (below the zero flow axis) illustrates the maximum inspiratory flow generated during a forced inspiration (called a *force inspiratory volume [FIV]*), plotted against the volume inhaled. This portion of the curve shows the flow generated between the RV and TLC. Depending on the sophistication of the equipment, the following information can be obtained from this test:

- Peak expiratory flow rate (PEFR)
- Peak inspiratory flow rate (PIFR)
- Forced vital capacity (FVC)
- Forced expiratory volume timed (FEV_T)
- Forced expiratory flow $_{25\%-75\%}$
- Forced expiratory flow $_{50\%}$ ($FEF_{50\%}$)
- Instantaneous flow at any given lung volume

In normal subjects, the expiratory flow rate decreases linearly with volume after the PEFR has been achieved (this portion of the curve represents approximately the last 70% to 80% of the FVC). In patients with obstructive lung disease, however, flow is frequently decreased at low lung volumes, and this causes a "cup-like" or "scooped out" appearance in the expira-

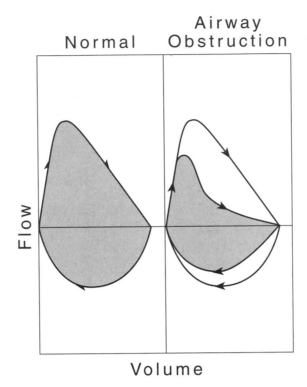

FIG 1-37
Flow-volume loop demonstrating the shape change that results from an obstructive lung disorder.

tory flow curve when 50% of the FVC has been exhaled. This portion of the flow curve is called the *forced expiratory flow$_{50\%}$ (FEF$_{50\%}$)* or $\dot{V}_{max_{50}}$ (Fig 1-37).

Forced Expiratory Time (FET).—With the growing concern over the appropriate use of high-cost medical technology, there has been a renewed interest in physical examination methods that are safe, reproducible, inexpensive, and accurate in detecting abnormalities. In the spirit of this trend, the forced expiratory time (FET) has recently been reintroduced in the literature. Although controversial in the past, the FET is now presented as a moderately good, simple, and inexpensive bedside test in the screening of obstructive airway disease.

The FET is defined as the time it takes an individual to forcefully exhale through an open mouth from total lung capacity until airflow is no longer audible. The FET is easily measured at the patient's bedside with only a stethoscope and a stopwatch. The patient is asked to take a deep breath in (to his/her TLC), and then to exhale as fast and as hard as possible. The cessation of airflow is determined by listening either at the mouth, or by stethoscope over the trachea. An FET of 4 seconds or less is normal. An FET of more than 6 seconds suggests airway obstruction.

The auscultated FET, combined with clinical history and physical examination and x-ray examination, permits the clinician to evaluate the patient's pulmonary function status at the bedside before resorting to more precise (and expensive) pulmonary function studies. The auscultated FET is simple to perform, inexpensive, fairly reproducible, and has the potential of providing the respiratory care practitioner with useful screening information in the assessment of obstructive airway disease. It may also be used to measure the effectiveness of bronchodilator therapy.

EXPIRATORY MANEUVER FINDINGS CHARACTERISTIC OF
RESTRICTIVE LUNG DISEASES

- Decreased forced vital capacity (FVC)
- Decreased forced expiratory flow $_{200\text{-}1,200}$ ($FEF_{200\text{-}1,200}$)
- Decreased forced expiratory flow $_{25\%\text{-}75\%}$ ($FEF_{25\%\text{-}75\%}$)
- Normal/Decreased forced expiratory volume, timed (FEV_T)
- Normal forced expiratory volume in 1 second/forced vital capacity ratio (FEV_1/FVC ratio)
- Decreased maximum voluntary ventilation (MVV)
- Decreased peak expiratory flow rate (PEFR)
- Decreased flow at 50% vital capacity ($\dot{V}_{max_{50}}$)

In restrictive lung disorders, flow and volume are reduced to about an equal extent. Clinically, this is referred to as "symmetrical" reduction in flows and volumes. The flow-volume loop, thus, is a "small version" of normal in restrictive pulmonary disease (Fig 1-38).

LUNG VOLUME AND CAPACITY FINDINGS CHARACTERISTIC OF
RESTRICTIVE LUNG DISEASES

- Decreased tidal volume (V_T)
- Decreased residual volume (RV)
- Decreased functional residual capacity (FRC)
- Normal residual volume/total lung capacity ratio (RV/TLC)
- Decreased total lung capacity (TLC)
- Decreased vital capacity (VC)
- Decreased inspiratory capacity (IC)
- Decreased expiratory reserve volume (ERV)

The above lung volumes and capacity abnormalities develop in response to pathologic conditions that alter the anatomic structures distal to the terminal bronchioles, i.e., the lung parenchyma. Such conditions include the following:

- Lung compression (e.g., secondary to kyphoscoliosis or pleural effusion)
- Atelectasis (e.g., secondary to pneumothorax or flail chest)
- Consolidation (e.g., pneumonia)
- Calcification (e.g., tuberculosis or asbestosis)
- Fibrosis (e.g., pneumonconiosis or chronic interstitial lung disease)
- Bronchogenic tumor (e.g., squamous cell carcinoma)
- Caseous tubercles (e.g., tuberculosis)
- Cavitations (e.g., tuberculosis or lung abscess)

These pathologic conditions cause increased lung rigidity. When lung rigidity increases, lung compliance decreases. Decreased lung compliance, in turn, causes a reduction in the patient's V_T, RV, RV/TLC, FRC, TLC, VC, IRV, and ERV (Fig 1-39). In addition, when lung compliance decreases, the patient's ventilatory rate increases while, at the same time, the V_T decreases (see Fig 1-19).

In pulmonary obstructive disease, the expiratory findings develop in response to patho-

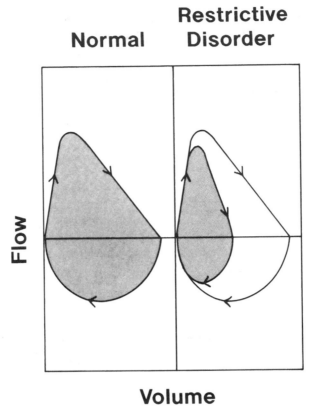

FIG 1-38
Flow-volume loop demonstrating the shape change that results from a restrictive lung disorder. Note the symmetrical loss of flow and volume.

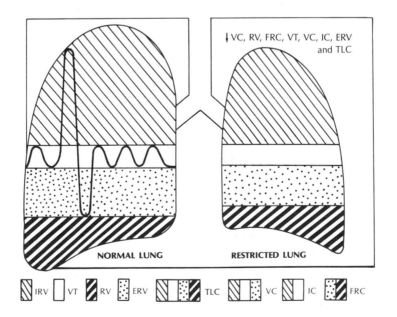

FIG 1-39
How restrictive lung disorders alter lung volumes and capacities. IRV = inspiratory reserve volume; V_T = tidal volume; RV = residual volume; ERV = expiratory reserve volume; TLC = total lung capacity; VC = vital capacity; IC = inspiratory capacity; FRC = functional residual capacity.

EXPIRATORY MANEUVER FINDINGS CHARACTERISTIC OF
OBSTRUCTIVE LUNG DISEASES

- Decreased forced vital capacity (FVC)
- Decreased forced expiratory flow $_{200-1,200}$ (FEF$_{200-1,200}$)
- Decreased forced expiratory flow $_{25\%-75\%}$ (FEF$_{25\%-75\%}$)
- Decreased forced expiratory volume, timed (FEV$_T$)
- Decreased forced expiratory volume in 1 second/forced vital capacity ratio (FEV$_1$/FVC ratio)
- Decreased maximum voluntary ventilation (MVV)
- Decreased peak expiratory flow rate (PEFR)
- Decreased flow at 50% vital capacity ($\dot{V}_{max_{50}}$)

---

logic conditions that alter the anatomic structures of the tracheobronchial tree. Such pathologic conditions include the following:

- Chronic inflammation and swelling of the peripheral airways (e.g., chronic bronchitis)
- Excessive mucus production and accumulation (e.g., cystic fibrosis)
- A tumor projecting into a bronchus (e.g., bronchogenic cancer)
- Destruction and weakening of the distal airways (e.g., emphysema)
- Bronchial smooth muscle constriction (e.g., asthma)

Because of the decreased expiratory flow rates seen in patients with obstructive pulmonary disease, the FEF$_{50\%}$ portion of the flow-volume loop usually has a "cuplike" or "scooped out" appearance (see Fig 1-37).

To fully appreciate how these pathologic conditions cause the expiratory findings seen in obstructive pulmonary disorders, an understanding of the following is essential:

- How activation of the dynamic compression mechanism affects respiratory function in obstructive pulmonary diseases
- Bernoulli's principle and the dynamic compression mechanism in obstructive pulmonary diseases
- How Poiseuille's law relates to respiratory function in obstructive pulmonary diseases
- How the airway resistance equation relates to respiratory function in obstructive pulmonary diseases

How activation of the dynamic compression mechanism affects respiratory function in obstructive pulmonary diseases.

The effort-dependent portion of a forced expiratory maneuver.—Normally, during approximately the first 20% to 30% of a forced vital capacity maneuver, the maximum (peak) flow rate is dependent on the amount of muscular effort exerted by the individual. Therefore, the first 20% to 30% of a forced expiratory maneuver is referred to as effort-dependent. In other words, the initial maximal flow rate during forced expiration depends on the muscular effort produced by the individual.

The effort-independent portion of a forced expiratory maneuver.—The flow rate during approximately the last 70% to 80% of a forced vital capacity maneuver is effort-independent, that is, once a maximum flow rate has been attained, the flow rate cannot be increased by further muscular effort.

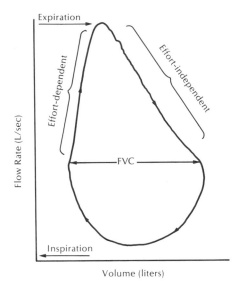

FIG 1-40
The effort-dependent and effort-independent portions of a forced expiratory maneuver in a flow-volume loop measurement. *FVC* = forced vital capacity.

The lung volume at which the patient initiates a forced expiratory maneuver also influences the maximum flow rate. As lung volumes decline, flow also declines. The reduced flow, however, is the maximum flow for that particular volume.

Figure 1-40 illustrates where the effort-dependent and effort-independent portions of a forced expiratory maneuver appear on a flow-volume loop.

Dynamic compression of the airways.—The limitation of the flow rate that occurs during approximately the last 70% to 80% of a forced vital capacity maneuver is due to the *dynamic compression* of the walls of the airways. As gas flows through the airways during passive expiration, the pressure within the airways diminishes to zero (Fig 1-41, A).

During a forced expiratory maneuver, however, as the airway pressure decreases from the alveolus to the atmosphere, there comes a point at which the pressure within the lumen of the airways equals the pleural pressure surrounding the airways. The transpulmonary pressure at this point is zero. This is called the *equal-pressure point.*

Downstream (i.e., toward the mouth) from the equal-pressure point, the lateral pressure within the airway becomes less than the surrounding pleural pressure. Consequently, the airways are compressed. As muscular effort and pleural pressure increase during a forced expiratory maneuver, the equal-pressure point moves upstream (i.e., toward the alveolus). Ultimately, the equal-pressure point becomes fixed where the individual's flow rate has achieved a maximum (see Fig 1-41, B). In essence, once dynamic compression occurs during a forced expiratory maneuver, increased muscular effort merely augments airway compression, which in turn increases airway resistance.

As the structural changes associated with obstructive pulmonary diseases intensify, the patient commonly responds by increasing intrapleural pressure during expiration to overcome the increased airway resistance produced by the disease. By increasing intrapleural pressure during expiration, however, the patient activates the dynamic compression mechanism, which in turn further reduces the diameter of the bronchial airways. This results in an even greater increase in airway resistance.

Bernoulli's principle and the dynamic compression mechanism in obstructive pulmonary diseases.—Bernoulli's principle states that when gas flowing through a tube encoun-

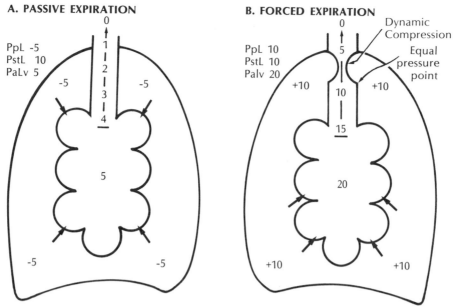

A. PASSIVE EXPIRATION

PpL -5
PstL 10
PaLv 5

B. FORCED EXPIRATION

PpL 10
PstL 10
Palv 20

Dynamic
Compression

Equal
pressure
point

FIG 1-41

The dynamic compression mechanism. **A,** during passive expiration, static elastic recoil pressure *(PstL)* is 10, pleural pressure *(PpL)* at the beginning of expiration is −5, and alveolar pressure *(Palv)* is +5. In order for gas to move from the alveolus to the atmosphere during expiration, the pressure must decrease progressively in the airways from +5 to 0. As **A** shows, PpL is always less than the airway pressure. **B,** during forced expiration, PpL becomes positive (+10 in this illustration). When this PpL is added to a PstL of +10, Palv becomes +20. As the pressure progressively decreases during forced expiration, there must be a point at which the pressures inside and outside the airway wall are equal. This point is the equal pressure point. Airway compression occurs downstream (toward the mouth) from this point because the lateral pressure in the lumen is less than the surrounding wall pressure.

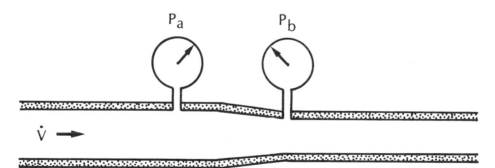

FIG 1-42

Illustration of Bernoulli's principle.

ters a narrowing or restriction, the velocity of the gas molecules increases. As a result, the gas molecules collide less frequently with the sides of the tube, and this causes the lateral pressure to drop (Fig 1-42).

This mechanism may play an insidious role in certain pulmonary disorders. In chronic obstructive pulmonary disease, for example, when the gas flow encounters bronchial narrowing during a forced expiratory maneuver, the decreased lateral pressure that results at the obstructed sites enhances dynamic compression.

How Poiseuille's law relates to respiratory function in obstructive pulmonary diseases.— During a normal inspiration, intrapleural pressure decreases from its normal resting level (about 2 to 3 cm H₂O pressure) and causes the bronchial airways to lengthen and to increase in diameter (passive dilation). During expiration, intrapleural pressure increases (or returns to its normal resting state) and causes the bronchial airways to decrease in length and in diameter (passive constriction) (Fig 1-43). These anatomic changes can affect bronchial gas flow and intrapleural pressure and can be expressed by Poiseuille's law.

*Poiseuille's law and its significance.—*Although the factors in Poiseuille's law are of little significance during normal, spontaneous breathing, they play a major role in obstructive pulmonary disorders. Poiseuille's law can be expressed for either flow or pressure.

*Poiseuille's law for flow.—*Poiseuille's law for flow states that when gas flows through a tube, the following applies:

$$\dot{V} = \frac{\Delta P \pi r^4}{8ln}$$

where *n* is the viscosity of a gas (or fluid), ΔP is the change of pressure from one end of the tube to the other, *r* is the radius of the tube, *l* is the length of the tube, and $\dot{V}$ is the gas (or fluid) flow through the tube; π and 8 are constants that will be excluded from the present discussion.

The equation states that flow is directly related to P and r^4 and indirectly related to *l* and *n*. In other words, flow will decrease in response to a decreased P and tube radius. Flow will increase in response to a decreased tube length and viscosity. Conversely, flow will increase in response to an increased P and tube radius and decrease in response to an increased tube length and viscosity.

It should be emphasized that flow is profoundly affected by the radius of the tube. As Poiseuille's law illustrates, $\dot{V}$ is a function of the fourth power of the radius (r^4). *In other*

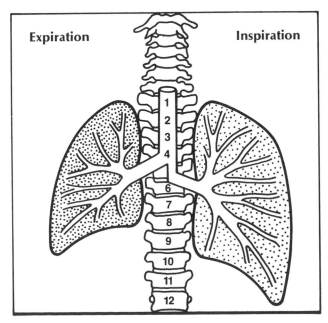

FIG 1-43
The normal change in size of the tracheobronchial tree during inspiration and expiration.

words, assuming pressure (ΔP) remains constant, decreasing the radius of a tube by one half reduces the gas flow to $\frac{1}{16}$ *of its original flow.*

For example, if the radius of a bronchial tube through which gas flows at a rate of 16 ml/sec is reduced to one half its original size because of mucosal swelling, the flow rate through the bronchial tube would decrease to 1 ml/sec ($\frac{1}{16}$ the original flow rate) (Fig 1-44).

Similarly, decreasing a tube radius by 16% decreases gas flow to one half its original rate. For instance, if the radius of a bronchial tube through which gas flows at a rate of 16 ml/sec is decreased by 16% (because of mucosal swelling, for example), the flow rate through the bronchial tube would decrease to 8 ml/sec (one half the original flow rate) (Fig 1-45).

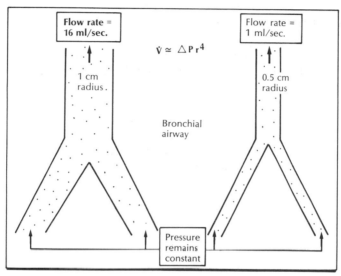

FIG 1-44
Poiseuille's law for flow applied to a bronchial airway with its radius reduced by 50%.

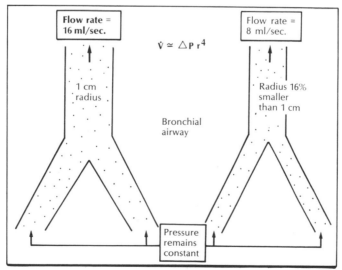

FIG 1-45
Poiseuille's law for flow applied to an airway with its radius reduced by 16%.

Poiseuille's law for pressure.—When Poiseuille's law is rearranged for pressure, it is written as follows:

$$P = \frac{\dot{V}8ln}{\pi r^4}$$

The equation now states that pressure is directly related to $\dot{V}$, l, and n and indirectly related to r^4. In other words, pressure increases in response to a decreased tube radius and decreases in response to decreased flow rate, tube length, or viscosity. The opposite is also true: pressure decreases in response to an increased tube radius and increases in response to increased flow rate, tube length, or viscosity.

Pressure is a function of the radius to the fourth power and therefore it is profoundly affected by the radius of a tube. In other words, if flow ($\dot{V}$) remains constant, decreasing a tube radius to one half of its previous size requires an increase in pressure to 16 times its original level.

For example, if the radius of a bronchus with a driving pressure of 1 cm H_2O is reduced to one half its original size because of mucosal swelling, the driving pressure through the bronchus would have to increase to 16 cm H_2O ($16 \times 1 = 16$) to maintain the same flow rate (Fig 1-46).

Similarly, decreasing the tube radius by 16% increases the pressure to twice its original level. For instance, if the radius of a bronchus with a driving pressure of 10 cm H_2O is decreased by 16% because of mucosal swelling, the driving pressure through the bronchus would have to increase to 20 cm H_2O (twice its original pressure) to maintain the same flow (Fig 1-47).

Poiseuille's law rearranged to simple proportionalities.—When Poiseuille's law is applied to the tracheobronchial tree during spontaneous breathing, the two equations can be rewritten as simple proportionalities:

$$\dot{V} \simeq Pr^4 \qquad P \simeq \frac{\dot{V}}{r^4}$$

where P is the intrapleural pressure, $\dot{V}$ is gas flow through the tracheobronchial tree, and r is the radius of the bronchus.

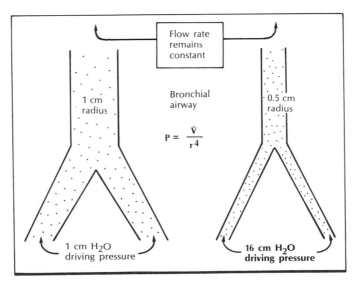

FIG 1-46
Poiseuille's law for pressure applied to an airway with its radius reduced by 50%.

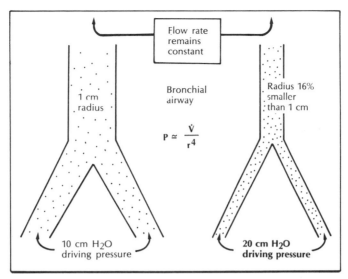

FIG 1-47

Poiseuille's law for pressure applied to an airway with its radius reduced by 16%.

Based on the proportionality for flow ($\dot{V} = Pr^4$), it can be stated that since gas flow varies directly with r^4 of the bronchial airway, flow must diminish during exhalation as the radius of the bronchial airways decreases. Stated differently, assuming that the pressure remains constant as the radius (r) of the bronchial airways decreases, the gas flow ($\dot{V}$) also decreases. During normal spontaneous breathing, the gas flow reduction during exhalation is negligible.

In terms of the proportionality for pressure ($P = \dot{V}/r^4$), if the gas flow is to remain constant during exhalation, the intrapleural pressure must vary indirectly with the fourth power of the radius of the airway. In other words, as the radius of the bronchial airways decreases during exhalation, the driving pressure must increase to maintain a constant gas flow. During normal spontaneous breathing, the need to increase intrapleural pressure during exhalation in order to maintain a certain gas flow is negligible.

In obstructive pulmonary diseases, however, both bronchial gas flow ($\dot{V}$) and intrapleural pressure (ΔP) may change substantially in response to the pathologic processes associated with the disorders.*

How the airway resistance equation relates to respiratory function in obstructive pulmonary diseases.—Changes in driving pressure (ΔP) and gas flow ($\dot{V}$) are used to measure airway resistance (R_{aw}). R_{aw} is measure in centimeters of water per liter per second, according to the following equation:

$$R_{aw} = \frac{\Delta P \ (cm \ H_2O)}{\dot{V} \ (L/sec)}$$

Normally, R_{aw} in the tracheobronchial tree is about 1.0 to 2.0 cm H_2O/L/sec. When the R_{aw} equation is applied to a normal ventilatory cycle, it can be seen that R_{aw} is greater during expiration than during inspiration. This is because the radius of the bronchial airways decreases during exhalation and—as Poiseuille's law for flow demonstrates—causes the gas flow ($\dot{V}$) to diminish.

Theoretically, during normal spontaneous breathing gas enters the alveoli during inspira-

*See a mathematic discussion of Poiseuille's law for flow and pressure in Appendix XVI.

tion (when the bronchial airways are dilated) more easily than it leaves the alveoli during expiration (when the caliber of the bronchial airways is smaller). Under normal circumstances, increased R_{aw} during expiration is of no significance. Because of the pathologic processes that develop in obstructive pulmonary diseases, however, R_{aw} may be quite high and may limit expiratory flow.

LUNG VOLUME AND CAPACITY FINDINGS CHARACTERISTIC OF
OBSTRUCTIVE LUNG DISEASES

- Increased tidal volume (V_T)
- Increased residual volume (RV)
- Increased functional residual capacity (FRC)
- Increased residual volume/total lung capacity ratio (RV/TLC)
- Increased/normal total lung capacity (TLC)
- Decreased/normal vital capacity (VC)
- Decreased inspiratory capacity (IC)
- Decreased expiratory reserve volume (ERV)

The changes in lung volumes and capacities listed above develop in response to pathologic conditions of the tracheofronchial tree. Some of the major pathologic conditions that alter the anatomic structures of the tracheobronchial tree are the following:

- Inflammation and swelling of the peripheral airways
- Excessive mucus production and accumulation
- Bronchial airway obstruction (e.g., from mucus or from a tumor projecting into a bronchus)
- Destruction and weakening of the distal airways
- Smooth muscle constriction of the airways (bronchospasm)

The above pathologic conditions cause increased airway resistance (R_{aw}) and airway closure during expiration. When R_{aw} becomes high, the patient's ventilatory rate decreases while, at the same time, the V_T increases. This ventilatory pattern is thought to be adopted to reduce the work of breathing (see Fig 1-19).

When bronchial closure develops during expiration, the gas that enters the alveoli during inspiration, when the bronchi are naturally wider, is prevented from leaving the alveoli during expiration. The alveoli then become overdistended with gas, a condition known as *air trapping*. Thus, excluding the V_T, bronchial closure and air trapping are the major mechanisms responsible for the abnormal lung volume and capacity findings seen in obstructive pulmonary diseases (Fig 1-48).

Pulmonary Diffusion Capacity

Trace gases are used to assess the adequacy of the pulmonary capillary membrane to transfer oxygen and carbon dioxide. Carbon monoxide (CO) is one such trace gas. The pulmonary diffusion capacity of carbon monoxide (D_{LCO}) measures the amount of CO that moves across the alveolar-capillary membrane. CO has an affinity for hemoglobin that is about 210 times greater than that of oxygen. Thus, when the patient has a normal hemoglobin concentration, pulmonary capillary blood volume, and ventilatory status, the only limiting factor to the diffusion of CO is the alveolar-capillary membrane (except in carboxyhemoglobinemia, where the carbon monoxide already combined with hemoglobin results in a reduced D_{LCO}).

The D_{LCO} decreases in response to lung disorders that affect the alveolar-capillary mem-

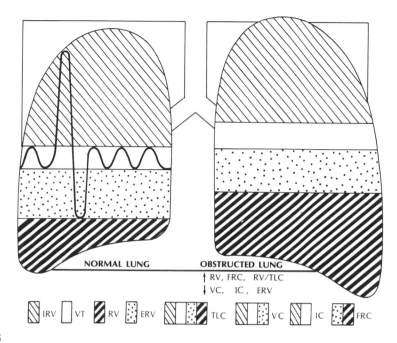

FIG 1-48

How obstructive lung disorders alter lung volumes and capacities. *IRV* = inspiratory reserve volume; V_T = tidal volume; *RV* = residual volume; *ERV* = expiratory reserve volume; *TLC* = total lung capacity; *VC* = vital capacity; *IC* = inspiratory capacity; *FRC* = functional residual capacity.

brane. For example, the D_{LCO} decreases in emphysema because of the alveolar-capillary de struction associated with the disease. The D_{LCO} also decreases in lung disorders such as the pneumonoconioses or other chronic interstitial lung diseases that cause pulmonary fibrosis.

Under normal conditions, the average D_{LCO} value for the resting male is 25 ml/min/mm Hg (STPD). This value is slightly lower in females, presumably because of their smaller nor mal lung volumes. The carbon monoxide *single-breath technique* is commonly used for this measurement.

PURSED-LIP BREATHING

Pursed-lip breathing is seen in patients during the advanced stages of obstructive pulmonary disease. It is a relatively simple technique that many patients learn without formal instruc tion. While pursed-lip breathing, the patient exhales through lips that are held in a position similar to that of whistling, kissing, or blowing through a flute. The positive pressure created by retarding the airflow through pursed lips provides the airways with some stability and an increased ability to resist surrounding intrapleural pressures. This action offsets early airway collapse and air trapping during exhalation. In addition, pursed-lip breathing has been shown to slow the patient's ventilatory rate and generates a ventilatory pattern that is more effective in gas mixing (Fig 1-49).

INCREASED ANTEROPOSTERIOR CHEST DIAMETER (BARREL CHEST)

Because of the air trapping and lung hyperinflation in obstructive pulmonary diseases, the natural tendency of the lungs to recoil is decreased, and the normal tendency of the chest to move outward prevails. This condition results in an increased anteroposterior diameter and is referred to as the "barrel chest" deformity. Normally, the anteroposterior diameter is about

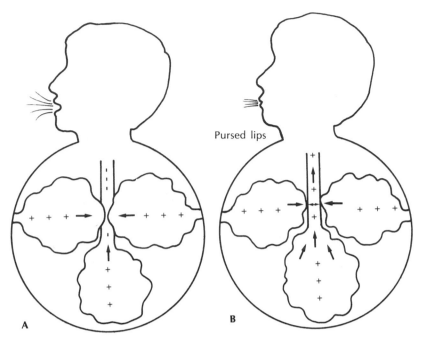

FIG 1-49
A, schematic illustration of alveoli compression of weakened bronchiolar airways during normal expiration in patients with chronic obstructive pulmonary disease (e.g., emphysema). **B,** effects of pursed-lip breathing. The weakened bronchiolar airways are kept open by the effects of positive pressure created by pursed lips during expiration.

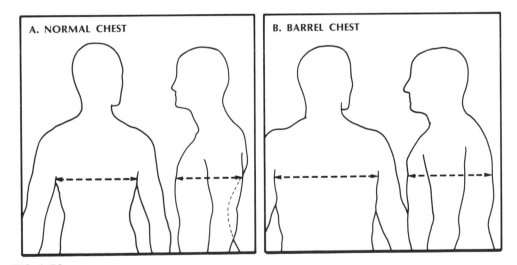

FIG 1-50
Normally, the ratio of the anteroposterior chest diameter to the lateral chest diameter is about 1:2 **(A).** In patients who have a barrel chest, however, a ratio nearer to 1:1 is present **(B).**

half the lateral diameter, or 1:2. When the patient has a barrel chest, the ratio may be nearer to 1:1. It should be noted that the anteroposterior diameter commonly increases with aging. Thus, older individuals may have a slight barrel chest appearance in the absence of any pulmonary disease. Normal newborn infants also usually have an anteroposterior ratio near 1:1 (Fig 1-50).

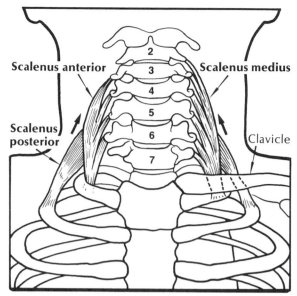

FIG 1-51
The scalene muscles

USE OF THE ACCESSORY MUSCLES OF INSPIRATION

During the advanced stages of chronic obstructive pulmonary disease, the accessory muscles of inspiration are activated when the diaphragm becomes significantly depressed by the increased residual volume and functional residual capacity. The accessory muscles assist or largely replace the diaphragm in creating subatmospheric pressure in the pleural space during inspiration. The major accessory muscles of inspiration are the following:

- Scalene
- Sternocleidomastoid
- Pectoralis major
- Trapezius

Scalene

The anterior, medial, and posterior scalene muscles are separate muscles that function as a unit. They originate on the transverse processes of the second to sixth cervical vertebrae and insert into the first and second ribs (Fig 1-51). These muscles normally elevate the first and second ribs and flex the neck. When used as accessory muscles for inspiration, their primary role is to elevate the first and second ribs.

Sternocleidomastoid

The sternocleidomastoid muscles are located on each side of the neck (Fig 1-52) where they rotate and support the head. They originate from the sternum and the clavicle and insert into the mastoid process and occipital bone of the skull.

Normally the sternocleidomastoid pulls from its sternoclavicular origin and rotates the head to the opposite side and turns it upward. When the sternocleidomastoid muscle functions as an accessory muscle of inspiration, the head and neck are fixed by other muscles,

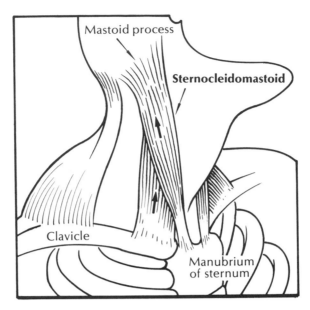

FIG 1-52
The sternocleidomastoid muscle.

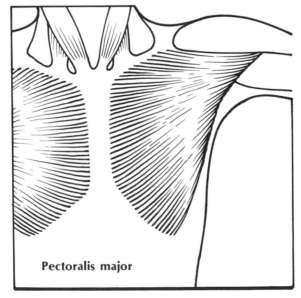

FIG 1-53
The pectoralis major muscles.

and the sternocleidomastoid pulls from its insertion on the skull and elevates the sternum. This action increases the anteroposterior diameter of the chest.

Pectoralis Major

The pectoralis majors are powerful, fan-shaped muscles that originate from the clavicle and the sternum and insert into the upper part of the humerus. The primary function of the pectoralis muscles is to pull the upper part of the arm to the body in a hugging motion (Fig 1-53).

When operating as an accessory muscle of inspiration, the pectoralis pulls from the hu-

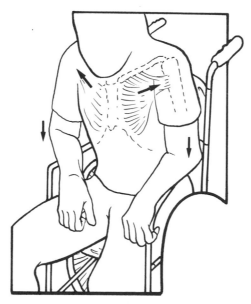

FIG 1-54
How a patient may appear when using the pectoralis major muscles for inspiration.

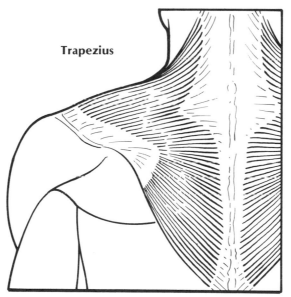

FIG 1-55
The trapezius muscles.

meral insertion and elevates the chest, thereby resulting in an increased anteroposterior diameter. Patients with chronic obstructive pulmonary disease usually secure their arms to something stationary and use the pectoralis major to increase the anteroposterior diameter of the chest (Fig 1-54).

Trapezius

The trapezius is a large, flat, triangular muscle that is situated superficially in the upper part of the back and the back of the neck. The muscle originates from the occipital bone, the ligamentum nuchae, and the spinous processes of the seventh cervical vertebra and all the

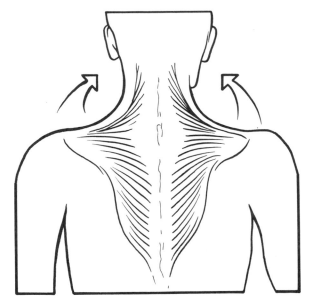

FIG 1-56
The action of the trapezius muscle is typified in shrugging the shoulders.

thoracic vertebrae. It inserts into the spine of the scapula, the acromion process, and the lateral third of the clavicle (Fig 1-55). The trapezius muscle rotates the scapula, raises the shoulders, and abducts and flexes the arm. Its action is typified in shrugging the shoulders (Fig 1-56).

When used as an accessory muscle of inspiration, the trapezius helps to elevate the thoracic cage.

USE OF ACCESSORY MUSCLES OF EXPIRATION

Because of the airway narrowing and collapse associated with chronic obstructive pulmonary disorders, the accessory muscles of exhalation are often recruited when airway resistance becomes significantly elevated. When these muscles actively contract, intrapleural pressure increases and offsets the increased airway resistance. The major accessory muscles of exhalation are the following:

- Rectus abdominis
- External oblique
- Internal oblique
- Transversus abdominis

Rectus Abdominis

A pair of rectus abdominis muscles extends the entire length of the abdomen. Each muscle forms a vertical mass about 4 in. wide, separated by the linea alba. It arises from the iliac crest and pubic symphysis and inserts into the xyphoid process and the fifth, sixth, and seventh ribs. When activated, the muscle assists in compressing the abdominal contents, which in turn push the diaphragm into the thoracic cage (Fig 1-57).

External Oblique

The broad, thin, external oblique muscle is on the anterolateral side of the abdomen. The muscle is the longest and most superficial of all the anterolateral muscles of the abdomen. It

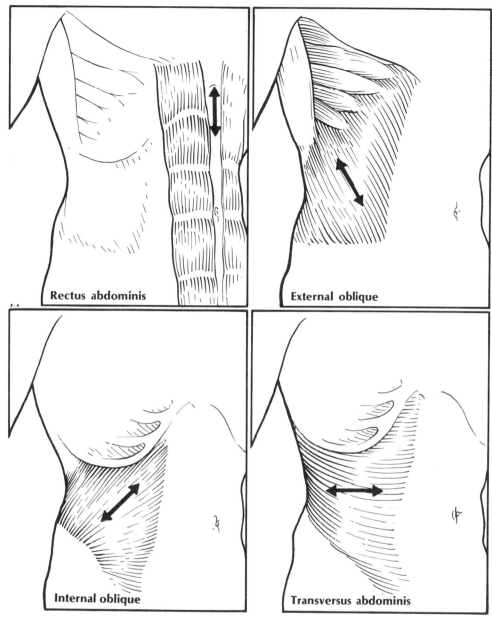

FIG 1-57
Accessory muscles of expiration.

arises by eight digitations from the lower eight ribs and the abdominal aponeurosis. It inserts in the iliac crest and into the linea alba. The muscle assists in compressing the contents of the abdomen. This action also pushes the diaphragm into the thoracic cage during exhalation (see Fig 1-57).

Internal Oblique

The internal oblique muscle is in the lateral and ventral part of the abdominal wall directly under the external oblique muscle. It is smaller and thinner than the external oblique. It arises from the inguinal ligament, the iliac crest, and the lower portion of the lumbar aponeurosis. It inserts into the last four ribs and into the linea alba. The muscle assists in

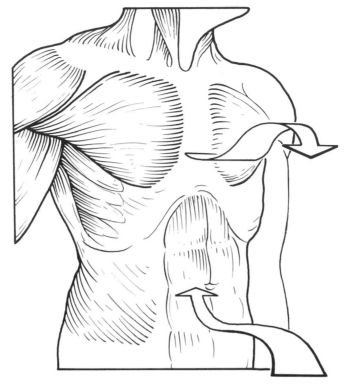

FIG 1-58
When the accessory muscles of expiration contract, intrapleural pressure increases, the chest moves outward, and airflow increases.

compressing the abdominal contents and in pushing the diaphragm into the thoracic cage (see Fig 1-57).

Transversus Abdominis

The transversus abdominis muscle is found immediately under each internal oblique muscle. It arises from the inguinal ligament, the iliac crest, the thoracolumbar fascia, and the lower six ribs. It inserts into the linea alba. When activated, it also serves to constrict the abdominal contents (see Fig 1-57).

When all four pairs of accessory muscles of exhalation contract, the abdominal pressure increases and drives the diaphragm into the thoracic cage. As the diaphragm moves into the thoracic cage during exhalation, the intrapleural pressure increases and enhances expiratory gas flow (Fig 1-58).

ABNORMAL BLOOD GAS FINDINGS

As the pathologic processes of a respiratory disorder intensify, the patient's arterial blood gas (ABG) values are usually altered to some degree. Table 1-8 lists normal ABG values.

Ventilatory Acid-Base Abnormalities

Ventilatory acid-base abnormalities associated with respiratory diseases are seen in (1) acute alveolar hyperventilation with hypoxemia, (2) acute ventilatory failure with hypoxemia, (3) chronic ventilatory failure with hypoxemia, (4) acute alveolar hyperventilation superimposed

Table 1-8 Normal Blood Gas Values		
Blood Gas Value*	**Arterial**	**Venous**
pH	7.35 to 7.45	7.30 to 7.40
P_{CO_2}	35 to 45 mm Hg (Pa_{CO_2})	42 to 48 mm Hg ($P\bar{v}_{CO_2}$)
HCO_3^-	22 to 28 mEq/L	24 to 30 mEq/L
P_{O_2}	80 to 100 mm Hg Pa_{O_2}	35 to 45 mm Hg ($P\bar{v}_{O_2}$)

*Technically, only the oxygen (P_{O_2}) and carbon dioxide (P_{CO_2}) pressure readings are "true" blood gas values. The pH indicates the balance between the bases and acids in the blood. The bicarbonate (HCO_3^-) reading is an indirect measurement that is calculated from the pH and P_{CO_2} levels.

on chronic ventilatory failure, and (5) acute ventilatory failure superimposed on chronic ventilatory failure.

ACUTE ALVEOLAR HYPERVENTILATION WITH **HYPOXEMIA**	
ABG Changes	**Example**
pH: increased	7.53
pa_{CO_2}: decreased	28 mm Hg
HCO_3^-: decreased	20 mM/L
Pa_{O_2}: decreased	63 mm Hg

When a patient is stimulated to breathe more and has the muscular power to do so, alveolar hyperventilation develops (i.e., the Pa_{CO_2} decreases below the normal value). When a decreased Pa_{CO_2} is accompanied by alkalemia (a pH above normal), *acute alveolar hyperventilation* (also called respiratory alkalosis) is said to exist. In respiratory disease, acute alveolar hyperventilation is usually accompanied by (and may be caused by) hypoxemia. The basic pathophysiologic mechanisms that produce the abnormal arterial blood gases in acute alveolar hyperventilation are as follows.

Decreased Pa_{O_2}, decreased Pa_{CO_2}.—The decreased Pa_{O_2} seen during acute alveolar hyperventilation usually develops from the decreased $\dot{V}/\dot{Q}$ ratio, capillary shunting (or a shuntlike effect), and venous admixture associated with the pulmonary disorder. The Pa_{O_2} will continue to drop as the pathologic effects of the disease intensify. Eventually, the Pa_{O_2} may decline to a point low enough (a Pa_{O_2} of about 60 mm Hg) to stimulate the peripheral chemoreceptors, which in turn causes the ventilatory rate to increase (Fig 1-59). Once this happens, the patients's Pa_{O_2} generally remains at a constant level. The increased ventilatory response, however, is often accompanied by a decrease in the Pa_{CO_2} (Fig 1-60).

The following pathophysiologic mechanisms may also contribute to an increased ventilatory rate and to a reduction the Pa_{CO_2}:

- Decreased lung compliance
- Stimulation of the central chemoreceptors
- Activation of the deflation reflex
- Activation of the irritant reflex

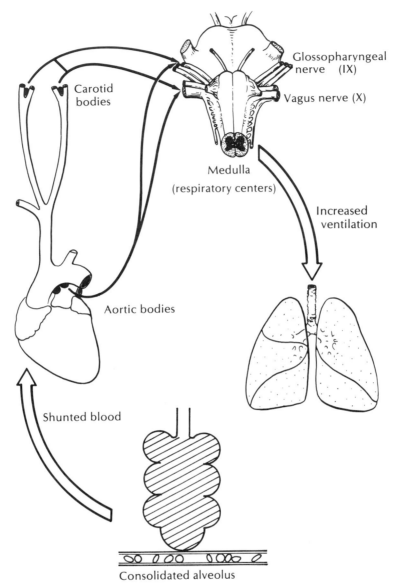

FIG 1-59
Relationship of venous admixture to stimulation of peripheral chemoreceptors in response to alveolar consolidation.

- Stimulation of the J receptors
- Pain/anxiety

Decreased HCO$_3^-$, increased pH.—Sudden changes in the patient's Pa$_{CO_2}$ level cause an immediate change in the HCO$_3^-$ and pH levels. The reason for this is the P$_{CO_2}$/HCO$_3^-$/pH relationship.

Review of the Pa$_{CO_2}$/HCO$_3^-$/pH relationship.—The bulk of the CO$_2$ is transported from the tissue cells to the lungs as HCO$_3^-$ (Fig 1-61). As the CO$_2$ level increases, the plasma P$_{CO_2}$, HCO$_3^-$, and H$_2$CO$_3$ levels increase. The converse is also true: as the level of CO$_2$ decreases, the plasma P$_{CO_2}$, HCO$_3^-$, and H$_2$CO$_3$ levels decrease.

Because the blood pH is dependent on the ratio between the plasma HCO$_3^-$ (base) and H$_2$CO$_3$ (acid), acute ventilatory changes will immediately alter the pH level. The normal

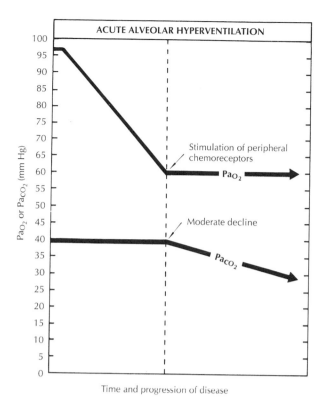

FIG 1-60

Pa_{O_2} and Pa_{CO_2} trends during acute alveolar hyperventilation.

HCO_3^--to-H_2CO_3 ratio is 20:1. Even though plasma HCO_3^- and plasma H_2CO_3 move in the same direction during acute ventilatory changes, acute changes in the H_2CO_3 level play a much more powerful role in altering the pH status than do acute changes in the HCO_3^- level. This is due to the 20:1 ratio between HCO_3^- to H_2CO_3.

In other words, for every H_2CO_3 molecule increase or decrease, 20 HCO_3^- molecules must also increase or decrease, respectively. If this does not happen, the normal 20:1 ratio between the HCO_3^- and H_2CO_3 will change. When the HCO_3^--to-H_2CO_3 ratio is less than 20:1, an *acidosis* exists. When the HCO_3^--to-H_2CO_3 ratio is greater than 20:1, an *alkalosis* exists.

In view of the above relationship, during periods of acute alveolar hyperventilation the PA_{CO_2} will decrease and allow more CO_2 to leave the pulmonary blood. This action necessarily decreases the blood Pa_{CO_2}, H_2CO_3, and HCO_3^- levels (Fig 1-62). Because acute changes in H_2CO_3 levels are more significant than are acute changes in HCO_3 levels, an increased HCO_3^--to-H_2CO_3 ratio develops (a ratio greater than 20:1). This action causes the patient's blood pH to increase, or become more alkaline. The normal buffer line on the PCO_2/ HCO_3^-/pH nomogram in Figure 1-63 illustrates the expected HCO_3^- and pH changes that develop in response to sudden CO_2 changes only.

ACUTE VENTILATORY FAILURE WITH **HYPOXEMIA**	
ABG Changes	**Example**
pH: decreased	7.21
Pa_{CO_2}: increased	79 mm Hg
HCO_3^-: increased (slightly)	28 mM/L
Pa_{O_2}: decreased	57 mm Hg

Ventilatory failure is defined as a condition in which the lungs are unable to meet the metabolic demands of the body in terms of carbon dioxide homeostasis. In other words, the patient is unable to provide the muscular, mechanical work necessary to move gas into and out of the lungs to meet the normal carbon dioxide metabolic demands of the body. This condition leads to an increased PA_{CO_2} and, subsequently, to an increased Pa_{CO_2} level. Ventilatory failure is not associated with a "typical ventilatory pattern." The patient may be apneic or have severe hyperpnea and tachypnea. The bottom line is that ventilatory failure will develop in response to any ventilatory pattern that does not provide adequate alveolar ventilation. When an increased Pa_{CO_2} is accompanied by acidemia (decreased pH), *acute ventilatory failure* (also called respiratory acidosis) is said to exist. Clinically, this is a medical emergency, and mechanical ventilation is indicated.

The basic pathophysiologic mechanisms that produce the abnormal arterial blood gas findings in acute ventilatory failure are as follows.

Decreased Pa_{O_2}, increased Pa_{CO_2}.—Whenever a respiratory disorder becomes critical over a relatively short period of time, acute ventilatory failure may develop. When this happens, the patient's overall $\dot{V}/\dot{Q}$ ratio decreases. This condition causes the PA_{O_2} to decrease and the PA_{CO_2} to increase. This action in turn causes the Pa_{O_2} to decrease and the Pa_{CO_2} to increase.

Increased HCO_3^-, decreased pH.—The sudden rise in the Pa_{CO_2} level causes the H_2CO_3 and HCO_3^- levels to increase (Fig 1-64). Because acute changes in H_2CO_3 are more significant than acute changes in HCO_3^-, a decreased HCO_3^--to-H_2CO_3 ratio develops (a ratio less than 20:1). This action causes the patient's blood pH to decrease, or become less alkaline.

CHRONIC VENTILATORY FAILURE WITH HYPOXEMIA	
ABG Changes	**Example**
pH: normal	7.38
Pa_{CO_2}: increased	66 mm Hg
HCO_3^-: increased (significantly)	35 mM/L
Pa_{O_2}: decreased	63 mm Hg

Chronic ventilatory failure is defined as a greater-than-normal Pa_{CO_2} level with a normal pH status. Clinically, chronic hypercarbia is most commonly seen in severe chronic obstructive pulmonary disease. Chronic ventilatory failure, however, is seen in other respiratory diseases. Table 1-9 lists some respiratory diseases associated with chronic ventilatory failure during the advanced stages of the disorder.

The basic pathophysiologic mechanisms that produce the abnormal arterial blood gas findings in chronic ventilatory failure are as follows:

Decreased Pa_{O_2}, increased Pa_{CO_2}.—As a respiratory disorder becomes progressively severe (e.g., chronic bronchitis or emphysema), the work of breathing may become so great and the pulmonary shunting so significant that more oxygen is consumed than is gained. Although the exact mechanism is unclear, the patient slowly develops a breathing pattern that uses the

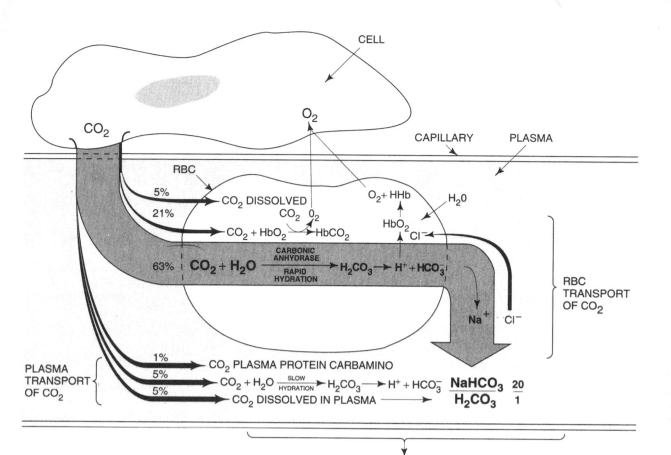

FIG 1-61

How CO_2 is converted to HCO_3^- at the tissue sites. Most of the CO_2 that is produced at the tissue cells is carried to the lungs in the form of HCO_3^-. CA = carbonic anhydrase. (From Des Jardins T: *Cardiopulmonary Anatomy and Physiology: Essentials for Respiratory Care,* 2nd ed, Albany, NY, Delmar Publishers Inc, 1993. Used by permission.)

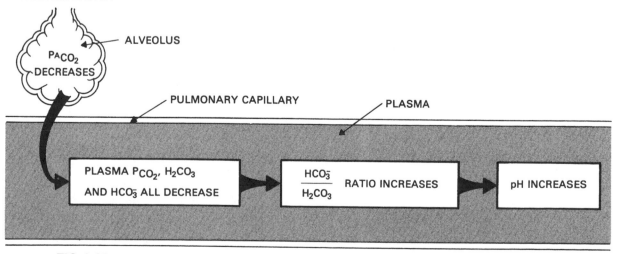

FIG 1-62

Alveolar hyperventilation causes the PA_{CO_2} and the plasma P_{CO_2}, H_2CO_3, and HCO_3^- to decrease. This action increases the HCO_3^-/H_2CO_3 ratio, which in turn increases the blood pH. (From Des Jardins T: *Cardiopulmonary Anatomy and Physiology: Essentials for Respiratory Care,* 2nd ed, Albany NY, Delmar Publishers Inc, 1993. Used by permission.)

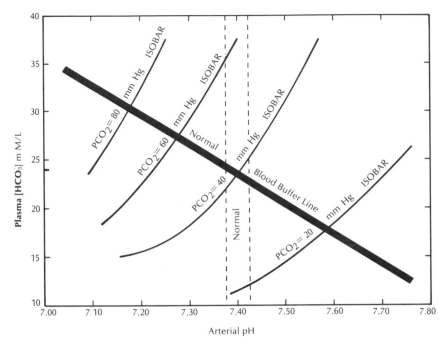

FIG 1-63

$P_{CO_2}/HCO_3^-/pH$ relationship.

Table 1-9 Respiratory Diseases Associated With Chronic Ventilatory Failure During the Advanced Stages	
Chronic Obstructive Pulmonary Diseases (Most Common)	**Other Respiratory Diseases**
Chronic bronchitis	Pneumoconiosis
Emphysema	Tuberculosis
Bronchiectasis	Fungal diseases
Cystic fibrosis	Kyphoscoliosis

least amount of oxygen for the energy expended. In essence, the patient selects a breathing pattern based on *work efficiency* rather than *ventilatory efficiency*.* As a result, the patient's alveolar ventilation slowly decreases, which in turn causes the Pa_{O_2} to decrease and the Pa_{CO_2} to increase (Fig 1-65).

Increased HCO_3^-, normal pH.—When an individual hypoventilates for a long time, the kidneys will try to correct the decreased pH by retaining HCO_3^- in the blood. Renal compensation in the presence of chronic hypoventilation can be shown when the calculated HCO_3^- and pH readings are higher than expected for a particular P_{CO_2} level. For example, in terms of the absolute $P_{CO_2}/HCO_3^-/pH$ relationship, when the P_{CO_2} level is about 80 mm Hg, the HCO_3^- level should be about 30 mM/L and the pH should be about 7.19, according to the normal blood buffer line (Fig 1-66). If the HCO_3^- and pH levels are greater than these val-

*See the discussion on altered airway resistance and its effect on the ventilatory patterns.

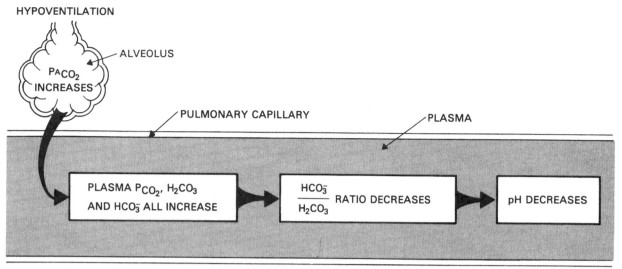

FIG 1-64

Alveolar hypoventilation causes the PA_{CO_2} and the plasma P_{CO_2}, H_2CO_3, and HCO_3^- to increase. This action decreases the HCO_3^-/H_2CO_3 ratio, which in turn decreases the blood pH. (From Des Jardins T: *Cardiopulmonary Anatomy and Physiology: Essentials for Respiratory Care,* ed 2, Albany, NY, 1993, Delmar Publishers Inc. Used by permission.)

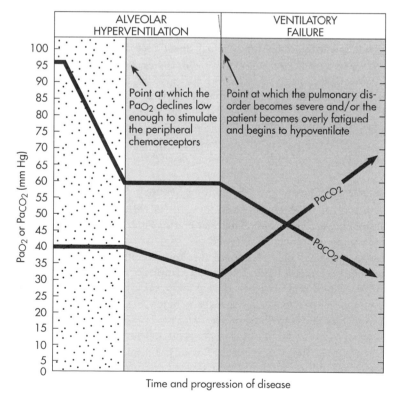

FIG 1-65

Pa_{O_2} and Pa_{CO_2} trends during acute or chronic ventilatory failure.

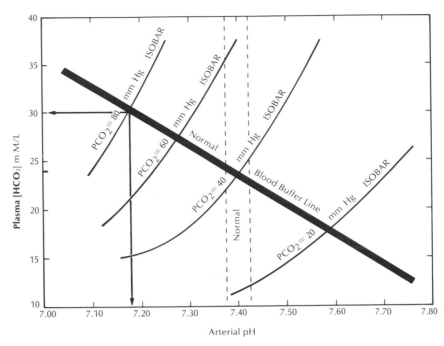

FIG 1-66
Expected pH and HCO_3^- levels when the Pa_{CO_2} is about 80 mm Hg.

ues (i.e., the pH and HCO_3^- readings cross a P_{CO_2} isobar* above the normal blood buffer line in the upper left-hand corner of the nomogram), renal retention of HCO_3^- (partial renal compensation) has occurred. When the HCO_3^- level increases enough to return the acidic pH to normal, *complete renal compensation* is said to have occurred (chronic ventilatory failure).

As a general rule, the kidneys do not overcompensate for an abnormal pH level, that is, should the patient's blood pH level become acidic for a long time due to hypoventilation, the kidneys will not retain enough HCO_3^- for the pH value to climb higher than 7.4. The opposite is also true: should the patient's blood pH become alkalotic for a long time due to hyperventilation, the kidneys will not excrete enough HCO_3^- to cause the pH level to fall below 7.4.

In persons who have been hypoventilating over a long period of time, however, it is not uncommon to find a pH level greater than 7.4. This is believed to be due to the water and chloride ion shifts between the intracellular and extracellular spaces that occur while the kidneys are compensating for a decreased blood pH.

To summarize, the lungs play an important role in maintaining the P_{CO_2}, HCO_3^-, and pH levels on a moment-to-moment basis. The kidneys, on the other hand, play an important role in maintaining the HCO_3^- and pH levels during long periods of hyperventilation or hypoventilation. It is a common error to assume that the maintenance of HCO_3^- levels in the body is solely under the influence of the kidneys.

Finally, it should be noted that blood gas analyzers determine HCO_3^- levels on the basis of the patient's in vitro buffer slope. Because of this, a nomogram such as the one shown in Figure 1-63 must be used to determine the expected HCO_3^- and pH values for a particular Pa_{CO_2} level.

---

*The isobars on the $PCO_2/HCO_3^-/pH$ nomogram illustrate the pH changes that develop in the blood as a result of (1) metabolic changes (i.e., HCO_3^- changes) or (2) a combination of metabolic and respiratory (CO_2) changes.

Acute Ventilatory Changes Superimposed on Chronic Ventilatory Failure

Because *acute ventilatory changes* are frequently seen in patients with *chronic ventilatory failure,* the respiratory care practitioner must be familiar with and be on the alert for (1) *acute alveolar hyperventilation superimposed on chronic ventilatory failure* and (2) *acute ventilatory failure superimposed on chronic ventilatory failure.*

ACUTE ALVEOLAR HYPERVENTILATION SUPERIMPOSED ON
CHRONIC VENTILATORY FAILURE

ABG Changes	Example
pH: increased	7.55
Pa_{CO_2}: increased	62 mm Hg
HCO_3^-: increased	38 mM/L
Pa_{O_2}: decreased	51 mm Hg

Similar to any other person (healthy or unhealthy), the patient with chronic ventilatory failure can acquire an acute shunt-producing disease such as pneumonia. Some of these patients have the mechanical reserve to significantly increase their alveolar ventilation in an attempt to maintain their baseline Pa_{O_2}. In some of these patients, however, the increased alveolar ventilation is excessive.

When this happens, the patient's PA_{CO_2} rapidly decreases. This action, in turn, causes the patient's Pa_{CO_2} to decrease from its normally high baseline level. As the Pa_{CO_2} decreases, the arterial pH increases. As this condition intensifies, the patient's baseline arterial blood gas values can quickly change from *chronic ventilatory failure* to *acute alveolar hyperventilation superimposed on chronic ventilatory failure* (Table 1-10).

It should be noted that without seeing or knowing the past history of the patient with acute alveolar hyperventilation superimposed on chronic ventilatory failure, the arterial blood gas values could initially be interpreted as *partially compensated metabolic alkalosis with severe hypoxemia* (see Table 1-10). The clinical manifestation that offsets this interpretation, however, is the presence of *marked hypoxemia*. This degree of hypoxemia is not commonly seen in patients with metabolic alkalosis. Another tip-off is the presence of a *wide alveolar-arterial oxygen tension difference* [$P(A-a)O_2$] in acute alveolar hyperventilation superimposed on chronic ventilatory failure (when measured on room air). A wide $P(A-a)O_2$ is not normally produced in the hypoventilation seen in partially compensated metabolic alkalosis.

Thus, whenever an arterial blood gas appears to reflect partially compensated metabolic alkalosis, but is accompanied by significant hypoxemia, the respiratory care practitioner should be alert to the possibility of *acute alveolar hyperventilation superimposed on chronic ventilatory failure.*

ACUTE VENTILATORY FAILURE SUPERIMPOSED ON
CHRONIC VENTILATORY FAILURE

ABG Changes	Example
pH: decreased	7.23
Pa_{CO_2}: increased	107 mm Hg
HCO_3^-: increased	41 mM/L
Pa_{O_2}: decreased	38 mm Hg

Some patients that acquire an acute shunt-producing disease like pneumonia do not have the mechanical reserve to meet the hypoxemic challenge of the increased shunt. When these patients attempt to maintain their baseline Pa_{O_2} by increasing alveolar ventilation, they begin to consume more oxygen than is gained with the increased alveolar ventilation. When this happens, the patient begins to breathe less. If the alveolar ventilation decreases too much, the patient's PA_{CO_2} rapidly increases. This action, in turn, causes the Pa_{CO_2} to increase from its normally high baseline level. As the Pa_{CO_2} increases, the arterial pH decreases. As this condition intensifies, the patient's baseline arterial blood gas values can quickly change from *chronic ventilatory failure* to *acute ventilatory failure superimposed on chronic ventilatory failure* (see Table 1-10).

It should be noted that if the respiratory care practitioner judges the severity of the ventilatory failure on the Pa_{CO_2} alone (in this case, 110 mm Hg), the patient would appear to be in severe ventilatory failure (see Table 1-10). As a general rule, however, when starting at normal baseline arterial blood gas values (e.g., a pH of 7.40, a Pa_{CO_2} of 40 mm Hg, and a HCO_3^- level of 24 mM/L), the pH will *decrease* by 0.05 unit and the HCO_3^- will *increase* by 1 mM/L for every 10 mm Hg increase in Pa_{CO_2}; for every 10 mm Hg *decrease* in Pa_{CO_2}, the pH will *increase* by 0.10 unit and the HCO_3^- will *decrease* by 2 mM/L (Table 1-11).

Because the pH of 7.21 in this example is not as low as expected for a Pa_{CO_2} level of 110 mm Hg (a pH of 7.05 is expected), the acute ventilatory failure is not as severe as the Pa_{CO_2} value of 110 mm Hg would lead one to believe (see Table 1-10). *The severity of acute ventilatory failure is based on the severity of acidemia.*

Thus, whenever the Pa_{CO_2} is high, and the pH is not as low as expected, the respiratory

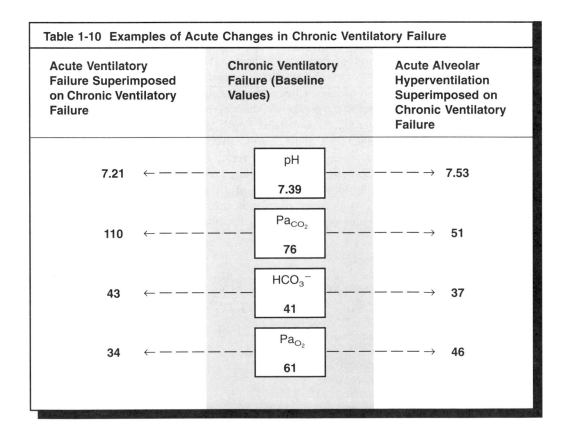

Table 1-10 Examples of Acute Changes in Chronic Ventilatory Failure		
Acute Ventilatory Failure Superimposed on Chronic Ventilatory Failure	**Chronic Ventilatory Failure (Baseline Values)**	**Acute Alveolar Hyperventilation Superimposed on Chronic Ventilatory Failure**
7.21	pH 7.39	7.53
110	Pa_{CO_2} 76	51
43	HCO_3^- 41	37
34	Pa_{O_2} 61	46

care practitioner should be alert to the possibility of *acute ventilatory failure superimposed on chronic ventilatory failure.*

METABOLIC ACIDOSIS

ABG Changes	Example
pH: decreased	7.26
Pa_{CO_2}: normal	37 mm Hg
HCO_3^-: decreased	18 mM/L
Pa_{O_2}: normal (or decreased when lactic acidosis is present)	94 mm Hg (or 52 mm Hg when lactic acidosis is present)

By using the isobars of the $P_{CO_2}/HCO_3^-/pH$ nomogram shown in Figure 1-63, the presence of other acids, not related to an increased Pa_{CO_2} level or renal compensation, can be identified. The presence of other acids is verified when the calculated HCO_3^- reading and pH level are both lower than expected for a particular Pa_{CO_2} level in terms of the absolute $P_{CO_2}/HCO_3^-/pH$ relationship. For example, according to the normal blood buffer line, a HCO_3^- reading of 15 mEq/L and a pH of 7.2 would both be less than expected in a patient who has a P_{CO_2} of 40 mm Hg (see Figure 1-63). This condition is referred to as *metabolic acidosis.* Clinically, there are a number of conditions that can cause metabolic acidosis (Table 1-12).

METABOLIC ALKALOSIS

ABG Changes	Example
pH: increased	7.56
Pa_{CO_2}: normal	44 mm Hg
HCO_3^-: increased	27 mM/L
Pa_{O_2}: normal	94 mm Hg

The presence of other bases, not related to either a decreased Pa_{CO_2} level or renal compensation, can also be identified by using the $P_{CO_2}/HCO_3^-/pH$ nomogram illustrated in Figure 1-63. The presence of metabolic alkalosis is verified when the calculated HCO_3^- and pH readings are both higher than expected for a particular Pa_{CO_2} level in terms of the absolute $P_{CO_2}/HCO_3^-/pH$ relationship. For example, according to the normal blood buffer line, a HCO_3^- reading of 35 mEq/L and a pH level of 7.54 would both be higher than expected in a patient who has a Pa_{CO_2} of 40 mm Hg (see Figure 1-63). This condition is a known as *metabolic alkalosis.* Clinically, there are a number of conditions that can cause metabolic alkalosis (see Table 1-12).

Table 1-11 Approximate Pa_{CO_2}/HCO_3^-/pH Relationship

pH	Pa_{CO_2} (mm Hg)	HCO_3^- (mM/L)
7.70	10	18
7.60	20	20
7.50	30	22
7.40	40	24
7.35	50	25
7.30	60	26
7.25	70	27
7.20	80	28
7.15	90	29
7.10	100	30
7.05	110	31
7.00	120	32
6.95	130	33

Table 1-12 Common Causes of Metabolic Acid-Base Abnormalities

Metabolic Acidosis	Metabolic Alkalosis
Lactic acidosis	Hypokalemia
Ketoacidosis	Hypochloremia
Renal failure	Gastric suctioning
Dehydration	Vomiting
Chronic diarrhea	Use of steroid medications
	Excess sodium bicarbonate

Assessment of the Hypoxic State

The assessment of the hypoxic state should always accompany the assessment of the patient's ventilatory and acid-base status. In adults, an acceptable therapeutic range for the Pa_{O_2} at sea level is greater than 80 mm Hg.* An acceptable Pa_{O_2} range for newborns is between 40 and 70 mm Hg.

In adults breathing room air, hypoxemia is defined as a Pa_{O_2} less than 80 mm Hg. Clinically, hypoxemia is often classified as either *mild, moderate,* or *severe.* Mild hypoxemia may be defined as a Pa_{O_2} less than 80 mm Hg; moderate hypoxemia is generally thought to be present when the Pa_{O_2} is less than 60 mm Hg. Severe hypoxemia is present when the Pa_{O_2} is less than 40 mm Hg.

CYANOSIS

Cyanosis is often seen in severe respiratory disorders. *Cyanosis* is the term used to describe the blue-gray or purplish discoloration of the mucous membranes, fingertips, and toes whenever the blood in these areas contains at least 5 g/dl of reduced hemoglobin. When the normal 14 to 15 g/dl of hemoglobin is fully saturated, the Pa_{O_2} will be about 97 to 100 mm Hg,

---

*In adults over 60 years of age, subtract 1 mm Hg from 80 mm Hg for each year over 60 years of age for the normal lower Pa_{O_2} limit at sea level.

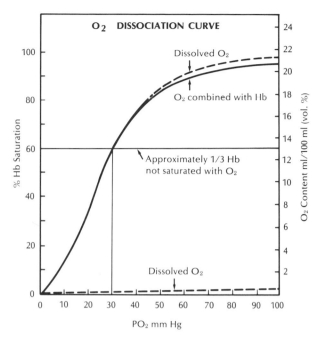

O₂ DISSOCIATION CURVE

FIG 1-67
Cyanosis is likely whenever the blood contains at least 5 g of reduced hemoglobin. In the normal individual who has about 15 g of hemoglobin per 100 ml of blood, a P_{O_2} of about 30 mm Hg will produce 5 g of reduced hemoglobin. The hemoglobin, however, is still approximately 60% saturated with oxygen.

and there will be about 20 vol% of oxygen in the blood. In a cyanotic patient with one third (5 g/dl) of the hemoglobin reduced, the Pa_{O_2} will be about 30 mm Hg and there will be 13 vol% of oxygen in the blood (Fig 1-67).

The detection and interpretation of cyanosis is difficult, and there are wide individual variations between observers. The recognition of cyanosis depends on the acuity of the observer, on the light conditions in the examining room, and on the pigmentation of the patient. Cyanosis of the nail beds is also influenced by temperature since vasoconstriction induced by cold may slow circulation to the point where the blood becomes bluish in the surface capillaries even though the arterial blood in the major vessels is not oxygen-poor.

Central cyanosis, as observed on the mucous membranes of the mouth, is almost always a sign of hypoxemia and so has a definite diagnostic value.

In severely anemic patients, cyanosis may never be seen since these patients could not remain alive with 5 g/dl reduced hemoglobin. In the patient with *polycythemia,** however, cyanosis may be present at a Pa_{O_2} well above 30 mm Hg since the amount of reduced hemoglobin is often greater than 5 g/dl in these patients—even when their total oxygen transport is within normal limits. In respiratory disease, cyanosis is the end result of (1) a decreased ventilation-perfusion ratio, (2) pulmonary shunting, and (3) venous admixture.

ABNORMAL OXYGENATION INDICES

There are a number of oxygen transport measurements available to assess the oxygenation status of the critically ill patient. Results from these studies can provide important information to adjust therapeutic interventions. The oxygen transport studies can be divided into the *oxygen-tension-based indices* and the *oxygen- saturation- and content-based indices.*†

*See the section on polycythemia, page 92.
†See Appendix XX for a representative example of a cardiopulmonary profile sheet used to monitor the oxygen transport status of the critically ill patient.

Oxygen-Tension-Based Indices
Arterial Oxygen Tension (Pa_{O_2})

The Pa_{O_2} has withstood the test of time as a good indicator of the patient's oxygenation status (see assessment of the hypoxic state). In general, an appropriate Pa_{O_2} on a low oxygen concentration almost always indicates good lung oxygenation function. The Pa_{O_2}, however, can be misleading in a number of clinical situations. For example, the Pa_{O_2} may give a "false-positive" oxygenation reading when the patient has (1) a low hemoglobin concentration, (2) a decreased cardiac output, (3) peripheral shunting, (4) hypothermia, or (5) been exposed to carbon monoxide or cyanide.

Alveolar-Arterial Oxygen Tension Difference [$P(A\text{-}a)_{O_2}$]

The $P(A\text{-}a)_{O_2}$ is the oxygen tension difference between the alveoli and arterial blood. The $P(A\text{-}a)_{O_2}$ is also known as the *alveolar-arterial oxygen tension gradient.* Clinically, the information required for the $P(A\text{-}a)_{O_2}$ is obtained from (1) the patient's alveolar oxygen tension (PA_{O_2}), which is derived from the *ideal alveolar gas equation,* and (2) the patient's Pa_{O_2} and Pa_{CO_2}, which is obtained from an arterial blood gas analysis.

The ideal alveolar gas equation is written as:

$$PA_{O_2} = (P_B - P_{H_2O})\, F_{I_{O_2}} - Pa_{CO_2}\ (1.25)$$

where P_B is the barometric pressure, PA_{O_2} is the partial pressure of oxygen within the alveoli, P_{H_2O} is the partial pressure of water vapor in the alveoli (which is 47 mm Hg), $F_{I_{O_2}}$ is the fractional concentration of inspired oxygen, Pa_{CO_2} is the partial pressure of arterial carbon dioxide, and the number 1.25 is a factor that adjusts for alterations in oxygen tension due to variations in the respiratory exchange ratio, or respiratory quotient (RQ). The respiratory quotient is the ratio of carbon dioxide production ($\dot{V}_{CO_2}$) divided by oxygen consumption ($\dot{V}_{O_2}$). Under normal circumstances, about 250 ml of oxygen are consumed by the tissue cells and about 200 ml of carbon dioxide are excreted into the lung. The RQ is normally about 0.8.

Thus, if a patient is receiving an $F_{I_{O_2}}$ of 0.30 on a day when the barometric pressure is 750 mm Hg, and if the patient's Pa_{CO_2} is 70 mm Hg and the Pa_{O_2} 60 mm Hg, the $P(A\text{-}a)_{O_2}$ can be calculated as follows:

$$PA_{O_2} = (P_B - P_{H_2O})\, F_{I_{O_2}} - Pa_{CO_2}\ (1.25)$$

$$= (750 - 47)\ .30 - 70\ (1.25)$$

$$= (703)\ .30 - 87.5$$

$$= 210.9 - 87.5$$

$$= 123.4 \text{ mm Hg}$$

Using the Pa_{O_2} obtained from the arterial blood gas, the $P(A\text{-}a)_{O_2}$ can now easily be calculated as follows:

$$123.4 \text{ mm Hg } (PA_{O_2})$$

$$\underline{-60.0 \text{ mm Hg } (Pa_{O_2})}$$

$$= 63.4 \text{ mm Hg } (P(A\text{-}a)_{O_2})$$

The normal $P(A\text{-}a)_{O_2}$ on room air at sea level ranges between 7 and 15 mm Hg, and it should not exceed 30 mm Hg. The $P(A\text{-}a)_{O_2}$ increases in response to (1) oxygen diffusion disorders (e.g., chronic interstitial lung diseases), (2) decreased ventilation/perfusion ratios disorders (e.g., chronic obstructive pulmonary diseases, (3) right-to-left intracardiac shunting (e.g., a patent ventricular septum), and (4) age.

While the $P(A-a)_{O_2}$ may be useful in patients breathing a low $F_{I_{O_2}}$, it loses some of its sensitivity in patients breathing a high $F_{I_{O_2}}$. The $P(A-a)_{O_2}$ increases at high oxygen concentrations. Because of this, the $P(A-a)_{O_2}$ has less value in the critically ill patient who is breathing a high oxygen concentration.

Finally, it should be mentioned that several variations of the $P(A-a)_{O_2}$ have been introduced over the years. Such oxygenation indices have included the *arterial-alveolar oxygen ratio* (Pa_{O_2}/PA_{O_2}) and the *arterial to inspired oxygen concentration ratio* $(Pa_{O_2}/F_{I_{O_2}})$. It is generally felt that these studies are not helpful and probably should be abandoned.

Oxygen Saturation- and Content-Based Indices

The oxygen saturation- and content-based indices can serve as excellent indicators of an individual's cardiac and ventilatory status. These oxygenation studies are derived from the patient's total oxygen content in the arterial blood (Ca_{O_2}), mixed venous blood $(C\bar{v}_{O_2})$, and pulmonary capillary blood (Cc_{O_2}). The Ca_{O_2}, $C\bar{v}_{O_2}$, and Cc_{O_2} are calculated by using the following formulas:

$$Ca_{O_2}: \text{Oxygen content of arterial blood}$$

$$(Hb \times 1.34 \times Sa_{O_2}) + (Pa_{O_2} \times 0.003)$$

$$C\bar{v}_{O_2}: \text{Oxygen content of mixed venous blood}$$

$$(Hb \times 1.34 \times S\bar{v}_{O_2}) + (P\bar{v}_{O_2} \times 0.003)$$

$$Cc_{O_2}: \text{Oxygen content of pulmonary capillary blood}$$

$$(Hb \times 1.34)\text{*} + (PA_{O_2}\dagger \times 0.003)$$

where Hb is grams percent hemoglobin (g% Hb), 1.34 is the approximate amount (ml) of oxygen each g% of Hb is capable of carrying, Sa_{O_2} is the arterial oxygen saturation, Pa_{O_2} is the arterial oxygen tension, 0.003 is the dissolved oxygen factor, $S\bar{v}_{O_2}$ is the venous oxygen saturation, $P\bar{v}_{O_2}$ is the venous oxygen tension, and PA_{O_2} is the alveolar oxygen tension.

Clinically, the most common oxygen saturation- and content-based indices are (1) total oxygen delivery, (2) arterial-venous oxygen content difference, (3) oxygen consumption, (4) oxygen extraction ratio, (5) mixed venous oxygen saturation, and (6) pulmonary shunt.

Total Oxygen Delivery

Total oxygen delivery (D_{O_2}) is the amount of oxygen delivered to the peripheral tissue cells. The D_{O_2} is calculated as follows:

$$D_{O_2} = \dot{Q}_T \times (Ca_{O_2} \times 10)$$

where $\dot{Q}_T$ is total cardiac output (L/min); Ca_{O_2} is oxygen content of arterial blood (ml oxygen/100 ml blood); and the factor 10 is used to convert the Ca_{O_2} to ml O_2/L blood.

Thus, if a patient has a cardiac output of 4 L/min and a Ca_{O_2} of 15 vol%, the D_{O_2} will be 600 ml of oxygen per minute:

$$D_{O_2} = \dot{Q}_T \times (Ca_{O_2} \times 10)$$

$$= 4 \text{ L/min} \times (15 \text{ vol\%} \times 10)$$

$$= 600 \text{ ml } O_2/\text{min}$$

---

*It is assumed that the hemoglobin saturation with oxygen in the pulmonary capillary blood is 100 percent or 1.0.
†See Ideal Alveolar Gas Equation, Appendix XIII.

Normally, the D_{O_2} is about 1,000 ml O_2 per minute. Clinically, a patient's D_{O_2} *decreases* when there is a decline in blood oxygen saturation, hemoglobin concentration, or cardiac output. The D_{O_2} *increases* in response to an increase in blood oxygen saturation, hemoglobin concentration, or cardiac output.

Arterial-Venous Oxygen Content Difference

The *arterial-venous oxygen content difference* ($C(a-\bar{v})_{O_2}$) is the difference between the Ca_{O_2} and the $C\bar{v}_{O_2}$ ($Ca_{O_2} - C\bar{v}_{O_2}$). Thus, if a patient's Ca_{O_2} is 15 vol% and the $C\bar{v}_{O_2}$ is 8 vol%, the $C(a-\bar{v})_{O_2}$ is 7 vol%:

$$C(a-\bar{v})_{O_2} = Ca_{O_2} - C\bar{v}_{O_2}$$
$$= 15 \text{ vol\%} - 8 \text{ vol\%}$$
$$= 7 \text{ vol\%}$$

Normally, the $C(a-\bar{v})_{O_2}$ is about 5 vol%. The $C(a-\bar{v})_{O_2}$ is useful in assessing the patient's cardiopulmonary status, since oxygen changes in the mixed venous blood ($C\bar{v}_{O_2}$) often occur earlier than oxygen changes in arterial blood gas. Clinically, the patient's $C(a-\bar{v})_{O_2}$ *increases* in response to such things as decreased cardiac output, exercise, seizures, and hyperthermia. The $C(a-\bar{v})_{O_2}$ *decreases* in response to increased cardiac output, skeletal relaxation (e.g., induced by drugs), peripheral shunting (e.g., sepsis), certain poisons (e.g., cyanide), and hypothermia.

Oxygen Consumption

Oxygen consumption ($\dot{V}_{O_2}$), also known as *oxygen uptake,* is the amount of oxygen consumed by the peripheral tissue cells during a one-minute period. The $\dot{V}_{O_2}$ is calculated as follows:

$$\dot{V}_{O_2} = \dot{Q}_T \, [C(a-\bar{v})_{O_2} \times 10]$$

where $\dot{Q}_T$ is the total cardiac output (L/min); $C(a-\bar{v})_{O_2}$ is the arterial-venous oxygen content difference ($Ca_{O_2} - C\bar{v}_{O_2}$); and the factor 10 is used to convert the $C(a-\bar{v})_{O_2}$ to ml O_2/L.

Thus, if a patient has a cardiac output of 4 L/min and a $C(a-\bar{v})_{O_2}$ of 6 vol%, the total amount of oxygen consumed by the tissue cells in one minute would be 240 ml:

$$\dot{V}_{O_2} = \dot{Q}_T \, [C(a-\bar{v})_{O_2} \times 10]$$
$$= 4 \text{ L/min} \times 6 \text{ vol\%} \times 10$$
$$= 240 \text{ ml } O_2/\text{min}$$

Normally, the $\dot{V}_{O_2}$ is about 250 ml of O_2 per minute. Clinically, the $\dot{V}_{O_2}$ *increases* in response to seizures, exercise, hyperthermia, and body size. The $\dot{V}_{O_2}$ *decreases* in response to skeletal muscle relaxation (e.g., induced by drugs), peripheral shunting (e.g., sepsis), certain poisons (e.g., cyanide), and hypothermia.

Oxygen Extraction Ratio

The *oxygen extraction ratio* (O_2ER), also known as the *oxygen coefficient ratio* or *oxygen utilization ratio,* is the amount of oxygen consumed by the tissue cells divided by the total amount of oxygen delivered. The O_2ER is calculated by dividing the $C(a-\bar{v})_{O_2}$ by the Ca_{O_2}. Thus, if a patient has a Ca_{O_2} of 15 vol% and a $C\bar{v}_{O_2}$ of 10 vol%, the O_2ER would be 33%:

$$O_2ER = \frac{Ca_{O_2} - C\bar{v}_{O_2}}{Ca_{O_2}}$$

$$= \frac{15 \text{ vol}\% - 10 \text{ vol}\%}{15 \text{ vol}\%}$$

$$= \frac{5 \text{ vol}\%}{15 \text{ vol}\%}$$

$$= .33$$

Normally, the O_2ER is about 25%. Clinically, the patient's O_2ER *increases* in response to (1) a decreased cardiac output, (2) periods of increased oxygen consumption (e.g., exercise, seizures, or hyperthermia), (3) anemia, and (4) decreased arterial oxygenation. The O_2ER *decreases* in response to (1) increased cardiac output, (2) skeletal muscle relaxation (e.g., induced by drugs), (3) peripheral shunting (e.g., sepsis), (4) certain poisons (e.g., cyanide), (5) hypothermia, (6) increased hemoglobin, and (7) increased arterial oxygenation.

Mixed Venous Oxygen Saturation

When a patient has a normal arterial oxygen saturation (Sa_{O_2}) and hemoglobin concentration, the *mixed venous oxygen saturation* ($S\bar{v}_{O_2}$) is often used as an early indicator of changes in the patient's $C(a\text{-}\bar{v})_{O_2}$, $\dot{V}_{O_2}$, and O_2ER. The $S\bar{v}_{O_2}$ can signal changes in the patient's $C(a\text{-}\bar{v})_{O_2}$, $\dot{V}_{O_2}$, and O_2ER earlier than arterial blood gases, since the Pa_{O_2} and Sa_{O_2} levels are often normal during early $C(a\text{-}\bar{v})_{O_2}$, $\dot{V}_{O_2}$, and O_2ER changes.

Normally, the $S\bar{v}_{O_2}$ is about 75%. Clinically, the $S\bar{v}_{O_2}$ *decreases* in response to (1) a decreased cardiac output, (2) exercise, (3) seizures, and (4) hyperthermia. The $S\bar{v}_{O_2}$ *increases* in response to (1) an increased cardiac output, (2) skeletal muscle relaxation (e.g., induced by drugs), (3) peripheral shunting (e.g., sepsis), (4) certain poisons (e.g., cyanide), and (5) hypothermia.

Finally, it should be noted that *over the past several years there has been a move away from the oxygen-tension-based indices to the oxygen-saturation-and content-based indices* when monitoring the oxygenation status of the critically ill patient. Table 1-13 summarizes how various clinical factors alter the patient's D_{O_2}, $\dot{V}_{O_2}$, $C(a\text{-}\bar{v})_{O_2}$, O_2ER, and $S\bar{v}_{O_2}$.

Pulmonary Shunting

Since pulmonary shunting and venous admixture are frequent complications in respiratory disorders, knowledge of the degree of shunting is desirable in developing patient care plans. The amount of intrapulmonary shunting can be calculated by using the *classic shunt equation:*

$$\frac{\dot{Q}s}{\dot{Q}_T} = \frac{Cc_{O_2} - Ca_{O_2}}{Cc_{O_2} - C\bar{v}_{O_2}}$$

where $\dot{Q}s$ is the cardiac output that is shunted, $\dot{Q}_T$ is the total cardiac output, Cc_{O_2} is the oxygen content of arterial blood, Ca_{O_2} is the oxygen content of arterial blood, and $C\bar{v}_{O_2}$ is the oxygen content of venous blood.

In order to obtain the data necessary to calculate the patient's intrapulmonary shunt, the following information must be gathered:

- BP (barometric pressure)
- Pa_{O_2} (partial pressure of arterial oxygen)
- Pa_{CO_2} (partial pressure of arterial carbon dioxide)
- $P\bar{v}_{O_2}$ (partial pressure of mixed venous oxygen)
- Hemoglobin (Hb) concentration

Table 1-13 Clinical Factors Affecting Various Oxygen Transport Study Values					
Clinical Factors	**Oxygenation Indices and Normal Values**				
	D_{O_2} (1,000 ml O_2/min)	$\dot{V}_{O_2}$ (250 ml O_2/min)	$C(a-\bar{v})_{O_2}$ (5 vol%)	O_2ER (25%)	$S\bar{v}_{O_2}$ (75%)
↑ O_2 consumption	~	↑	↑	↑	↓
↓ O_2 consumption	~	↓	↓	↓	↑
↓ Cardiac output	↓	~	↑	↑	↓
↑ Cardiac output	↑	~	↓	↓	↑
↓ Pa_{O_2}	↓	~	~	↑	↓
↑ Pa_{O_2}	↑	~	~	↓	↑
↓ Hb	↓	~	~	↑	↓
↑ Hb	↑	~	~	↓	↑
Peripheral shunting	~	↓	↓	↓	↑

↑ = increase
↓ = decrease
~ = unchanged

- PA_{O_2} (partial pressure of alveolar oxygen*
- $F_{I_{O_2}}$ (fractional concentration of inspired oxygen)

An example of the shunt calculation follows:

Case Study: Shunt Study Calculation in an Automobile Accident Victim

A 22-year-old man is on a volume-cycled mechanical ventilator on a day when the barometric pressure is 755 mm Hg. The patient is receiving an $F_{I_{O_2}}$ of .60. The following clinical data are obtained:

- Hb: 15 g/dl
- Pa_{O_2}: 65 mm Hg (Sa_{O_2} = 90%)
- Pa_{CO_2}: 56 mm Hg
- $P\bar{v}_{O_2}$ 35 mm Hg ($S\bar{v}_{O_2}$ = 65%)

With this information, the patient's PA_{O_2}, Cc_{O_2}, Ca_{O_2}, and $C\bar{v}_{O_2}$ can now be calculated. (Remember that P_{H_2O} represents alveolar water vapor pressure and is always 47 mm Hg.)

$$1.\ PA_{O_2} = (PB - P_{H_2O})\ F_{I_{O_2}} - Pa_{CO_2}\ (1.25)$$

$$= (755 - 47)\ .60 - 56\ (1.25)$$

$$= (708)\ .60 - 70$$

*See Ideal Alveolar Gas Equation, Appendix XIII.

$$= (424.8) - 70$$

$$= 354.8$$

2. $Cc_{O_2} = (Hb \times 1.34) + (Pa_{O_2} \times 0.003)$

$$= (15 \times 1.34) + (354.8 \times 0.003)$$

$$= (20.1) + 1.064$$

$$= 21.164 \ (vol\% \ O_2)$$

3. $Ca_{O_2} = (Hb \times 1.34 \times Sa_{O_2}) + (Pa_{O_2} \times 0.003)$

$$= (15 \times 1.34 \times .90) + (65 \times 0.003)$$

$$= (18.09) + (0.195)$$

$$= 18.285 \ (vol\% \ O_2)$$

4. $C\bar{v}_{O_2} = (Hb \times 1.34 \times S\bar{v}_{O_2}) + P\bar{v}_{O_2} \times 0.003)$

$$= (15 \times 1.34 \times .65) + (35 \times 0.003)$$

$$= (13.065) + (0.105)$$

$$= 13.17 \ (vol\% \ O_2)$$

With the information, the patient's intrapulmonary shunting can now be calculated.

$$\frac{\dot{Q}s}{\dot{Q}_T} = \frac{Cc_{O_2} - Ca_{O_2}}{Cc_{O_2} - C\bar{v}_{O_2}}$$

$$= \frac{21.164 - 18.285}{21.164 - 13.17}$$

$$= \frac{2.879}{7.994}$$

$$= 0.36$$

Thus, 36% of the patient's pulmonary blood flow is perfusing lung tissue that is not being ventilated.

With the proliferation of inexpensive personal computers, much of the shunt equation is now being written in simple programs. What was once a rather esoteric, error-prone procedure is now readily and accurately available to respiratory therapy practitioners.

Table 1-14 shows the clinical significance of pulmonary shunting. Table 1-15 summarizes how specific respiratory diseases alter oxygen-saturation-and content-based indices.

ABNORMAL CARDIOVASCULAR SYSTEM FINDINGS

Because the transport of oxygen to the tissue cells and the delivery of carbon dioxide to the lungs is a function of the cardiovascular system, a basic knowledge and understanding of (1) normal heart sounds, (2) normal electrocardiogram (ECG) pattern, (3) common heart arrhythmias, (4) noninvasive hemodynamic monitoring assessments, (5) invasive hemodynamic monitoring assessments, and (6) determinants of cardiac output are essential components of patient assessment.*

*See Appendix XX for an example of a cardiopulmonary profile sheet used to monitor the hemodynamic status of the critically ill patient.

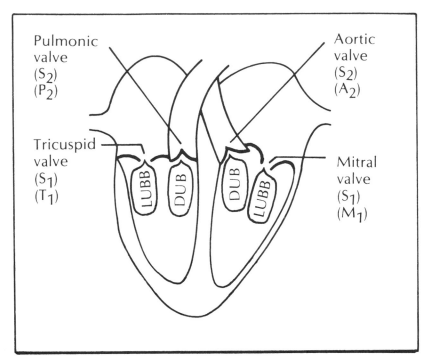

FIG 1-68
Origin of the "lubb-dub" sound of the heart.

Table 1-14 Clinical Significance of Pulmonary Shunting	
Degree of Pulmonary Shunting (%)	**Clinical Significance**
Below 10%	Normal lung status
10% to 20%	Indicates a pulmonary abnormality, but not significant in terms of cardiopulmonary support
20% to 30%	May be life-threatening, and cardiopulmonary support may be needed
Greater than 30%	Serious life-threatening condition, and cardiopulmonary support is almost always required

Normal Heart Sounds

Although there is still disagreement as to their exact origin, it is generally accepted that heart sounds develop in response to sudden changes in blood flow inside the heart that cause the walls of the heart chamber, the valves, and the great vessels to vibrate. It is the vibration of these structures that produces the heart sounds.

When the valves of the heart close, a "lubb-dub" sound is produced. The "lubb" sound is the first heart sound, or S_1. The "dub" sound is the second heart sound, or S_2.

S_1 is associated with the closure of the atrioventricular (AV) valves, i.e., the mitral and tricuspid valves (Fig 1-68). The mitral and the tricuspid valves produce separate sounds within S_1, these are referred to as M_1 and T_1. S_1 corresponds to the onset of systole and is louder, longer, and lower pitched than S_2 at the apex. Normally, closure of the mitral valve precedes closure of the tricuspid valve by about 0.02 seconds as the ventricles begin to contract. Be-

Table 1-15 Oxygen-, Saturation-, and Content-based Index Changes Commonly Seen in Respiratory Diseases

Pulmonary Disorder	Oxygenation Indices					
	$\dot{Q}_s/\dot{Q}_T$	D_{O_2}*	$\dot{V}_{O_2}$	$C(a\text{-}\overline{v})_{O_2}$	O_2ER	$S\overline{v}_{O_2}$

Obstructive Airway Diseases
  Chronic bronchitis
  Emphysema
  Bronchiectasis
  Asthma
  Cystic fibrosis
  Croup syndrome
	↑	↓	~	~	↑	↓

Infectious Pulmonary Diseases
  Pneumonia
  Lung abscess
  Fungal disorders
  Tuberculosis
	↑	↓	~	~	↑	↓

Pulmonary Edema	↑	↓	~	↑†	↑	↓
Pulmonary Embolism	↑	↓	~	↑†	↑	↓

Lung Collapse
  Flail chest
  Pneumothorax
  Pleural disease (e.g., hemothorax)
	↑	↓	~	↑†	↑	↓

Kyphoscoliosis	↑	↓	~	~	↑	↓
Pneumoconiosis	↑	↓	~	~	↑	↓
Cancer of the lung	↑	↓	~	~	↑	↓
Adult Respiratory Distress Syndrome	↑	↓	~	~	↑	↓
Idiopathic (Infant) Respiratory Distress Syndrome	↑	↓	~	~	↑	↓
Chronic Interstitial Lung Disease	↑	↓	~	~	↑	↓
Sleep Apnea	↑	↓	~	↑†	↑	↓
Smoke Inhalation Without surface burns	↑ ↑	↓	~	~	↑	↓
With surface burns	↑	↓	↑	↑	↑	↓
Near Drowning (Wet)	↑	↓	↑	↑	↑	↓

↑ = increase
↓ = decrease
~ = unchanged

*The D_{O_2} may be normal in patients with an increased cardiac output, an increased hemoglobin level (polycythemia), or a combination of both. For example, a normal D_{O_2} is often seen in patients with chronic obstructive pulmonary disease and polycythemia. When the D_{O_2} is normal, the patient's O_2 ER is usually normal.

†The increased $C(a\text{-}\overline{v})_{O_2}$ is associated with a decreased cardiac output.

cause the left ventricle is larger and more powerful than the right, however, the mitral valve closes with greater force than the tricuspid valve and therefore is the major source of the S_1 under normal circumstances.

S_2 results from closure of the semilunar valves, i.e., the aortic and pulmonic valves. The aortic and pulmonic valves each generate a separate sound within S_2; these are referred to as A_2 and P_2 (see Fig 1-68). Normally, the A_2 and P_2 sounds are about 0.03 seconds apart, aortic valve closure preceding pulmonary valve closure. A more distinct (wider) split is heard during inspiration as the intrathoracic pressure drops, which allows more blood to return to the right side of the heart. The increased blood volume in the right ventricle causes a delayed pulmonic valve closure. At the same time, the increase in negative intrapleural pressure causes blood vessels in the lungs to dilate and retain blood. This action reduces left ventricular stroke volume and left ventricular systole. As a result, the aortic valve closes earlier. Finally, even though the closure of the aortic valve still precedes closure of the pulmonic valve during expiration, the closure sequence is so rapid that A_2 and P_2 are generally heard as a single sound.

Abnormal Heart Sounds

Wide Split First Sound (S_1)

Under certain conditions, an abnormally wide or split first sound can be auscultated over the fourth intercostal space to the left of the sternum (patient's left). A wide split first sound can be produced by electrical or mechanical causes which cause asynchrony of the two ventricles. Some of the electrical causes include right bundle branch block, premature ventricular beats, and ventricular tachycardia.

Wide Split Second Sound (S_2)

The normal split second sound (A_2 and P_2) can be accentuated by conditions that cause an abnormal delay in pulmonic valve closure. Such a delay may be caused by (1) an increased volume in the right ventricle as compared to the left ventricle (e.g., atrial septal defect or ventricle septal defect), (2) chronic right ventricular outflow obstruction (e.g., pulmonic stenosis), (3) acute or chronic dilatation of the right ventricle due to sudden rise in pulmonary artery pressure (e.g., pulmonary embolism), or (4) electrical delay in activation of the right ventricle (right bundle branch block). The wide split has a duration of 0.04 to 0.05 seconds compared to the normal physiologic split of 0.03 seconds. It can be heard during inspiration and expiration and is best auscultated over the left base of the heart (second intercostal space to the left of the sternum [patient's left]).

Paradoxical Split Second Sound (S_2)

A paradoxical split of the S_2 occurs when there is a reversal of the normal closure sequence with pulmonic (P_2) closure occurring before aortic (A_2) closure. The paradoxical split S_2 may be heard when aortic closure is delayed as in marked volume or pressure loads on the left ventricle (e.g., aortic stenosis) or with conduction defects that delay left ventricular depolarization (e.g., left bundle branch block). The paradoxical split S_2 is best heard during expiration over the left base of the heart (the second intercostal space to the left of the sternum [patient's left]).

Fixed Splitting of the Second Sound (S_2)

Fixed splitting of the second sound refers to a split which displays little or no respiratory variation. The fixed splitting of the second sound occurs when the ventricles are unable to change their volumes with respirations. Such conditions include congestive heart failure, cardiomyopathy, atrial septal defect, or ventricular septal defect. The fixed split is best heard over the left base of the heart (the second intercostal space to the left of the sternum [patient's left]).

Fourth Heart Sound

The fourth heart sound is a low-frequency sound heard just before the first heart sound. It is also known as an "atrial gallop," a "presystolic gallop," and an "S_4 gallop." The S_4 is a diastolic sound that occurs during the late diastolic filling phase at the time the atria contract. When the ventricles have a decreased compliance or are receiving an increased diastolic volume, they generate a low-frequency vibration—the S_4. The S_4 may be normal in the young, but is seldom considered normal in persons older than 20 years of age. The S_4 may have its origin in either the left or right side of the heart.

The S_4 of *left ventricular origin* may be auscultated during inspiration or expiration and is best heard at the apex of the heart (the fifth intercostal space in the midclavicular line). Common causes include severe hypertension, aortic stenosis, cardiomyopathies, and left ventricular myocardial infarction.

The S_4 of right ventricular origin is best heard during inspiration over the left lateral sternal border (the fourth intercostal space to the left of the sternum [patient's left]). Common causes include pulmonary valve obstruction, pulmonary stenosis, pulmonary hypertension, or right ventricular myocardial infarction.

Third Heart Sound (S_3)

The third heart sound is a low-frequency sound heard just after the second heart sound. It is also known as "S_3," "S_3 gallop," or "ventricular gallop." The S_3 occurs in early diastole during rapid ventricular filling, about 0.14 to 0.16 seconds after the second sound (S_2), and reflects decreased ventricular compliance or an increased ventricular diastolic volume.

The S_3 is normal in children and young adults who have increased diastolic volumes. When normal it is called a *physiological third heart sound*. The abnormal S_3 is often heard in patients with coronary artery disease, cardiomyopathies, incompetent valves, left to right shunts, or patient ductus arteriosus. The S_3 may have its origin in either the left or right side of the heart. The S_3 of *left ventricular origin* is best heard during expiration over the apex (the fifth intercostal space to the left of the sternum at the midclavicular line). The S_3 of *right ventricular origin* is best heard during inspiration over the left lateral sternal border (the fourth intercostal space to the left of the sternum [patient's left]). Third heart sounds are often associated with sharp outward precordial movements which frequently can be seen or felt.

Ejection Sounds

Ejection sounds are high-frequency "clicky" sounds that occur just after the first sound with the onset of ventricular ejection. They are caused by the opening of the semilunar valves (aortic or pulmonic), e.g., when one of the valves is diseased or when ejection is rapid through a normal valve.

Ejection sounds of *aortic origin* are best heard over the right base of the heart (second intercostal space to the right of the sternum [patient's right]). Aortic ejection sounds are heard in patients with valvular aortic stenosis, aortic insufficiency, coarctation of the aorta, or aneurysm of the ascending aorta. Ejection sounds of pulmonic origin are best heard over the left base of the heart (second intercostal space to the left of the sternum [patient's left]). Pulmonic ejection sounds are heard in pulmonic stenosis, pulmonary hypertension, atrial septal defects, pulmonary embolism, hyperthyroidism, or in conditions that cause enlargement of the pulmonary artery.

Midsystolic Clicks

"Clicks" are high-frequency sounds that occur in early, mid, or late systole. The click occurs at least 0.14 seconds after the first sound. The most common cause of a click is mitral valve prolapse. The clicks of mitral origin are best heard at the apex or toward the left lateral sternal border.

Opening Snap

The opening snap is a short, high-frequency sound that occurs about 0.06 to 0.10 seconds after the second heart sound in early diastole. It is best heard between the apex and the left lateral sternal border. The opening snap is commonly caused by the audible opening of the mitral valve due to stiffening (i.e., mitral stenosis) or increased blood flow (i.e., ventricular septal defect or patent ductus arteriosus).

Murmurs

Murmurs are defined as sustained noises (e.g., blowing, harsh, rough, or rumbling sounds) that can be heard during systole, diastole, or both. Murmurs are caused by five major factors: (1) backward regurgitation through a leaking valve, septal defect, or arteriovenous connection, (2) forward flow through a narrowed or deformed valve, (3) high rate of blood flow through a normal or abnormal valve, (4) vibration of the loose structures within the heart—i.e., chordae tendineae, or (5) continuous flow through an arteriovenous shunt. Murmurs that occur when the ventricles are contracting are referred to as *systolic murmurs*. Murmurs that occur when the ventricles are relaxed are referred to as *diastolic murmurs*.

Systolic Murmurs

Systolic murmurs are defined as sustained noises that are audible during systole, or the period between S_1 and S_2. Forward flow across the aortic or pulmonic valves or regurgitant flow from the mitral or tricuspid valve may produce a systolic murmur. Systolic murmurs may be normal and can represent normal blood flow—e.g., thin chest, infants and children, or increased blood flow in pregnant women. Systolic murmurs are further classified as *early systolic murmurs, midsystolic murmurs,* and *late systolic murmurs.*

Early Systolic Murmurs

Early systolic murmurs begin with the first sound and peak in the first third of systole. Early murmurs have the greatest intensity in the early part of ventricular contraction. They are commonly caused by a small ventricular septal defect (VSD). The early systolic murmur of a small VSD stops before midsystole because as ejection continues and the ventricular size decreases, the small defect is sealed shut, causing the murmur to soften or cease.

Midsystolic Murmurs

A *midsystolic murmur* begins just after the first sound, peaks in the middle of systole, and does not quite extend to the second sound. It is a crescendo-decrescendo murmur that builds up and decreases symmetrically. It is also called an "ejection" murmur. This type of murmur is often heard in normal individuals, especially in the young who usually have increased blood volumes flowing over normal valves. In this setting, it is designated as an "innocent murmur." A midsystolic murmur may be caused by the forward blood flow through a normal, narrow, or irregular valve (i.e., aortic or pulmonic stenosis).

Late Systolic Murmur

A *late systolic murmur* is heard during the latter half of the systole, peaks in the latter third of systole, and extends to the second sound. It is a modified regurgitant murmur with a backward flow through an incompetent valve. It is commonly heard in patients with a mitral valve prolapse or tricuspid valve defect.

Diastolic Murmurs

Diastolic murmurs are defined as sustained noises that are audible between S_2 and the next S_1. Unlike systolic murmurs, diastolic murmurs are always considered pathologic. Common causes of diastolic murmurs include aortic regurgitation, pulmonic regurgitation, mitral stenosis, and tricuspid stenosis. Diastolic murmurs are further classified as early, mid, late, or pan in nature.

Early Diastolic Murmur

An *early diastolic murmur* begins with the second sound and peaks in the first third of diastole. An early diastolic murmur is commonly caused by aortic regurgitation and pulmonic regurgitation. The early diastolic murmur of *aortic regurgitation* has a high-frequency blowing quality and is best heard over the apex of the heart along the left sternal border. The murmur of *pulmonic regurgitation* occurs after a slight delay after S_2. It has a rough sound and is best heard over the left base of the heart.

Mid-Diastolic Murmur

A *mid-diastolic murmur* begins after the second sound and peaks in the mid-diastole. It is commonly caused by mitral stenosis and tricuspid stenosis. The murmur of *mitral stenosis* is a low-frequency, crescendo-decrescendo rumble heard at the apex. Mitral stenosis normally causes three distinct abnormal heart sounds: a loud first sound, an opening snap, and a mid-diastolic rumble with a late diastolic accentuation. The diastolic murmur of *tricuspid stenosis* is similar to that of mitral stenosis, except that it is best heard over the left lateral sternal border.

Late Diastolic Murmur

A *late diastolic murmur* begins in the latter half of diastole, peaks in the latter third of diastole, and extends to the first sound. It is often a component of the murmur of mitral stenosis or tricuspid stenosis. A late diastolic murmur is low in frequency and rumbling in quality.

Pandiastolic Murmur

A *pandiastolic murmur* begins with the second sound and extends throughout the diastolic period. There are four major causes of a pandiastolic murmur: (1) abnormal communication between an artery and vein, (2) abnormal communication between the aorta and the right side of the heart or with the left atrium, (3) an abnormal increase in flow or constriction in an artery, and (4) increased or turbulent blood flow through veins. A pandiastolic murmur is commonly heard in infants with *patent ductus arteriosus*. It is best heard over the left base of the heart (second intercostal space to the left of the sternum [patient's left]).

The Normal Electrocardiogram (ECG)

Because the respiratory care practitioner frequently works with critically ill patients who are on cardiac monitors, a basic understanding of the normal and common abnormal ECG pat-

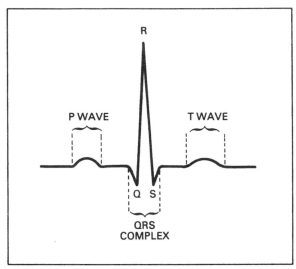

FIG 1-69
ECG pattern of a normal cardiac cycle.

terns is important. An ECG monitors, both visually and on recording paper, the electrical activity of the heart. Figure 1-69 illustrates the ECG pattern of a normal cardiac cycle. The P wave reflects the depolarization of the atria. The QRS complex represents the depolarization of the ventricles, and the T wave represents ventricular repolarization.

In normal adults, the heart rate is between 60 and 100 beats per minute. In normal infants, the heart rate is between 130 and 150 beats per minute. There are a number of methods that can be used to calculate the heart rate. For example, when the rhythm is regular, the heart rate can be determined at a glance by counting the number of large boxes (on the ECG strip) between two QRS complexes, and then dividing this number into 300. Thus, if an ECG strip consistently shows four large boxes between each QRS complex, the heart rate would be 75 beats per minute (300 ÷ 4 = 75). When the rhythm is irregular, the heart rate can be determined by counting the QRS complexes in a six-second strip and multiplying by 10. The following are heart arrhythmias commonly seen by the respiratory care practitioner.

Common Heart Arrhythmias

Sinus Bradycardia

In *sinus bradycardia,* the heart rate is less than 60 beats per minute. *Bradycardia* means "slow heart." Sinus bradycardia has a normal P-QRS-T pattern, and the rhythm is regular (Fig 1-70). Athletes often normally demonstrate this finding, due to increased cardiac stroke volume and other poorly understood mechanisms. Common pathologic causes of sinus bradycardia include a weakened or damaged sinoatrial (SA) node, severe or chronic hypoxemia, increased intracranial pressure, obstructive sleep apnea, and certain drugs (most notably the beta-blockers). Sinus bradycardia may lead to a decreased cardiac output and blood pressure. In severe cases, sinus bradycardia may lead to a decreased perfusion state and tissue hypoxia. The patient may demonstrate a weak or absent pulse, poor capillary refill, cold and clammy skin, and a depressed sensorium.

Sinus Tachycardia

In *sinus tachycardia,* the heart rate is greater than 100 beats per minute. *Tachycardia* means "fast heart." Sinus tachycardia has a normal P-QRS-T pattern, and the rhythm is regular (Fig

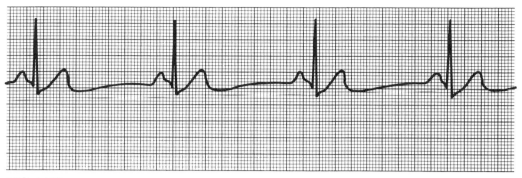

FIG 1-70
Sinus bradycardia. Rate is about 37 beats/min.

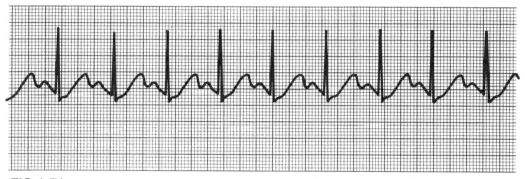

FIG 1-71
Sinus tachycardia. Rate is about 100 beats/min.

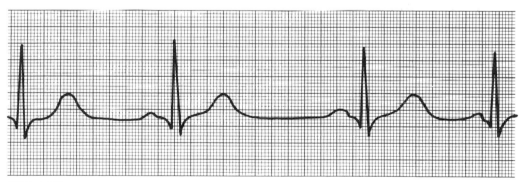

FIG 1-72
Sinus arrhythmia.

1-71). Sinus tachycardia is the normal physiologic response to stress and exercise. Common causes of sinus tachycardia include hypoxemia, severe anemia, hyperthermia, massive hemorrhage, pain, fear, anxiety, hyperthyroidism, and sympathomimetic or parasympatholytic drug administration.

Sinus Arrhythmia

In *sinus arrhythmia,* the heart rate varies by more than 10 percent from beat-to-beat. The P-QRS-T pattern is normal (Fig 1-72), but the interval between groups of complexes, e.g., the R-R interval, will vary. A sinus arrhythmia is a normal rhythm in children and young adults. The patient's pulse will often increase during inspiration and decrease during expiration. No treatment is required unless there is a significant alteration in the patient's arterial blood pressure.

Atrial Flutter

In *atrial flutter,* the normal P wave is absent and replaced by two or more regular sawtooth waves. The QRS complex is normal and the ventricular rate may be regular or irregular, depending on the relationship of the atrial to ventricular beats. Figure 1-73 shows an atrial flutter with a regular rhythm with a 4:1 conduction ratio (i.e., four atrial beats for every ventricular beat). Commonly, the atrial rate is constant between 250 and 350 beats per minute while the ventricular rate is in the normal range. Causes of atrial flutter include hypoxemia, a damaged sinoatrial (SA) node, and congestive heart failure.

Atrial Fibrillation

In *atrial fibrillation,* the atrial contractions are disorganized and ineffective, and the normal P wave is absent (Fig 1-74). The atrial rate ranges between 350 and 700 beats per minute. The QRS complex is normal, and the ventricular rate ranges between 100 and 200 beats per minute. Causes of atrial fibrillation include hypoxemia and a damaged sinoatrial (SA) node. Atrial fibrillation may reduce the cardiac output by 20 percent, due to a loss of atrial filling (the so-called "atrial kick").

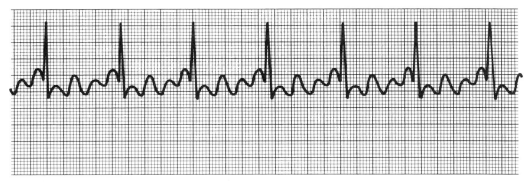

FIG 1-73
Atrial flutter. Atrial rate is greater than 300 beats/min; ventricular rate is about 60 beats/min.

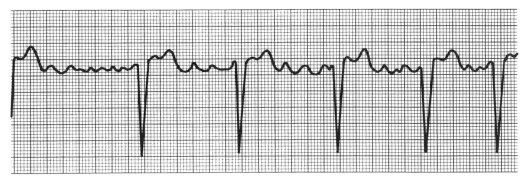

FIG 1-74
Atrial fibrillation.

Premature Ventricular Contractions

The premature ventricular contraction (PVC) is not preceded by a P wave. The QRS complex is wide, bizarre, and unlike the normal QRS complex (Fig 1-75). The regular heart rate is altered by the PVC. The heart rhythm may be very irregular when there are many PVCs. PVCs can occur at any rate. They often occur in pairs, after every normal heartbeat (bigeminal PVCs), and after every two normal heartbeats (trigeminal PVCs). Common causes of PVCs include intrinsic myocardial disease, hypoxemia, acidemia, hypokalemia, and congestive heart failure. PVCs may also be a sign of theophylline or alpha- or beta-agonist toxicity.

Ventricular Tachycardia

In *ventricular tachycardia,* the P wave is generally indiscernible, and the QRS complex is wide and bizarre in appearance (Fig 1-76). The T wave may not be separated from the QRS complex. The ventricular rate ranges between 150 and 250 beats per minute, and the rate is regular or slightly irregular. The patient's blood pressure is often decreased during ventricular tachycardia.

Ventricular Flutter

In *ventricular flutter,* the QRS complex has the appearance of a wide sine wave (regular, smooth, rounded ventricular wave) (Fig 1-77). The rhythm is regular or slightly irregular. The rate is 250 to 350 beats per minute. There is usually no discernible peripheral pulse associated with ventricular flutter.

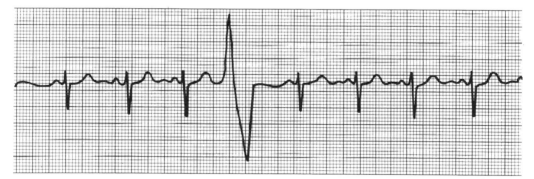

FIG 1-75
Premature ventricular contraction.

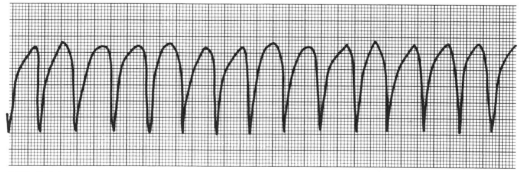

FIG 1-76
Ventricular tachycardia.

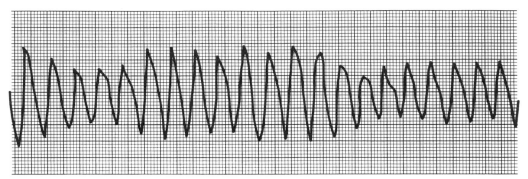

FIG 1-77
Ventricular flutter.

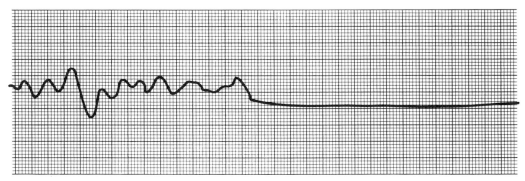

FIG 1-78
Ventricular fibrillation and asystole.

Ventricular Fibrillation

Ventricular fibrillation is characterized by chaotic electrical activity and cardiac activity. The ventricles literally quiver out of control with no perfusion beat-producing rhythm (Fig 1-78). During ventricular fibrillation, there is no cardiac output or blood pressure and, without treatment, the patient will die in minutes.

Asystole (Cardiac Standstill)

Asystole is the complete absence of electrical and mechanical activity. As a result, the cardiac output stops and the blood pressure falls to zero. The ECG tracing appears as a flat line and indicates severe damage to the heart's electrical conduction system (see Fig 1-78). Occasionally, periods of disorganized electrical and mechanical activity may be generated during long periods of asystole; this is referred to as an *agonal rhythm* or a *dying heart.*

Noninvasive Hemodynamic Monitoring Assessments

Hemodynamics are defined as forces that influence the circulation of blood. The general hemodynamic status of the patient can be monitored noninvasively at the bedside by assessing the heart rate (via an ECG monitor or auscultation), pulse, blood pressure, and perfusion state. During the acute stages of respiratory disease, the patient frequently demonstrates the following noninvasive hemodynamic changes:

Increased Heart Rate (Pulse), Cardiac Output, and Blood Pressure

Increased heart rate, pulse, and blood pressure develop frequently during the acute stages of pulmonary disease. This can be due to indirect response of the heart to the hypoxic stimulation of the peripheral chemoreceptors, primarily the carotid bodies. When the carotid bodies are stimulated, reflex signals are sent to the respiratory muscles, which in turn activate the so-called *pulmonary reflex,* which triggers tachycardia and an increased cardiac output and blood pressure. The increased cardiac output is a compensatory mechanism that, at least partially, counteracts the hypoxemia produced by the pulmonary shunting in respiratory disorders.

This process is perhaps best understood by assuming that the body's oxygen utilization remains relatively constant over a period of time. When the cardiac output increases during a period of steady metabolic requirements, oxygen transport increases, and the amount of oxygen extracted from each 100 ml of blood decreases. This results in an increase in the oxygen saturation of the returning venous blood, which in turn reduces the hypoxemia produced by the shunted blood. In other words, venous blood that perfuses underventilated alveoli will have less of a shunt effect if the oxygen content of the venous blood is 13 vol% as compared with, say, 10 vol%.

Other causes of increased heart rate, pulse, and blood pressure include severe anemia, high fever, anxiety, massive hemorrhage, certain cardiac arrhythmias, and hyperthyroidism. Finally, it should be noted that when the heart rate increases beyond 150 to 175 beats per minute, cardiac output and blood pressure begin to decline (the Starling relationship).

Decreased Perfusion State

The perfusion status can be evaluated by examining the patient's color, capillary refill, skin, and sensorium. Under normal conditions, the patient's nail beds and oral mucosa are pink. If these areas appear cyanotic or mottled, poor perfusion and tissue hypoxia are likely present. When the nail beds are compressed to expel blood, they should normally refill quickly and turn pink when the pressure is released. If the nail beds remain white, inadequate perfusion is present. Under normal conditions, a patient's skin should be dry and warm. When the skin is diaphoretic (wet), cool, or clammy, local perfusion is inadequate. Finally, when the patient is disoriented as to person, place, and time, a decreased perfusion state and cerebral hypoxia may be present.

Invasive Hemodynamic Monitoring Assessments

Invasive hemodynamic monitoring is used in the assessment and treatment of critically ill patients. Invasive hemodynamic monitors include the measurement of (1) intracardiac pressures and flows, via the pulmonary artery catheter, (2) arterial pressure, via an arterial catheter, and (3) central venous pressure, via a central venous catheter. These monitors provide rapid and precise measurements (assessment data) of the patient's cardiovascular function—which, in turn, are used to "down-regulate" or "up-regulate" the patient's treatment plan in a timely manner.

Pulmonary Artery Catheter

The *pulmonary artery catheter* (Swan-Ganz) is a balloon-tipped, flow-directed catheter that is inserted at the patient's bedside while monitoring the pressure waveform as the catheter, with the balloon inflated, is guided by blood flow through the right atrium, the right ventricle, and into the pulmonary artery (Fig 1-79). The pulmonary artery catheter is used to directly measure the *right atrial pressure* (via the proximal port), *pulmonary artery pressure* (via the distal port), *left atrial pressure* (indirectly via the pulmonary capillary wedge pressure), and *cardiac output* (via the thermodilution technique).

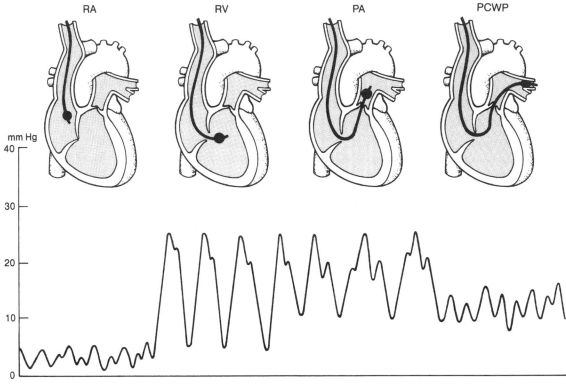

FIG 1-79

Insertion of the pulmonary catheter. The insertion site of the pulmonary catheter may be the basilic, brachial, femoral, subclavian, or internal jugular veins. The latter two are the most common insertion sites. As the catheter advances, pressure readings and waveforms are monitored to determine the catheter's position as it moves through the right atrium (RA), right ventricle (RV), pulmonary artery (PA), and finally into a pulmonary capillary "wedge" pressure (PCWP) position. Immediately after a PCWP reading, the balloon is deflated to allow blood to flow past the tip of the catheter. When the balloon is deflated, the catheter continuously monitors the pulmonary artery pressure. (From Des Jardins T: *Cardiopulmonary Anatomy and Physiology: Essentials for Respiratory Care,* Albany, NY, Delmar Publishers Inc, 1993. Used by permission.)

Arterial Catheter

The *arterial catheter* (line) is the most commonly used mode of invasive hemodynamic monitoring. It is generally inserted in the radial artery for patient comfort and convenient access reasons. The indwelling arterial catheter allows (1) continuous and precise measurements of systolic, diastolic, and mean blood pressure, (2) accurate information regarding fluctuations in blood pressure, and (3) guidance in the decision to "up-regulate" or "down-regulate" therapy for hypotension or hypertension. The arterial catheter is also useful in patients who require frequent or repeated arterial blood gas samples (e.g., the patient being mechanically ventilated). The blood samples are readily available, and the patient is not subjected to the pain of repeated arterial punctures.

Central Venous Pressure Catheter

The *central venous pressure catheter* readily measures the central venous pressure (CVP) and right ventricular filling pressure. It serves as an excellent monitor of right ventricular function. An increased CVP reading is commonly seen in patients who (1) have left ventricular heart failure (e.g., pulmonary edema), (2) are receiving excessively high positive pressure

Table 1-16 Hemodynamic Values Measured Directly

Hemodynamic Value	Abbreviation	Normal Range
Central venous pressure	CVP	0-8 mm Hg
Right atrial pressure	RAP	0-8 mm Hg
Mean pulmonary artery pressure	$\overline{PA}$	10-20 mm Hg
Pulmonary capillary wedge pressure (also called pulmonary artery wedge; pulmonary artery occlusion)	PCWP PAW PAO	4-12 mm Hg
Cardiac output	CO	4-6 L/min

Table 1-17 Hemodynamic Values Calculated from Direct Hemodynamic Measurements

Hemodynamic Value	Abbreviation	Normal Range
Stroke volume	SV	40-80 ml
Stroke volume index	SVI	$40 \pm$ ml/beat/m^2
Cardiac index	CI	3.0 ± 0.5 L/min/m^2
Right ventricular stroke work index	RVSWI	7-12 g/m^2
Left ventricular stroke work index	LVSWI	40-60 g/m^2
Pulmonary vascular resistance	PVR	50-150 dynes $\times$ sec $\times$ cm^{-5}
Systemic vascular resistance	SVR	800-1500 dynes $\times$ sec $\times$ cm^{-5}

mechanical breaths, (3) have cor pulmonale, or (4) have a severe flail chest, pneumothorax, or pleural effusion.

Table 1-16 summarizes the hemodynamic parameters that can be measured directly. Table 1-17 lists the hemodynamic parameters that can be calculated from results obtained from the direct measurements.*

Hemodynamic Monitoring in Respiratory Diseases

Because respiratory disorders can have a profound effect on the structure and function of the pulmonary vascular bed, right side of the heart, left side of the heart, or a combination of all three, the results generated by the above invasive hemodynamic monitors are commonly used in the assessment and treatment of these patients. For example, respiratory diseases associated with severe or chronic hypoxemia, acidemia, or pulmonary vascular obstruction can increase the pulmonary vascular resistance (PVR) significantly. An increased PVR, in turn, can lead to a variety of secondary hemodynamic changes such as increased CVP, RAP, $\overline{PA}$, RVSWI, and decreased CO, SV, SVI, CI, and LVSWI. Table 1-18 lists common hemodynamic changes seen in pulmonary diseases known to alter the patient's hemodynamic status.

Determinants of Cardiac Output

The cardiac output measured directly by the pulmonary artery catheter is a function of ventricular preload, ventricular afterload, and myocardial contractility.

*See Appendix XVIII for discussion of hemodynamic calculations.

Table 1-18 Hemodynamic Changes Commonly Seen in Respiratory Diseases

Disorder	Hemodynamic Indices											
	CVP	RAP	$\overline{PA}$	PCWP	CO	SV	SVI	CI	RVSWI	LVSWI	PVR	SVR
COPD Chronic bronchitis Emphysema Bronchiectasis Cystic fibrosis	↑	↑	↑	~	~	~	~	~	↑	~	↑	~
Pulmonary Edema	↑	↑	↑	↑↑	↓	↓	↓	↓	↑	↓	↑	↓
Pulmonary Embolism	↑	↑	↑↑	↓	↓	↓	↓	↓	↑	↓	↑	~
Adult Respiratory Distress Syndrome (ARDS)— Severe	~↑	~↑	~↑	~	~	~	~	~	~↑	~	~↑	~
Lung Collapse Flail chest Pneumothorax Pleural disease (e.g., hemothorax)	↑	↑	↑	↓	↓	↓	↓	↓	↑	↓	↑	↓
Kyphoscoliosis	↑	↑	↑	~	~	~	~	~	↑	~	↑	~
Pneumoconiosis	↑	↑	↑	~	~	~	~	~	↑	~	↑	~
Chronic Interstitial Lung Diseases	↑	↑	↑	~	~	~	~	~	↑	~	↑	~
Cancer of the lung (tumor mass)	↑	↑	↑	↓	↓	↓	↓	↓	↑	↓	↑	~
Hypovolemia (burns)	↓	↓	↓	↓	↓	↓	↓	↓	↓	↓	~	↑

↑ = increase
↓ = decrease
~ = unchanged

Ventricular preload.—The ventricular preload refers to the degree the muscle fibers of the ventricle are stretched prior to contraction (end-diastole). Within normal physiologic limits, the greater the preload, the stronger the ventricular muscle fibers will contract during systole, which in turn leads to a greater force of contraction. This mechanism enables the heart to increase cardiac output in response to an increased venous return.

Because ventricular preload is a function of the pressure generated by volume of blood returning to the heart, the *ventricular end-diastolic pressure* (VEDP), in essence, reflects the *ventricular end-diastolic volume* (VEDV). Thus, as the VEDP increases or decreases, the VEDV increases or decreases, respectively. The relationship between the VEDP (force) and VEDV (stroke volume) is known as the *Frank-Starling relationship*. Clinically, the patient's ventricular preload is reflected in (1) the degree of neck vein distention, (2) central venous pressure (CVP) measurements, and (3) pulmonary capillary wedge pressure (PCWP) measurements.

Ventricular afterload.—The ventricular afterload is defined as the resistance (opposing forces) against which the ventricles must work to eject blood.

The *right ventricular afterload* is reflected in the pulmonary vascular resistance (PVR). Thus, as the PVR increases or decreases, the right ventricular afterload increases or decreases, respectively. Clinically, conditions that increase PVR include (1) pulmonary vasoconstriction (e.g., caused by alveolar hypoxia), (2) destruction of the pulmonary capillaries (e.g., emphysema), (3) blockage of major pulmonary arteries (e.g., pulmonary emboli), or (4) excessive positive pressure mechanical ventilation.

The *left ventricular afterload* is reflected in the systemic vascular resistance (SVR). Thus, as the SVR increases or decreases, the left ventricular afterload increases or decreases, respectively. The arterial diastolic blood pressure best reflects the left ventricular afterload. For example, as the arterial diastolic pressure increases, the resistance (against which the left side of the heart must work to eject blood) also increases. Clinically, conditions that increase SVR include peripheral vasoconstriction, excessive blood volume, or increased blood viscosity.

Myocardial contractility.—Myocardial contractility refers to the *forcefulness* of myocardial contraction—independent of preload and afterload. An adequate myocardial contraction is absolutely essential for an adequate cardiac output. For example, when the myocardial contractility is weak or inadequate, the cardiac output will be poor, even when the ventricles fill appropriately with blood (preload) and the resistance to outflow is optimal (afterload). An increase in myocardial contractility is called positive inotropism. Common positive inotropic drugs include isoproterenol, dopamine, dobutamine, and amrinone. A decrease in myocardial contractility is called negative inotropism.

Clinically, there is no single invasive measurement that reflects myocardial contractility. However, the general status of a patient's myocardial contractility can be inferred through various clinical assessments such as pulse, blood pressure, skin temperature, and serial hemodynamic measurements. Myocardial contractility (specifically cardiac ejection fraction) can be measured using an MUGA scan, and cardiac wall motion can be assessed with two-dimensional echocardiography. A decreased cardiac contractility is commonly accompanied by an increased systemic vascular resistance, ventricular preload, pulmonary capillary wedge pressure, and central venous pressure.

INCREASED CENTRAL VENOUS PRESSURE/DECREASED SYSTEMIC BLOOD PRESSURE

In patients with a severe flail chest, pneumothorax, or pleural effusion, the major veins of the chest that return blood to the right heart may be compressed. When this happens, venous return decreases, and the central venous pressure (CVP) increases. This condition is mani-

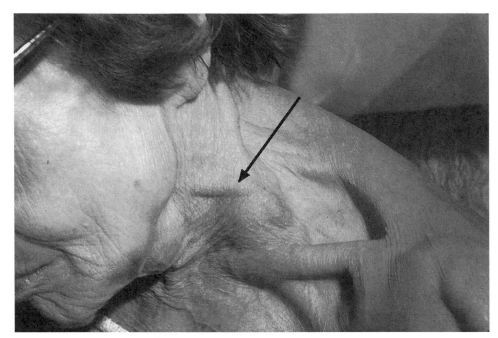

FIG 1-80
Distended neck veins (arrow).

fested by distended neck veins (Fig 1-80). The reduced venous return may also cause the patient's cardiac output and systemic pressure to decrease.

POLYCYTHEMIA, COR PULMONALE

- Distended neck veins
- Enlarged and tender liver
- Pitting edema

When pulmonary disorders produce chronic hypoxia, the hormone erythropoietin responds by stimulating the bone marrow to increase red blood cell (RBC) production. RBC production is known as *erythropoiesis.* An increased level of RBCs is called polycythemia. The polycythemia that results from hypoxia is an adaptive mechanism that increases the oxygen-carrying capacity of the blood.

Cor pulmonale is the term used to denote pulmonary arterial hypertension, right ventricular hypertrophy, increased right ventricular work, and ultimately, right ventricular failure. The three major mechanisms involved in producing cor pulmonale in chronic pulmonary disease are (1) the increased viscosity of the blood that is associated with polycythemia, (2) the increased pulmonary vascular resistance caused by hypoxic vasoconstriction, and (3) obliterating the pulmonary capillary bed, particularly in emphysema.

Increased Viscosity in Polycythemia

Unfortunately, the advantage of the increased oxygen-carrying capacity in polycythemia is at least partially offset by the increased viscosity of the blood when the hematocrit reaches 50% to 60%. Because of the increased viscosity of the blood, a greater driving pressure is needed to maintain a given flow. The work of the right ventricle must increase in order to generate the pressure needed to overcome the increased viscosity. This can ultimately lead to right ventricular hypertrophy, or cor pulmonale.

Hypoxic Vasoconstriction of the Pulmonary Vascular System

The decreased PA_{O_2} in chronic respiratory disorders causes the smooth muscles of the pulmonary arterioles to constrict. The exact mechanism of this phenomenon is unclear. It is known, however, that it is the partial pressure of oxygen in the alveoli (PA_{O_2}) and not the partial pressure of the arterial oxygen (Pa_{O_2}) that chiefly controls this response.

The effect of hypoxic vasoconstriction is to direct blood away from the hypoxic regions of the lungs and, thereby, offset the shunt effect. However, when the number of hypoxic regions becomes significant—as during the advanced stages of emphysema—a generalized pulmonary vasoconstriction may develop that may substantially increase pulmonary vascular resistance. The increased pulmonary vascular resistance, in turn, leads to pulmonary hypertension, increased work of the right side of the heart, right ventricular hypertrophy, and cor pulmonale.

To summarize, the cor pulmonale associated with chronic respiratory disorders may develop from the combine effects of polycythemia and pulmonary vasoconstriction. Both of these conditions occur as a result of hypoxia. Clinically, cor pulmonale leads to the accumulation of venous blood in the large veins. *This condition causes the neck veins to become distended, the liver to become enlarged and tender, and the extremities to show signs of peripheral edema and pitting edema.* It should also be noted that a loud pulmonic valve (P_2) closure is commonly heard during auscultation when pulmonary hypertension and cor pulmonale are present. In addition, an ECG often reveals right-axis deviation when cor pulmonale is present. In lead I, the right-axis deviation is demonstrated as a negative (downward) deflection of the QRS complex.

Pitting Edema

Bilateral, dependent, pitting edema is commonly seen in patients with congestive heart failure, cor pulmonale, and hepatic cirrhosis. To assess the presence and severity of pitting edema, firmly depress the skin over the tibia or the medial malleolus (2 to 4 inches above the foot) for 5 seconds and release. Normally, this procedure leaves no indentation, although a pit is often seen if the person has been standing all day or is pregnant. If pitting is present, it is graded on the following subjective scale: 1^+ (mild, slight depression) to 4^+ (severe, deep depression).

DIGITAL CLUBBING

Digital clubbing is sometimes noticed in patients with chronic respiratory disorders. Clubbing is characterized by a bulbous swelling of the terminal phalanges of the fingers and toes. The contour of the nail becomes rounded both longitudinally and transversely, and this results in an increase in the angle between the surface of the nail and the terminal phalanx (Fig 1-81).

The specific cause of clubbing is unknown. It is a normal hereditary finding in some families without any known history of cardiopulmonary disease. It is believed that the following factors may be causative: (1) circulating vasodilators, such as bradykinin and the prostaglandins, that are released from normal tissues but are not degraded by the lungs because of intrapulmonary shunting; (2) chronic infection; (3) unspecified toxins; (4) capillary stasis from increased venous backpressure; (4) arterial hypoxemia; and (5) local hypoxia. Successful treatment of the underlying disease may result in resolution of the clubbing and return of the digits to normal.

COUGH, SPUTUM PRODUCTION, AND HEMOPTYSIS

Cough

A cough is the sudden, audible expulsion of air from the lungs and is very common in respiratory diseases, especially in disorders that cause inflammation of the tracheobronchial tree.

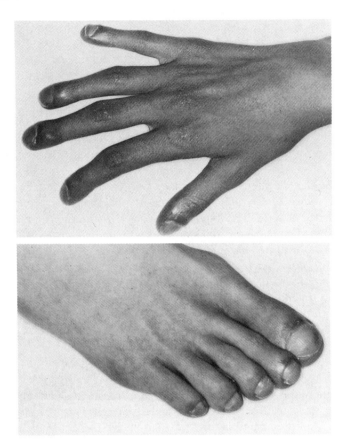

FIG 1-81
Digital clubbing.

In general, a cough is preceded by (1) a deep inspiration, (2) partial closure of the glottis, and (3) forceful contraction of the accessory muscles of expiration to expel air from the lungs. In essence, a cough is a protective mechanism that serves to clear the lungs, bronchi, or trachea of irritants and secretions. A cough also serves to prevent the aspiration of foreign materials into the lung. For example, cough is a common symptom with chronic sinusitis and postnasal drip. The effectiveness of a cough depends largely on (1) the depth of the preceding inspiration and (2) the extent of dynamic compression of the airways (see Fig 1-41, B).

A cough may be initiated voluntarily or, to some extent, suppressed voluntarily. Under most circumstances, however, a cough is a reflex that arises from stimulation of the cough or irritant receptors (also called subepithelial mechanoreceptors), which are located in the pharynx, larynx, trachea, and large bronchi. When stimulated, the irritant receptors send a signal by way of the glossopharyngeal (cranial nerve IX) and vagus (cranial nerve X) nerves to the cough reflex center located in the medulla. The medulla in turn causes the glottis to close and the accessory muscles of expiration to contract.

Some factors that stimulate the irritant receptors are as follows:

- Inflammation
- Mucus accumulation
- Noxious gases (e.g., cigarette smoke, chemical inhalation)
- Very hot or very cold air
- Mechanical stimulation (e.g., endotracheal suctioning, or compression of the airways).

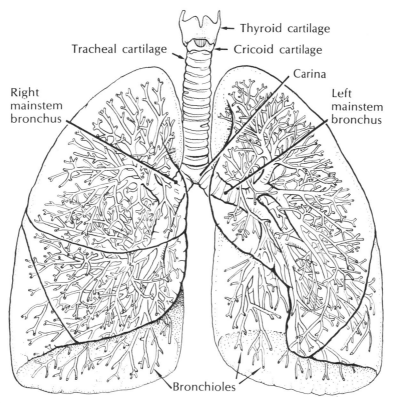

FIG 1-82
The tracheobronchial tree.

Sputum Production

Excessive sputum production is commonly seen in respiratory diseases that cause an acute or chronic inflammation of the tracheobronchial tree (Fig 1-82).

Histology of the tracheobronchial tree

The wall of the tracheobronchial tree is composed of three major layers: an epithelial lining, the lamina propria, and a cartilaginous layer (Fig 1-83).

The *epithelial lining,* which is separated from the lamina propria by a basement membrane, is predominantly composed of pseudostratified, ciliated, columnar epithelium interspersed with numerous mucus- and serum-secreting glands. The ciliated cells extend from the beginning of the trachea to—and sometimes including—the respiratory bronchioles. As the tracheobronchial tree becomes progressively smaller, the columnar structure of the ciliated cells gradually decreases in height. In the terminal bronchioles the epithelium appears more cuboidal than columnar. These cells flatten even more in the respiratory bronchioles (see Fig 1-83).

A mucous layer, commonly referred to as the mucous blanket, covers the epithelial lining of the tracheobronchial tree (Fig 1-84). The viscosity of the mucous layer progressively increases from the epithelial lining to the inner luminal surface, and there are two distinct layers: (1) the sol layer, which is adjacent to the epithelial lining, and (2) the gel layer, which is the more viscous layer adjacent to the inner luminal surface. The mucous blanket is 95% water. The remaining 5% consists of glycoproteins, carbohydrates, lipids, DNA, some cellular debris, and foreign particles.

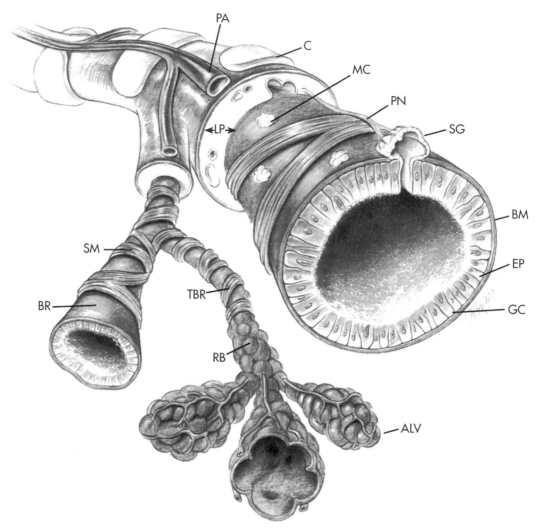

FIG 1-83

The normal lung. *PA* = pulmonary artery; *C* = cartilage; *LP* = lamina propria; *PN* = para-sympathetic nerve; *SG* = submucosal gland; *SM* = smooth muscle; *MC* = mast cell; *BM* = basement membrane; *EP* = epithelium; *GC* = goblet cell; *BR* = bronchioles; *TBR* = terminal bronchioles; *RB* = respiratory bronchioles; *ALV* = alveoli.

The mucus blanket is produced by the *goblet cells* and the *submucosal,* or *bronchial, glands.* The goblet cells are located intermittently between the pseudostratified, ciliated columnar cells and have been identified as distal the terminal bronchioles.

Most of the mucus blanket is produced by the submucosal glands, which extend deeply into the lamina propria and are composed of several different cell types: serous cells, mucous cells, collecting duct cells, mast cells, myoepithelial cells, and clear cells, which are probably lymphocytes. The submucosal glands are particularly numerous in the medium-sized bronchi and disappear in the bronchioles. These glands are innervated by parasympathetic (cholinergic) nerve fibers and normally produce about 100 ml of clear, thin bronchial secretions per day.

The mucus blanket is an important cleansing mechanism of the tracheobronchial tree. Inhaled particles stick to the mucus. The distal ends of the cilia continually strike the innermost portion of the gel layer and propel the mucus layer, along with any foreign particles, toward the larynx. At this point, the cough mechanism moves secretions beyond the larynx

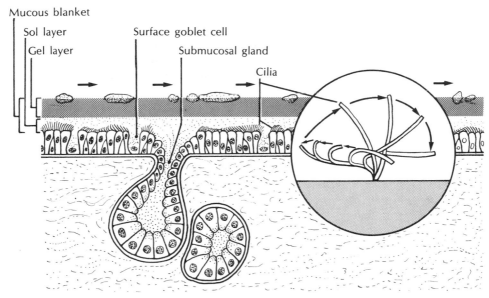

FIG 1-84
The epithelial lining of the tracheobronchial tree.

and into the oropharynx. This mucociliary mechanism is commonly referred to as the *muco-ciliary transport* or the *mucociliary escalator.* It is estimated that the cilia move the mucous blanket at an average rate of 2 cm/min.

The submucosal layer of the tracheobronchial tree is the *lamina propria.* Within the lamina propria is a loose, fibrous tissue that contains tiny blood vessels, lymphatic vessels, and branches of the vagus nerve. A circular layer of smooth muscle is also found within the lamina propria. It extends from the trachea down to and including the terminal bronchioles.

The *cartilaginous* structures that surround the tracheobronchial tree progressively diminish in size as the airways extend into the lungs. The cartilaginous layer is completely absent in bronchioles less than 1 mm in diameter (see Fig 1-83).

Types of sputum production

Depending on the severity and nature of the respiratory disease, sputum production may take several forms. For example, during the early stages of tracheobronchial tree inflammation, the sputum is usually clear, thin, and odorless. As the disease intensifies, the sputum becomes yellow-green and opaque. The yellow-green appearance results from an enzyme (myeloperoxidase) that is released during the cellular breakdown of leukocytes. It should be noted that the yellow-green color may be caused by retained or stagnant secretions or secretions caused by an acute infection.

Thick and tenacious sputum is commonly seen in patients suffering from chronic bronchitis, bronchiectasis, cystic fibrosis, and asthma. Patients with pulmonary edema expectorate a thin, frothy, pinkish sputum. Technically, this fluid is not true sputum. It results from the movement of plasma and red blood cells across the alveolar-capillary membrane into the alveoli.

Hemoptysis

Hemoptysis is the coughing up of blood or blood-tinged sputum from the tracheobronchial tree. In true hemoptysis, the sputum is usually bright red and interspersed with air bubbles.

Clinically, hemoptysis may be confused with hematemesis, which is blood that originates from the upper gastrointestinal tract and usually has a dark, coffee-ground appearance.

Repeated expectoration of blood-streaked sputum is seen in chronic bronchitis, bronchiectasis, cystic fibrosis, pulmonary embolism, lung cancer, necrotizing infections, tuberculosis, and fungal diseases. A small amount of hemoptysis is common following bronchoscopy, particularly when biopsies are taken.

Massive hemoptysis is defined as coughing up 400 to 600 ml of blood within a 24-hour period. Death from exsanguination due to hemoptysis is rare.

SUBSTERNAL/INTERCOSTAL RETRACTIONS

Substernal and intercostal retractions may be seen in patients with severe restrictive lung disorders such as pneumonia or adult respiratory distress syndrome. In an effort to overcome the low lung compliance, the patient must generate a greater-than-normal negative intrapleural pressure during inspiration. This greater negative intrapleural pressure in turn causes the tissues between the ribs and the substernal area to retract inward during inspiration (Fig 1-85). Because the thorax of the newborn is very flexible (due to the large amount of cartilage found in the skeletal structure), substernal and intercostal retractions are seen in infants with idiopathic respiratory distress syndrome (IRDS).

CHEST PAIN/DECREASED CHEST EXPANSION

Chest pain is one of the most frequent complaints of patients with cardiopulmonary problems. Chest pain can be divided into two categories: pleuritic and nonpleuritic.

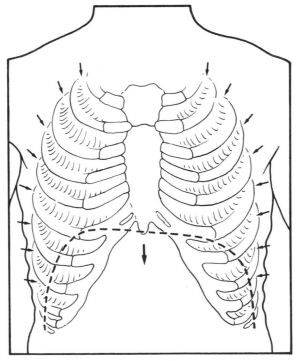

FIG 1-85
Intercostal retraction of soft tissues during inspiration.

Pleuritic Chest Pain

Pleuritic chest pain is usually described as a sudden, sharp, or stabbing pain. The pain generally intensifies during deep inspiration and coughing, and diminishes during breath holding or "splinting." The origin of the pain may be the chest wall, muscles, ribs, parietal pleura, diaphragm, mediastinal structures, or intercostal nerves. Since the visceral pleura, which covers the lungs, does not have any sensory nerve supply, pain originating in the parietal region signifies extension of inflammation from the lungs to the contiguous parietal pleura that lines the inner surface of the chest wall. This condition is known as *pleurisy* (Fig 1-86). When a patient with pleurisy inhales, the lung expands, irritates the inflamed parietal pleura, and causes pain.

Because of the nature of the pleuritic pain, a patient will usually prefer to lie on the side affected to allow greater expansion of the uninvolved lung and to help splint the chest on the involved side. Pleuritic chest pain is a characteristic feature of the following respiratory diseases:

- Pneumonia
- Pleural effusion
- Pneumothorax
- Pulmonary embolism
- Lung cancer
- Pneumonconiosis
- Fungal diseases
- Tuberculosis

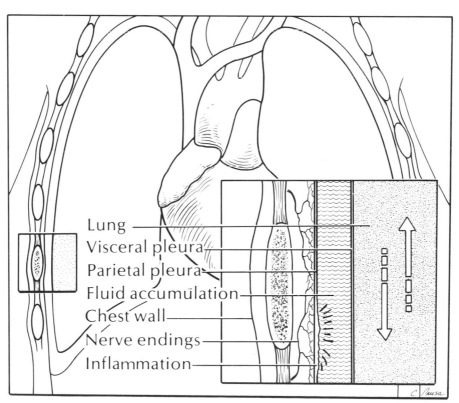

FIG 1-86
When the parietal pleura is irritated and inflamed, the nerve endings located in the parietal pleura send pain signals to the brain.

Nonpleuritic Chest Pain

Nonpleuritic chest pain is usually described as a constant pain that is located centrally. The pain may also radiate. Nonpleuritic chest pain is associated with the following disorders:

* Myocardial ischemia
* Pericardial inflammation
* Systemic hypertension
* Esophagitis
* Local trauma or inflammation of the chest cage, muscles, bones, or cartilage
* Pulmonary hypertension

ABNORMAL HEMATOLOGY, BLOOD CHEMISTRY, AND ELECTROLYTE FINDINGS

Abnormal *hematology, blood chemistry,* or *electrolyte* values assist the respiratory care practitioner and physician in the assessment of cardiopulmonary disorders. Knowledge of these laboratory tests provides a greater understanding of the clinical manifestations of a particular cardiopulmonary disorder.

Hematology

The most frequent laboratory hematology test is the *complete blood count* (CBC). The CBC provides important information about the patient's diagnosis, prognosis, response to treatment, and recovery. The CBC includes the *red blood cell* (RBC) *count, hemoglobin hematocrit,* the *total white blood count,* and at least an estimate of the *platelet count.*

Red Blood Cell Count

The RBC (erythrocytes) constitute the major portion of the blood cells. In the healthy adult male, there are about 5 million RBCs in each cubic millimeter of blood. The healthy adult female has about 4 million RBCs in each cubic millimeter of blood. Clinically, the total number of RBCs and its indices are useful in assessing the patient's overall oxygen-carrying capacity. The RBC indices are helpful in the identification of specific RBC deficiencies.

Red Blood Cell Indices

Hematocrit (Hct).—The hematocrit is the volume of RBCs in 100 ml of blood and is expressed as a percentage of the total volume. In the healthy adult male, the hematocrit is about 45%; in the healthy adult female, the hematocrit is about 42%. In the healthy newborn, the hematocrit ranges between 45% and 60%.

Hemoglobin (Hb).—Most of the oxygen that diffuses into the pulmonary capillary blood rapidly moves into the RBCs and chemically attaches to the hemoglobin. Each RBC contains approximately 280 million hemoglobin molecules. The hemoglobin value is reported in grams per 100 ml of blood (also referred to as grams percent of hemoglobin [g% Hb]). The normal hemoglobin value for the adult male is 14 to 16 g%. The normal adult female hemoglobin value is 12 to 15 g%. Hemoglobin constitutes about 33 percent of the RBC weight.

Mean cell volume (MCV).—The MCV is the actual size of the RBCs and is used to classify anemias. It is an index that expresses the volume occupied by a single red cell and is a measure in cubic microns of the mean volume. The normal MCV is 87 to 103 cubic microns for both men and women.

Mean corpuscular hemoglobin concentration (MCHC).—The MCHC is a measure of the concentration or proportion of hemoglobin in an average (mean) RBC. The MCHC is derived by dividing the g% Hb by the hematocrit. For example, if a patient has 15 g% Hb and a Hct of 45%, the MCHC would be 33%. The normal MCHC for men and women ranges between 32% and 36%. The MCHC is most useful in assessing the degree of anemia because the two most accurate hematologic components (hemoglobin and hematocrit—not RBC) are used for the test.

Mean cell hemoglobin (MCH).—The MCH is a measure of weight of hemoglobin in a single RBC. This value is derived by dividing the total hemoglobin (g% Hb) by the RBC count. The MCH is useful in diagnosing severely anemic patients, but not as good as MCHC because the RBC is not always accurate. The normal range for the MCH is 27 to 32 picograms per RBC.

Assessing the RBC count and its indices are useful in the identification of the following types of anemias:

Normochromic (normal hemoglobin) and normocytic (normal cell size) anemia.—This type of anemia is most commonly caused by excessive blood loss. The amount of hemoglobin and the number of RBCs are decreased, but the individual size and content remain normal. Clinically, the laboratory report reveals the following:

- Hct: below normal
- Hb: below normal
- MCV: below normal
- MCHC: normal
- MCH: normal

Hypochromic (decreased hemoglobin) microcytic (small cell size) anemia.—In this form of anemia, the size of the RBCs and the hemoglobin content are decreased. This form of anemia is commonly seen in patients with chronic blood loss, iron deficiencies, chronic infections, and malignancies. Clinically, the laboratory report reveals the following:

- Hct: below normal
- Hb: below normal
- MCV: below normal
- MCHC: below normal
- MCH: below normal

Macrocytic (large cell size) anemia.—This form of anemia is commonly caused by folic acid and vitamin B_{12} deficiencies. Patients with macrocytic anemia produce less RBCs, but the RBCs that are present are larger than normal. Clinically, the laboratory report reveals the following:

- Hct: below normal
- Hb: below normal
- MCV: above normal (due to the larger RBC size)
- MCHC: above normal (due to the larger RBC size)

White Blood Cell Count

The major functions of the WBCs (leukocytes) are to (1) fight against infection, (2) defend the body by phagocytosis against foreign organisms, and (3) to produce (or at least transport and distribute) antibodies in the immune response. The WBCs are far less numerous than the RBCs, averaging between 5,000 to 10,000 cells per cubic millimeter of blood. There are two types of WBCs; *granular* and *nongranular leukocytes.* Because the general function of the leukocytes is to combat inflammation and infection, the clinical diagnosis of an injury or infection often entails what is called a *differential count,* which is the determination of the number of each type of cell in 100 WBCs. Table 1-19 shows a normal differential count.

Granular Leukocytes

The granular leukocytes (also called *granulocytes*) are so classified because of the granules present in their cytoplasm. The granulocytes are further divided into the following three types according to the staining properties of the granules: *neutrophils, eosinophils,* and *basophils.* Because these cells have distinctive multilobar nuclei, they are often referred to as *polymorphonuclear leukocytes.*

Neutrophils.—The *neutrophils* comprise about 60% to 70% of the total number of WBCs. They have granules that are neutral and, thus, do not stain with an acid or a basic dye. The neutrophils are the first WBCs to arrive at the site of inflammation, usually appearing within 90 minutes of the injury. They represent the primary defense against bacterial organisms through the process of phagocytosis. The neutrophils are one of several types of cells called *phagocytes* that ingest and destroy bacterial organisms and particulate matter. The neutrophils also release an enzyme called *lysozyme,* which destroys certain bacteria. An increased neutrophil count is associated with (1) bacterial infection, (2) physical and emotional stress, (3) tumors, (4) inflammatory or traumatic disorders, (5) some leukemias, (6) myocardial infarction, and (7) burns.

Early forms of neutrophils are nonsegmented and are often called *band* forms. They almost always signify infection if elevated above 10% of the differential. More mature forms of neutrophils have segmented nuclei. They may increase even in the absence of infection, e.g., with stress (exercise) or with the use of corticosteroid medication.

Eosinophils.—The cytoplasmic granules of the eosinophils stain red with the acid dye eosin. These leukocytes comprise 2% to 4% of the total number of WBCs. Although the precise function of the eosinophils is unknown, they are thought to play a role in the breakdown of protein material. It is known, however, that the eosinophils are activated by allergies (such as an allergic asthmatic episode) and parasitic infections. Eosinophils are thought to detoxify the agents or chemical mediators associated with allergic reactions. An increased eosinophil count may also be associated with lung cancer, chronic skin infections (e.g., psoriasis or scabies), polycythemia, and tumors.

Basophils.—The *basophils* comprise only about 0.5% to 1% of the total white blood count. The granules of the basophils stain blue with a basic dye. The precise function of the ba-

Table 1-19 Normal Differential White Blood Cell Count	
Granular Leukocytes	**Nongranular Leukocytes**
Neutrophils 60% to 70%	Lymphocytes 20% to 25%
Eosinophils 2% to 4%	Monocytes 3% to 8%
Basophils 0.5% to 1%	

sophils is not clearly understood. It is thought that the basophils are involved in allergic and stress responses. They are also considered to be phagocytic and to contain heparin, histamines, and serotonin.

Nongranular Leukocytes

There are two groups of nongranular leukocytes, the *monocytes* and *lymphocytes*. The term *mononuclear leukocytes* is also used to describe these cells, since they do not contain granules, but have spherical nuclei.

Monocytes.—The *monocytes* are the second order of cells to arrive at the inflammation site, usually appearing about five hours or more after the injury. After 48 hours, however, the monocytes are usually the predominant cell type in the inflamed area. The monocytes are the largest of the WBCs and comprise about 3% to 8% of the total leukocyte count. The monocytes are short-lived, phagocytic WBCs, with a half-life of approximately one day. They circulate in the bloodstream from which they move into tissues—at which point they may mature into long-living *macrophages* (also called *histiocytes*). The macrophages are large wandering cells that engulf larger and greater quantities of foreign material than the neutrophils. When the foreign material cannot be digested by the macrophages, the macrophages may proliferate to form a capsule that surrounds and encloses the foreign material (e.g., fungal spores). Although the monocytes and macrophages do not respond as quickly to an inflammatory process as the neutrophils, they are considered one of the first lines of inflammatory defense. Thus, an elevated number of monocytes suggests infection and inflammation. The monocytes play an important role in chronic inflammation and are also involved in the immune response.

Lymphocytes.—The *lymphocytes* are involved in the production of *antibodies*, which are special proteins that inactivate antigens. To appreciate the importance of the lymphocytes, and the clinical significance of their destruction or depletion (e.g., *acquired immunodeficiency syndrome [AIDS]*), a brief review of the role and function of the lymphocytes in the immune system is in order.

The lymphocytes can be divided into two categories: the B cells and T cells. T and B cells can be identified with an electron microscope according to certain distinguishing surface marks, called *rosettes:* T cells have a smooth surface; B cells have projections. B cells compose 10% to 30% of the total lymphocytes; T cells compose 70% to 90% of the total lymphocytes.

The B cells, which are formed in the bone marrow, further divide into either *plasma cells* or *memory cells.* The plasma cells secrete antibodies in response to foreign antigens. The memory cells retain the ability to recognize specific antigens long after the initial exposure and, thus, contribute to long-term immunity against future exposures to invading pathogens.

The T cells, which are formed in the thymus, are further divided into four functional categories: (1) cytotoxic T cells (also called killer lymphocytes or natural killer cells), which attack and kill foreign or infected cells, (2) helper T cells, which recognize foreign antigens and help to activate cytotoxic T cells and plasma cells (B cells), (3) inducer T cells, which stimulate the production of the different T cell subsets, and (4) suppressor T cells, which work to suppress the responses of the other cells and help to provide feedback information to the system.

The T cells may also be classified according to their surface antigens, i.e., the T cells may display either T4 antigen or T8 antigen. The T4 surface antigen subset, which comprises between 60% and 70% of the circulating T cells, consists mainly of the helper and inducer cells. The T8 surface antigen subset consists mainly of the cytotoxic and suppressor cells.

Sequence of Lymphocyte Responses to Infection

Initially, the macrophages attack and engulf the foreign antigens. This activity, in turn, stimulates the production of T cells and, ultimately, the antibody-producing B cells (plasma cells). The T4 cells play a pivotal role in the overall modulation of this immune response by (1) secreting a substance called lymphokine, which is a potent stimulus to T-cell growth and differentiation, (2) recognizing foreign antigens, (3) causing clonal proliferation of T cells, (4) mediating cytotoxic and suppressor functions, and (5) enabling B cells to secrete specific antibodies.

Because T cells (especially the T4 lymphocytes) have such a central role in this complex immune response, it should not be difficult to imagine the devastating effect that would ultimately follow from the systematic depletion of T lymphocytes. For example, virtually all the infectious complications of AIDS may be explained with reference to the effect that the *human immunodeficiency virus (HIV)* has on the T cells. A decreased number of T cells increases the patient's susceptibility to a wide range of opportunistic infections and neoplasms. In the healthy, noninfected HIV subject, the T4/T8 ratio is about 2.0. In the HIV-infected patient with AIDS, the T4/T8 ratio is usually 0.5 or less.

Platelet Count

Platelets (also called thrombocytes) are the smallest of the formed elements in the blood. They are round or oval, flattened and disk-shaped in appearance. Platelets are produced in the bone marrow and possibly in the lungs. Platelet activity is essential for blood clotting. The normal platelet count is 150,000 to 350,000/mm^3.

A deficiency of platelets leads to prolonged bleeding time or impaired clot retention. A low platelet count (thrombocytopenia) is associated with (1) massive blood transfusion, (2) pneumonia, (3) cancer chemotherapy, (4) infection, (5) allergic conditions, and (6) toxic effects of certain drugs (e.g., heparin, isoniazid, penicillins, prednisone, and streptomycin). A high platelet count (thrombocythemia) is associated with (1) cancer, (2) trauma, (3) asphyxiation, (4) rheumatoid arthritis, (5) iron deficiency, (6) acute infections, (7) heart disease, and (8) tuberculosis.

A platelet count of less than 20,000/mm^3 is associated with spontaneous bleeding, prolonged bleeding time, and poor clot retraction. The precise platelet count necessary for hemostasis is not firmly established. Generally, platelet counts of greater than 50,000/mm^3 are not associated with spontaneous bleeding. Thus, various diagnostic or therapeutic procedures such as bronchoscopy or the insertion of an arterial catheter are usually safe when the platelet count is greater than 50,000/mm^3.

Blood Chemistry

A basic knowledge of the blood chemistry, the normal values, and common health problems that alter these values is an important cornerstone of patient assessment. Table 1-20 lists the blood chemistry tests usually monitored in respiratory care.

Electrolytes

In order for the cells of the body to function properly, a normal concentration of electrolytes must be maintained. Thus, the monitoring of the electrolytes is extremely important in the patient whose body fluids are being endogenously or exogenously manipulated (e.g., intrave-

Table 1-20 Blood Chemistry Tests Commonly Monitored in Respiratory Care

Chemical	Normal Value	Common Abnormal Findings
Glucose	70 to 110 mg/dl	Hyperglycemia (excess glucose level) Diabetes mellitus Acute infection Myocardial infarction Thiazide and "loop" diuretics Hypoglycemia (low glucose level) Pancreatic tumors or liver disease Pituitary or adrenocortical hyperfunction
Lactic Dehydrogenase (LDH)	80 to 120 Wacker Units	Increases are associated with: Myocardial infarction Chronic hepatitis Pneumonia Pulmonary infarction
Serum Glutamic Oxaloacetic Transaminase (SGOT)	8 to 33 U/ml	Increases are associated with: Myocardial infarction Congestive heart failure Pulmonary infarction
Bilirubin	Adult: 0.1 to 1.2 mg/dl Newborn: 1 to 12 mg/dl	Increases are associated with: Massive hemolysis Hepatitis
Blood Urea Nitrogen (BUN)	8 to 18 mg/dl	Increases are associated with: Acute or chronic renal failure
Serum Creatinine	0.6 to 1.2 mg/dl	Increases are associated with: Renal failure

nous therapy, renal disease, or diarrhea). Table 1-21 lists electrolytes monitored in respiratory care.

ABNORMAL BRONCHOSCOPY FINDINGS

The *fiberoptic bronchoscope* is a well-established diagnostic and therapeutic tool used by a number of medical specialists, including those in the intensive care units, special procedure rooms, and outpatient settings. With minimal risk to the patient—and without interrupting the patient's ventilation—the flexible fiberoptic bronchoscope allows direct visualization of the upper airways (nose, oral cavity, and pharynx), larynx, vocal cords, subglottic area, trachea, bronchi, lobar bronchi, and segmental bronchi down to the third or fourth generation. Under fluoroscopic control, more peripheral areas can be examined or treated.

Table 1-21 Electrolytes Commonly Monitored in Respiratory Care

Electrolyte	Normal Value	Common Abnormal Findings	Clinical Manifestations
Sodium (Na$^+$)	136 to 142 mEq/L	Hypernatremia (excess Na$^+$) Dehydration	Desiccated mucous membranes Flushed skin Great thirst Dry tongue
		Hyponatremia (low Na$^+$) Sweating Burns Loss of gastrointestinal secretions Use of some diuretics Excessive water intake	Abdominal cramps Muscle twitching Poor perfusion Vasomotor collapse Confusion Seizures
Potassium (K$^+$)	3.8 to 5.0 mEq/L	Hyperkalemia (excess K$^+$) Renal failure Muscle tissue damage Hypokalemia (low K$^+$) Diuretic therapy Endocrine disorder Diarrhea Reduced intake or loss of K$^+$ Chronic stress	Irritability Nausea Diarrhea Weakness Ventricular fibrillation Metabolic alkalosis Muscular weakness Malaise Cardiac arrhythmias Hypotension
Chloride (Cl$^-$)	95 to 103 mEq/L	Hyperchloremia (excess Cl$^-$) Renal tubular acidosis Hypochloremia (low Cl$^-$) Alkalosis	Deep, rabid breathing Weakness Disorientation Metabolic alkalosis Muscle hypertonicity Tetany Depressed ventilation (respiratory compensation)
Calcium (Ca^{++})	4.5 to 5.4 mEq/L	Hypercalcemia (excess Ca^{++}) Malignant tumors Bone fractures Diuretic therapy Excessive use of antacids or milk consumption Vitamin-D intoxication Hyperparathyroidism	Lethargy, weakness Hyporeflexia Constipation, anorexia, renal stones Mental deterioration

Table 1-21 Electrolytes Commonly Monitored in Respiratory Care

Hypocalcemia (low Ca^{++})
Respiratory alkalosis
Pregnancy
Vitamin-D deficiency
Diuretic therapy
Hypoparathyroidism

Paresthesia, cramping of muscles, stridor, convulsions, mental disturbance, Chvostek's sign, Jrousseau's sign

Diagnostic bronchoscopy is indicated for a number of clinical conditions, including further inspection and assessment of (1) abnormal radiographic findings (e.g., question of bronchogenic carcinoma or the extent of a bronchial tumor or mass lesion), (2) persistent atelectasis, (3) excessive bronchial secretions, (4) acute smoke inhalation injuries, (5) intubation damage, (6) bronchiectasis, (7) foreign bodies, (8) hemoptysis, (9) lung abscess, (10) major thoracic trauma, (11) stridor or localized wheezing, and (12) unexplained cough. When abnormalities are found, additional diagnostic procedures include brushings, biopsies, needle aspirations, and washings. A videotape or colored polaroid photograph may also be used to record any abnormalities.

Therapeutic bronchoscopy includes (1) suctioning of excessive secretions/retained secretions/mucus plugs, (2) removal of foreign bodies, (3) selective lavage (with normal saline or mucolytic agents), (4) management of life-threatening hemoptysis, and (5) endotracheal intubation. While the merits of fiberoptic bronchoscopy are well documented, routine respiratory therapy modalities at the patient's bedside (e.g., chest physical therapy, postural drainage, deep breathing and coughing techniques, and positive expiratory pressure [PEP] therapy) are considered the first line of defense in the treatment of atelectasis from pooled secretions. Therapeutic bronchoscopy is commonly used in the management of bronchiectasis, lung abscess, smoke inhalation and thermal injuries, and lung cancer.

SELF-ASSESSMENT QUESTIONS

Multiple Choice
1. Which of the following respiratory diseases are classified as a restrictive lung disorder?
    I. Tuberculosis
    II. Fungal diseases
    III. Chronic interstitial lung disease
    IV. Pneumothorax
        a. I and III only
        b. II and IV only
        c. III and IV only
        d. II, III, and IV only
        e. I, II, III, and IV
2. During the patient interview, an open-ended question
    I. Elicits "cold facts."
    II. Is used for narrative information.
    III. Builds and enhances rapport.
    IV. Calls for short one- or two-word answers.
        a. I only
        b. IV only
        c. I and IV only
        d. II and III only
        e. II, III, and IV only
3. Which of the following pathologic conditions increases vocal fremitus?
    I. Atelectasis
    II. Pleural effusion
    III. Pneumothorax
    IV. Pneumonia
        a. III only
        b. IV only
        c. II and III only
        d. I and IV only
        e. I, III, and IV only
4. A dull or soft percussion note would likely be heard in which of the following pathologic conditions?
    I. Chronic obstructive pulmonary disease
    II. Pneumothorax
    III. Pleural thickening
    IV. Atelectasis
        a. I only
        b. II only
        c. III only
        d. II and III only
        e. III and IV only
5. Bronchial breath sounds are likely to be heard in which of the following pathologic conditions?
    I. Alveolar consolidation
    II. Chronic obstructive pulmonary disease
    III. Atelectasis
    IV. Fluid accumulation in the tracheobronchial tree
        a. III only
        b. IV only
        c. I and III only
        d. II and IV only
        e. I, III, and IV only

6. Wheezing is
    I. Produced by bronchospasm.
    II. Generally auscultated during inspiration.
    III. A cardinal finding of bronchial asthma.
    IV. Usually heard as high-pitched sounds.
       a. I only
       b. I and III only
       c. II and IV only
       d. I, III, and IV only
       e. I, II, III, and IV

7. In which of the following pathologic conditions is transmission of the whispered voice of a patient through a stethoscope unusually clear?
    I. Chronic obstructive pulmonary disease
    II. Alveolar consolidation
    III. Atelectasis
    IV. Pneumothorax
       a. I only
       b. II and III only
       c. I and IV only
       d. I, II, and III only
       e. II, III, and IV only

8. An individual's ventilatory pattern is composed of a/an
    I. Inspiratory and expiratory force.
    II. Ventilatory rate.
    III. Tidal volume
    IV. Inspiratory and expiratory ratio.
       a. I and III only
       b. II and III only
       c. II, III, and IV only
       d. I, II, and III only
       e. I, II, III, and IV

9. Which of the following abnormal breathing patterns is commonly associated with diabetic acidosis?
       a. Orthopnea
       b. Kussmaul's respiration
       c. Biot's respiration
       d. Hypoventilation
       e. Cheyne-Stokes respiration

10. What is the average compliance of the lungs and chest wall combined?
       a. 0.05 L/cm H_2O
       b. 0.1 L/cm H_2O
       c. 0.2 L/cm H_2O
       d. 0.3 L/cm H_2O
       e. 0.4 L/cm H_2O

11. When lung compliance decreases, the patient's
    I. Ventilatory rate usually decreases.
    II. Tidal volume usually decreases
    III. Ventilatory rate usually increases.
    IV. Tidal volume usually increases.
       a. I only
       b. II only
       c. III only
       d. II and III only
       e. I and IV only

12. What is the normal airway resistance in the tracheobronchial tree?
    a. 0.5 to 1.0 cm H_2O/L/sec
    b. 1.0 to 2.0 cm H_2O/L/sec
    c. 2.0 to 3.0 cm H_2O/L/sec
    d. 3.0 to 4.0 cm H_2O/L/sec
    e. 4.0 to 5.0 cm H_2O/L/sec

13. What is the normal ventilation/perfusion ratio ($\dot{V}/\dot{Q}$ ratio)?
    a. 0.2
    b. 0.4
    c. 0.6
    d. 0.8
    e. 1.0

14. When venous admixture occurs, which of the following occur(s)?
    I. P_{O_2} of the nonreoxygenated blood increases
    II. Ca_{O_2} of the reoxygenated blood decreases
    III. P_{O_2} of the reoxygenated blood increases
    IV. Ca_{O_2} of the nonreoxygenated blood decreases
    a. I only
    b. IV only
    c. II and III only
    d. III and IV only
    e. I and II only

15. The pathophysiology of some respiratory disorders cause a shuntlike effect, some cause a capillary shunt, and some cause a combination of both. Which of the following respiratory diseases causes a shuntlike effect?
    I. Pneumonia
    II. Asthma
    III. Pulmonary edema
    IV. Adult respiratory distress syndrome
    a. II only
    b. III only
    c. I and III only
    d. II, III, and IV only
    e. I, II, III, and IV

16. What percentage is the normal anatomic shunt?
    a. 2 to 5
    b. 6 to 8
    c. 9 to 10
    d. 11 to 15
    e. 15 to 20

17. When the systemic blood pressure increases, the aortic and carotid sinus baroreceptors initiate reflexes that cause
    I. Increased heart rate.
    II. Decreased ventilatory rate.
    III. Increased ventilatory rate.
    IV. Decreased heart rate.
    a. I only
    b. II only
    c. III only
    d. II and IV only
    e. I and III only

18. What is the PEFR in the normal healthy female between 20 and 30 years of age?
    a. 250 L/min
    b. 350 L/min
    c. 450 L/min
    d. 550 L/min
    e. 650 L/min

19. Which of the following can be obtained from a flow-volume loop study?
    I. MEFV
    II. PEFR
    III. FEV_T
    IV. $FEF_{25\%-75\%}$
        a. IV only
        b. I and II only
        c. II and III only
        d. I, III, and IV only
        e. I, II, III, and IV

20. Which of the following expiratory maneuver findings is/are characteristic of a restrictive lung disease?
    I. Normal FVC
    II. Decreased $FEF_{25\%-75\%}$
    III. Normal PEFR
    IV. Decreased FEV_T
        a. I and III only
        b. II and IV only
        c. III and IV only
        d. II and III only
        e. I, II, III, and IV

21. The effort-independent portion of a forced vital capacity consists of the
    a. First 20% to 30% of the forced vital capacity maneuver.
    b. Last 70% to 80% of the forced vital capacity maneuver.
    c. Middle portion of the forced vital capacity maneuver.
    d. First 50% of the forced vital capacity maneuver.
    e. Entire vital capacity maneuver.

22. Bernoulli's principle states that when gas flow through a tube encounters a restriction, the
    I. Velocity of the gas molecules decreases.
    II. Lateral gas pressure decreases.
    III. Velocity of the gas molecules increases.
    IV. Velocity of the gas molecules remains the same.
        a. II and V only
        b. II and IV only
        c. I and IV only
        d. II and III only
        e. IV and V only

23. When arranged for flow ($\dot{V}$), Poiseuille's law states that $\dot{V}$ is
    I. Indirectly related to r^4.
    II. Directly related to P.
    III. Indirectly related to π.
    IV. Directly related to 1.
        a. I only
        b. II only
        c. II and III only
        d. III and IV only
        e. II, III, and IV only

24. In an obstructive lung disorder, the
    I. FRC is decreased.
    II. RV is increased.
    III. VC is decreased.
    IV. IRV is increased.
        a. I and III only
        b. II and III only
        c. II and IV only
        d. II, III, and IV only
        e. I, II, and III

25. What is the anteroposterior-transverse chest diameter ratio in the normal adult?
    a. 1:05
    b. 1:1
    c. 1:2
    d. 1:3
    e. 1:4
26. Under normal conditions, the average DL_{CO} value for the resting male is
    a. 10 ml/min/mm Hg.
    b. 15 ml/min/mm Hg.
    c. 20 ml/min/mm Hg.
    d. 25 ml/min/mm Hg.
    e. 30 ml/min/mm Hg.
27. Which of the following muscles originate from the clavicle?
    I. Scalene muscles
    II. Sternocleidomastoid muscles
    III. Pectoralis major muscles
    IV. Trapezius muscles
    a. I only
    b. II only
    c. IV only
    d. I and IV only
    e. II and III only
28. Which of the following muscles inserts into the xyphoid process and into the fifth, sixth, and seventh ribs?
    a. Rectus abdominis muscle
    b. External oblique muscle
    c. Internal oblique muscle
    d. Transversus abdominis muscle
29. During acute alveolar hyperventilation, the
    I. HCO_3^- decreases.
    II. Pa_{CO_2} increases.
    III. H_2CO_3 decreases.
    IV. PA_{CO_2} increases.
    a. I only
    b. II only
    c. III only
    d. I and III only
    e. II and IV only
30. When lactic acidosis is present, the
    I. pH will likely be lower than expected for a particular Pa_{CO_2}.
    II. HCO_3^- will likely be higher than expected for a particular PA_{CO_2}.
    III. pH will likely be higher than expected for a particular Pa_{CO_2}.
    IV. HCO_3^- will likely be lower than expected for a particular Pa_{CO_2}.
    a. I only
    b. II only
    c. III only
    d. II and III only
    e. I and IV only
31. What is the clinical interpretation of the following arterial blood gas values (in addition to hypoxemia)?
    • pH: 7.17
    • Pa_{CO_2}: 77 mm Hg
    • HCO_3^-: 27 mM/L
    • Pa_{O_2}: 54 mm Hg
    a. Chronic ventilatory failure
    b. Acute alveolar hyperventilation superimposed on chronic ventilatory failure
    c. Acute ventilatory failure

    d. Acute alveolar hyperventilation

    e. Acute ventilatory failure superimposed on chronic ventilatory failure

32. A 74-year-old male with a long history of emphysema and chronic bronchitis enters the emergency room in respiratory distress. His respiratory rate is 34 breaths per minute and labored. His heart rate is 115 beats per minute, and his blood pressure is 170/120. His arterial blood gas values are as follows:

- pH: 7.57
- Pa_{CO_2}: 68 mm Hg
- HCO_3^-: 37 mM/L
- Pa_{O_2}: 49 mm Hg

What is the clinical interpretation of the above arterial blood gas values (in addition to hypoxemia)?

    a. Chronic ventilatory failure

    b. Acute alveolar hyperventilation superimposed on chronic ventilatory failure

    c. Acute ventilatory failure

    d. Acute alveolar hyperventilation

    e. Acute ventilatory failure superimposed on chronic ventilatory failure

33. Which of the following is classified as metabolic acidosis?

    a. pH 7.23; Pa_{CO_2} 63; HCO_3^- 26; Pa_{O_2} 52

    b. pH 7.16; Pa_{CO_2} 38; HCO_3^- 16; Pa_{O_2} 86

    c. pH 7.56; Pa_{CO_2} 27; HCO_3^- 21; Pa_{O_2} 101

    d. pH 7.64; Pa_{CO_2} 49; HCO_3^- 31; Pa_{O_2} 91

    e. pH 7.37; Pa_{CO_2} 66; HCO_3^- 29; Pa_{O_2} 73

34. Which of the following cause metabolic acidosis?

  I. Hypokalemia

  II. Renal failure

  III. Dehydration

  IV. Hypokalemia

    a. I only

    b. II only

    c. IV only

    d. I and IV only

    e. II and III only

35. According to the $Pa_{CO_2}/HCO_3^-/pH$ relationship, if the Pa_{CO_2} suddenly increased to 90 mm Hg in a patient who normally has a pH of 7.4, a Pa_{CO_2} of 40 mm Hg, and a HCO_3^- of 24 mM/L, the pH will decrease to approximately

    a. 7.15.

    b. 7.10.

    c. 7.05.

    d. 7.00.

    e. 6.95.

36. The lowest acceptable Pa_{O_2} for an 80-year-old patient is about

    a. 55 mm Hg.

    b. 60 mm Hg.

    c. 65 mm Hg.

    d. 70 mm Hg.

    e. 80 mm Hg.

37. The Pa_{O_2} may give a "false-positive" oxygenation reading when the patient has

  I. Hypothermia.

  II. Cyanide poisoning.

  III. A decreased cardiac output.

  IV. Carbon monoxide poisoning.

  V. Peripheral shunting.

    a. I and II only

    b. II and IV only

    c. III, IV, and V only

    d. I, II, III, IV, and V only

    e. I, II, III, IV, and V

38. If a patient is receiving an $F_{I_{O_2}}$ of 40% on a day when the barometric pressure is 745 mm Hg, and if the patient's Pa_{CO_2} is 65 mm Hg and the Pa_{O_2} is 45 mm Hg, the $P(A-a)_{O_2}$ is about
    a. 153 mm Hg.
    b. 198 mm Hg.
    c. 230 mm Hg
    d. 267 mm Hg.
    e. 343 mm Hg.

39. A 46-year-old female with severe asthma presents in the emergency room with the following clinical data:
    - Hb: 11 g%
    - Pa_{O_2}: 46 mm Hg
    - Sa_{O_2}: 70%

    Based on the above clinical data, the patient's Ca_{O_2} is about
    a. 6.75 vol% O_2.
    b. 10.50 vol% O_2.
    c. 12.30 vol% O_2.
    d. 15.25 vol% O_2.
    e. 18.85 vol% O_2.

40. If a patient has a cardiac output of 6 L/min and a Ca_{O_2} of 12 vol%, what is the D_{O_2}?
    a. 210 ml O_2/min
    b. 345 ml O_2/min
    c. 540 ml O_2/min
    d. 720 ml O_2/min
    e. 930 ml O_2/min

41. If a patient's Ca_{O_2} is 11 vol% and the $C\bar{v}_{O_2}$ is 7 vol%, the $C(a-\bar{v})_{O_2}$ is
    a. 4 vol%
    b. 7 vol%
    c. 11 vol%
    d. 15 vol%
    e. 18 vol%

42. Clinically, the patient's $C(a-\bar{v})_{O_2}$ increases in response to
    I. Hypothermia.
    II. A decreased cardiac output.
    III. Seizures.
    IV. Cyanide poisoning.
    a. II only
    b. IV only
    c. II and III only
    d. I and IV only
    e. II, III, and IV only

43. If a patient has a cardiac output of 6 L/min and a $C(a-\bar{v})_{O_2}$ of 4 vol%, the $\dot{V}_{O_2}$ is
    a. 120 ml O_2/min.
    b. 160 ml O_2/min.
    c. 180 ml O_2/min.
    d. 200 ml O_2/min.
    e. 240 ml O_2/min.

44. Clinically, the $\dot{V}_{O_2}$ decreases in response to
    I. Exercise.
    II. Hyperthermia.
    III. Body size.
    IV. Peripheral shunting.
    a. II only
    b. IV only
    c. I and III only
    d. II, III, and IV only
    e. I, II, III, and IV

45. If a patient has a Ca_{O_2} of 12 vol% and a $C\bar{v}_{O_2}$ of 7 vol%, the O_2ER is about
    a. 0.27.

b. 0.33.

c. 0.42.

d. 0.53.

e. 0.75.

46. Clinically, the O_2ER increases in response to

I. A decreased cardiac output.

II. Hyperthermia.

III. Anemia.

IV. Exercise.

a. I only

b. III only

c. II and IV only

d. II, III, and IV only

e. I, II, III, and IV

47. Clinically, the $S\bar{v}_{O_2}$ decreases in response to

I. An increased cardiac output.

II. Peripheral shunting.

III. Hypothermia.

IV. Seizures.

a. I only

b. IV only

c. II and III only

d. I, II, and III only

e. I, II, III, and IV

48. In the patient with severe emphysema, the oxygenation indices are commonly as follows:

I. Decreased $S\bar{v}_{O_2}$

II. Increased $\dot{V}_{O_2}$

III. Decreased $C(a-\bar{v})_{O_2}$

IV. Increased O_2ER

a. I only

b. III only

c. I and IV only

d. II and III only

e. I, II, and III only

49. In the patient with pulmonary edema, the oxygenation indices are commonly as follows:

I. Increased O_2ER

II. Decreased $S\bar{v}_{O_2}$

III. Increased $C(a-\bar{v})_{O_2}$

IV. Decreased $\dot{V}_{O_2}$

a. II only

b. IV only

c. I and III only

d. I, II, and III only

e. I, II, III, and IV

50. A 48-year-old woman is on a volume-cycled mechanical ventilator on a day when the barometric pressure is 745 mm Hg. She is receiving intermittent mandatory ventilation of 7 breaths per minute and an $F_{I_{O_2}}$ of 0.70. The following clinical values are obtained:

• Pa_{CO_2}: 46 mm Hg

• Pa_{O_2}: 60 mm Hg (90% saturated)

• $P\bar{v}_{O_2}$: 38 mm Hg (75% saturated)

• Hb: 11 g/dl

Based on the above clinical information, how much intrapulmonary shunting does the patient have?

a. PA_{O_2} = _____

b. Cc_{O_2} = _____

c. Ca_{O_2} = _____

d. $C\bar{v}_{O_2}$ = _____

e. $\dot{Q}_S/\dot{Q}_T$ = _____

51. In which of the following arrhythmias is there no cardiac output or blood pressure?
    a. Ventricular flutter
    b. Atrial fibrillation
    c. Ventricular flutter
    d. Premature ventricular contractions
    e. Ventricular fibrillation

52. The general hemodynamic status of the patient can be monitored noninvasively at the patient's bedside by assessing the
    I. Perfusion state.
    II. Heart rate.
    III. Pulse.
    IV. Blood pressure.
    a. I only
    b. IV only
    c. II and III only
    d. II, III, and IV only
    e. I, II, III, and IV

53. Cardiac output and blood pressure begin to decline when the heart rate increases beyond
    a. 100 to 125 beats per minute.
    b. 125 to 150 beats per minute.
    c. 150 to 175 beats per minute.
    d. 175 to 200 beats per minute.
    e. 200 to 250 beats per minute.

54. An increased central venous pressure (CVP) reading is commonly seen in the patient who
    I. Has a severe pneumothorax.
    II. Is receiving high positive pressure breaths.
    III. Has cor pulmonale.
    IV. Is in left heart failure.
    a. I only
    b. III only
    c. IV only
    d. II, III, and IV only
    e. I, II, III, and IV

55. The normal range of the mean pulmonary artery pressure is
    a. 0 to 5 mm Hg.
    b. 5 to 10 mm Hg.
    c. 10 to 20 mm Hg.
    d. 20 to 30 mm Hg.
    e. 30 to 40 mm Hg.

56. Clinically, a patient's left ventricular afterload increases in response to
    I. Excessive blood volume.
    II. Decreased blood viscosity.
    III. Pulmonary emboli.
    IV. Pulmonary capillary destruction.
    a. I only
    b. III only
    c. II and IV only
    d. III and IV only
    e. I and II only

57. In respiratory disease, cor pulmonale is partly caused by pulmonary vasoconstriction. The pulmonary vasoconstriction is chiefly caused by a/an
    a. Decreased PA_{O_2}.
    b. Increased Pa_{CO_2}.
    c. Decreased pH.
    d. Increased PA_{CO_2}.
    e. Decreased Pa_{O_2}.

58. Which of the following is associated with digital clubbing?
    I. Chronic infection
    II. Local hypoxia
    III. Circulating vasodilators
    IV. Arterial hypoxia
        a. II only
        b. IV only
        c. II and IV only
        d. II, III, and IV only
        e. I, II, III, and IV

59. Blood-streaked sputum is associated with
    I. Cystic fibrosis.
    II. Bronchiectasis.
    III. Lung cancer.
    IV. Pulmonary embolism.
        a. II only
        b. IV only
        c. II and III only
        d. I, III, and IV only
        e. I, II, III, and IV

60. Which of the following is (are) associated with pleuritic chest pain?
    I. Lung cancer
    II. Pneumonia
    III. Myocardial ischemia
    IV. Tuberculosis
        a. I only
        b. II only
        c. III only
        d. I and III only
        e. I, II, and IV only

61. In the healthy adult female, the hematocrit is about
        a. 31%.
        b. 38%.
        c. 42%.
        d. 45%.
        e. 50%.

62. The normal hemoglobin value for the adult male is
        a. 10 to 12 g%.
        b. 12 to 14 g%.
        c. 14 to 16 g%.
        d. 16 to 18 g%.
        e. 18 to 20 g%.

63. Which of the following represent the primary defense against bacterial organisms through phago-cytosis?
        a. Eosinophils
        b. Neutrophils
        c. Monocytes
        d. Basophils
        e. Lymphocytes

64. Various clinical procedures, such as bronchoscopy or the insertion of an arterial catheter, are generally safe when the platelet count is no lower than
        a. 150,000/mm^3.
        b. 100,000/mm^3.
        c. 75,000/mm^3.
        d. 50,000/mm^3.
        e. 20,000/mm^3.

65. Hypokalemia is associated with
    I. Cardiac arrhythmias.
    II. Metabolic alkalosis.
    III. Hypertension.
    IV. Diuretic therapy.
        a. I only
        b. II only
        c. IV only
        d. III and IV only
        e. I, III, and IV only

Answers appear in Appendix XXI.

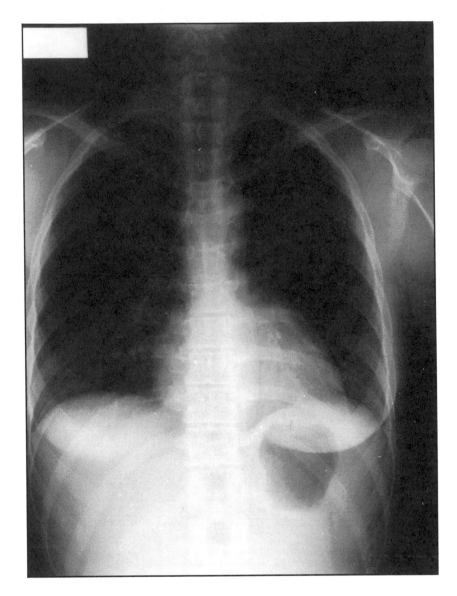

FIG 2-1
Standard posteroanterior (PA) chest radiograph with the patient's lungs in full inspiration.

CHAPTER 2

Radiologic
Examination
of the Chest

Radiography is the making of a photographic image of the internal structures of the body, created by passing x-rays through the body to an x-ray film, or radiograph. In patients with respiratory disease, radiography plays an important role in the diagnosis of lung disorders, in the assessment of the extent and location of the disease, and in the evaluation of the subsequent progress of the disease.

FUNDAMENTALS OF RADIOGRAPHY

X-rays are created when fast-moving electrons with sufficient energy collide with matter in any form. Clinically, x-rays are produced by an electronic device called an x-ray tube.

The x-ray tube is a vacuum-sealed glass tube that contains a cathode and a rotating anode. A tungsten plate about ½-inch square is fixed to the end of the rotating anode at the center of the tube. This tungsten block is called the *target*. Tungsten is an effective target metal because of its high melting point, which can withstand the extreme heat to which it is subjected, and its high atomic number, which makes it more effective in the production of x-rays.

When the cathode is heated, electrons "boil off." When a high voltage (70 to 150 kV) is applied to the x-ray tube, the electrons are driven to the rotating anode where they strike the tungsten target with tremendous energy. The sudden deceleration of the electrons at the tungsten plate converts energy to x-rays. Although most of the electron energy is converted to heat, a small amount (less than 1 percent) is transformed to x-rays and allowed to escape from the tube through a set of lead shutters called a *collimator.* From the collimator, the x-rays travel through the patient to the x-ray film.

The ability of the x-rays to penetrate matter depends on the density of the matter. For chest radiographs, the x-rays may pass through bone, air, soft tissue, or fat. Dense objects such as bone absorb more x-rays (prevent penetration) than objects that are not as dense, such as the air-filled lungs.

After passing through the patient, the x-rays strike the x-ray film. X-rays that pass through low-density objects strike the film at full force and produce a black image on the film. X-rays that are absorbed by high-density objects (such as bone) either do not reach the film at all or strike the film with less force. Relative to the density of the object, these objects appear as light gray to white on the film.

STANDARD POSITIONS AND TECHNIQUES OF CHEST RADIOGRAPHY

Clinically, the standard radiograph of the chest includes two views: a posteroanterior (PA) projection and a lateral projection (either a left or right lateral radiograph) with the patient in the standing position. When the patient is seriously ill or immobilized, an upright radiograph may not be possible. In such cases, a supine anteroposterior (AP) radiograph is obtained at the patient's bedside. A lateral radiograph is rarely obtainable under such circumstances.

Posteroanterior Radiograph

The standard posteroanterior (PA) chest radiograph is obtained by having the patient stand (or sit) in the upright position. The anterior aspect of the patient's chest is pressed against a film cassette holder, with the shoulders rotated forward to move the scapulae away from the lung fields. The distance between the x-ray tube and the film is six feet. The x-ray beam travels from the x-ray tube, through the patient and then to the x-ray film.

The x-ray is usually taken with the patient's lungs in full inspiration to show the lung fields and related structures to their greatest possible extent. At full inspiration, the diaphragm is lowered to about the level of the ninth to eleventh ribs posteriorly (Fig 2-1). For certain clinical conditions, radiographs are sometimes taken at the end of both inspiration and expiration. For example, in patients with obstructive lung disease, an expiratory radiograph may be made to evaluate diaphragmatic excursion and the symmetry, or asymmetry, of such excursion (Fig 2-2).

Anteroposterior Radiograph

The supine anteroposterior (AP) radiograph may be taken in patients who are debilitated, immobilized, or too young to tolerate the PA procedure. The AP radiograph is usually taken with a portable x-ray machine at the patient's bedside. The film is placed behind the patient's back, with the x-ray machine positioned in front of the patient about 48 inches from the film.

Compared to the PA radiograph, the AP radiograph has a number of disadvantages. For example, the heart and superior portion of the mediastinum are significantly magnified in the AP radiograph. This is because the heart is positioned in front of the thorax as the x-ray beams pass through the chest from the anterior to posterior direction, causing the image of the heart to be enlarged (Fig 2-3).

Other disadvantages are that the AP radiograph often has less resolution and more distortion. Since the patient is often unable to sustain a maximal inspiration, the lower lung lobes frequently appear hazy, erroneously suggesting pulmonary congestion or pleural effusion. Finally, because the AP radiograph is often taken in the intensive care unit, extraneous shadows, such as ventilator tubing and indwelling lines, are often present (Fig 2-4).

Lateral Radiograph

The lateral radiograph is obtained to complement the PA radiograph. It is taken with the side of the patient's chest compressed against the cassette. The patient's arms are raised with the forearms resting on the head.

To view the right lung and heart, the patient's right side is placed against the cassette. To view the left lung and heart, the patient's left side is placed against the cassette. Thus, a right lateral radiograph would be selected to view a density or lesion that is known to be in the right lung. If neither lung is of particular interest, a left lateral radiograph is usually selected to reduce the magnification of the heart. The lateral radiograph provides a view of the structures behind the heart and diaphragmatic dome. It can also be combined with the PA radiograph to give a three-dimensional view of the structures or of any abnormal densities (Fig 2-5).

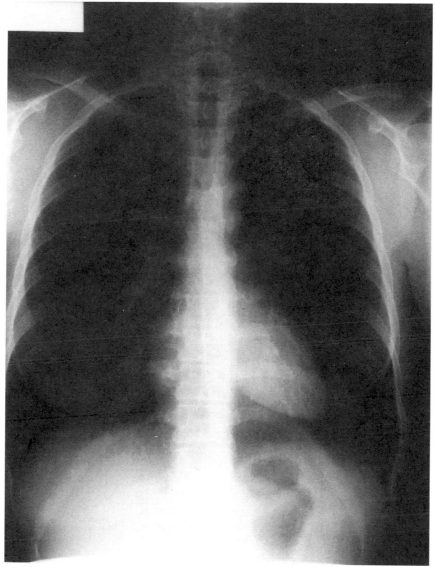

FIG 2-2

A posteroanterior (PA) chest radiograph of the same patient shown in Figure 2-1 during expiration.

Lateral Decubitus Radiograph

The lateral decubitus radiograph is obtained by having the patient lie on the left side or the right side rather than standing or sitting in the upright position. The naming of the decubitus radiograph is determined by the side on which the patient lies; thus, a "right lateral" decubitus radiograph means that the patient's right side is down.

The lateral decubitus radiograph is useful in the diagnosis of a suspected or known fluid accumulation in the pleural space (pleural effusion) that is not easily seen in the PA radiograph. A pleural effusion, which is usually more thinly spread out over the diaphragm in the upright position, collects in the gravity-dependent areas while the patient is in the lateral decubitus position, allowing the fluid to be more readily seen (Fig 2-6).

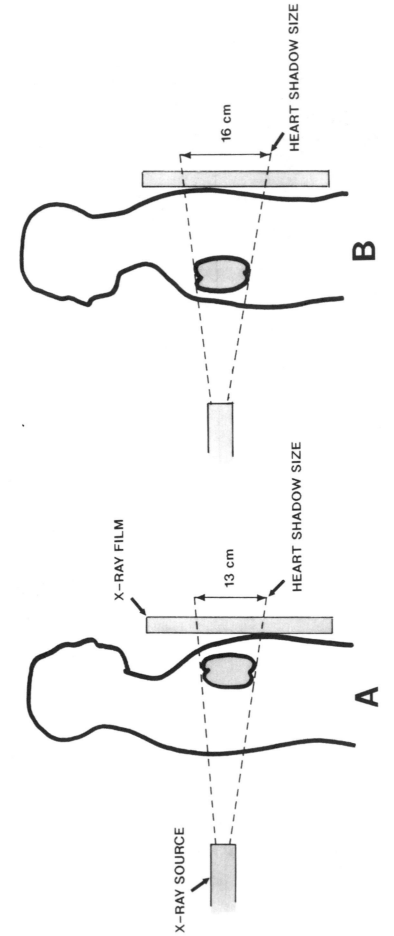

Chest against film

Back against film

X–RAY FILM

13 cm

16 cm

HEART SHADOW SIZE

HEART SHADOW SIZE

X–RAY SOURCE

A

B

Posteroanterior

Anteroposterior

FIG 2-3

Compared to the posteroanterior (PA) chest radiograph, the heart is significantly magnified in the anteroposterior (AP) chest radiograph. In the PA radiograph, the ratio of the width of the heart to the width of the thorax is normally less than 1:2. The reason the heart appears larger in the AP radiograph is because the heart is positioned in front of the thorax as the x-ray beams pass through the chest from the anterior to posterior direction. This allows more space for the heart shadow to "fan out" before it reaches the x-ray film.

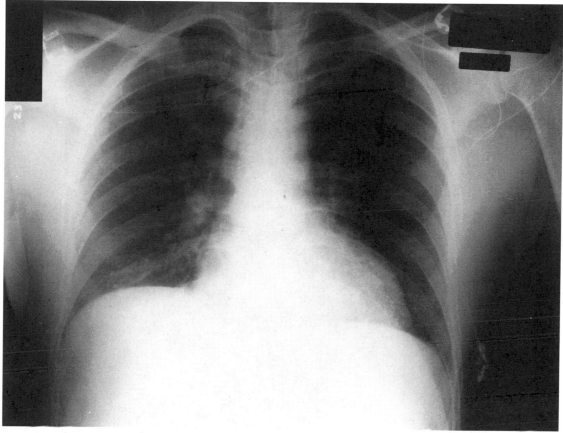

FIG 2-4

Anteroposterior (AP) chest radiograph. Note that the diaphragms are elevated, the lower lung lobes appear hazy, the ratio of the width of the heart to the thorax is less than 2 : 1, and the extraneous lines on the patient's left side.

INSPECTING THE CHEST RADIOGRAPH

Before the respiratory care practitioner can effectively identify abnormalities on a chest radiograph, it is important to recognize the normal anatomic structures. Figure 2-7 represents a normal PA chest radiograph with identification of important anatomic landmarks. Figure 2-8 labels the anatomic structures seen on a lateral chest radiograph. Table 2-1 lists some of the more important radiologic terms used to describe abnormal lung findings.

Technical Quality of the Radiograph

The *first* step in examining a chest radiograph is to evaluate the *technical quality* of the radiograph itself. Was the patient in the correct position when the radiograph was taken? To verify the proper position, check the relationship of the medial ends of the clavicles to the vertebral column. For the PA radiograph, the vertebral column should be precisely in the center between the medial ends of the clavicles, and the distance between the right and left costophrenic angles and the spine should be equal. Even a small degree of patient rotation relative to the film can create a false image, erroneously suggesting tracheal deviation, cardiac displacement, or cardiac enlargement.

Second, the exposure quality of the radiograph should be evaluated. Normal exposure is verified by determining if the spinal processes of the vertebrae are visible to the fifth or sixth

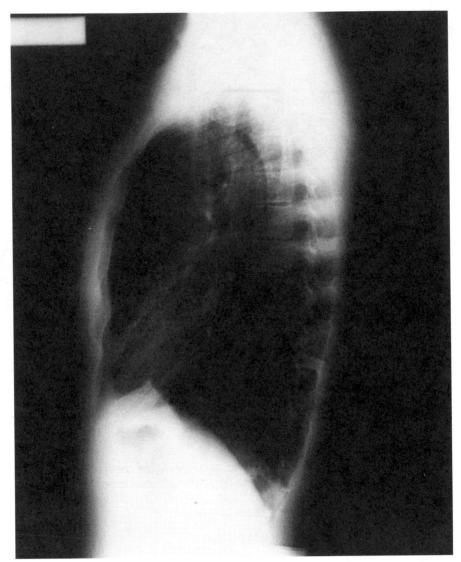

FIG 2-5
Lateral radiograph.

thoracic level (T5-T6). X-ray equipment now available allows the vertebrae to be seen down to the level of the cardiac shadow. The degree of exposure can be further evaluated by comparing the relative densities of the heart and lungs. For example, since the heart has a greater density than the airfilled lungs, the heart appears "whiter" than the lung fields. The heart and lungs become more radiolucent (darker) with greater exposure of the radiograph. A radiograph that has been overexposed is said to be "heavily penetrated" or "burned-out." Conversely, the heart and lungs on an underexposed radiograph may appear denser and whiter. The lungs may erroneously appear to have infiltrates and there may be little or no visibility of the thoracic vertebrae.

Third, the level of inspiration at the moment the radiograph was taken should be evaluated. At full inspiration the diaphragmatic domes should be at the level of the ninth to eleventh ribs posteriorly. On radiographs taken during expiration, the lungs appear denser, the diaphragm is elevated, and the heart appears wider and enlarged.

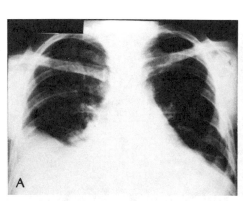

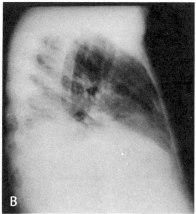

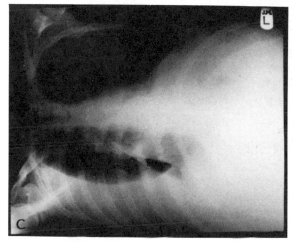

FIG 2-6
Lateral decubitus radiograph showing large amounts of free pleural
fluid. (From Light RL: *Pleural Diseases,* Philadelphia, 1983, Lea &
Febiger. Used by permission.)

Sequence of Examination

While the precise sequence in examining a chest radiograph is not important, the inspection
should be done in a systematic fashion. Some practitioners prefer an "inside-out" approach to
inspecting the chest radiograph, which entails beginning with the mediastinum and proceed-
ing outward to the extrathoracic soft tissue. Some practitioners prefer the reverse. The following is an "inside-out" method.

Mediastinum

The mediastinum should be inspected for width, contour, and shifts from the midline. Inspect
the anatomy of the mediastinum, including the trachea, carina, cardiac borders, aortic arch,
and superior vena cava (see Fig 2-7).

Trachea.—On the PA projection, the trachea should appear as a translucent band overlying
the vertebral column. The diameter of the bronchi progressively tapers a short distance beyond the carina, and then disappear (see Fig 2-7). There are a number of clinical conditions
that can cause the trachea to shift from its normal position. For example, fluid or gas accumulation in the pleural space causes the trachea to shift *away* from the affected area. Lung
collapse or fibrosis usually causes the trachea to shift *toward* the affected area. The trachea
may also be displaced by tumors of the upper lung regions.

It is helpful to realize that anatomic structures in the chest (e.g., the trachea) move out of

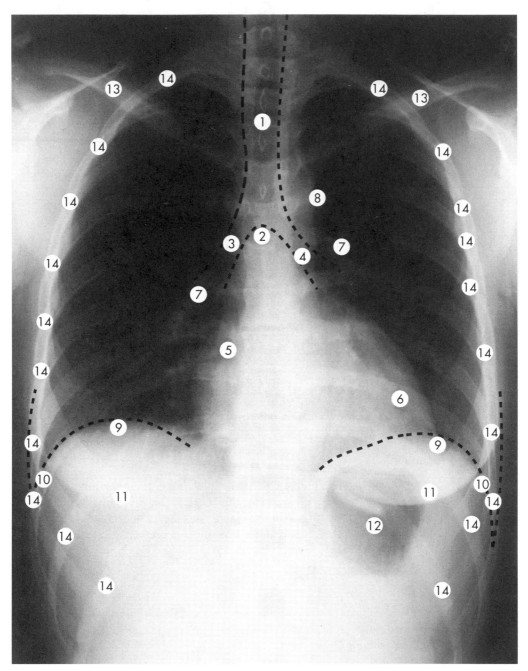

FIG 2-7

Normal PA chest radiograph. (1) Trachea (note vertebral column in middle of trachea. (2) Carina. (3) Right mainstem bronchus. (4) Left mainstem bronchus. (5) Right atrium. (6) Left ventricle. (7) Hilar vasculature. (8) Aortic knob. (9) Diaphragm. (10) Costopheric angles. (11)
Breast shadows. (12) Gastric air bubble. (13) Clavicle. (14) Rib.

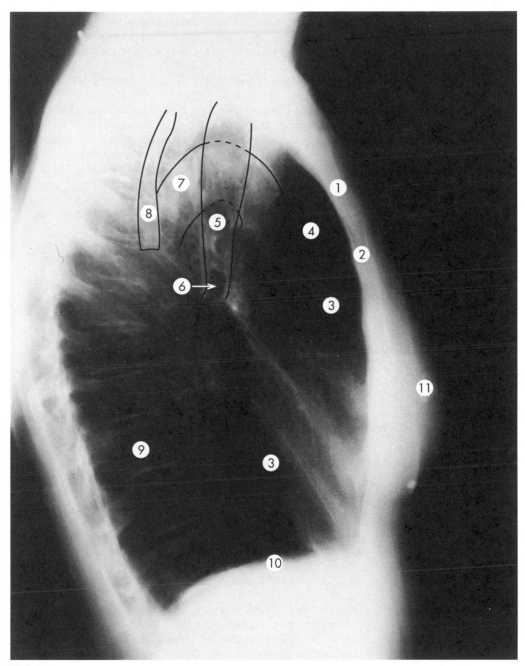

FIG 2-8
Normal lateral chest radiograph. (1) Manubrium. (2) Sternum. (3) Cardiac shadow. (4) Retro-sternal air space in the lung. (5) Trachea. (6) Bronchus, on end. (7) Aortic arch (ascending and descending). (8) Scapulae. (9) Vertebral column. (10) Diaphragm. (11) Breast shadow.

Table 2-1 Common Radiologic Terms

Air Cyst	A thin-walled radiolucent area surrounded by normal lung tissue.
Bleb	Refers to a superficial air cyst protruding into the pleura. Also called bulla.
Bulla	A large thin-walled radiolucent area surrounded by normal lung tissue.
Bronchogram	An outline of air-containing bronchi beyond the normal point of visibility. An air bronchogram develops as a result of an infiltration or consolidation that surrounds the bronchi, producing a contrasting air column on the radiograph. That is, the bronchi appear as dark tubes surrounded by a white area produced by the infiltration or consolidation.
Cavity	A radiolucent (dark) area surrounded by dense tissue (white). A cavity is the hallmark of a lung abscess. A fluid level may be seen inside a cavity.
Consolidation	The act of becoming solid. Commonly used to describe the solidification of the lung due to a pathologic engorgement of the alveoli as occurs in acute pneumonia.
Homogeneous density	Refers to a uniformly dense lesion (white area). Commonly used to describe solid tumors, fluid-containing cavities, or fluid in the pleural space.
Honeycombing	A coarse reticular (netlike) density. Commonly seen in pneumoconiosis.
Infiltration	A general term used to describe any poorly defined radiodensity (white area). Commonly used to describe an inflammatory lesion.
Interstitial density	Used to describe a density caused by interstitial thickening.
Lesion	Any pathologic or traumatic alteration of tissue or loss of function of a part.
Opacity	State of being opaque (white). An opaque area or spot. Impervious to light rays, or by extension, x-rays. Opposite of translucent or radiolucent.
Pleural density	A radiodensity caused by fluid, tumor, inflammation, or scarring.
Pulmonary mass	Refers to a lesion that is 6 cm or more in diameter. Commonly used to describe a pulmonary tumor.
Pulmonary nodule	Refers to a lesion that is less than 6 cm in diameter and composed of dense tissue. Also called a solitary pulmonary nodule or "coin" lesion, because of its rounded coinlike appearance.
Radiodensity	Refers to dense areas that appear white on the radiograph. The opposite of radiolucency.
Radiolucency	The state of being radiolucent. The property of being partly or wholly permeable to x-rays. Commonly used to describe darker areas on a radiograph, such as emphysematous lung or a pneumothorax.
Translucent	Refers to permitting the passage of light. Commonly used to describe darker areas of the radiograph.

their normal position because they are either *pushed* or *pulled* in a given direction. In other words, they may be moved up or down or from side to side by lesions pulling or pushing in that direction. Table 2-2 lists examples of factors that push or pull the trachea out of its normal position in the chest radiograph.

Heart.—On the PA projection, the ratio of the width of the heart to the thorax (the cardiothoracic ratio) is normally less than 1:2. A small portion of the heart should be seen on the right side of the vertebral column. Two bulges should be seen on the right border of the heart. The upper bulge is the superior vena cava; the lower bulge is the right atrium. Three bulges are normally seen on the left side of the heart. The superior bulge is the aorta, the middle bulge is the main pulmonary artery, and the inferior bulge is the left ventricle (see Fig 2-7). See Table 2-2 for examples of factors that push or pull the heart out of its normal position in the chest radiograph.

Hilar Region

The right and left hilar regions should be evaluated for change in size or position. Normally, the left hilum is about 2 cm higher that the right (see Fig 2-7). An increased density of the hilar region may indicate engorgement of hilar vessels caused by increased pulmonary vascular resistance. Vertical displacement of the hilum suggests volume loss from one or more upper lobes of the lung on the affected side. In infectious lung disorders, such as histoplasmosis or tuberculosis, the lymph nodes around the hilar region are often enlarged and/or calcified. Malignant pulmonary lesions, including hilar malignant lymphadenopathy, may also be seen. See Table 2-2 for additional factors that push or pull the hilar region out of its normal position in the chest radiograph.

Table 2-2 Examples of Factors that Pull or Push Anatomic Structures out of their Normal Position in the Chest Radiograph		
Structure	**Examples of Abnormal Position**	**Lesion**
Mediastinum • Trachea • Carina • Heart • Major vessels	Leftward shift	Pulled left by upper lobe tuberculosis, atelectasis, or fibrosis Pushed left by right upper lobe emphysematous bulla, fluid, gas, or tumor
Left Diaphragm	Upward shift	Pulled up by left lower lobe atelectasis or fibrosis Pushed up by distended gastric air bubble
Horizontal Fissure • Right lung • Right hilum	Downward shift	Pulled down by right middle lobe or right lower lobe atelectasis Pushed down by right upper lobe neoplasm
Left Lung	Rightward shift	Pulled right by right lung collapse, atelectasis, or fibrosis Pushed right by left-sided tension pneumothorax or hemothorax

Lung Parenchyma (Tissue)

The lungs should be examined systematically from top to bottom, comparing one lung with the other. Normally, tissue markings can be seen throughout the lungs (see Fig 2-7). The absence of tissue markings may suggest a pneumothorax, recent pneumonectomy, or chronic obstructive lung disease (e.g., emphysema) or may be the result of an overexposed radiograph. An excessive amount of tissue markings may indicate fibrosis, interstitial or alveolar edema, lung compression, or an underexposed radiograph. The periphery of the lung fields should be inspected for abnormalities that obscure the lung's interface with the pleural space, mediastinum, or diaphragm. See Table 2-2 for additional examples of factors that push or pull the lung tissue out of its normal position in the chest radiograph.

Pleura

The peripheral borders of the lungs should be examined for pleural thickening, presence of fluid (pleural effusion) or air (pneumothorax) in the pleural space, or for mass lesions (see Fig 2-7). The costophrenic angles should be inspected. Blunting of the costophrenic angle suggests the presence of fluid. A lateral decubitus radiograph may be required to confirm the presence of fluid (see Fig 2-6).

Diaphragm

Both the right and left hemidiaphragm should have a upwardly convex, dome-shaped contour. The right and left costophrenic angles should be clear. Normally, the right diaphragm is about 2 cm higher than the left, because of the liver below it (see Fig 2-7). Chronic obstructive pulmonary diseases (e.g., emphysema) and diseases that cause gas or fluid to accumulate in the pleural space flatten and depress the normal curvature of the diaphragm. Abnormal elevation of one diaphragm may be due to excessive gas in the stomach, collapse of the middle or lower lobe on the affected side, pulmonary infection at the lung bases, phrenic nerve damage, or spinal curvature. See Table 2-2 for additional examples of factors that push or pull the diaphragm out of its normal position in the chest radiograph.

Gastric Air Bubble

The area below the diaphragm should be inspected. A stomach bubble is commonly seen under the left hemidiaphragm (see Fig 2-7). Free air may appear under either diaphragm following abdominal surgery or in patients with peritoneal abscess.

Bony Thorax

The ribs, vertebrae, clavicles, sternum, and scapulae should be inspected. The intercostal space should be symmetrical and equal over each lung field (see Fig 2-7). Intercostal spaces too close together suggest a loss of muscle tone, commonly seen in patients with paralysis involving one side of the chest. In chronic obstructive pulmonary disease, the intercostal spaces are generally far apart, due to alveolar hyperinflation. Finally, the ribs should be inspected for deformities or fractures. If a rib fracture is suspected but not seen on the standard chest radiograph, a special *rib series* (radiographs that focus on the ribs) may be necessary.

Extrathoracic Soft Tissues

The soft tissue external to the bony thorax should be closely inspected. If the radiograph is that of a female, the outer boundaries of the breast shadows should be identified (see Fig

2-7). If the patient has undergone a mastectomy, there will be a relative hyperlucency on the side of the mastectomy. Large breasts can create a significant amount of haziness over the lower lung fields, giving the false appearance of pneumonia or pulmonary congestion. While nipple shadows are easily identified when they are bilaterally symmetrical, one may become less visible when the patient is slightly rotated. The other nipple then appears abnormally opaque and may be mistaken for a pulmonary nodule. After a tracheostomy or pneumothorax, subcutaneous air bubbles (called subcutaneous emphysema) often form in the soft tissue, especially if the patient is on a positive pressure ventilator.

OTHER RADIOLOGIC TECHNIQUES
Fluoroscopy

Fluoroscopy is a technique by which x-ray motion pictures of the chest are taken. Fluoroscopy subjects the patient to a larger dose of x-rays than does standard radiography. Thus, it is only used in selected cases, as in the assessment of abnormal diaphragmatic movement (e.g., unilateral paralysis) or for localization of lesions to be biopsied during fiberoptic bronchoscopy.

Bronchography

Bronchography entails the instillation of a radiopaque material into the lumen of the tracheobronchial tree. A chest radiograph is then taken, providing a film called a bronchogram. The contrast material provides a clear outline of the trachea, carina, right and left main stem bronchi, and segmental bronchi. Bronchography is occasionally used to diagnose bronchogenic carcinoma and to determine the presence or extent of bronchiectasis (Fig 2-9). Computerized tomography of the chest has largely replaced this technique.

Computerized Tomography

Computerized tomography (CT) scanning provides a series of cross-sectional (transverse) pictures (called tomograms) of the structures within the body at multiple levels. Each pulmonary tomogram provides an image of what a "slice" through the chest would look like at a specific point. Similar to the radiograph, dense structures such as bone appear white on the tomogram, while structures with a relatively low density such as the lungs appear dark or black. Thus, a dense tumor in the lungs would appear as a white object surrounded by dark lungs (Fig 2-10).

For poorly defined lesions noticed on the standard radiograph, the CT scan is a useful supplement in determining the precise location, size, and shape of the lesion. The CT scan is especially helpful in confirming the presence of a mediastinal mass, small pulmonary nodules, small lesions of the bronchi, pulmonary cavities, a small pneumothorax, pleural disease, and small tumors (as small as 0.3 to 0.5 cm).

Magnetic Resonance Imaging

Magnetic resonance imaging (MRI) uses magnetic resonance as its source of energy to take cross-sectional (transverse, sagittal, or coronal) images of the body. It uses no ionizing radiation. The patient is placed in the cylindrical-shaped imager, and the body part in question is exposed to a magnetic field and radiowave transmission. The MRI produces a high-contrast image that can detect subtle lesions (Fig 2-11).

The MRI is superior to CT scanning for identifying complex congenital heart disorders, bone marrow diseases, adenopathy, and lesions of the chest wall. The MRI is an excellent

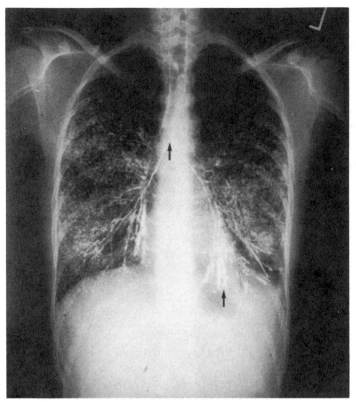

FIG 2-9
Bronchogram obtained using contrast medium in a patient with a history of bronchiectasis. *Arrows* indicate the carina and the bronchi leading to the posterior basilar segment of the left lower lobe. (From Rau JL Jr, Pearce DJ: *Understanding Chest Radiographs,* Denver, 1984, Multi-Media Publishing Inc. Used by permission.)

supplement to CT scanning to study the mediastinum and hilar region. For most abnormalities of the chest, however, CT scanning is generally better than MRI for motion (patient motion causes loss of resolution), spatial resolution, and cost reasons.

Because the MR imager generates an intense magnetic field, objects made of *ferromagnetic* material are strongly attracted to it. Thus, patients with ferromagnetic cerebral aneurysm clips or ferromagnetic prosthetic cardiac valves should not undergo MRI, since the magnetic force of the MR image can cause these devices to shift and harm the patient. The magnetic force of the MR imager can also interfere with the normal function of cardiac pacemakers.

Pulmonary Angiography

Pulmonary angiography is useful in identifying pulmonary emboli or arteriovenous malformations and involves the injection of a radiopaque contrast medium through a catheter that has been passed through the right side of the heart and into the pulmonary artery. The injection of the contrast material into the pulmonary circulation is followed by rapid serial pulmonary angiograms. The pulmonary vessels are filled with radiopaque contrast material and, therefore, will appear white. Figure 2-12 shows an abnormal angiogram in which the major blood vessels appear dark distal to pulmonary emboli.

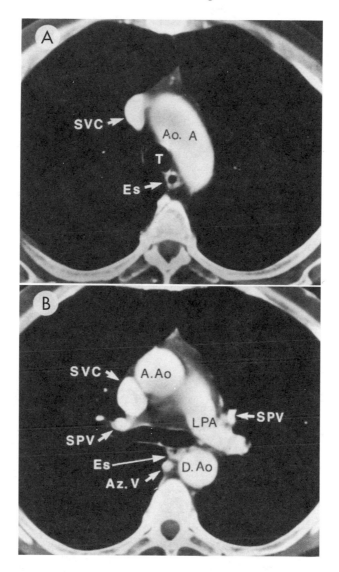

FIG 2-10

Anatomy of mediastinum on contrast-enhanced CT scan. (A) Ao A = aortic arch, SVC = superior vena cava, T = trachea, Es = esophagus. (B) A Ao = ascending aorta, SVC = superior vena cava, LPA = left pulmonary artery, SPV = superior pulmonary vein, Es = esophagus, D Ao = descending aorta, Az V = azygos vein. (From Armstrong P, Wilson AG, Dee P: *Imaging of Diseases of the Chest,* St. Louis, 1990, Mosby-Year Book. Used by permission.)

Ventilation/Perfusion Scan

A ventilation/perfusion scan is useful in determining the presence of pulmonary embolism. The *perfusion scan* is obtained by injecting small particles of albumin, called macroaggregates, tagged with a radioactive material such as iodine 131 or technetium 99m. Following injection, the radioactive particles are carried in the blood to the right side of the heart, from which they are distributed throughout the lungs by the blood flow in the pulmonary arteries. The radioactive particles that travel through unobstructed arteries become trapped in the pul-

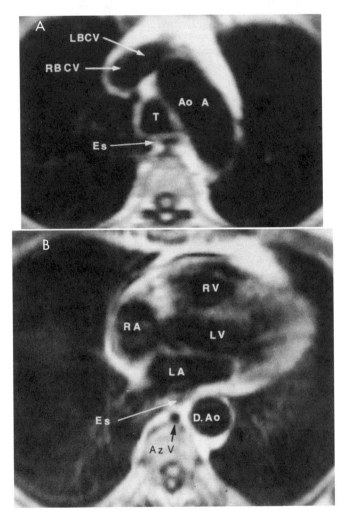

FIG 2-11

Anatomy of mediastinum on MRI. (A) LBCV = left brachiocephalic vein, RBCV = right bra-chiocephalic vein, Ao A = aortic arch, T = trachea, Es = esophagus. (B) RV = right ven-tricle, LV = left ventricle, RA = right atrium, LA = left atrium, D Ao = descending aorta, Es = esophagus, Az V = azygos vein. (From Armstrong P, Wilson AG, Dee P: *Imaging of Dis-eases of the Chest*, St. Louis, 1990, Mosby-Year Book. Used by permission.)

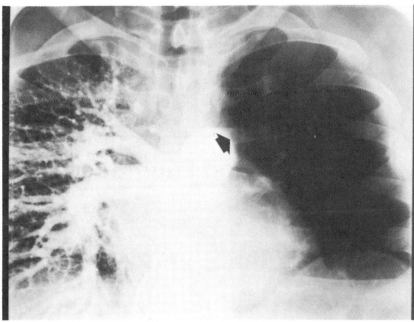

FIG 2-12

Abnormal pulmonary angiogram. Radiopaque material injected into the blood is prevented from flowing past the pulmonary embolism *(arrow)*. This causes the angiogram to appear dark distal to the obstruction.

monary capillaries, since they are between 20 to 50 μm in diameter and the diameter of the average pulmonary capillary is about 8 to 10 μm.

The lungs are then scanned with a gamma camera that produces a picture of the radioactive distribution throughout the pulmonary circulation. The *dark areas* show good blood flow, and the *white* or *light areas* represent decreased or complete absence of blood flow. The macroaggregates eventually break down, pass through the pulmonary circulation, and are excreted by the liver. The injection of these radioactive particles has no significant effect on the patient's hemodynamics, since the patent pulmonary capillaries far outnumber those "embolized" by the radioactive particles. In addition to pulmonary emboli, a perfusion scan defect (white or light areas) may be caused by a lung abscess, lung compression, loss of the pulmonary vascular system (e.g., emphysema), atelectasis, or alveolar consolidation.

The perfusion scan is supplemented with the *ventilation scan*. During the ventilation scan the patient breathes a radioactive gas, such as xenon 133, from a closed-circuit spirometer. A gamma camera is used to create a picture of the gas distribution throughout the lungs. A normal ventilation scan shows a uniform distribution of the gas, with the *dark* areas reflecting the presence of the radioactive gas and, therefore, good ventilation. *White or light areas* represent decreased or complete absence of ventilation. Figure 2-13 shows an abnormal perfusion scan and a normal ventilation scan of a patient with a severe pulmonary embolism. An abnormal ventilation scan may also be caused by airway obstruction (e.g., mucus plug), bronchospasm, loss of alveolar elasticity (e.g., emphysema), alveolar consolidation, or pulmonary edema.

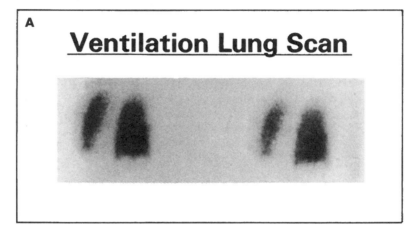

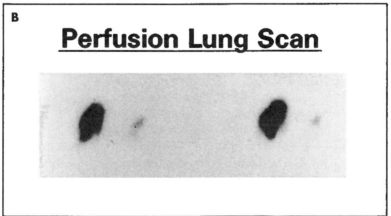

FIG 2-13

A normal ventilation lung scan and an abnormal perfusion lung scan are commonly seen in patients with severe pulmonary embolism. **A,** A normal ventilation scan shows a uniform distribution of gas, with the dark areas reflecting the presence of the radioactive gas and, therefore, good ventilation (right lung is on viewer's left). **B,** An abnormal perfusion scan. The dark area shown in the right lung represents good blood flow. The white or light areas shown in the left lung represent a decreased or complete absence of blood flow (right lung is on viewer's left).

SELF-ASSESSMENT QUESTIONS

Multiple Choice

1. Clinically, the standard radiograph of the chest includes the following:
   - I. Anteroposterior (AP) radiograph
   - II. Lateral decubitus radiograph
   - III. Lateral radiograph
   - IV. Posteroanterior (PA) radiograph
     - a. I only
     - b. IV only
     - c. III and IV only
     - d. I and II only
     - e. I, III, and IV only

2. Compared to the PA radiograph, the AP radiograph
   - I. Magnifies the heart.
   - II. Is usually more distorted.
   - III. Frequently appears more hazy.
   - IV. Often has extraneous shadows.
     - a. I only
     - b. II only
     - c. III and IV only
     - d. I, III, and IV only
     - e. I, II, III, and IV

3. To view the right lung and heart in the lateral radiograph, the
   - a. Left side of the patient's chest is placed against the cassette.
   - b. Anterior portion of the patient's chest is pressed against the cassette.
   - c. Right side of the patient's chest is placed against the cassette.
   - d. Posterior portion of the patient's chest is placed against the cassette.

4. A "right lateral" decubitus radiograph means that the
   - a. Right side of the chest is down.
   - b. Posterior side of the chest is up.
   - c. Left side of the chest is down.
   - d. Anterior side of the chest is up.

5. A leftward shift of the mediastinum is commonly seen on the chest radiograph in response to
   - I. Left upper lobe atelectasis.
   - II. Right upper lobe gas.
   - III. Left upper lobe fibrosis.
   - IV. Right upper lobe tumor.
     - a. I and III only
     - b. III and IV only
     - c. II, III, and IV only
     - d. I, II, III, and IV

6. The normal exposure of the radiograph is verified by determining if the spinal processes of the vertebrae are visible to the
   - a. C1 to C3 level.
   - b. C3 to C5 level.
   - c. T2 to T4 level.
   - d. T5 to T6 level.
   - e. T10 to T12 level.

7. A radiograph that is described as being "heavily penetrated" is
   - I. Darker in appearance.
   - II. More translucent.
   - III. Whiter in appearance.
   - IV. More opaque in appearance.
     - a. I only
     - b. III only

    c. IV only

    d. III and IV only

    e. I and II only

8. When the radiograph is taken at full inspiration, the diaphragmatic domes should be at the level of the

    a. First to fourth ribs posteriorly.

    b. Fourth to sixth ribs posteriorly.

    c. Sixth to ninth ribs posteriorly.

    d. Ninth to eleventh ribs posteriorly.

    e. Eleventh to twelfth ribs posteriorly.

9. Which of the following involves x-ray motion pictures of the chest?

    a. Bronchography

    b. Fluoroscopy

    c. Magnetic resonance imaging

    d. Computerized tomography

    e. Pulmonary angiography

10. The MRI is superior to CT scanning for identifying

    I. Lesions of the chest.

    II. Bone marrow diseases.

    III. Congenital heart disorders.

    IV. Adenopathy.

    a. I and II only

    b. III and IV only

    c. II and III only

    d. II, III, and IV only

    e. I, II, III and IV

Answers appear in Appendix XXI.

RECORDING SKILLS—THE BASIS FOR DATA COLLECTION, ORGANIZATION, ASSESSMENT SKILLS (CRITICAL THINKING), AND TREATMENT PLANS

Because all health care workers share information through written communication, it is essential for the respiratory care practitioner to understand how to document and use the patient's medical records effectively and efficiently. The process of adding written information to the patient's chart is called *charting, recording,* or *documenting.* Good charting should provide the basic clinical information necessary for **critical thinking,** or **assessment skills**—i.e., good charting should be an effective way to summarize pertinent clinical data, analyze and assess it (i.e., determine the cause of the clinical data), record the formulation of an appropriate treatment plan, and document the adjustments of the treatment plan (in response to its effectiveness) once it has been implemented.

Good charting enhances communication and continuity of care among all members of the health care team. There is a definite and direct relationship between effective charting (communication) and the quality of patient care. Good charting also provides a permanent record of past and current assessment data, treatment plans, therapy given, and the patient's response to various therapeutic modalities. This information may be used by various governmental agencies and accreditation teams to evaluate the hospital's patient care and to prove that care was given appropriately for cost reimbursement. Accurate and legible records are the only means hospitals have to prove that they are providing appropriate care and meeting established standards.

In addition, many health care reimbursement plans (e.g., Medicare and Medicaid) are based on diagnosis related groups (DRGs). Under this plan, remuneration is based on disease diagnoses. Many private insurance companies use similar illness categories when setting hospital payment rates. Prior to reimbursement, these insurance companies carefully review the patient's medical record when assessing whether appropriate and efficient care was given.

Finally, the patient's chart is a legal document that can be called into court. Even though the physician or hospital owns the original record, the patient, lawyers, and courts can gain access to it. Thus, as an instrument of continuous patient care, and as a legal document, the patient's chart should contain all pertinent respiratory care assessments, planning, interventions, and evaluations for that patient.

TYPES OF PATIENT RECORDS

There are three basic methods used to record assessment data: the traditional chart, the problem-oriented medical record (POMR), and computer documentation.

Traditional Chart

The *traditional record* (also called *block chart* or *source-oriented record*) is divided into distinct areas of blocks, with emphasis placed on specific information. The traditional record is commonly seen in the patient's chart as full colored sheets of block information. Typical blocks of information include the *admission sheet, physician's order sheet, progress notes, history and physical examination data, medication sheet, nurses' admission information, nursing care plans, nursing notes, graph/flowsheets, laboratory and x-ray reports,* and *discharge summary.* The order, content, and number of blocks vary among institutions. The traditional chart makes recording easier, but it also makes it more difficult to readily and efficiently review a particular event or to follow the overall progress of the patient.

Problem-Oriented Medical Record

The organization of the *problem-oriented medical record* (POMR) is based on an objective, scientific problem-solving method. The POMR is, perhaps, one of the most important medical records used by the health care practitioner to (1) systematically gather clinical data, (2) formulate an assessment (i.e., the cause of the clinical data), and (3) develop an appropriate treatment plan. There are a number of good POMR methods available for recording assessment data. *Regardless of which method is selected, it is essential that one method be adopted and used consistently.*

A good POMR method should include a systematic approach that documents the following:

- The subjective and objective information collected
- An assessment based on the subjective and objective data
- The treatment plan (which has measurable outcomes)
- An evaluation of the patient's response to the treatment plan
- A section to record any adjustments made to the original treatment plan.

One of the most common POMR methods is the SOAPIER progress note—often abbreviated in the clinical setting to a SOAP progress note. SOAPIER is an acronym for seven specific aspects of charting that systematically review one health problem.

S: *Subjective* information refers to information about the patient's feelings, concerns, or sensations presented by the patient. For example:

- "I coughed hard all night long."
- "My chest feels very tight."
- "I feel very short of breath."

Only the patient can provide subjective information. Some cases may not have subjective information. For instance, a comatose, intubated patient on a mechanical ventilator would not be able to provide subjective data.

O: *Objective* information are the data the respiratory therapy care practitioner can measure, factually describe, or obtain from other professional reports or test results. Objective data include the following:

* heart rate
* respiratory rate
* blood pressure
* temperature
* breath sounds
* cough effort
* sputum production (volume, consistency, color, and odor)
* arterial blood gas and pulse oximetry data
* pulmonary function study results
* x-rays
* hemodynamic data
* chemistry results.

A: *Assessment* refers to the practitioner's professional conclusion about what is the "cause" of the subjective and objective data presented by the patient. In the patient with a respiratory disorder, the *cause* is most commonly due to a specific anatomic alteration of the lung. The assessment, moreover, is the specific reason as to "why" the respiratory care practitioner is working with the patient. For example, the presence of wheezes would be objective data (the clinical indicator) to verify the assessment (the cause) of bronchial smooth muscle constriction; an arterial blood gas with a pH of 7.18, a Pa_{CO_2} of 80 mm Hg, an HCO_3^- of 29 mEq/L, and a Pa_{O_2} of 54 mm Hg would be the objective data to verify the assessment of acute ventilatory failure with moderate hypoxemia; or the presence of rhonchi would be a clinical indicator to verify the assessment of secretions in the large airways.

P: *Plan* is the therapeutic procedure(s) selected to remedy the cause identified in the assessment that is responsible for the subjective and objective data demonstrated by the patient. For example, an assessment of bronchial smooth muscle constriction would justify the administration of a bronchodilator; the assessment of acute ventilatory failure would justify mechanical ventilation.

I: *Implementation is the actual administration of the specific therapy plan.*

E: *Evaluation* is the collection of measurable data regarding the patient's response to and effectiveness of the therapy plan. For example, an arterial blood gas may reveal that the patient's Pa_{O_2} did not increase to a safe level in response to oxygen therapy.

R: *Revision* refers to any changes that may be made to the original therapy plan in response to the evaluation. For example, if the Pa_{O_2} does not increase appropriately after the implementation of oxygen therapy, the respiratory care practitioner might continue to increase the patient's FI_{O_2} until the desired Pa_{O_2} is reached.

For the new practitioner, a pre-designed SOAP form is especially useful in (1) the rapid collection and systematic organization of important clinical data, (2) the formulation of an assessment (i.e., the cause of the clinical data), and (3) the development of a treatment plan. For example, consider the following case example and SOAP progress note (Fig. 3-1):

CASE EXAMPLE (Subjective and Objective Data Presented in Bold)

A **26-year-old male** presented in the emergency room with a **severe asthmatic episode.** On observation, his arms were fixed to the bed rails, he was using his **accessory muscles of**

inspiration, and he was **pursed-lip breathing.** The patient stated that. . . **"It feels like some-one is standing on my chest. I just can't seem to take a deep breath."** His **heart rate** was **111 beats per minute** and his **blood pressure** was **170/110.** His **respiratory rate** was **28 and shallow. Hyperresonant notes** were produced upon percussion. **Auscultation** revealed **expiratory wheezing** and **rhonchi bilaterally.** His **chest x-ray** revealed a **severely depressed diaphragm** and **alveolar hyperinflation.** His **peak expiratory flow** was **165 L/min.** Even though his **cough effort** was **weak,** he produced a **large amount** of **thick white secretions.** His **arterial blood gases** showed a **pH of 7.27,** a **Pa_{CO_2} of 62,** an **HCO_3^- of 25,** and a **Pa_{O_2} of 49** (on room air) (see Fig. 3-1).

While the SOAP form shown in Fig. 3-1 may, initially, appear long and time-consuming, the experienced respiratory care practitioner—and assessor—can typically condense and abbreviate SOAP information in a few minutes (primarily at the patient's bedside), and in just a few short statements. Typically, a written SOAP only uses 1 to 3 inches of space in the patient's chart. For example, the information presented in Fig. 3-1 may actually be documented in the patient's chart in the following abbreviated form:

S—"It feels like someone is standing on my chest. I can't take a deep breath."
O—Use of acc. mus. of insp.; pursed-lip; hyperresonance; exp. whz; ↓ diaph. & alv. hyper-infl.; PEFR 165; wk. cough; lg. amt. thick/white sec., pH 7.27; Pa_{CO_2} 62; HCO_3^- 25; Pa_{O_2} 49.
A—bronchospasm; hyperinflation; poor ability to mob. tk. sec.; acute vent. fail. with severe hypox.
P—bronchodilator Tx/pro., CPT & PD/pro., mucolytic/pro., mech. vent/pro., ABG 30 min.

After the treatment has been administered, another abbreviated SOAP note should be made to determine if the treatment plan needs to be "up-regulated" or "down-regulated." For example, if the arterial blood gas obtained after the implementation of the above *Plan* (outlined in the SOAP) showed that the patient's Pa_{O_2} was still too low, it would be appropriate to "revise" the original treatment plan by increasing the $F_{I_{O_2}}$ on the mechanical ventilator. Figure 3-2 illustrates objective data, assessments, and treatment plans commonly associated with respiratory disorders.

Computer Documentation

Computer documentation (the so-called "paperless medical record") is increasing in popularity in the hospital setting. This technology can save time in storage and retrieval of patient information. Common uses of computer documentation include ordering supplies and services for the patient; storing admission data; writing and storing patient care plans; listing medications, treatments, and procedures; and storing and retrieving diagnostic test results.

Computer documentation allows easy access to patient data. It eliminates phone calls to other departments to order patient supplies or services; reading through the entire chart to review data such as medication listings, treatments, diagnostic test results, and procedures; or reading through the entire chart to evaluate patient progress. The patient's clinical information is permanently recorded, and other health care departments can review it and communicate with one another.

Basic computer knowledge and skills are usually taught through the hospital's in-service education. Each nursing station usually has a computer screen to display information, a keyboard to enter or retrieve data, and possibly a printer to produce printed copy. The entire patient record or just a part of it may be retrieved and printed.

To summarize, good charting skills are essential to critical thinking and patient assessment—they provide the basic means to collect clinical data, analyze it, assess it, and formulate a treatment plan. Furthermore, good charting skills document the effectiveness of patient

RESPIRATORY ASSESSMENT FLOW CHART

Subjective →	Objective →	Assessment →	Plan →
"It feels like someone is standing on my chest."	**Vital signs:** RR **28** HR **111** BP **170/110**		PRESENT PLAN
	Temp. ___ On antipyretic agent? ☐Yes ☐No		
	Chest assessment:		None
"I just can't seem to take a deep breath."	Insp. **Use of accessory muscles of inspiration and pursed-lip breathing**		
	Palp. **—**		
	Perc. **Hyperresonant**		PLAN MODIFICATIONS
	Ausc. **Expiratory wheezing and rhonchi bilaterally**	**Bronchospasm**	
		Large airway secretions	
			Bronchodilator Tx per protocol
Anterior	Radiography **Severely depressed diaphragm**	**Airtrapping**	
R L			
	Bedside splr.: PEFR ā **165** p̄ **—** Tx		
	SVC ___ FVC ___ NIF ___		
Posterior	**Cough:** ☐Strong **X** Weak	**Poor ability to mobilize**	**CPT & PD per protocol**
L R	Sputum production: **X** Yes ☐No	**thick secretions**	
	Sputum char. **Large amt, thick/white secretions**		
			Mucolytics per protocol
Pt. name	**ABG:** pH **7.27** PaCO₂ **62** HCO₃⁻ **25**	**Acute ventilatory failure**	**Mechanical ventilation per protocol**
Age Male Female	PaO₂ **49** SaO₂ **—** SpO₂ **—**	**with severe hypoxemia**	
26 **X**	Neg. O₂ transport factors		
Date Time	Other: **—**		
— **—**			
Admitting diagnosis **Asthma**			
Therapist **—**			**ABG in 30 minutes & reassess**
Hospital **—**			

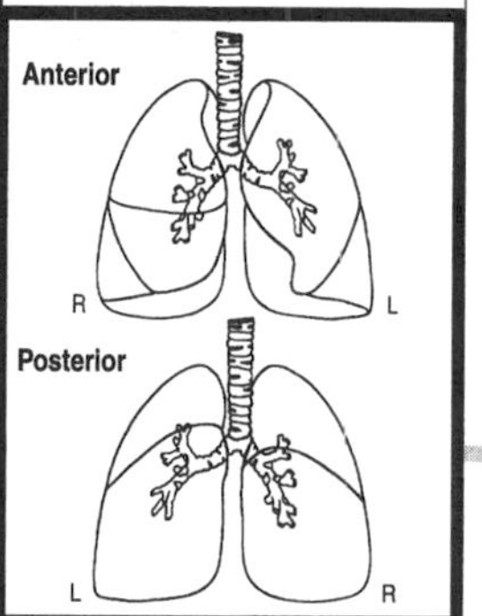

FIG 3-1
Pre-designed SOAP form.

RESPIRATORY CARE PROTOCOL GUIDE — A

Objective Data						Assessment	Plan
Chest Assessment				**Chest Radiograph**	**Bedside Spirometry**	**Common Causes of Clinical Indicators**	**Treatment Selection** (physician ordered[†])
Inspection	Palpation	Percussion	Auscultation				
Usually normal	Usually normal	May be hyperresonant	Wheezes	Usually normal	↓PEFR ↓FVC SVC > FVC	Bronchospasm Ex: Asthma; Bronchial secretions; mucus plugs Ex: Bronchitis/Cystic Fibrosis; Laryngeal edema Ex: Croup/Postextubation Edema; Bronchial tumor	Bronchodilator therapy; Bronchial hygiene therapy; Cool, bland aerosol therapy; General management/comfort
May be normal	May be normal	May be normal	Rhonchi	May be normal	↓PEFR ↓FVC	Large airway secretions Ex: Bronchitis/Cystic Fibrosis	Bronchial hygiene therapy
• Use of accessory muscles of inspiration • Pursed-lip breathing • Barrel chest	↓Tactile and vocal fremitus	Hyperresonant	• ↓Breath sounds • ↓Heart sounds	• ↓↓Diaphragm • Translucency • Over expanded	↓PEFR ↓FVC ↓FEV$_1$/FVC	Airtrapping and hyperinflation Ex: COPD • Emphysema • Bronchitis	Treat underlying cause, if possible. Ex: • Bronchospasm • Airway secretions
Usually normal	↑Tactile and vocal fremitus	Dull	• Bronchial breath sounds • Crackles • Whispered pectoriloquy	• Opacity	↓VC	Atelectasis/Consolidation/Infiltration Ex: Parenchymal disorders • Pneumonia • ARDS, IRDS, TB • Fibrosis • Postoperative atelectasis	• Antibiotic agents[†] • Lung hyperinflation therapy • Bronchial hygiene therapy — when atelectasis is caused by mucus accumulation/mucus plugs.
Usually normal	Usually normal	Dull	• Crackles • May be: wheezes/rhonchi	• Enlarged heart • Infiltrates "Butterfly"	↓VC	Pulmonary edema • Left heart failure	• Positive inotropic agents[†] • Diuretics[†]
• Distended neck veins • Enlarged liver • Peripheral edema • Pitting edema	Usually normal	Usually normal	S$_3$ and S$_4$ gallop	Enlarged right heart	Not specific	Right heart failure	Treat underlying cause. Ex: • Pulmonary vascular obstruction • Hypoxemia
• May be asymetrical chest shape	• Usually normal • Tracheal shift	Hyperresonant	Absent or ↓breath sounds	• Pneumothorax • Translucency • Mediastinum shift • ↓↓Diaphragm	Not indicated	Air pressure in intrapleural space greater than atmosphere • Tension pneumothorax	Chest tube to evacuate air (If > 20%),[†] followed by hyperinflation therapy
May be asymetrical chest shape	Usually normal	Hyperresonant	Absent or ↓breath sounds	• Pneumothorax • Translucency	Not indicated	Air in intrapleural space • Non Tension pneumothorax	Chest tube to evacuate air (If > 20%),[†] followed by hyperinflation therapy
Usually normal	• Usually normal • May be tracheal shift	Dull	• ↓Breath sounds	• Opacity • ↓Diaphragm	↓VC	Fluid in intrapleural space • Pleural effusion	Treat underlying cause • Thoracentesis[†] • Lung hyperinflation therapy
Paradoxical chest movement	Tender	Not indicated	Varies	• Rib fractures • Opacity (e.g., ARDS and/or atelectasis)	Not possible	Double fractures of three or adjacent ribs • Flail chest	• Stabilization of chest — mechanical ventilation • Lung hyperinflation therapy

Clinical manifestations (clinical indicators) that commonly develop in response to respiratory disease

FIG 3-2
Respiratory care protocol guides.

B | RESPIRATORY CARE PROTOCOL GUIDE

Objective Data (clinical manifestations or clinical indicators)	Assessment (common causes of clinical indicators)	Plan (treatment selection)
Cough effort: ☐ Strong ☐ Weak **Sputum production:** ☐ No ☐ Yes **Sputum characteristics:** • Amount • Clean, thin, odorless • Thick and tenacious • Frothy • Green/yellow/opaque • Red (hemoptysis)	**Patient's ability to mobilize secretions:** ☐ Adequate ☐ Inadequate ☐ Large ☐ Small • Early bronchial inflammation • Dehydration/↓ mucillary transport • Pulmonary edema • Acute infection • TB, tumor, trauma, pulmonary infarction	Bronchial hygiene therapy
Arterial blood gas status — Ventilatory • pH↑, $PaCO_2$↓, HCO_3↓ • pH normal, $PaCO_2$↓, HCO_3↓↓	• Acute alveolar hyper-ventilation • Chronic alveolar hyperventilation	• Treat the underlying cause, if possible. Ex: pneumonia, pain. • Generally none (occurs normally at high altitude)
• pH↓, $PaCO_2$↑, HCO_3↑ • pH normal, $PaCO_2$↑, HCO_3↑↑	• Acute ventilatory failure • Chronic ventilatory failure	• Mechanical ventilation[†] • General maintenance (e.g., low flow oxygen), bronchial hygiene
Sudden ventilatory changes on chronic ventilatory failure: • pH↑, $PaCO_2$↑, HCO_3↑↑, PaO_2↓	• Acute alveolar hyperventilation on chronic ventilatory failure	• Treat the underlying cause, if possible. Ex: pneumonia
• pH↓, $PaCO_2$↑↑, HCO_3↑, PaO_2↓	• Acute ventilatory failure on chronic ventilatory failure	• Mechanical ventilation[†]
Metabolic • pH↑, $PaCO_2$ normal or ↑, HCO_3↑, PaO_2 normal	• Metabolic alkalosis: • Hypokalemia • Hypochloremia	• Potassium administration[†] • Chloride administration[†]
• pH↓, $PaCO_2$ normal or ↓, HCO_3↓, PaO_2 normal • pH↓, $PaCO_2$ normal or ↓, HCO_3↓, PaO_2 normal • pH↓, $PaCO_2$ normal or ↓, HCO_3↓, PaO_2 normal	• Metabolic acidosis: • Lactic-acidosis • Keto-acidosis • Renal failure	• Oxygen administration, cardiovascular support[†] • Insulin administration[†] • Renal failure management[†]
Ventilatory and metabolic: • pH↓, $PaCO_2$↑, HCO_3↓	• Combined metabolic and respiratory acidosis	• Mechanical ventilation[†] • Treat the underlying cause of metabolic acidosis (see above)
• pH↑, $PaCO_2$↓, HCO_3↑	• Combined metabolic and respiratory alkalosis	• Treat the underlying cause for acute alveolar hyperventilion • Treat the underlying cause for metabolic alkalosis (see above)
Indicators for mechanical ventilation: • pH↑, $PaCO_2$↓, HCO_3↓, PaO_2↓, but patient is becoming fatigued • pH↓, $PaCO_2$↑, HCO_3↑, PaO_2↓, but patient still has ventilatory pattern • pH↓, $PaCO_2$↑, HCO_3↑, PaO_2↓, and patient has no ventilatory pattern	• Impending ventilatory failure • Ventilatory failure • Apnea	• Mechanical ventilation[†]
Oxygenation status: • PaO_2 < 80 mm Hg • PaO_2 < 60 mm Hg • PaO_2 < 40 mm Hg	• Mild hypoxemia • Moderate hypoxemia • Severe hypoxemia	• Oxygen therapy • Treat the underlying cause of hypoxemia
Negative oxygen transport indicators: ☐ ↓PaO_2 ☐ Anemia ☐ Blood loss ☐ ↓Cardiac output ☐ CO poisoning ☐ abnormal Hb	**Oxygen transport status:** ☐ Adequate ☐ Inadequate	Treat the underlying cause, if possible. Ex: ☐ Oxygen therapy ☐ Blood replacement[†] ☐ Positive inotropic agents[†]

FIG 3-2 (Cont'd)

care and adjustments of the treatment plan in response to its effectiveness. Without good charting skills, the practitioner merely administers health care without a predetermined (and recorded) goal.

Historically, respiratory care practitioners have focused on treating patients with specific disease entities and implementing physician's orders. Little planning was done by respiratory care practitioners to individualize their treatments for a specific patient. Today, a systematic problem-solving approach to respiratory care, based on a broad theoretical knowledge—combined with technical expertise and communication skills—is critical.

SELF-ASSESSMENT QUESTIONS

1. The process of adding written information to the patient's chart is called
   I. Recording.
   II. Critical thinking.
   III. Documenting.
   IV. Charting.
   a. II only
   b. IV only
   c. I and III only
   d. I, III and IV only
   e. I, II, III and IV

2. Good charting should be an effective way to do the following:
   a. _____
   _____
   b. _____
   _____
   c. _____
   _____
   d. _____
   _____

3. The admission sheet, physician's order sheet, and history sheet are all what type of patient records?
   I. Source-orientated record
   II. Problem-oriented medical record
   III. Block chart
   IV. Traditional chart
   a. I only
   b. II only
   c. IV only
   d. III and IV only
   e. I, III and IV only

4. Which of the following is based on an objective, scientific problem-solving method?
   I. Source-orientated record
   II. Problem-oriented medical record
   III. Block chart
   IV. Traditional chart
   a. I only
   b. II only
   c. IV only
   d. III and IV only
   e. I, III and IV only

5. A good problem-oriented medical record (POMR) should include a systematic approach that documents the following:
   a. _____
   _____
   b. _____
   _____
   c. _____
   _____
   d. _____
   _____
   e. _____
   _____

6. One of the most common POMR methods is the SOAPIER progress note, often abbreviated in the clinical setting to a SOAP progress note. Define the following components of a SOAP progress note and given one of more examples.

S: _____
_____
_____
_____
_____
_____

Example(s): _____
_____
_____
_____
_____
_____

O: _____
_____
_____
_____
_____
_____

Example(s): _____
_____
_____
_____
_____
_____

A: _____
_____
_____
_____
_____
_____

Example(s): _____
_____
_____
_____
_____
_____

P: _____
_____
_____
_____
_____
_____

Example(s): _____
_____
_____
_____
_____
_____

7. Bronchial breath sounds and dull percussion notes are associated with which of the following clinical assessments?
   I. Air trapping
   II. Bronchospasm

III. Atelectasis

IV. Consolidation

    a. I only

    b. II only

    c. III only

    d. I and II only

    e. III and IV only

8. List the three major indicators for mechanical ventilation.

    a. _____

        _____

    b. _____

        _____

    c. _____

        _____

9. A patient is placed on a mechanical ventilator with arterial blood gas values that reveal a pH of 7.56, a Pa_{CO_2} of 24, an HCO_3^- of 20, and a Pa_{O_2} of 52. Write the indicators for mechanical ventilation that justify placing the patient on a mechanical ventilator with these arterial blood gas values.

    Answer: _____

    _____

10. CASE:

    A 36-year-old female is in the emergency room in respiratory distress. Her heart rate is 136 beats per minute and her blood pressure is 165/120. Her respiratory rate is 32 and labored. The patient states that. . ."It feels like a rope is around my neck." Expiratory wheezing and rhonchi are auscultated bilaterally. Her arterial blood gas values reveal a pH of 7.56, a Pa_{CO_2} of 28, HCO_3^- of 21, and a Pa_{O_2} of 47 mm Hg (on room air). Her cough effort is strong and she is producing a moderate amount of thin white secretions. Her peak expiratory flow rate is 185 L/min, and her chest x-ray demonstrates a moderately depressed diaphragm and alveolar hyperinflation. With the above clinical information, SOAP the patient (use Figure 3-2 for assistance).

    S: _____

    _____

    _____

    _____

    O: _____

    _____

    _____

    _____

    _____

    _____

    _____

    A: _____

    _____

    _____

    _____

    _____

    P: _____

    _____

    _____

    _____

    _____

    _____

Answers appear in Appendix XXI.

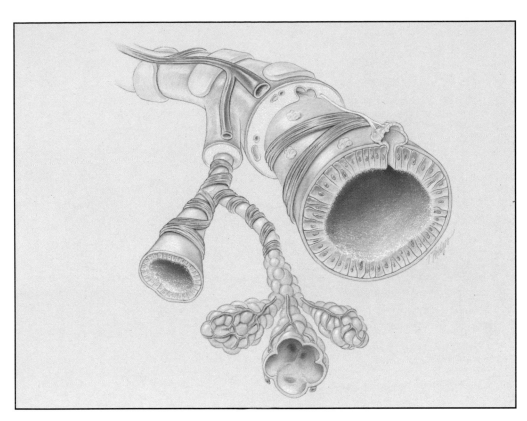

PLATE 1 Normal lung (*see* Fig. 1-83).

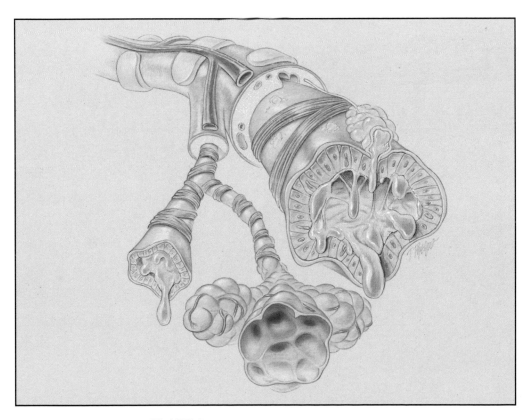

PLATE 2 Chronic bronchitis (*see* Fig. 4-1).

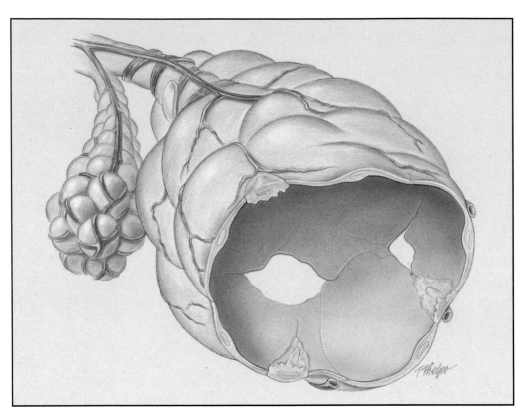

PLATE 3   Panlobular emphysema (*see* Fig. 5-1).

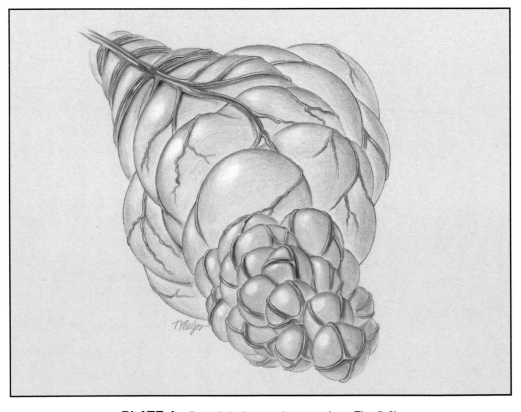

PLATE 4   Centrilobular emphysema (*see* Fig. 5-2).

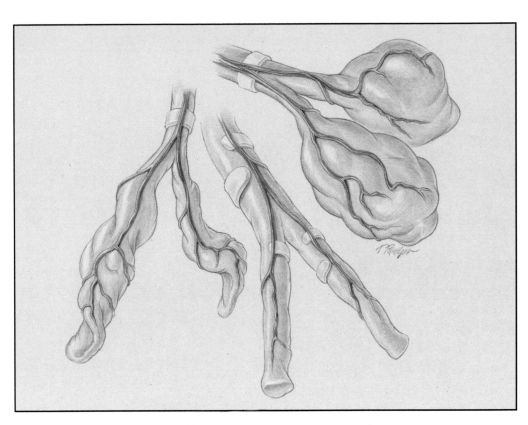

PLATE 5   Bronchiectasis (*see* Fig. 6-1).

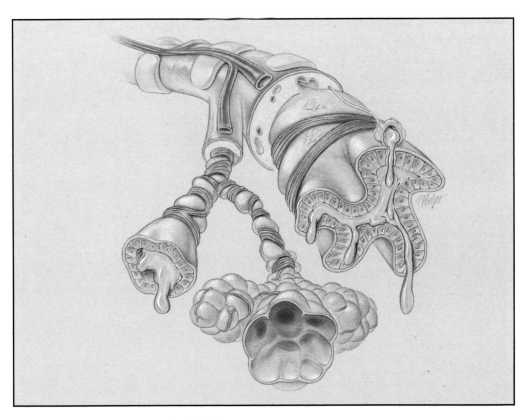

PLATE 6   Asthma (*see* Fig. 7-1).

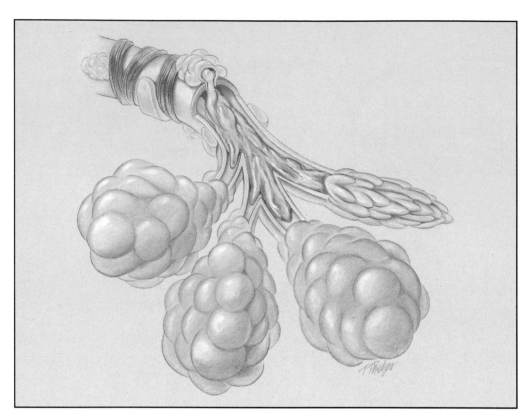

PLATE 7 Cystic fibrosis (*see* Fig. 8-1).

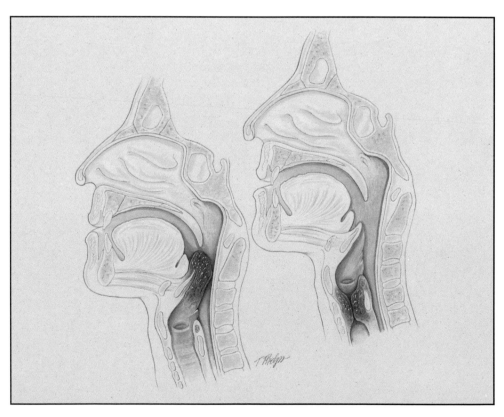

PLATE 8 Croup syndrome: Laryngotracheobronchitis and acute epiglottitis (*see* Fig. 9-1).

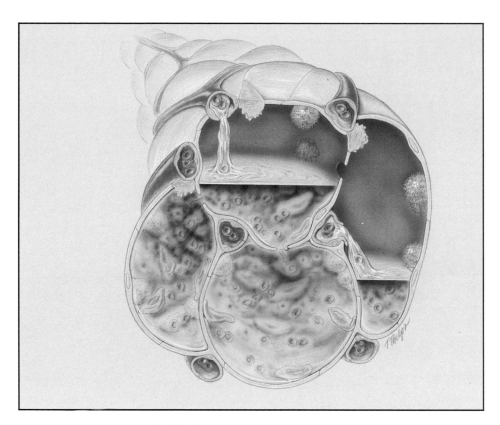

PLATE 9 Pneumonia (*see* Fig. 10-1).

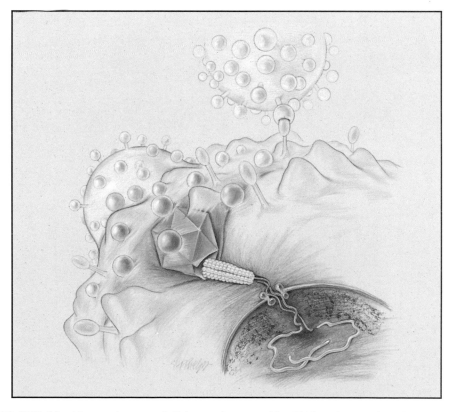

PLATE 10 Human immunodeficiency virus attacking T4 lymphocyte (*see* Fig. 11-1).

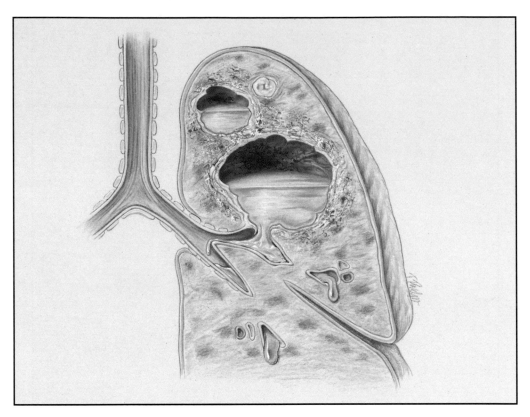

PLATE 11 Lung abscess (*see* Fig. 12-1).

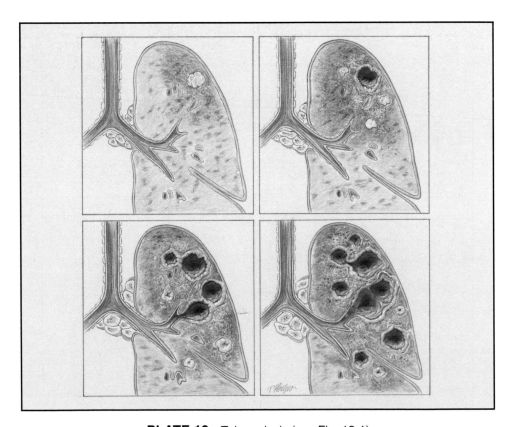

PLATE 12 Tuberculosis (*see* Fig. 13-1).

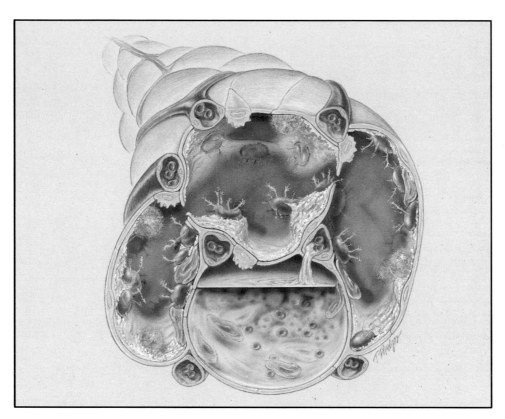

PLATE 13 Fungal disorder of the lung (*see* Fig. 14-1).

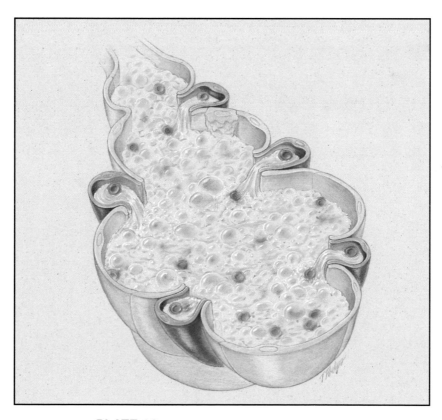

PLATE 14 Pulmonary edema (*see* Fig. 15-1).

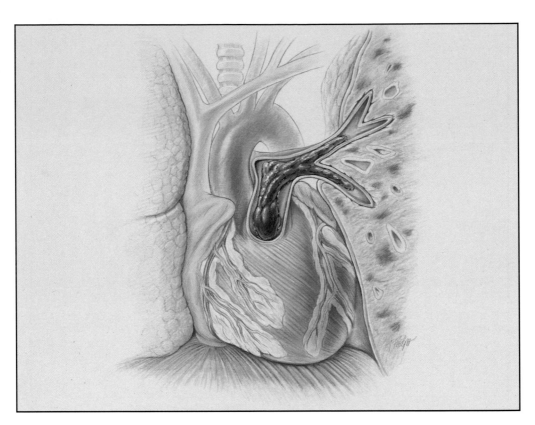

PLATE 15 Pulmonary embolism (*see* Fig. 16-1).

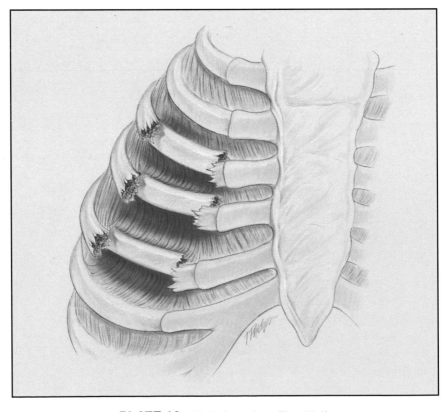

PLATE 16 Flail chest (*see* Fig. 17-1).

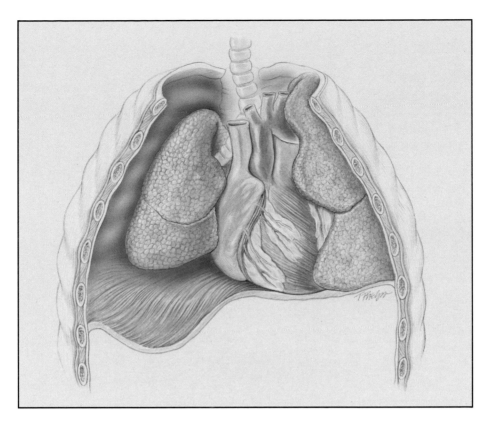

PLATE 17 Pneumothorax (*see* Fig. 18-1).

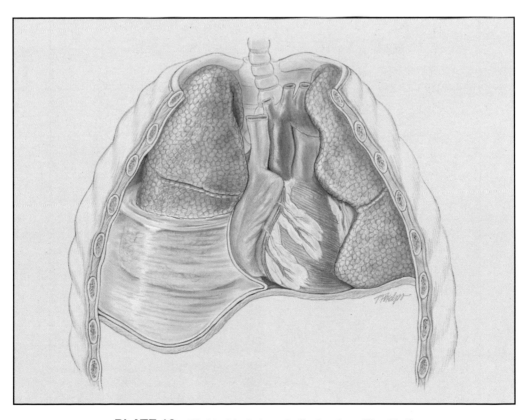

PLATE 18 Right-sided pleural effusion (*see* Fig. 19-1).

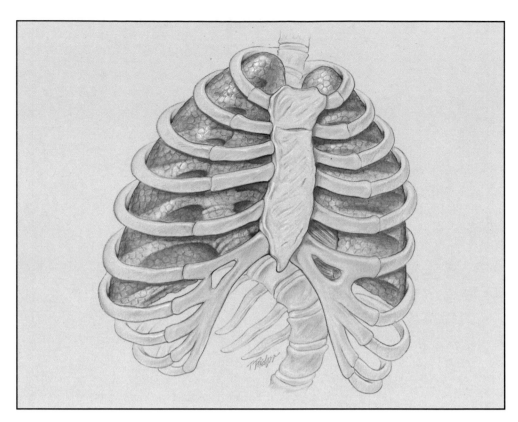

PLATE 19 Kyphoscoliosis (*see* Fig. 20-1).

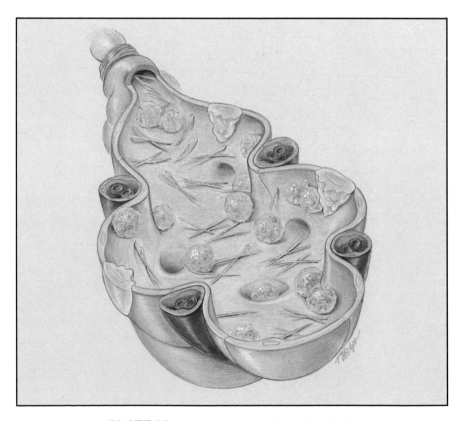

PLATE 20 Pneumoconiosis (*see* Fig. 21-1).

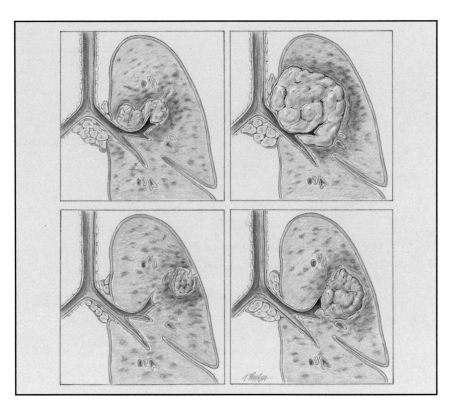

PLATE 21   Cancer of the lung (*see* Fig. 22-1).

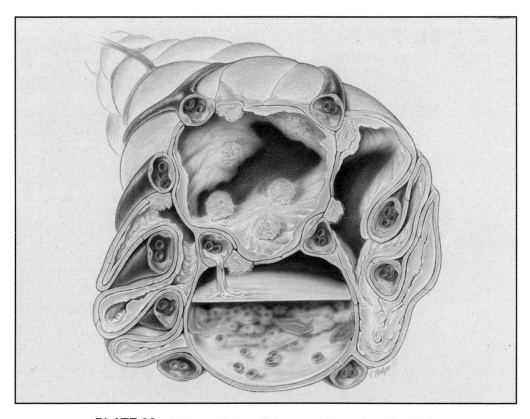

PLATE 22   Adult respiratory distress syndrome (*see* Fig. 23-1).

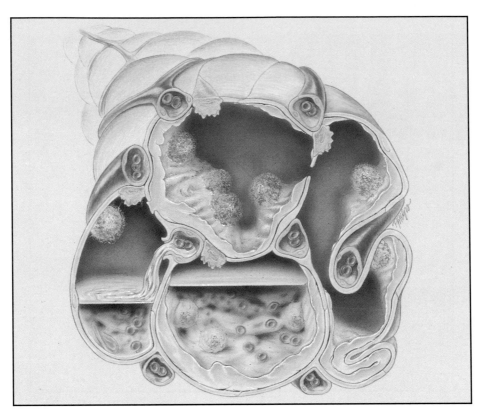

PLATE 23 Idiopathic (infant) respiratory distress syndrome (*see* Fig. 24-1).

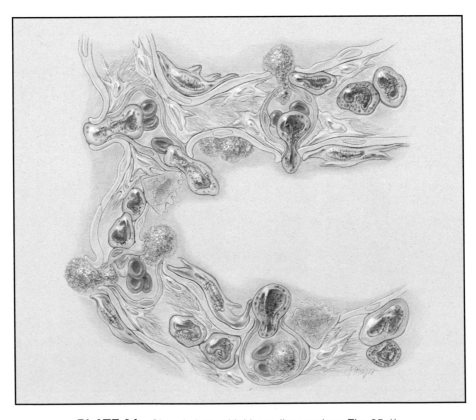

PLATE 24 Chronic interstitial lung disease (*see* Fig. 25-1).

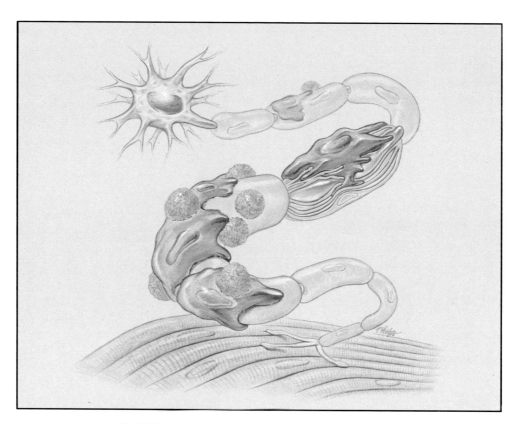

PLATE 25 Guillain-Barré syndrome (*see* Fig. 26-1).

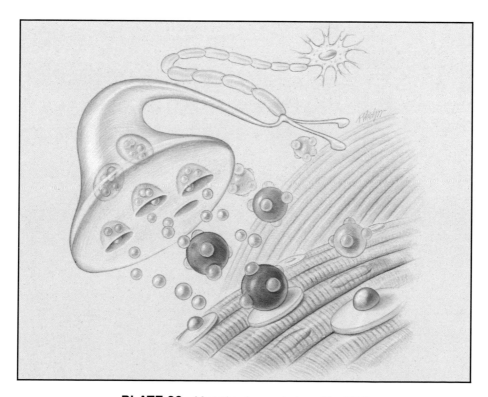

PLATE 26 Myasthenia gravis (*see* Fig. 27-1).

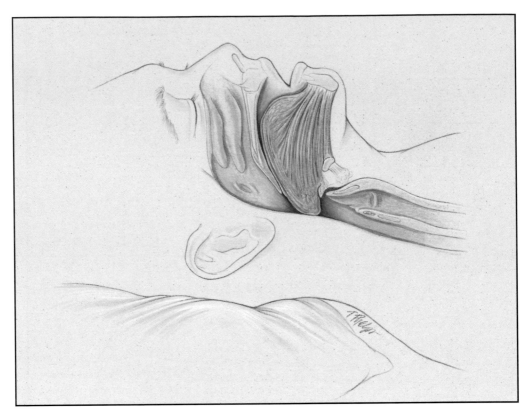

PLATE 27 Sleep apnea (*see* Fig. 28-1).

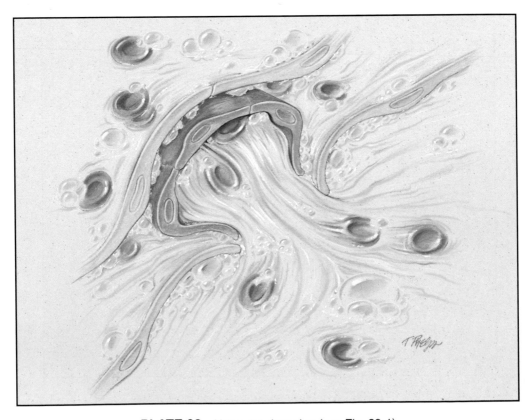

PLATE 28 Near wet-drowning (*see* Fig. 29-1).

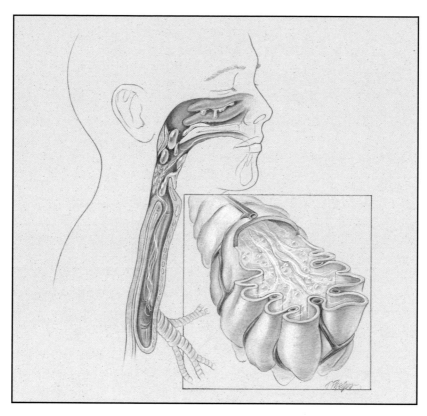

PLATE 29 Smoke inhalation and thermal injuries (*see* Fig. 30-1).

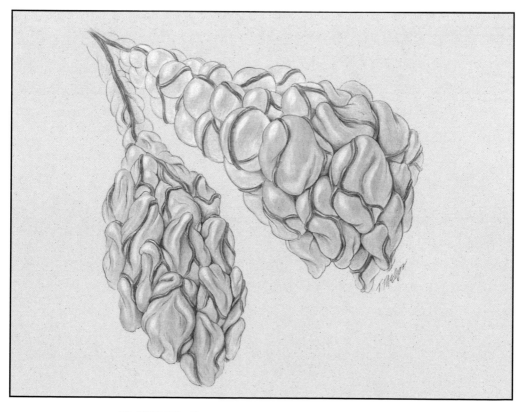

PLATE 30 Postoperative atelectasis (*see* Fig. 31-1).

PART

II

OBSTRUCTIVE
AIRWAY DISEASES

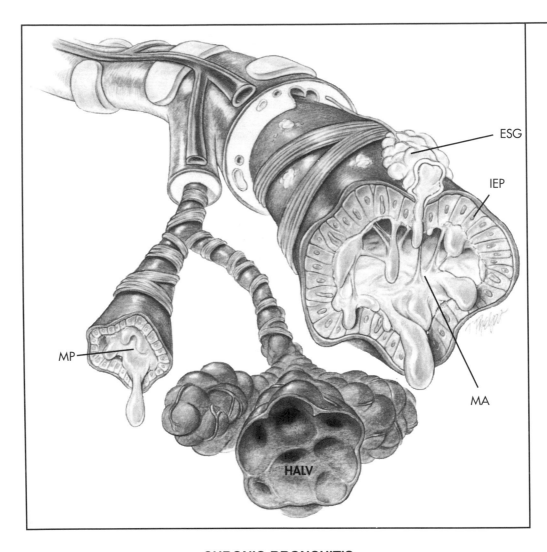

CHRONIC BRONCHITIS

FIG 4-1

Chronic bronchitis (one of the most common airway diseases). *ESG* = enlarged submucosal gland; *IEP* = inflammation of epithelium; *MA* = mucus accumulation; *MP* = mucus plug; *HALV* = hyperinflation of alveoli (distal to airway obstruction). (See also Plate 2.)

CHRONIC BRONCHITIS

ANATOMIC ALTERATIONS OF THE LUNGS

The conducting airways are the primary structures that undergo change in chronic bronchitis. This is particularly true for the peripheral airways. Due to chronic inflammation the bronchial walls are narrowed by vasodilation, congestion, and mucosal edema. This condition often leads to "secondary bronchial smooth muscle constriction." In addition, continued bronchial irritation causes the submucosal bronchial glands to enlarge and the number of goblet cells to increase, resulting in excessive mucus production. The number and function of cilia lining the tracheobronchial tree is diminished, and the peripheral bronchi are often partially or totally occluded by inflammation and mucus plugs, which in turn leads to hyperinflated alveoli (Fig 4-1).

To summarize, the following major pathologic or structural changes are associated with chronic bronchitis:

* Chronic inflammation and swelling of the peripheral airways
* Excessive mucus production and accumulation
* Smooth muscle constriction of bronchial airway (bronchospasm)
* Bronchial airway obstruction
* Hyperinflated alveoli distal to obstructed airway

ETIOLOGY

Although the exact cause of chronic bronchitis is not known, the following are thought to be important etiologic factors.

Cigarette smoking.—Cigarette smoking clearly plays a major etiologic role in chronic bronchitis. Individuals who smoke are much more prone to develop chronic bronchitis than nonsmokers. Inhaled cigarette smoke contains thousands of particles, many of which are irritants that cause bronchial inflammation and destruction of ciliary activity. The excess mucus that accumulates due to decreased ciliary activity increases the patient's vulnerability to secondary bronchial infections, which may further compromise already inflamed bronchial mucosae.

Atmospheric pollutants.—Common atmospheric pollutants such as sulfur dioxide, the nitrogen oxides, and ozone are believed to play a significant etiologic role in chronic bronchitis.

Prolonged exposure to sulfur dioxide is known to increase airway resistance, and ozone, present in smog, is a well-known respiratory tract irritant. Epidemiologic data reveal an increased morbidity from lung disease in areas of high air pollution.

Infection.—Although the role of infection is uncertain, there is evidence that individuals who have repeated respiratory tract infections during childhood are likely to develop chronic bronchitis later in life. Because of the inability of the tracheobronchial tree to clear the excess mucus associated with chronic bronchitis, additional infections compromise the already damaged bronchial tree, and a vicious cycle develops.

OVERVIEW

OF THE CARDIOPULMONARY CLINICAL MANIFESTATIONS ASSOCIATED WITH
CHRONIC BRONCHITIS*

❏ **INCREASED RESPIRATORY RATE**
Several pathophysiologic mechanisms operating simultaneously may lead to an increased ventilatory rate. These are (see page 17)
  • Stimulation of peripheral chemoreceptors
  • Anxiety

❏ **PULMONARY FUNCTION STUDY FINDINGS**

Expiratory Maneuver Findings (see page 41)

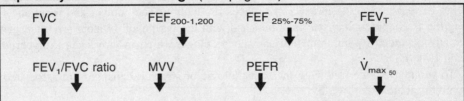

Lung Volume and Capacity Findings (see page 48)

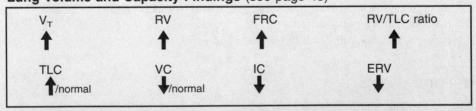

❏ **INCREASED HEART RATE (PULSE), CARDIAC OUTPUT, AND BLOOD PRESSURE** (see page 86)
❏ **INCREASED ANTEROPOSTERIOR CHEST DIAMETER (BARREL CHEST)** (see page 49)
❏ **PURSED-LIP BREATHING** (see page 49)
❏ **USE OF ACCESSORY MUSCLES DURING INSPIRATION** (see page 51)
❏ **USE OF ACCESSORY MUSCLES DURING EXPIRATION** (see page 54)

---

*Chronic bronchitis and pulmonary emphysema frequently occur together as a disease complex referred to as chronic obstructive pulmonary disease (COPD). Patients with COPD typically demonstrate clinical manifestations related to both chronic bronchitis and emphysema.

❑ **ARTERIAL BLOOD GASES**

Mild to Moderate Chronic Bronchitis

Acute Alveolar Hyperventilation with Hypoxemia (see page 57)

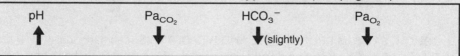

pH	Pa_{CO_2}	HCO_3^-	Pa_{O_2}
↑	↓	↓(slightly)	↓

Severe Chronic Bronchitis

Chronic Ventilatory Failure with Hypoxemia (see page 60)

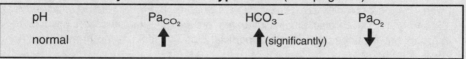

pH	Pa_{CO_2}	HCO_3^-	Pa_{O_2}
normal	↑	↑(significantly)	↓

Acute Ventilatory Changes Superimposed on Chronic Ventilatory Failure (see page 65)

Because acute ventilatory changes are frequently seen in patients with chronic ventilatory failure, the respiratory care practitioner must be familiar with and be on alert for (1) acute alveolar hyperventilation superimposed on chronic ventilatory failure and (2) acute ventilatory failure superimposed on chronic ventilatory failure.

❑ **CYANOSIS** (see page 68)
❑ **OXYGENATION INDICES** (see page 69)

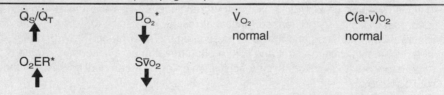

$\dot{Q}_S/\dot{Q}_T$	D_{O_2}*	$\dot{V}_{O_2}$	$C(a-v)_{O_2}$
↑	↓	normal	normal
O_2ER*	$S\bar{v}_{O_2}$		
↑	↓		

*The D_{O_2} may be normal in patients who have compensated to the decreased oxygenation status with (1) an increased cardiac output, (2) an increased hemoglobin level, or (3) a combination of both. When the D_{O_2} is normal, the O_2ER is usually normal.

❑ **HEMODYNAMIC INDICES (SEVERE CHRONIC BRONCHITIS)** (see page 87)

CVP	RAP	$\overline{PA}$	PCWP
↑	↑	↑	normal
CO	SV	SVI	CI
normal	normal	normal	normal
RVSWI	LVSWI	PVR	SVR
↑	normal	↑	normal

❑ **POLYCYTHEMIA, COR PULMONALE** (see page 92)
- Elevated hemoglobin concentration and hematocrit
- Distended neck veins
- Enlarged and tender liver
- Peripheral edema
- Pitting edema

❏ **CHEST ASSESSMENT FINDINGS** (see page 6)
  • Decreased tactile and vocal fremitus
  • Hyperresonant percussion note
  • Diminished breath sounds
  • Diminished heart sounds
  • Crackles/rhonchi/wheezing

❏ **COUGH, SPUTUM PRODUCTION, AND HEMOPTYSIS** (see page 93)
The American Thoracic Society's definition of chronic bronchitis is based on a major clinical manifestation of the disease. The defintion states that chronic bronchitis is characterized by a daily, productive cough for at least three consecutive months each year for two years in a row. Common bacteria found in the bronchial secretions of patients with chronic bronchitis are *Streptococcus pneumoniae* and *Haemophilus influenzae*. Because of the chronic airway inflammation, cough, and infection associated with chronic bronchitis, rupture of the superficial blood vessels of the bronchi and hemoptysis may be seen.

❏ **RADIOLOGIC FINDINGS**
Chest radiograph
  • Translucent (dark) lung fields
  • Depressed or flattened diaphragms
  • Long and narrow heart (pulled downward by diaphragms)
  • Enlarged heart
  There may be no radiograph abnormalities in chronic bronchitis if only the large bronchi are affected. If the more peripheral bronchi are involved, however, there may be substantial air trapping. In the advanced stages of chronic bronchitis, the density of the lungs decreases, and, consequently, the resistance to x-ray penetration is not as great. This is revealed on x-ray film as areas of translucency or areas that are darker in appearance. Due to the increased functional residual capacity, the diaphragms may be depressed or flattened and are seen as such on the radiograph (Fig 4-2). Finally, since right ventricular enlargement and failure often develop as a secondary problem during the advanced stages of chronic bronchitis, an enlarged heart may be seen on the chest radiograph.
BRONCHOGRAM
  • Small spikelike protrusions
  Small spikelike protrusions ("railroad tracks" appearance of airways) from the larger bronchi are often seen on bronchograms of persons with chronic bronchitis. It is believed that the spikes result from pooling of the radiopaque medium in the enlarged ducts of the mucous glands (Fig 4-3).

GENERAL MANAGEMENT OF CHRONIC BRONCHITIS
Patient and Family Education

Both the patient and the patient's family should be instructed on the disease and its effects on the body. They should also be instructed in home care therapies, the objectives of these therapies, and how to administer medications. As with emphysema patients, the services of a pulmonary rehabilitation team are sometimes necessary in the management of patients with chronic bronchitis. Such teams include a respiratory care practitioner, physical therapist, respiratory nurse specialist, occupational therapist, dietitian, social worker, and psychologist. A physician trained in respiratory rehabilitation usually outlines and orchestrates the patient's therapeutic program.

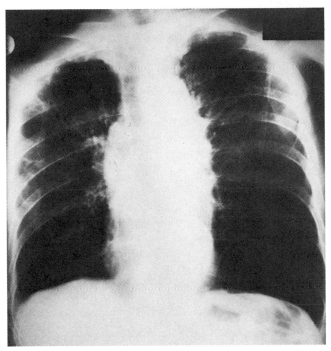

FIG 4-2
Chest x-ray film of a patient with chronic bronchitis. Note the translucent (dark) lung fields, depressed diaphragms, and long and narrow heart.

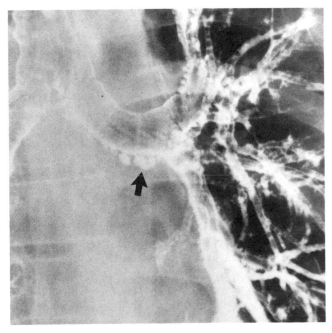

FIG 4-3
Chronic bronchitis. Bronchogram with localized view of left hilum. Rounded collections of contrast lie adjacent to bronchial walls and are particularly well seen below the left main stem bronchus *(arrows)*. They are caused by contrast in dilated mucous gland ducts (From Armstrong P, Wilson AG, Dee P: *Imaging of Diseases of the Chest,* St. Louis, 1990, Mosby-Year Book. Used by permission.)

Behavioral Management

Avoidance of Smoking and Inhaled Irritants.—Patients with chronic bronchitis must be strongly encouraged to stop smoking. A "stop-smoking" clinic with techniques designed to disrupt and break the patient's smoking behaviors (e.g., nicotine polacrilex [nicotine gum] and transdermal nicotine patches combined with counseling) may be helpful. Patients with chronic bronchitis should be instructed to avoid inhaled irritants such as dust, fumes, mist, and toxic gases.

Avoidance of infections.—Patients with chronic bronchitis should avoid people with contagious respiratory tract infections, especially influenza. Annual immunization against influenza is usually performed, as is onetime immunization with pneumococcal vaccine.

Mobilization of Bronchial Secretions

Because of the excessive mucus production and accumulation associated with chronic bronchitis, a number of respiratory therapy modalities may be used to enhance the mobilization of bronchial secretions (see Appendix XI).

Medications

Mucolytic agents.—Mucolytic agents may be used to break down the large amounts of thick tenacious mucus (see Appendix VI).

Sympathomimetics.—Sympathomimetic drugs are commonly prescribed for patients with chronic bronchitis to offset bronchial smooth muscle spasm (see Appendix II).

Parasympatholytics.—Parasympatholytic agents are also used to offset bronchial smooth muscle constriction (see Appendix III).

Xanthines.—Xanthines are used to enhance bronchial smooth muscle relaxation (see Appendix IV).

Expectorants.—Expectorants are often used when water alone is not sufficient to facilitate expectoration (see Appendix VII).

Antibiotics.—Antibiotics are commonly administered to prevent or combat secondary respiratory tract infections (see Appendix VIII).

Supplemental Oxygen

Because hypoxemia is often associated with chronic bronchitis, supplemental oxygen may be required. The hypoxemia that develops in chronic bronchitis is usually caused by the hypoventilation and shuntlike effect associated with the disorder. Hypoxemia caused by a shuntlike effect can generally be corrected by oxygen therapy. It should be noted, however, that when the patient demonstrates chronic ventilatory failure during the advanced stages of chronic bronchitis, caution must be taken not to eliminate the patient's hypoxic ventilatory drive.

Continuous Mechanical Ventilation

Because acute ventilatory failure (superimposed on chronic ventilatory failure) is often seen in patients with severe chronic bronchitis, continuous mechanical ventilation may be required to maintain an adequate ventilatory status. Continuous mechanical ventilation is justified when the acute ventilatory failure is thought to be reversible.

● ● ● ● | CHRONIC BRONCHITIS CASE STUDY | ● ● ● ●

ADMITTING HISTORY AND PHYSICAL EXAMINATION

This 58-year-old male has worked in a cotton mill in South Carolina for the past 37 years. He has a 100 pack-year history of cigarette smoking, and he also chews tobacco regularly. He sought medical assistance because of a chronic cough. He describes it as a "smoker's cough" and states that it is present about four to five months of the year. For the past three years his cough produced grayish-yellow sputum during the winter months. The sputum was mostly mucoid in nature, and only occasionally was it thicker and yellow. He stated that he was slightly shorter of breath than in the past, but attributed this to "getting older."

At physical examination the patient was in no distress. He was obese. He generated a strong cough occasionally during the visit, but the cough was not productive. The expiratory phase of respiration was prolonged. Auscultation of the chest revealed occasional moist rhonchi. The chest radiograph was read as "suggestive of increased markings in the lower lung fields bilaterally." Some pulmonary hyperinflation was noticed. Pulmonary function studies showed a decrease in FVC (70% of predicted), FEV_1 (50% of predicted), and PEFR (30% of predicted). The respiratory therapist's assessment at this time was documented in the patient's chart as follows:

RESPIRATORY ASSESSMENT AND PLAN

S: "Smoker's cough," Episodic mucopurulent sputum production.

O: Few rhonchi at lung bases. Strong cough. Chest radiograph: increased markings at bases and hyperinflation. PFTs: decreased FVC, FEV_1, & PEFR.

A: • Probable mild chronic bronchitis (history & physical exam)

  • Obstructive pathology (decreased FVC, FEV_1, & PEFR)

  • Mild to moderate airway secretions (rhonchi)

  • Good ability to mobilize secretions (strong cough)

P: Patient education on smoking. Refer to Smoking Cessation Clinic.

The patient was advised to stop smoking and to seek medical assistance if the sputum became thick and yellow. The physician also prescribed a pneumococcal vaccine. Two weeks later, influenza prophylaxis was performed (vaccine). The Smoking Cessation Clinic prescribed slow-release nicotine patches, and he attended a week-long smoking cessation program. Anti-anxiety medication for prn use was also prescribed. The patient did well, and at 16-month follow-up was no longer smoking. The patient stated that he had not had his "smoker's cough" or produced any sputum in weeks. The patient was scheduled for another routine follow-up appointment in six months.

DISCUSSION

This case suggests a very probable role for the respiratory care practitioner of the future. He may well be working in outpatient settings that will necessitate his evaluation and treatment of patients such as this one.

The history of productive cough and the findings of expiratory prolongation and rhonchi in a smoker who is not seriously ill are rightly suggestive of a diagnosis of chronic bronchitis. The pulmonary function data and chest x-ray confirm this suspicion.

The physician's prescription of influenza prophylaxis, pneumococcal vaccine, and slow-release nicotine patches speaks to the key part of therapy in chronic bronchitis, namely, avoidance of irritant fumes and particles; influenza and pneumococcal vaccines for hopeful avoidance of those two common complicating diseases; and the need for continued follow-up.

Note that *no* specific respiratory therapy was prescribed at this time by the respiratory care practitioner who was truly practicing in a cost-effective manner.

SELF-ASSESSMENT QUESTIONS

Multiple Choice

1. In chronic bronchitis
   I. The bronchial walls are narrowed due to vasoconstriction.
   II. The bronchial glands are enlarged.
   III. The number of goblet cells is decreased.
   IV. The number of cilia lining the tracheobronchial tree is increased.
       a. I only
       b. II only
       c. III only
       d. III, and IV only
       e. II, III, and IV only

2. Which of the following is/are believed to play a major etiologic role in chronic bronchitis?
   I. Ozone
   II. Nitrous oxide
   III. Sulfur dioxide
   IV. Nitrogen oxides
       a. I only
       b. II only
       c. III only
       d. II and IV only
       e. I, III, and IV only

3. Common bacteria found in the tracheobronchial tree of patients with chronic bronchitis is/are
   I. *Staphylococcus.*
   II. *Haemophilus influenzae.*
   III. *Klebsiella.*
   IV. *Streptococcus.*
       a. I only
       b. II only
       c. III and IV only
       d. II and IV only
       e. I, II, and IV only

4. In chronic bronchitis, the patient commonly demonstrates
   I. Increased FVC.
   II. Decreased ERV.
   III. Increased VC.
   IV. Decreased RV.
       a. II only
       b. III only
       c. I and III only
       d. III and IV only
       e. I, III, and IV only

5. The patient with severe chronic bronchitis usually presents with the following arterial blood gas values:
   I. Decreased pH
   II. Increased HCO_3^-
   III. Decreased Pa_{CO2}
   IV. Increased Pa_{O2}
       a. I only
       b. II only
       c. III only
       d. I and II only
       e. III and IV only

6. Sympathomimetic agents are commonly prescribed for patients with chronic bronchitis to offset bronchial smooth muscle spasm. What is the trade name of the sympathomimetic agent called albuterol?
    I. Proventil
    II. Ventolin
    III. Vanceril
    IV. Brethine
        a. I only
        b. IV only
        c. I and II only
        d. II and IV only
        e. II, III, and IV only

7. The patient with severe chronic bronchitis commonly demonstrates the following oxygenation indices:
    I. Decreased $C(a-\bar{v})o_2$
    II. Increased O_2ER
    III. Decreased $\dot{D}o_2$
    IV. Increased $\dot{V}o_2$
        a. I only
        b. III only
        c. IV only
        d. II and III only
        e. I, III, and IV only

8. The patient with severe chronic bronchitis commonly demonstrates the following hemodynamic indices:
    I. Increased PCWP
    II. Decreased RAP
    III. Increased $\overline{PA}$
    IV. Decreased CO
        a. I only
        b. III only
        c. IV only
        d. I and III only
        e. I, III, and IV only

9. Parasympatholytic agents are often used to offset the bronchial smooth muscle constriction associated with chronic bronchitis. The trade name of the parasympatholytic agent called ipratropium bromide is
        a. Theophylline.
        b. Atropine sulfate.
        c. Atrovent.
        d. Guaifenesin.
        e. Erythromycin.

10. Patients with severe chronic bronchitis commonly demonstrate
    I. Peripheral edema.
    II. Distended neck veins.
    III. An elevated hemoglobin concentration.
    IV. An enlarged liver.
        a. I only
        b. III only
        c. II and IV only
        d. II, III, and IV only
        e. I, II, III, and IV

Answers appear in Appendix XXI.

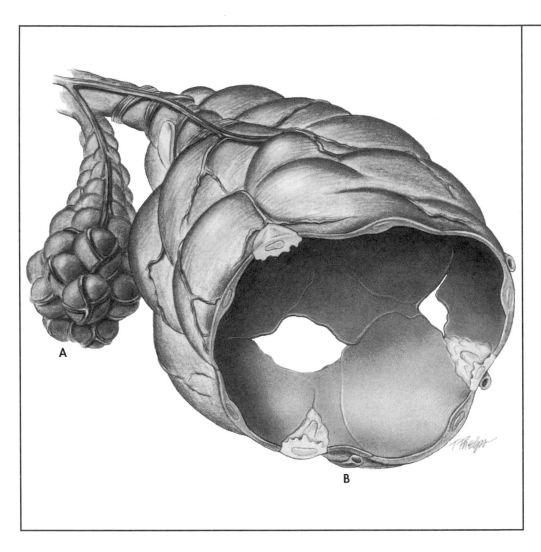

PANLOBULAR EMPHYSEMA

FIG 5-1

A, normal alveoli (for comparison purposes only). **B,** panlobular emphysema: abnormal weakening and enlargement of all air spaces distal to the terminal bronchioles. (See also Plate 3.)

CHAPTER 5

EMPHYSEMA

ANATOMIC ALTERATIONS OF THE LUNGS

Emphysema is characterized by a weakening and permanent enlargement of the air spaces distal to the terminal bronchioles and by destruction of the alveolar walls. As these structures enlarge and the alveoli coalesce, many of the adjacent pulmonary capillaries are also affected, and this results in a decreased area for gas exchange. Furthermore, the distal airways, weakened by emphysema, collapse during expiration in response to increased intrapleural pressure. This action traps gas in the distal alveoli. There are two major types of emphysema: panacinar (panlobular) emphysema and centriacinar (centrilobular) emphysema.

In *panlobular emphysema* there is an abnormal weakening and enlargement of all air spaces distal to the terminal bronchioles, including the respiratory bronchioles, alveolar ducts, alveolar sacs, and alveoli. The alveolar-capillary surface area is significantly decreased (Fig 5-1). Panlobular emphysema is commonly found in the lower parts of the lungs and is usually associated with a deficiency of α_1-*protease inhibitor* (previously called α_1-antitrypsin).

Centrilobular emphysema primarily involves the respiratory bronchioles in the proximal portion of the acinus. The respiratory bronchiolar walls enlarge, become confluent, and are then destroyed. There is usually a rim of parenchyma that remains relatively unaffected (Fig 5-2). Centrilobular emphysema is the most common form of emphysema and is often associated with chronic bronchitis.

To summarize, the following are the major pathologic or structural changes associated with emphysema:

- Permanent enlargement and deterioration of the air spaces distal to the terminal bronchioles
- Destruction of pulmonary capillaries
- Weakening of the distal airways, primarily the respiratory bronchioles
- Air trapping

ETIOLOGY

The main etiologic factors of emphysema are cigarette smoking, genetic predisposition, infection, and inhaled irritants. The clinical manifestations typically appear after the age of 50, and males are affected about four times more often than females.

Cigarette smoking.—Although the exact mechanism is unknown, cigarette smoking is thought to be one of the most important etiologic factors in emphysema. Cigarette smoke contains numerous irritants that stimulate mucus production and ultimately impair or destroy

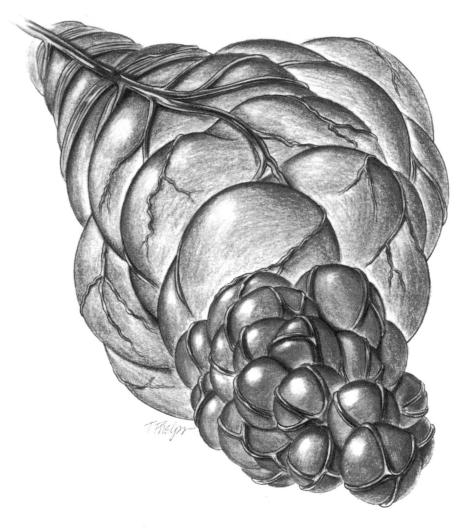

CENTRILOBULAR EMPHYSEMA

FIG 5-2

Centrilobular emphysema. Abnormal weakening and enlargement of the respiratory bronchioles in the proximal portion of the acinus. (See also Plate 4.)

ciliary transport. The excess mucus that accumulates as a result of decreased ciliary activity increases the patient's vulnerability to respiratory tract infections. Cigarette smoking also causes bronchoconstriction, which in turn increases airway resistance and further impedes tracheobronchial clearance.

Genetic predisposition.—It has been known for many years that panlobular emphysema occurs with unusual frequency in certain families, where it primarily affects young adults. It is now known that genetic α_1-*protease inhibitor* (α_1PI) deficiency is the key to the high incidence of panlobular emphysema in some families. α_1PI is a serum glycoprotein that inhibits several proteolytic enzymes. It is synthesized and secreted by the liver. When old white blood cells are destroyed in the lungs, an *elastase* is released that in turn destroys elastic tissue. α_1PI is the enzyme responsible for inactivating the elastase.

The normal level of α_1PI is 200 to 400 mg/dl and is genetically referred to as an MM or simply an M phenotype (homozygote). The phenotype associated with the lower serum concentration is ZZ, or simply Z. The heterozygous offspring of parents with the M and Z phenotypes have the phenotype MZ. The MZ phenotype results in an intermediate deficiency of α_1PI. The precise role of the intermediate level of α_1PI is unclear. It is strongly recommended, however, that these individuals not smoke or work in areas having significant air pollution.

Infection.—There is increasing epidemiologic evidence that repeated respiratory tract infections during childhood may cause permanent airway damage, which may eventually develop into chronic obstructive pulmonary disease in adult life.

Inhaled irritants.—Common atmospheric pollutants such as sulfur dioxide, the nitrogen oxides, and ozone may have an etiologic role in emphysema. Sulfur dioxide is known to increase airway resistance, and ozone, present in urban air pollution (smog), is a respiratory tract irritant. Epidemiologic data support the observation that in areas of high air pollution there is an increased incidence of obstructive lung disease.

OVERVIEW

OF CARDIOPULMONARY CLINICAL MANIFESTATIONS ASSOCIATED WITH
EMPHYSEMA*

❑ **INCREASED RESPIRATORY RATE**

Several pathophysiologic mechanisms operating simultaneously may lead to an increased ventilatory rate. These are (see page 17)
- Stimulation of peripheral chemoreceptors
- Anxiety

❑ **PULMONARY FUNCTION STUDY FINDINGS**

Expiratory Maneuver Findings (see page 41)

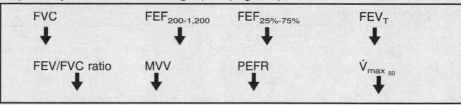

Lung Volume and Capacity Findings (see page 48)

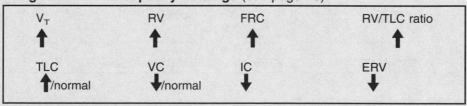

❑ **DECREASED DIFFUSION CAPACITY** (see page 48)
❑ **INCREASED HEART RATE (PULSE), CARDIAC OUTPUT, AND BLOOD PRESSURE** (see page 86)

---

*Pulmonary emphysema and chronic bronchitis frequently occur together as a disease complex referred to as chronic obstructive pulmonary disease (COPD); therefore, patients with COPD typically demonstrate clinical manifestations related to both emphysema and chronic bronchitis.

❑ **INCREASED ANTEROPOSTERIOR CHEST DIAMETER (BARREL CHEST)** (see page 49)
❑ **PURSED-LIP BREATHING** (see page 49)
❑ **USE OF ACCESSORY MUSCLES DURING INSPIRATION** (see page 51)
❑ **USE OF ACCESSORY MUSCLES DURING EXPIRATION** (see page 54)
❑ **ARTERIAL BLOOD GASES**

Mild to Moderate Emphysema

Acute Alveolar Hyperventilation with Hypoxemia (see page 57)

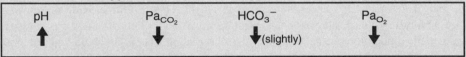

pH	Pa_{CO_2}	HCO_3^-	Pa_{O_2}
↑	↓	↓ (slightly)	↓

Severe Emphysema (End-Stage)

Chronic Ventilatory Failure with Hypoxemia (see page 60)

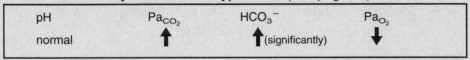

pH	Pa_{CO_2}	HCO_3^-	Pa_{O_2}
normal	↑	↑ (significantly)	↓

Acute Ventilatory Changes Superimposed on Chronic Ventilatory Failure (see page 65)

Because acute ventilatory changes are frequently seen in patients with chronic ventilatory failure, the respiratory care practitioner must be familiar with and be on alert for (1) acute alveolar hyperventilation superimposed on chronic ventilatory failure and (2) acute ventilatory failure superimposed on chronic ventilatory failure.

❑ **CYANOSIS** (see page 68)
❑ **OXYGENATION INDICES** (see page 69)

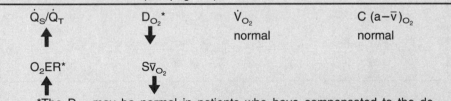

$\dot{Q}_S/\dot{Q}_T$	D_{O_2}*	$\dot{V}_{O_2}$	$C(a-\bar{v})_{O_2}$
↑	↓	normal	normal

O_2ER*	$S\bar{v}_{O_2}$
↑	↓

*The D_{O_2} may be normal in patients who have compensated to the decreased oxygenation status with (1) an increased cardiac output, (2) an increased hemoglobin level, or (3) a combination of both. When the D_{O_2} is normal, the O_2ER is usually normal.

❑ **HEMODYNAMIC INDICES (SEVERE EMPHYSEMA)** (see page 87)

CVP	RAP	$\overline{PA}$	PCWP
↑	↑	↑	normal
CO	SV	SVI	CI
normal	normal	normal	normal
RVSWI	LVSWI	PVR	SVR
↑	normal	↑	normal

❏ **POLYCYTHEMIA, COR PULMONALE** (see page 92)
  * Elevated hemoglobin concentration and hematocrit
  * Distended neck veins
  * Enlarged and tender liver
  * Peripheral edema
  * Pitting edema

❏ **DIGITAL CLUBBING** (see page 93)
❏ **CHEST ASSESSMENT FINDINGS** (see page 6)
  * Hyperresonant percussion note
  * Wheezing
  * Diminished breath sounds
  * Diminished heart sounds
  * Decreased tactile and vocal fremitus (when compromised by chronic bronchitis)
  * Crackles/rhonchi (when accompanied by acute or chronic bronchitis)

❏ **RADIOLOGIC FINDINGS**
  Chest radiograph
  * Translucent (dark) lung fields
  * Depressed or flattened diaphragms
  * Long and narrow heart (pulled downward by diaphragms)
  * Right ventricular enlargement
  * Increased retrosternal airspace (lateral radiograph)

Because of the decreased lung recoil and air trapping in emphysema, the functional residual capacity increases. This decreases the density of the lungs. Consequently, the resistance to x-ray penetration is not as great. This is revealed on x-ray films as areas of translucency or areas that are darker in appearance. Because of the increased functional residual capacity, the diaphragm is depressed or flattened and the heart is often long and narrow (Fig 5-3). The lateral chest radiograph characteristically shows an increased retrosternal airspace (more than 3.0 cm from the anterior surface of the aorta to the back of the sternum measured 3.0 cm below the manubriosternal junction) and flattened diaphragms (Fig 5-4). Finally, since right ventricular enlargement and failure often develop as a secondary problem during the advanced stages of emphysema, an enlarged heart may be seen on the chest radiograph (Fig 5-5).

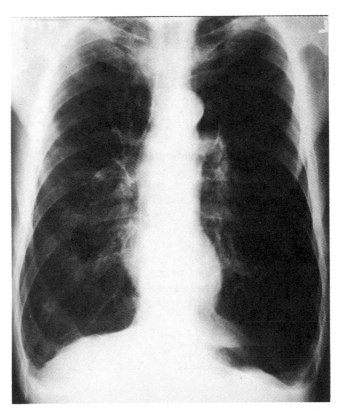

FIG 5-3
Chest x-ray film of a patient with emphysema. As shown, the heart often appears long and narrow as a result of being drawn downward by the descending diaphragm.

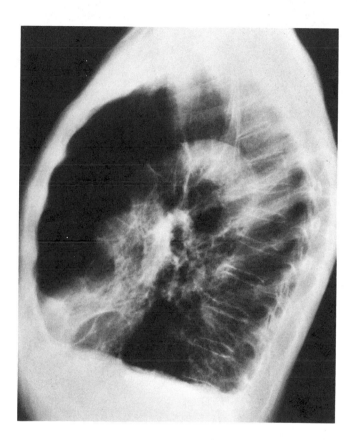

FIG 5-4

Emphysema. Lateral chest radiograph demonstrating a characteristically large retrosternal radiolucency with increased separation of aorta and sternum measuring 4.6 cm, 3 cm below the angle of Louis and extending down to within 3 cm of the diaphragm anteriorly. Both costophrenic angles are obtuse and both hemidiaphragms flat. (From Armstrong P, Wilson AG, Dee P: *Imaging of Diseases of the Chest,* St. Louis, 1990, Mosby-Year Book. Used by permission.)

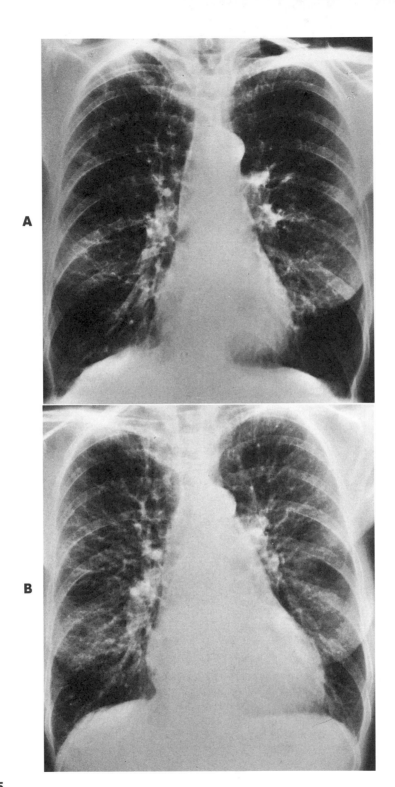

FIG 5-5

Cor pulmonale. **A,** 50-year-old male with chronic airflow obstruction. Lungs are large in volume, the diaphragm is flat, and there is vascular attenuation at the right apex. These features suggest emphysema, and this was supported by a low carbon monoxide diffusion capacity. Lung "markings" are increased peripherally, particularly in the left midzone. **B,** the patient became chronically hypoxic and, with respiratory infections, hypercapnic. One of these episodes was associated with cor pulmonale when the patient became edematous, the heart enlarged, and the hilar and pulmonary parenchymal vessels enlarged. Note that the emphysematous right upper zone shows less vascular markings and is relatively transradiant. Note also that the diaphragm is less depressed and more curved than before. (From Armstrong P, Wilson AG, Dee P: *Imaging of Diseases of the Chest,* St. Louis, 1990, Mosby-Year Book. Used by permission.)

GENERAL MANAGEMENT OF EMPHYSEMA

The general management of emphysema is essentially the same as that of chronic bronchitis—especially since emphysema commonly appears as a disease complex with chronic bronchitis. The patient with emphysema should receive (1) patient and family education, (2) behavioral management in regard to the avoidance of smoking, inhaled irritants, and infection, and (3) proper nutrition instruction.

While sympathomimetic, parasympatholytic, and xanthine agents are commonly prescribed to offset bronchial smooth muscle spasm, it should be noted that these agents do not affect the obstruction produced by airway deterioration and weakening associated with emphysema. When excessive bronchial secretions are present (e.g., emphysema coupled with chronic bronchitis), expectorants, mucolytics, and a variety of respiratory therapy modalities (e.g., chest physical therapy) may be used to enhance the mobilization of the secretions. However, it should be pointed out that bronchial secretions are often absent in the patient with "pure emphysema," without the complication of chronic bronchitis. Antibiotics are commonly administered to prevent or combat secondary respiratory tract infections.*

A new, promising, and expensive intravenous drug, called Prolastin, may be helpful in patients suffering from $\alpha_1 PI$ deficiency. The long-term benefits of Prolastin, however, are yet to be demonstrated.

Finally, when hypoxemia is present, supplemental oxygen may be required. As with the patient with chronic bronchitis, however, caution must be taken not to eliminate the patient's hypoxic drive when chronic ventilatory failure is present. Because acute ventilatory failure (superimposed on chronic ventilatory failure) is often seen in patients with severe emphysema, continuous mechanical ventilation may be required to maintain an adequate ventilatory status. Continuous mechanical ventilation is justified when the acute ventilatory failure is reversible.

*See General Management of Chronic Bronchitis for further discussion and Appendix references for the above medications and treatment modalities.

● ● ● ● EMPHYSEMA CASE STUDY ● ● ● ●

ADMITTING HISTORY AND PHYSICAL EXAMINATION

This 27-year-old male was admitted to the hospital with the chief complaint of dyspnea on exertion. He had a three-year history of recurrent respiratory problems that had required several hospitalizations of several days' duration. Recently, his respiratory status deteriorated to the point where he had to stop working. He had been employed for several years as a cook in a fast-food restaurant where he was continuously exposed to a smoky environment. He had never smoked.

On questioning, the patient related that he had been very short of breath for the past six weeks. During the week prior to admission, he was unable to walk up one flight of stairs without stopping, and his walking tolerance had decreased to about 100 yards. Two days prior to admission he noticed swelling of his ankles, and that he had gained 8 pounds in one week.

On physical examination, an anxious, profusely sweating male in moderate respiratory distress had the following vital signs: regular heart rate of 120/minute, blood pressure of 140/70, respiratory rate of 32/minute, and an oral temperature of 100° F. Inspection of the chest revealed suprasternal notch retraction, with some use of the accessory muscles of inspiration. There was an increased A-P diameter of the chest, and the nail beds were moderately cyanotic. Pitting edema (+3) was noticed on the ankles. The patient was slightly confused. The patient was not able to cooperate well and was unable to concentrate. The lungs were mildly hyperresonant to percussion, and his breath sounds were diminished.

The chest x-ray showed a generalized increase in pulmonary markings and slight hyperinflation of the lungs. There were some infiltrates in the lower lung regions, and possible infiltrates in the right upper lobe. The radiology report suggested the presence of a pneumonic process superimposed on chronic lung disease, and mild signs of cor pulmonale.

On his third attempt, the patient was able to perform a relatively good PEFR effort, with results of 180 L/min. His arterial blood gases, while on a 3 L/min. O_2 nasal cannula were pH 7.27, Pa_{CO_2} 82, HCO_3^- 43, and Pa_{O_2} of 48. Laboratory studies revealed a hemoglobin of 16.5 g/dl, and a white blood count of 15,000/mm^3. Sputum cultures were positive for a variety of pathogenic and nonpathogenic organisms. The serum $\alpha_1 PI$ level was 30 mg/dl (N = 200 to 400 mg/dl). The remainder of the physical examination was not remarkable. The respiratory assessment read as follows:

RESPIRATORY ASSESSMENT AND PLAN

S: "I'm short of breath with any exercise at all." Cough for past six weeks.

O: HR 120, BP 140/70, RR of 32, and Temp. of 100° F. Use of accessory muscles of inspiration, increased A-P diameter, cyanosis, and pitting edema of ankles. Hyperresonant percussion note and diminished breath sounds. Infiltrates, hyper-inflation of lungs, and mild cor pulmonale on CXR. PEFR 180. ABGs: pH 7.27, Pa_{CO_2} 82, HCO_3^- 43, Pa_{O_2} 48. Elevated WBC and gram-positive organisms in sputum. $\alpha_1 PI$ = 30 mg/dl.

A: • Panacinar emphysema ($\alpha_1 PI$ deficiency)
   • Air flow obstruction & air trapping (PEFR & x-ray)
   • Probable pneumonitis (x-ray)
   • Mild cor pulmonale (leg edema, x-ray)
   • Acute on chronic ventilatory failure with moderate hypoxemia (ABGs)

P: Place on continuous oximetry. Trial of bronchodilator therapy per protocol. Trial period of oxygen by HAFOE mask at $F_{I_{O_2}}$ 0.28. Have ventilator on standby.

The hospital course was relatively smooth. Intravenous antibiotics were prescribed. The low-flow oxygen was enough to increase the patient's Pa_{O_2} to an acceptable level and to correct the acute on chronic ventilatory failure. Within an hour after the low-flow oxygen was started, the patient's arterial blood gases were pH 7.36, Pa_{CO_2} 64, HCO_3^- 37, and Pa_{O_2} 81.

The patient's heart rate, respiratory rate, and blood pressure returned to normal. Blood serologies suggest *Mycoplasma pneumoniae* infection. He was managed conservatively and improved steadily. When he appeared to have had the maximum benefit from the hospitalization, he was discharged. Arrangements were made to have him enroll in an α_1-antitrypsin therapy trial and attend pulmonary rehabilitation classes. He was urged to seek alternate employment.

DISCUSSION

This fascinating, but fortunately rare, form of emphysema is one in which "pure" emphysema is the dominant pathology. In patients with α_1-protease inhibitor deficiency, chronic bronchitis may be present, but it is much less common than in usual, cigarette smoking-induced "chronic obstructive pulmonary disease." In this condition, the patient's lack of the protease inhibitor α_1-antitrypsin resulted in WBC-mediated protease destruction of his pulmonary parenchyma. Note the slow, insidious onset of his symptoms.

The selection of a good program of oxygen supplementation for his cor pulmonale and a trial of bronchodilator therapy are certainly indicated. Note the selection of a HAFOE mask because of his initial significant carbon dioxide retention. Pneumococcal and influenza prophylaxis are certainly indicated in this case. Smoking cessation and frequent intravenous administration of α_1-antitrypsin replacement represent modern therapy of this unusual disease, as does counseling that he should not knowingly be exposed to irritants in situations such as the smoky environment of his previous workplace.

SELF-ASSESSMENT QUESTIONS

Multiple Choice

1. The type of emphysema that creates an abnormal enlargement of all structures distal to the terminal bronchioles is called
   a. Centrilobular emphysema.
   b. α_1-protease inhibitor deficiency emphysema.
   c. ZZ phenotype emphysema.
   d. Terminal bronchiole emphysema.
   e. Panlobular emphysema.

2. What is the normal level of α_1-protease inhibitor?
   a. 0 to 200 mg/dl
   b. 200 to 400 mg/dl
   c. 400 to 600 mg/dl
   d. 600 to 800 mg/dl
   e. 800 to 900 mg/dl

3. The diffusion capacity of patients with emphysema is
   a. Increased.
   b. Decreased.
   c. Normal.

4. Patients with severe emphysema commonly demonstrate the following oxygenation indices:
   I. Decreased $S\bar{v}_{O_2}$
   II. Increased O_2ER
   III. Decreased D_{O_2}
   IV. Increased $C(a - \bar{v})_{O_2}$
   a. I only
   b. III only
   c. IV only
   d. I, II, and III only
   e. I, II, III, and IV only

5. The phenotype associated with a low serum concentration of α_1-protease inhibitor is
   a. MM phenotype.
   b. MZ phenotype.
   c. ZZ phenotype.
   d. M phenotype.
   e. ZM phenotype.

6. Which of the following pulmonary function study findings are associated with severe emphysema?
   I. Increased FRC
   II. Decreased PEFR
   III. Increased RV
   IV. Decreased FVC
   a. I and III only
   b. III and IV only
   c. II and III only
   d. II, III, and IV only
   e. I, II, III, and IV only

7. The patient with severe emphysema commonly demonstrates the following hemodynamic indices:
   I. Decreased CVP
   II. Increased $\overline{PA}$
   III. Decreased RVSWI
   IV. Increased PVR
   a. I only
   b. III only
   c. II and IV only
   d. I and II only
   e. II, III, and IV only

8. Because *acute ventilatory changes* are often seen in patients with chronic ventilatory failure, the respiratory care practitioner must be on alert for this problem in patients with severe emphysema. Which of the following arterial blood gas values represent acute alveolar hyperventilation superimposed on chronic ventilatory failure?

    I. Increased pH

    II. Increased Pa_{CO_2}

    III. Increased HCO_3^-

    IV. Increased Pa_{O_2}

      a. II only

      b. II and IV only

      c. I and III only

      d. I, II, and III only

      e. I, II, III, and IV only

9. The chest radiograph of a patient with emphysema is

    I. Opaque.

    II. Whiter in appearance.

    III. More translucent.

    IV. Darker in appearance.

      a. I only

      b. II only

      c. I and III only

      d. II and III only

      e. III and IV only

10. The single most important etiologic factor in emphysema is thought to be

      a. α_1-protease inhibitor deficiency.

      b. Cigarette smoking.

      c. Infection.

      d. Sulfur dioxide.

      e. Ozone.

Answers appear in Appendix XXI.

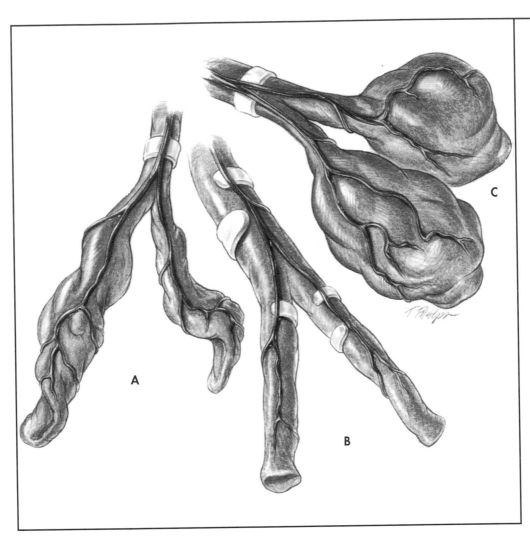

BRONCHIECTASIS

FIG 6-1

Bronchiectasis. **A,** varicose bronchiectasis. **B,** cylindrical bronchiectasis. **C,** saccular bronchiectasis. (See also Plate 5.)

CHAPTER 6

Bronchiectasis

ANATOMIC ALTERATIONS OF THE LUNGS

Bronchiectasis is characterized by chronic dilation and distortion of one or more bronchi due to extensive inflammation and destruction of the bronchial wall cartilage, blood vessels, elastic tissue, and smooth muscle components. Either or both lungs may be involved. Bronchiectasis is commonly limited to a lobe or a segment and is frequently found in the lower lobes. The smaller bronchi, with less supporting cartilage, are predominantly affected.

Because of bronchial wall destruction, the mucociliary clearing mechanism is impaired. This results in the accumulation of copious amounts of bronchial secretions that often become foul-smelling due to secondary colonization with anaerobic organisms. This condition often leads to "secondary bronchial smooth muscle constriction." The small bronchi and bronchioles distal to the affected areas become partially or totally obstructed with secretions. This condition leads to either or both of the following anatomic alterations: (1) hyperinflation of the distal alveoli as a result of expiratory check-valve obstruction, or (2) atelectasis, consolidation, and parenchymal fibrosis as a result of complete bronchial obstruction.

Three forms—or anatomic varieties—of bronchiectasis have been described: *varicose (fusiform), cylindrical (tubular),* and *saccular (cystic).*

Varicose Bronchiectasis

The bronchi are dilated and constricted in an irregular fashion similar to varicose veins, ultimately resulting in a distorted, bulbous shape (Fig. 6-1, *A*).

Cylindrical Bronchiectasis

The bronchi are dilated and have regular outlines similar to a tube. The dilated bronchi fail to taper for six to ten generations and then in the bronchogram appear to end squarely because of mucus obstruction (Fig. 6-1, *B*).

Saccular Bronchiectasis

The bronchi progressively increase in diameter until they end in large, cystlike sacs in the lung parenchyma. This form of bronchiectasis causes the greatest damage to the tracheobronchial tree. The bronchial walls become composed of fibrous tissue alone—cartilage, elastic tissue, and smooth muscle are all absent (Fig. 6-1, *C*).

To summarize, the following are the major pathologic or structural changes associated with bronchiectasis:

- Chronic dilation and distortion of bronchial airways
- Excessive production of often foul-smelling sputum
- Smooth muscle constriction of bronchial airways
- Hyperinflated alveoli
- Atelectasis, consolidation, and parenchymal fibrosis

ETIOLOGY

The etiology of bronchiectasis is not always clear, but there is evidence that indicates that the disease may be either acquired or congenital.

Acquired Bronchiectasis

Pulmonary Infection.—Bronchiectasis is commonly seen in individuals who have repeated and prolonged episodes of respiratory tract infections. Children who have frequent bouts of bronchopneumonia—due to the respiratory complications of measles, chickenpox, pertussis, or influenza, for example—may acquire some form of bronchiectasis later in life.

Bronchial Obstruction.—Bronchial obstruction caused by tumor masses, enlarged hilar lymph nodes, or aspirated foreign bodies may result in bronchiectasis distal to the obstruction. It is felt that these conditions impair the mucociliary clearing mechanism, and this impairment, in turn, favors the development of necrotizing bacterial infections.

Pulmonary tuberculosis.—Because of the inflammatory process and bronchial wall destruction associated with pulmonary tuberculosis, bronchiectasis is a not uncommon secondary complication.

Congenital Bronchiectasis

Kartagener's syndrome.—Kartagener's syndrome is a triad consisting of bronchiectasis, dextrocardia (having the heart on the right side of the body), and paranasal sinusitis. Kartagener's syndrome accounts for as much as 20% of all congenital bronchiectasis.

Hypogammaglobulinemia.—Bronchiectasis is commonly seen in individuals who have inadequate regional or systemic defense mechanisms because of inherited or acquired immune deficiency disorders. These individuals have a high predisposition for recurrent episodes of respiratory infections.

Cystic Fibrosis.—Because of impairment of the mucociliary clearing mechanism and the abundance of stagnant, thick mucus associated with cystic fibrosis, bronchial obstruction due to mucus plugging and bronchial infections frequently results. The necrotizing inflammations that develop under these conditions often lead to secondary bronchiectasis.

Depending on the amount of bronchial secretions and the degree of bronchial destruction and fibrosis associated with bronchiectasis, the disease may create an obstructive or a restrictive lung disorder—or a combination of both. If the majority of the bronchial airways are only partially obstructed, the bronchiectasis will manifest primarily as an obstructive lung disorder. If, on the other hand, the majority of the bronchial airways are completely obstructed, the distal alveoli will collapse, and the bronchiectasis will manifest primarily as a restrictive disorder. Finally, it should be emphasized that if the disease is limited to a relatively small portion of the lung—as it often is—the patient may not have any of the following clinical manifestations.

❑ **INCREASED RESPIRATORY RATE**

Several pathophysiologic mechanisms operating simultaneously may lead to an increased ventilatory rate. These are (see page 17)
- Stimulation of peripheral chemoreceptors
- Decreased lung compliance/increased ventilatory rate relationship
- Anxiety

❑ **PULMONARY FUNCTION STUDY FINDINGS**
When Primarily Obstructive in Nature, Expiratory Maneuver Findings (see page 41)

FVC	FEF$_{200-1,200}$	FEF$_{25\%-75\%}$	FEV$_T$
↓	↓	↓	↓
FEV$_1$/FVC ratio	MVV	PEFR	$\dot{V}_{max_{50}}$
↓	↓	↓	↓

Lung Volume and Capacity Findings (see page 48)

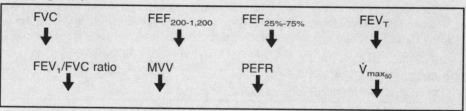

V$_T$	RV	FRC	RV/TLC ratio
↑	↑	↑	↑
TLC	VC	IC	ERV
↑/normal	↓/normal	↓	↓

When Primarily Restrictive in Nature, Lung Volume and Capacity Findings (see page 39)

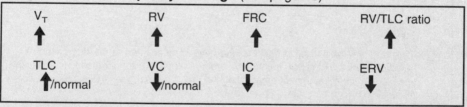

V$_T$	RV	RV/TLC	FRC
↓	↓	normal	↓
TLC	VC	IC	ERV
↓	↓	↓	↓

❑ **INCREASED HEART RATE (PULSE), CARDIAC OUTPUT, AND BLOOD PRESSURE** (see page 86)
❑ **INCREASED ANTEROPOSTERIOR CHEST DIAMETER (BARREL CHEST)** (see page 49)
❑ **PURSED-LIP BREATHING** (see page 49)

- ❑ **USE OF ACCESSORY MUSCLES DURING INSPIRATION** (see page 51)
- ❑ **USE OF ACCESSORY MUSCLES DURING EXPIRATION** (see page 54)
- ❑ **ARTERIAL BLOOD GASES**

Mild to Moderate Bronchiectasis

Acute Alveolar Hyperventilation with Hypoxemia (see page 57)

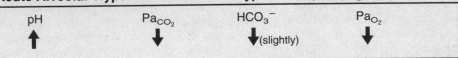

pH	Pa_{CO_2}	HCO_3^-	Pa_{O_2}
↑	↓	↓(slightly)	↓

Severe Bronchiectasis

Chronic Ventilatory Failure with Hypoxemia (see page 60)

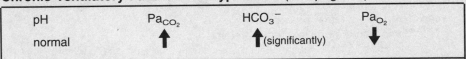

pH	Pa_{CO_2}	HCO_3^-	Pa_{O_2}
normal	↑	↑(significantly)	↓

Acute Ventilatory Changes Superimposed on Chronic Ventilatory Failure (see page 65)

Because acute ventilatory changes are frequently seen in patients with chronic ventilatory failure, the respiratory care practitioner must be familiar with and be on the alert for (1) acute alveolar hyperventilation superimposed on chronic ventilatory failure and (2) acute ventilatory failure superimposed on chronic ventilatory failure.

- ❑ **CYANOSIS** (see page 68)
- ❑ **OXYGENATION INDICES** (see page 69)

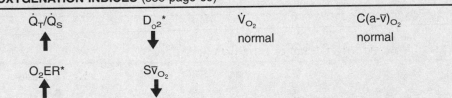

$\dot{Q}_T/\dot{Q}_S$	D_{O_2}*	$\dot{V}_{O_2}$	$C(a-\bar{v})_{O_2}$
↑	↓	normal	normal

O_2ER*	$S\bar{v}_{O_2}$		
↑	↓		

*The D_{O_2} may be normal in patients who have compensated to the decreased oxygenation status with (1) an increased cardiac output, (2) an increased hemoglobin level, or (3) a combination of both. When the D_{O_2} is normal, the O_2ER is usually normal.

- ❑ **HEMODYNAMIC INDICES (SEVERE BRONCHIECTASIS)** (see page 87)

CVP	RAP	$\overline{PA}$	PCWP
↑	↑	↑	normal

CO	SV	SVI	CI
normal	normal	normal	normal

RVSWI	LVSWI	PVR	SVR
↑	normal	↑	normal

- ❑ **POLYCYTHEMIA, COR PULMONALE** (see page 92)
  - Elevated hemoglobin concentration and hematocrit
  - Distended neck veins

- Enlarged and tender liver
- Peripheral edema
- Pitting edema

❏ **CHEST ASSESSMENT FINDINGS** (see page 6)
When primarily obstructive in nature
- Decreased tactile and vocal fremitus
- Hyperresonant percussion note
- Diminished breath sounds
- Crackles/rhonchi/wheezing

When primarily restrictive in nature (over areas of atelectasis and consolidation)
- Increased tactile and vocal fremitus
- Bronchial breath sounds
- Whispered pectoriloquy
- Dull percussion note

❏ **COUGH, SPUTUM PRODUCTION AND HEMOPTYSIS** (see page 93)
A chronic cough with production of large quantities of foul-smelling sputum is a hall-mark of bronchiectasis. A 24-hour collection of sputum is usually voluminous and tends to settle into several different layers. Streaks of blood are seen frequently in the sputum, presumably originating from necrosis of the bronchial walls and erosion of bronchial blood vessels. Frank hemoptysis may also occur from time to time, but is rarely life-threatening. Because of the excessive bronchial secretions, secondary bacterial infections are frequent. *Haemophilus influenzae, streptococcus, Pseudomonas aeruginosa*, and various anaerobic organisms are commonly cultured from the sputum of patients with bronchiectasis.

The productive cough in bronchiectasis is triggered by the large amount of secretions that fill the tracheobronchial tree. The stagnant secretions stimulate the subepithelial mechanoreceptors, which in turn produce a vagal reflex that triggers a cough. The subepithelial mechanoreceptors are found in the trachea, bronchi, and bronchioles, but they are predominantly located in the upper airways.

❏ **RADIOLOGIC FINDINGS**
Chest radiograph
When primarily obstructive in nature
- Translucent (dark) lung fields
- Depressed or flattened diaphragms
- Long and narrow heart (pulled downward by diaphragms)
- Right ventricular enlargement

When the pathophysiology of bronchiectasis is primarily obstructive in nature, the lungs become hyperinflated, the functional residual volume increases, and the density of the lungs decreases. As a result of this condition, the resistance to x-ray penetration is not as great and is revealed on the chest radiograph as areas of translucency or areas that are darker in appearance. Because of the increased functional residual capacity, the diaphragms may be depressed and are seen in this position on the radiograph. Finally, since right ventricular enlargement and failure often develop as a secondary problem during the advanced stages of bronchiectasis, an enlarged heart may be seen on the chest radiograph.

When primarily restrictive in nature
- Increased opacity
- Atelectasis and consolidation

When atelectasis and consolidation develop as a result of bronchiectasis, an increased opacity will be seen in these areas on the radiograph.

Bronchogram

Bronchography (the injection of an opaque contrast material into the tracheobronchial tree) is occasionally performed on patients with bronchiectasis. The bronchogram obtained from this procedure may be useful in diagnosing bronchiectasis and delineating the extent and type of tracheobronchial involvement.

In *cylindrical bronchiectasis,* the bronchogram shows dilated, cylinder-shaped bronchioles. There may be increased bronchial markings and adjacent emphysema (Fig. 6-2). In *saccular bronchiectasis,* the bronchogram shows large, saclike structures; fibrotic markings; associated atelectasis; and adjacent emphysema (Fig. 6-3). In *varicose bronchiectasis,* the bronchogram may show bronchi that are dilated and constricted in an irregular fashion and terminate in a distorted, bulbous shape (Fig. 6-4). Computerized tomography of the chest has largely replaced this technique.

CT scan

- Increased bronchial wall opacity will often be seen. The bronchial walls may appear as:
  - Thick
  - Dilated
  - Ring lines or clusters
  - Signet ring-shaped
  - Flame-shaped

The CT scan changes may include many signs that are similar to the chest radiograph findings. The bronchial walls may appear thick, dilated, or as rings of opacities arranged in lines or clusters (Fig. 6-5). A characteristic appearance in bronchiectasis is the "signet ring" opacity produced by the ring shadow of a dilated airway with its accompanying artery. Airways that are filled with secretions produce rounded or "flame-shaped" opacities that can be identified by following them through adjacent sections to unfilled airways. Bullae and cystic bronchiectasis are difficult to distinguish on the CT scan. The CT scan also confirms atelectasis, consolidation, and hyperinflation.

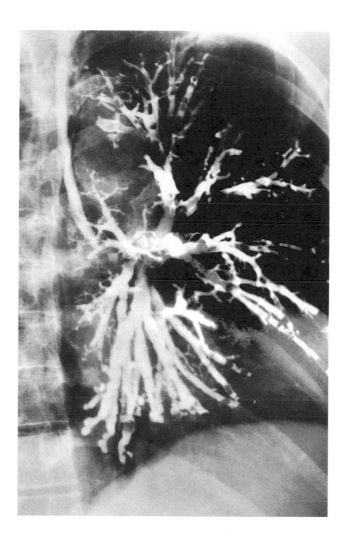

FIG 6-2

Cylindrical bronchiectasis. Left posterior oblique projection of a left bronchogram showing cylindrical bronchiectasis affecting the whole of the lower lobe except for the superior segment. Few side branches fill. Basal airways are crowded together, indicating volume loss of the lower lobe, a common finding in bronchiectasis. (From Armstrong P, Wilson AG, Dee P: *Imaging of Diseases of the Chest,* St. Louis, 1990, Mosby-Year Book. Used by permission.)

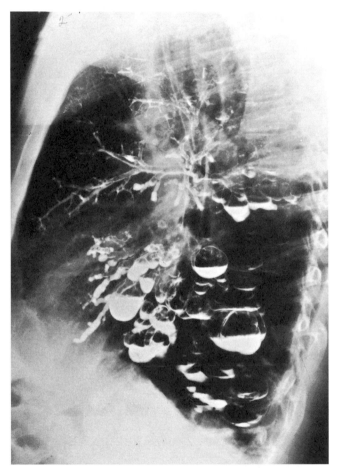

FIG 6-3
Saccular bronchiectasis. Right lateral bronchogram showing saccular bronchiectasis affecting mainly the lower lobe and posterior segment of the upper lobe. (From Armstrong P, Wilson AG, Dee P: *Imaging of Diseases of the Chest,* St. Louis, 1990, Mosby-Year Book. Used by permission.)

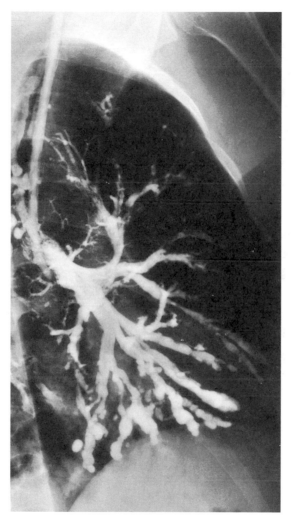

FIG 6-4
Varicose bronchiectasis. Left posterior oblique projection of left bronchogram in a patient with the ciliary dyskinesia syndrome. All basal bronchi are affected by varicose bronchiectasis. (From Armstrong P, Wilson AG, Dee P: *Imaging of Diseases of the Chest,* St. Louis, 1990, Mosby-Year Book. Used by permission.)

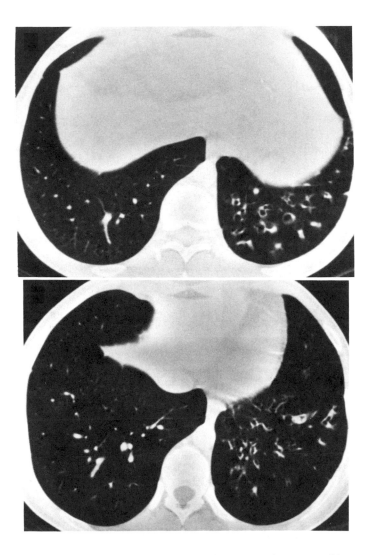

FIG 6-5
Bronchiectasis. High-resolution thin-section (1.5-mm) computed tomographic scan showing multiple oval and rounded ring opacities in the left lower lobe. The right lung appears normal. The fact that the airways tend to be arranged in a linear fashion and to have walls of more than hairline thickness helps to distinguish these bronchiectatic airways from cysts or bullae. (From Armstrong P, Wilson AG, Dee P: *Imaging of Diseases of the Chest,* St. Louis, 1990, Mosby-Year Book. Used by permission.)

GENERAL MANAGEMENT OF BRONCHIECTASIS
Mobilization of Bronchial Secretions

Because of the excessive mucus production and accumulation associated with bronchiectasis, a number of respiratory therapy modalities may be used to enhance the mobilization of bronchial secretions (see Appendix XI).

Medications

Mucolytic Agents.—Mucolytic agents may be used to break down the large amounts of thick tenacious mucus (see Appendix VI).

Sympathomimetics.—Sympathomimetic drugs are commonly prescribed for patients with bronchiectasis to offset bronchial smooth muscle spasm (see Appendix II).

Parasympatholytics.—Parasympatholytic agents are also used to offset bronchial smooth muscle constriction (see Appendix III).

Xanthines.—Xanthines are used to enhance bronchial smooth muscle relaxation (see Appendix IV).

Expectorants.—Expectorants are often used when water alone is not sufficient to facilitate expectoration (see Appendix VII).

Antibiotics.—Antibiotics are commonly administered to prevent or combat secondary respiratory tract infections (see Appendix VIII).

Supplemental Oxygen

Because hypoxemia is often associated with bronchiectasis, supplemental oxygen may be required. The hypoxemia that develops in bronchiectasis is caused by the pulmonary shunting associated with the disorder. It should be noted, however, that when the patient demonstrates chronic ventilatory failure during the advanced stages of bronchiectasis, caution must be taken not to eliminate the patient's hypoxic ventilatory drive.

Continuous Mechanical Ventilation

Because acute ventilatory failure (superimposed on chronic ventilatory failure) is often seen in patients with severe bronchiectasis, continuous mechanical ventilation may be required to maintain an adequate ventilatory status. Continuous mechanical ventilation is justified when the acute ventilatory failure is thought to be reversible.

• • • •   BRONCHIECTASIS CASE STUDY   • • • •

ADMITTING HISTORY AND PHYSICAL EXAMINATION

A 31-year-old patient consulted his physician concerning an increasingly productive cough. He reported a "bad case" of pneumonia seven years ago and several episodes of pulmonary infection since that time. On such occasions, he was usually prescribed an antibiotic and, until six months ago, the infections responded readily to treatment. Six months ago, he noticed increasing severity of his chronic cough and, for the first time, his cough became productive. Most recently, he produced up to a cup of thick, tenacious, yellow-white sputum per day. Within the past two to three days he had noticed some dark blood mixed with the sputum. He also noticed some dyspnea on exertion, but this had not been particularly troublesome. The past medical history revealed chronic sinusitis, present since adolescence, but was otherwise unremarkable.

Physical examination revealed a well-developed adult male in no apparent distress. Vital signs were within normal limits. He coughed frequently during the examination and did produce a moderate amount of yellow, blood-streaked sputum. There were crackles and rhonchi heard over the right lower lung fields posteriorly.

Laboratory results showed a mild leukocytosis, but were otherwise normal. Sputum culture produced *M. influenzae*. A CT scan revealed saccular dilations of the right lower lobe bronchus. The respiratory therapist assigned to assess and treat the patient at this time recorded the following in the patient's chart:

RESPIRATORY ASSESSMENT AND PLAN

S: Productive cough, hemoptysis, worse in past 5 months. Mild dyspnea on exertion.

O: Observed moderate amount of mucopurulent, blood-streaked sputum. Crackles and rhonchi over R.L.L. Sputum culture: *H. influenzae.* CT scan: suggests saccular dilation of R.L.L. bronchi.

A: • Postpneumonic bronchiectasis R.L.L. (history & CT scan)
 • Excessive airway secretions & sputum production (rhonchi & sputum expectoration)
 • Acute bronchial infection & hemoptysis (yellow & blood-streaked sputum)

P: Bronchial hygiene and aerosol therapy per protocols, to include postural drainage and a short trial of aerosolized mucolytic (acetylcysteine).

The patient was treated vigorously with chest physiotherapy and mucolytic therapy. The physician prescribed antibiotics, and pneumonia vaccine was given. The patient was discharged from the hospital after three days, considerably improved. He was instructed to seek prompt medical attention with all pulmonary infections. His wife was instructed in postural drainage techniques.

DISCUSSION

The main problem facing the respiratory care practitioner caring for bronchiectasis is one of efficient removal of excessive bronchopulmonary secretions. Over the years, postural drainage and percussion, good systemic hydration, and judicious use of antibiotics have been the hallmarks of therapy. In more recent times, intermittent use of mucolytics has been more important. Pneumococcal prophylaxis is, of course, important, as is prompt attention to parenchymal pulmonary infections.

The clinical distinction between chronic bronchiectasis and cystic fibrosis is a subtle one, and this latter condition must always be ruled out in bronchiectatic patients.

The goal of long-term therapy in bronchiectasis is prevention of lung parenchyma-destroying pulmonary infections, and avoidance of frequent hospitalizations. Hemoptysis is often a sign of more deep-seated infection requiring antibiotic therapy.

Note that in this case, patient and family instruction in the techniques of percussion and postural drainage was not overlooked.

SELF-ASSESSMENT QUESTIONS

Multiple Choice

1. In which of the following forms of bronchiectasis are the bronchi dilated and constricted in an irregular fashion?
   - I. Fusiform
   - II. Saccular
   - III. Varicose
   - IV. Cylindrical
     - a. I only
     - b. II only
     - c. III only
     - d. II and IV only
     - e. I and III only

2. Which of the following are common causes of acquired bronchiectasis?
   - I. Hypogammaglobulinemia
   - II. Pulmonary tuberculosis
   - III. Kartagener's syndrome
   - IV. Cystic fibrosis
     - a. I only
     - b. II only
     - c. III only
     - d. III and IV only
     - e. I, III, and IV only

3. In the primarily obstructive form of bronchiectasis, the patient commonly demonstrates
   - I. Decreased FRC.
   - II. Increased $FEF_{25\%-75\%}$.
   - III. Decreased PEFR.
   - IV. Increased $\dot{V}_{max\ 50}$.
     - a. I only
     - b. III only
     - c. I and III only
     - d. II and IV only
     - e. III, and IV only

4. Mucolytic agents are commonly used to enhance the mobilization of secretions in patients with bronchiectasis. Which of the following is/are classified as a mucolytic agent(s)?
   - I. Acetylcysteine
   - II. Cromolyn sodium
   - III. Beclomethasone
   - IV. rhDNase
     - a. I only
     - b. II only
     - c. IV only
     - d. II and III only
     - e. I and IV only

5. Which of the following is considered the hallmark of bronchiectasis?
   - a. Chronic cough and large quantities of foul-smelling sputum
   - b. Abnormal bronchogram
   - c. Acute ventilatory failure superimposed on chronic ventilatory failure
   - d. Presents as both a restrictive and obstructive pulmonary disorder
   - e. Acute alveolar hyperventilation superimposed on chronic ventilatory failure

6. Which of the following is/are commonly cultured in the sputum of patients with bronchiectasis?
   - I. *Staphylococcus*
   - II. *Pseudomonas aeruginosa*
   - III. *Haemophilus influenzae*

IV. *Klebsiella*
   a. I only
   b. III only
   c. IV only
   d. I, II, and III only
   e. I, II, III, and IV

7. When the pathophysiology of bronchiectasis is primarily obstructive in nature, the patient demonstrates the following clinical manifestations:
   I. Decreased tactile and vocal fremitus
   II. Bronchial breath sounds
   III. Dull percussion note
   IV. Crackles/rhonchi/wheezing
   a. II only
   b. III only
   c. I and IV only
   d. II, and IV only
   e. II, III, and IV

8. Which of the following is/are used to diagnose bronchiectasis?
   I. Arterial blood gases
   II. Bronchography
   III. Oxygen indices
   IV. Computerized tomography
   a. II only
   b. III only
   c. I and III only
   d. II and IV only
   e. I, II, III, and IV

9. Which of the following is/are congenital causes of bronchiectasis?
   I. Pertussis
   II. Cystic fibrosis
   III. Chickenpox
   IV. Measles
   a. I only
   b. II only
   c. III and IV only
   d. I and III only
   e. I, III, and IV only

10. Which of the following hemodynamic indices are associated with bronchiectasis?
   I. Decreased CVP
   II. Increased $\overline{PA}$
   III. Decreased RVSWI
   IV. Increased RAP
   a. II only
   b. III only
   c. II and IV only
   d. I and III only
   e. I, II, III, and IV

Answers appear in Appendix XXI.

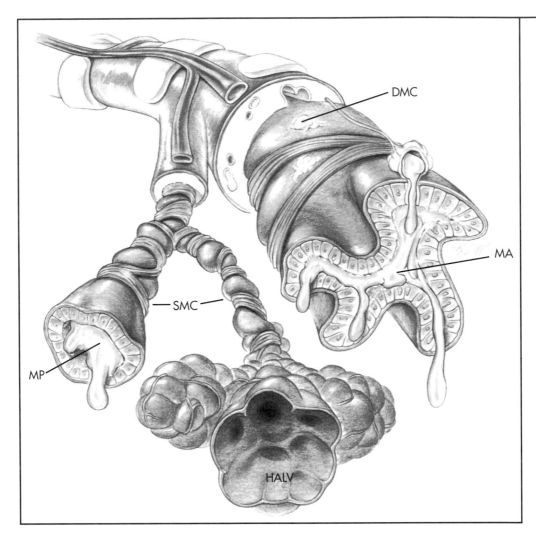

ASTHMA

FIG 7-1

Asthma. *DMC* = degranulation of mast cell; *SMC* = smooth muscle constriction; *MA* = mucus accumulation; *MP* = mucus plug; *HALV* = hyperinflation of alveoli. (See also Plate 6.)

Asthma

ANATOMIC ALTERATIONS OF THE LUNGS

During an asthma attack, the smooth muscles surrounding the small airways of the lungs constrict in response to a particular stimulus. In time the smooth muscle layers hypertrophy and may increase to three times their normal size. There is a proliferation of goblet cells, and the bronchial mucous glands enlarge. The airways become filled with thick, tenacious mucus, and extensive mucus plugging may develop. The bronchial mucosa is edematous and infiltrated with eosinophils and other inflammatory cells. The cilia are damaged, and the basement membrane of the mucosa is thicker than normal. As a result of smooth muscle constriction, bronchial mucosal edema, and mucus hypersecretion, air trapping and alveolar hyperinflation develop. A remarkable feature of bronchial asthma is that the anatomic alterations that occur during an asthmatic attack are completely absent between the asthmatic episodes (Fig. 7-1).

To summarize, the major pathologic or structural changes observed during an asthmatic episode are as follows:

- Smooth muscle constriction of bronchial airways (bronchospasm)
- Excessive production of thick, tenacious tracheobronchial secretions
- Mucus plugging
- Hyperinflation of alveoli

ETIOLOGY

Asthma is divided into two major types according to the precipitating factors: *extrinsic asthma,* or asthma caused by external or environmental agents, and *intrinsic asthma,* or asthma that occurs in the absence or lack of evidence of an antigen-antibody reaction. While some authorities believe that the distinction between these terms is of minimal clinical value, the terms are nevertheless widely used.

Extrinsic Asthma (Allergic or Atopic Asthma)

When an asthmatic episode can be clearly associated with exposure to a specific antigenic agent (e.g., pollen, grass and weeds, house dust, house mites, animal dander, or feathers), the patient is said to have *extrinsic asthma* (also called allergic or atopic asthma). Extrinsic asthma is an *immediate* (Type I) *anaphylaxis* hypersensitivity reaction. Extrinsic asthma occurs in individuals who have **atopy,** which is a hypersensitivity condition associated with (1) a genetic predisposition and (2) an excessive amount of IgE antibody production in response to a variety of antigens.

About 10% to 20% of the general population are atopic and, therefore, have a tendency to develop an IgE-mediated allergic reaction such as asthma, hay fever, allergic rhinitis, or eczema. Such individuals develop a wheal and flare reaction to a variety of skin test allergens. Extrinsic asthma is family-related and usually appears in children and in adults under the age of 30 years. It often disappears after puberty.

Because extrinsic asthma is associated with an antigen-antibody-induced bronchospasm, an immunologic mechanism plays an important role. Like other organs, the lungs are protected against infection by certain immunologic mechanisms. Under normal circumstances, these mechanisms function without any apparent clinical evidence of their activity. In patients susceptible to extrinsic or allergic asthma, however, it is the hypersensitivity of the immune response itself that actually creates the disease.

The Immunologic Mechanism

1. When a susceptible individual is exposed to a certain antigen, lymphoid tissue cells form specific IgE (reaginic) antibodies. The IgE antibodies attach themselves to the surface of mast cells in the bronchial walls (Fig. 7-2, *A*).

2. Reexposure or continued exposure to the same antigen creates an antigen-antibody reaction on the surface of the mast cell, which in turn causes the mast cell to degranulate and release chemical mediators such as histamine, eosinphil chemotactic factor of anaphylaxis (ECF-A), neutrophil chemotactic factors (NCF), leukotrienes (formerly known as slow-reacting substance of anaphylaxis [SRS-A]), prostaglandins, and platelet-activating factor (PAF) (Fig. 7-2, *B*).

3. The release of these chemical mediators stimulates parasympathetic nerve endings in the bronchial airways, leading to a reflex bronchoconstriction. Moreover, these chemical mediators increase the permeability of capillaries, which results in the dilation of blood vessels and tissue edema (Fig. 7-2, *C*).

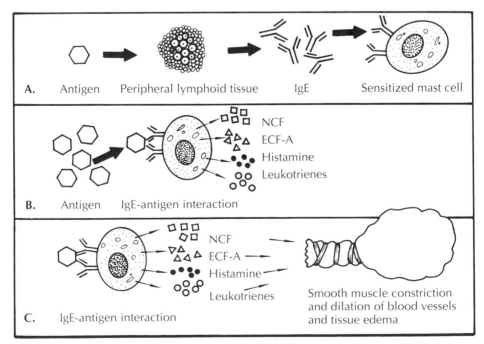

FIG 7-2
The immunologic mechanism in asthma.

The patient with extrinsic asthma may demonstrate an early asthmatic response, a late asthmatic response, or a dual asthmatic response. The *early asthmatic response* begins within minutes of exposure to an inhaled antigen and resolves in approximately one hour. A *late asthmatic response* begins several hours after the exposure of an inhaled antigen, but lasts much longer. The late asthmatic response may or may not follow an early asthmatic response. An early asthmatic response followed by a late asthmatic response is called a *dual asthmatic response*.

Intrinsic Asthma (Nonallergic or Nonatopic Asthma)

When an asthmatic episode cannot be directly linked to a specific antigen, it is referred to as intrinsic asthma (also called nonallergic or nonatopic asthma). The etiologic factors responsible for intrinsic asthma are elusive. Individuals with intrinsic asthma are not hypersensitive or atopic to environmental antigens and have a normal serum IgE level. The onset of intrinsic asthma usually occurs after the age of 40 years, and there is typically no strong family history of allergy.

In spite of the general distinction between extrinsic and intrinsic asthma, a significant overlap exists. Clinically, it is often impossible to distinguish between the two. Precipitating factors known to cause intrinsic asthma are referred to as *nonspecific stimuli*. Some of the more common nonspecific stimuli associated with intrinsic asthma include the following (Fig. 7-3):

Infections.—While bacterial infections may cause asthma, viral upper airway infection is more predominate. For example, intrinsic asthma is commonly seen in children with a respiratory syncytial virus, rhinovirus, and influenza virus.

Exercise and Cold Air.—It has long been known that asthma is associated with vigorous exercise. The asthmatic episode typically occurs about 5 to 10 minutes after, rather than during, the exercise. Exercise in cold dry air (e.g., jogging, ice skating, or cross country skiing) is more likely to provoke an asthmatic response.

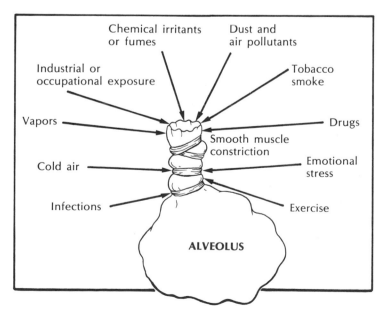

FIG 7-3
Intrinsic factors triggering asthma.

Industrial Pollutants or Occupational Exposure.—Numerous industrial pollutants or occupational exposure are associated with asthma. Atmospheric industrial pollutants known to provoke asthma include smoke, sulfur dioxide, nitrous oxide, ozone, dust, and noxious gases. Common occupational substances include isocyanate (found in polyurethane, plastics, varnish, and car spray paints), trimellitic anhydride (found in epoxy resins), and organic dusts (found in various woods, plants). It may also be included here that the inhalation of cigarette (or marijuana) smoke is associated with airway inflammation and bronchoconstriction.

Drugs, Food Additives, and Food Preservatives

Asthma is associated with aspirin and other nonsteroidal anti-inflammatory drugs (NSAIDs). It is estimated that as much as 20% of the asthmatic population is sensitive to aspirin and NSAIDs. Various beta-adrenergic blocking agents used to treat hypertension and some cardiac disorders (e.g., propranolol or metoprolol) may provoke an asthmatic episode. In regard to food additives, the yellow food-coloring agent called *tartrazine* may provoke an asthmatic episode. The ingestion of tartrazine is especially contraindicated in patients sensitive to aspirin. *Bisulfites* and *metabisulfites,* commonly used as preservatives and antioxidants in restaurant food (e.g., salad bars, certain wines, beers, and dried fruits), are known to provoke bronchoconstriction. It is estimated that about 5% of the asthmatic population is sensitive to food and drink that contain sulfites.

Gastroesophageal Reflux.—Gastroesophageal reflux (GER) (regurgitation), which occurs to some extent even in normal individuals, appears to contribute significantly to the stimulation of bronchoconstriction in some patients. The precise mechanism of this relationship is not known.

Sleep (Nocturnal Asthma).—Patients with asthma often have more difficulty late at night or in the early morning hours. Precipitating factors associated with nocturnal asthma include gastroesophageal reflux, retained airway secretions (caused by a suppressed cough reflex during sleep), exposure to irritants or allergens in the bedroom, and prolonged time between medications.

Emotional Stress.—In some patients, the exacerbation of asthma appears to correlate with emotional, stress, or psychological factors.

OVERVIEW
OF THE CARDIOPULMONARY CLINICAL MANIFESTATIONS ASSOCIATED WITH
AN ASTHMATIC EPISODE

❏ **INCREASED RESPIRATORY RATE**
Several pathophysiologic mechanisms operating simultaneously may lead to an increased ventilatory rate. These are (see page 17)
• Stimulation of peripheral chemoreceptors
• Decreased lung compliance/increased ventilatory rate relationship
• Anxiety

❏ **PULMONARY FUNCTION STUDY FINDINGS**

Expiratory Maneuver Findings (see page 41)

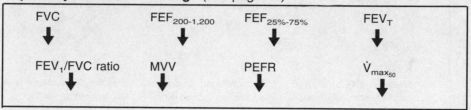

Lung Volume and Capacity Findings (see page 48)

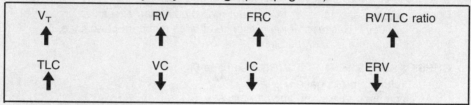

❏ **INCREASED HEART RATE (PULSE), CARDIAC OUTPUT, AND BLOOD PRESSURE** (see page 86)
❏ **INCREASED ANTEROPOSTERIOR CHEST DIAMETER (BARREL CHEST)** (see page 49)
❏ **PURSED-LIP BREATHING** (see page 49)
❏ **USE OF ACCESSORY MUSCLES DURING INSPIRATION** (see page 51)
❏ **USE OF ACCESSORY MUSCLES DURING EXPIRATION** (see page 54)
❏ **SUBSTERNAL INTERCOSTAL RETRACTIONS** (see page 98)
Substernal, supraclavicular, and intercostal retractions during inspiration may be seen, particularly in children.

❏ **ARTERIAL BLOOD GASES**

Mild to Moderate Asthmatic Episode

Acute Alveolar Hyperventilation with Hypoxemia (see page 57)

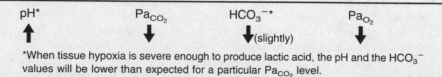

*When tissue hypoxia is severe enough to produce lactic acid, the pH and the HCO_3^- values will be lower than expected for a particular Pa_{CO_2} level.

Severe Asthmatic Episode (Status Asthmaticus)

Acute Ventilatory Failure with Hypoxemia (see page 59)

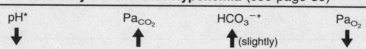

*When tissue hypoxia is severe enough to produce lactic acid, the pH and the HCO_3^- values will be lower than expected for a particular Pa_{CO_2} level.

❑ **CYANOSIS** (see page 68)
❑ **OXYGENATION INDICES** (see page 69)

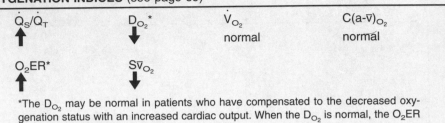

$$\dot{Q}_S/\dot{Q}_T \uparrow \qquad D_{O_2}{}^* \downarrow \qquad \dot{V}_{O_2} \text{ normal} \qquad C(a\text{-}\bar{v})_{O_2} \text{ normal}$$

$$O_2ER^* \uparrow \qquad S\bar{v}_{O_2} \downarrow$$

*The D_{O_2} may be normal in patients who have compensated to the decreased oxygenation status with an increased cardiac output. When the D_{O_2} is normal, the O_2ER is usually normal.

❑ **COUGH AND SPUTUM PRODUCTION** (see page 93)

During an asthmatic episode, the patient may produce an excessive amount of thick, tenacious mucus. Because of the presence of large numbers of eosinophils and other WBCs, the sputum is often purulent.

❑ **CHEST ASSESSMENT FINDINGS** (see page 6)

- Expiratory prolongation
- Decreased tactile and vocal fremitus
- Hyperresonant percussion note
- Diminished breath sounds
- Diminished heart sounds
- Wheezing/rhonchi

❑ **PULSUS PARADOXUS**

When an asthmatic episode produces severe alveolar air trapping and hyperinflation, pulsus paradoxus is a classic clinical manifestation. Pulsus paradoxus is defined as a systolic blood pressure that is more than 10 mm Hg lower on inspiration than on expiration. This exaggerated waxing and waning of arterial blood pressure can be detected by using a sphygmomanometer or, in severe cases, by palpating the pulse. Pulsus paradoxus during an asthmatic attack is believed to be due to the major intrapleural pressure differences during inspiration and expiration.

Decreased blood pressure during inspiration

During inspiration, the patient frequently recruits accessory muscles of inspiration. The accessory muscles help to produce a greater negative intrapleural pressure, which in turn enhances intrapulmonary gas flow. The increased negative intrapleural pressure, however, also causes blood vessels in the lungs to dilate and to pool blood. Consequently, the volume of blood returning to the left ventricle decreases. This causes a reduction in cardiac output and arterial blood pressure during inspiration.

Increased blood pressure during expiration

During expiration, the patient often activates the accessory muscles of expiration in an effort to overcome the increased R_{aw}. The increased power produced by these accessory muscles of expiration generates a greater positive intrapleural pressure. Although increased positive intrapleural pressure helps to offset R_{aw}, it also works to narrow or squeeze the blood vessels of the lung. This increased pressure on the pulmonary blood vessels enhances left ventricular filling and results in an increased cardiac output and arterial blood pressure during expiration.

❏ **RADIOLOGIC FINDINGS**

Chest radiograph
- Translucent (dark) lung fields
- Depressed or flattened diaphragms

As the alveoli become enlarged during an asthmatic attack, the residual volume and functional residual capacity increase. This condition decreases the density of the lungs. Consequently, the radiograph is translucent or darker than normal in appearance. Because of the increased residual volume and functional residual capacity, the diaphragm is depressed and flattened (Fig. 7-4).

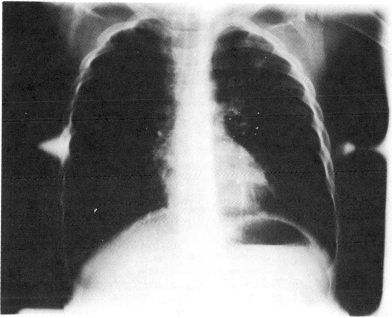

FIG 7-4
Chest x-ray film of a 2-year-old patient during an asthmatic attack.

GENERAL MANAGEMENT OF ASTHMA
Environmental Control

The patient should make every effort to eliminate common household factors that may trigger an asthmatic episode. For example, rugs, drapes, furniture, and bed linen should be aired frequently. Foam rubber pillows should replace pillows made of feathers, and damp areas such as the basement should be well ventilated and kept dry. Other household members or visitors should not be allowed to smoke in the house. The heating system should be cleaned at least once a year, and temperature and humidity should be maintained at a comfortable level.

Medications

Sympathomimetics.—Sympathomimetic drugs are the most popular agents used in the treatment of asthma to offset bronchial smooth muscle spasm. They are currently thought of as first-line agents during an acute exacerbation (see Appendix II).

Parasympatholytics.—Parasympatholytic agents are also used to offset bronchial smooth muscle constriction (see Appendix III).

Xanthines.—Xanthines are used to enhance bronchial smooth muscle relaxation (see Appendix IV).

Corticosteroids.—Although the exact mode of action of corticosteroids is not known, they have been shown to be highly effective in treating asthma when other measures have failed. They are currently thought of as first-line agents (see Appendix V).

Other Antiinflammatory Agents.—Inhaled antiinflammatory agents such as cromolyn sodium (Intal) and nedocromil sodium (Tilade) are helpful and are also considered first-line agents.

Mobilization of Bronchial Secretions

Because of the excessive mucus production and accumulation associated with asthma, a number of respiratory therapy modalities may be used to enhance the mobilization of bronchial secretions (see Appendix XI).

Supplemental Oxygen

Because hypoxemia is associated with asthma, supplemental oxygen may be required. The hypoxemia that develops in asthma is most commonly caused by the hypoventilation and shuntlike effect associated with the disorder. Hypoxemia caused by a shuntlike effect can at least partially be corrected by oxygen therapy. The hypoxemia associated with true alveolar hypoventilation cannot be corrected by oxygen therapy.

Monitoring

Arterial blood gas determinations, pulse oximetry, and pulmonary function measurements such as PEFR or FEV_1 are used to assess the severity and progression of the asthmatic episode. These measurements are made periodically to assess the patient's response to treatment. Vital signs must also be monitored closely, and a chest radiograph should be obtained as soon as possible to help evaluate the degree of air trapping.

Continuous Mechanical Ventilation (Status Asthmaticus)

Because acute ventilatory failure is associated with status asthmaticus, continuous mechanical ventilation may be required to maintain an adequate ventilatory status. Status asthmaticus is defined as a severe asthmatic episode that does not respond to correctional pharmacologic therapy (see above). When the patient becomes fatigued, the ventilatory rate decreases. Clinically, the patient demonstrates a progressive decrease in Pa_{O_2} and pH and a steady increase in Pa_{CO_2} (acute ventilatory failure). If this trend is not reversed, mechanical ventilation becomes necessary.

● ● ● ● | ASTHMA CASE STUDY | ● ● ● ●

ADMITTING HISTORY AND PHYSICAL EXAMINATION

A five-year-old female was admitted to the emergency room in severe respiratory distress. Her respiratory symptoms dated back to age one month, when she first developed wheezing. She was hospitalized in different hospitals on a number of occasions and was usually managed satisfactorily with aerosolized epinephrine and IV-administered aminophylline. On two occasions, steroids were required to break the bronchospasm. She developed a cough and wheezing the night prior to admission and became progressively worse during the night. At 8 AM she was brought to the emergency department.

Physical examination revealed an extremely anxious, well-developed female in acute respiratory distress. Pulse was 220 per minute and respirations were 62 per minute. Her temperature was 100° F rectally. She had enlarged, infected tonsils and moderate cervical adenopathy. She was retracting. There was dullness to percussion and absent breath sounds over the left upper lobe. Coarse crackles were heard over the left lower lobe, and generalized, sibilant expiratory wheezes with a markedly prolonged expiratory phase were noticed. The PEFR was 50 L/min (normal about 100 to 150 L/min). Blood gases on room air were pH 7.17, Pa_{CO_2} 61, HCO_3^- 16, and Pa_{O_2} 56. Other physical findings were normal. At this time, the respiratory care practitioner documented the following:

RESPIRATORY ASSESSMENT AND PLAN

S: Acute respiratory distress and anxiety

O: P = 220, RR = 62. Breath sounds absent over LUL. Wheezes throughout. PEFR: 50 L/min. Crackles LLL. Room air ABGs pH 7.17, Pa_{CO_2} 61, HCO_3^- 16, and Pa_{O_2} 56. No CXR yet.

A: • Asthma—bronchospasm (wheezing, decreased PEFR)

• Possible pneumonitis (dullness & crackles over LLL)

• Acute ventilatory failure with moderate hypoxemia (ABG) and metabolic acidosis (pH & HCO_3^- lower than expected for a Pa_{CO_2} of 61)

P: O_2 per nasal cannula at 2 lpm. Monitor O_2 saturation. Monitor PEFR. Med. neb. every 30 minutes with albuterol 0.15 ml in 2.0 ml normal saline. Beclovent inhaler 4 puffs now and 2 every 30 minutes × 4 via mask. Be sure intubation equipment and ventilator are readily available. Repeat ABG in 30 minutes. Therapist to remain at bedside.

The patient was treated vigorously with IV-administered aminophylline, low flow oxygen, and steroids. She seemed to improve slightly, but 30 minutes later her Pa_{CO_2} had risen to 67. At this time she was paralyzed (Norcuron), intubated, and ventilated. The next morning on an FI_{O_2} of 0.4 and a mechanical ventilator rate of 12 per minute, her blood gases were pH 7.38, Pa_{CO_2} 37, HCO_3^- 21, and Pa_{O_2} 124. Her wheezes had diminished, but were still present. At this point, the following was recorded:

RESPIRATORY ASSESSMENT AND PLAN

S: N/A (patient sedated and paralyzed)

O: Sedated, paralyzed, less wheezes, ABG: pH 7.38, Pa_{CO_2} 37, HCO_3^- 21, Pa_{O_2} 124 (on CMV 12, FI_{O_2} 0.4)

A: • Improved bronchospasm (decreased wheezing)

• Adequately ventilated and oxygenated on present ventilator settings (ABGs)

P: Discuss with physician: D/C Norcuron. Continue in-line med. nebs. IMV wean and O_2 wean as per protocols. Continue to monitor O_2 saturation.

She remained intubated for another 24 hours, at which time the lungs were clear, and suctioning returned scant but clear secretions. She was weaned from the ventilator with ease and was extubated shortly thereafter. The patient was discharged the following day.

DISCUSSION

Asthma is a potentially fatal disease, largely because its severity is unrecognized in the home or outpatient setting. This patient received optimal emergent treatment of her resistant asthma, but required intubation and mechanical ventilation nonetheless. Among the basic lessons to be learned here are that some asthmatic patients' conditions worsen despite vigorous inpatient therapy. Almost continuous assessment by the respiratory care practitioner is necessary if more aggressive therapy (including induced sedation, paralysis and mechanical ventilation) is to be effective.

This acutely ill patient illustrates the necessity for almost continuous monitoring by the respiratory care practitioner as well as the need for almost continuous "SOAP" notes if the patient care team is to be apprised of the patient's progress. The two such notes recorded here are but a small portion of the more than 30 such notes that we found on analysis of her final medical record after discharge!

SELF-ASSESSMENT QUESTIONS

Multiple Choice

1. During an asthmatic episode, the smooth muscle of the bronchi may hypertrophy as much as
   a. 2 times normal size.
   b. 3 times normal size.
   c. 4 times normal size.
   d. 5 times normal size.
   e. 6 times normal size.

2. Asthma causes a/an
   I. Increase in goblet cells.
   II. Decrease in cilia.
   III. Increase in bronchial gland size.
   IV. Decrease in eosinophils
      a. I and III only
      b. II and IV only
      c. I, II, and III only
      d. II, III, and IV only
      e. I, II, III, and IV

3. During an extrinsic-type asthma attack, the lymphoid tissue cells form which antibody?
      a. IgA
      b. IgM
      c. IgG
      d. IgE

4. When chemical mediators of the mast cells are released,
   I. Bronchial dilation occurs.
   II. Blood constriction occurs.
   III. Blood vessels constrict.
   IV. Tissue edema occurs.
      a. I only
      b. II only
      c. II and IV only
      d. I and III only
      e. I, III, and IV only

5. Which of the following are associated with intrinsic asthma?
   I. NSAIDs
   II. Respiratory syncytial virus
   III. Gastroesophageal reflux
   IV. Bisulfites
      a. I and IV only
      b. II and III only
      c. III and IV only
      d. II, III, and IV only
      e. I, II, III, and IV

6. When pulsus paradoxus appears during an asthma attack,
   I. Left ventricle filling is increased during inspiration.
   II. Cardiac output decreases during expiration.
   III. Left ventricle filling increases during expiration.
   IV. Cardiac output increases during inspiration.
      a. I only
      b. II only
      c. III only
      d. I and II only
      e. III and IV only

7. During an asthmatic episode, the following abnormal lung volume and capacity findings are found:
   I. Increased FRC
   II. Decreased ERV
   III. Increased FEV_1
   IV. Decreased RV
      a. I only
      b. II only
      c. I and II only
      d. III and IV only
      e. II, III, and IV only

8. During mast cell degranulation, which of the following chemical mediators are released?
   I. NCF
   II. ECF-A
   III. Histamine
   IV. Leukotrienes
      a. I only
      b. II only
      c. III only
      d. II and IV only
      e. I, II, III, and IV

9. Patients commonly present with these arterial blood gas values during an acute asthmatic episode:
   I. Increased pH
   II. Increased Pa_{CO_2}
   III. Decreased HCO_3^-
   IV. Decreased Pa_{O_2}
      a. IV only
      b. I and III only
      c. II and IV only
      d. I, II, and III only
      e. I, III, and IV only

10. The onset of intrinsic asthma usually occurs after
      a. 20 years of age.
      b. 30 years of age.
      c. 40 years of age.
      d. 50 years of age.
      e. 60 years of age.

True or False

1. Pathologic alterations of the lungs are absent between asthmatic episodes.   True _____ False _____
2. A patient with extrinsic asthma generally demonstrates symptoms after the age of 30 years.   True _____ False _____
3. There is generally an absence of an antigen-antibody reaction in intrinsic asthma.   True _____ False _____
4. Extrinsic asthma is also known as an allergic disorder.   True _____ False _____
5. A partial beta-blockade may be responsible for the occurrence of asthma in some individuals.   True _____ False _____
6. During an asthmatic attack, wheezing occurs more frequently during expiration.   True _____ False _____

Matching

Directions: On the line next to the trade name in column A, match the generic name from column B. Items in column B may be used once, more than once, or not at all.

A
TRADE NAME

1. _____Vanceril
2. _____Alupent
3. _____Bronkosol
4. _____Atrovent
5. _____Proventil
6. _____Beclovent
7. _____Brethine
8. _____Metaprel
9. _____Ventolin
10. _____Intal

B
GENERIC NAME

a. Terbutaline
b. Isoetharine
c. Metaproterenol
d. Racemic vaponefrin
e. Beclomethasone
f. Theophylline
g. Albuterol
h. Dexamethasone
i. Ipratopium bromide
j. Cromolyn sodium

Answers appear in Appendix XXI.

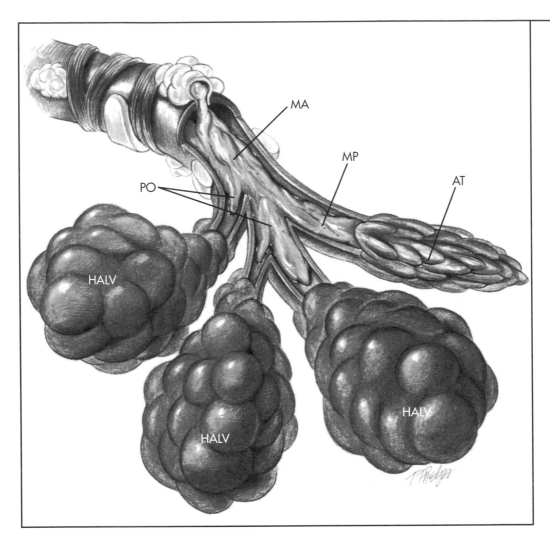

CYSTIC FIBROSIS

FIG 8-1

Cystic fibrosis. *MA* = mucus accumulation; *MP* = mucus plug; *AT* = atelectasis; *PO* = partial obstruction; *HALV* = hyperinflation of alveoli. (See also Plate 7.)

CHAPTER 8

Cystic Fibrosis

ANATOMIC ALTERATIONS OF THE LUNGS*

Although the lungs of patients with cystic fibrosis appear normal at birth, abnormal structural changes develop quickly. Initially there are bronchial gland hypertrophy and metaplasia of goblet cells, which secrete large amounts of thick, tenacious mucus. Because the mucus is particularly tenacious, impairment of the normal mucociliary clearing mechanism ensues, and many small bronchi and bronchioles become partially or totally obstructed (mucus plugging). Partial obstruction leads to overdistention of the alveoli, and complete obstruction leads to patchy areas of atelectasis. Bronchial obstruction and hyperinflation of the lungs are the predominant features of cystic fibrosis in the advanced stages.

The abundance of stagnant mucus in the tracheobronchial tree also serves as an excellent culture medium for bacteria, particularly *Staphylococcus aureus, Haemophilus influenzae,* and *Pseudomonas aeruginosa.* The infection stimulates additional mucus production and further compromises the mucociliary transport system. This condition may lead to "secondary bronchial smooth muscle constriction." Finally, as the disease progresses, the patient may develop signs and symptoms of chronic bronchitis, bronchiectasis, and lung abscesses (Fig. 8-1).

To summarize, the major pathologic or structural changes associated with cystic fibrosis are as follows:

* Excessive production and accumulation of thick, tenacious mucus in the tracheobronchial tree
* Bronchial smooth muscle constriction
* Partial or total bronchial obstruction (mucus plugging)
* Atelectasis
* Hyperinflation of the alveoli

ETIOLOGY

Cystic fibrosis is genetically transmitted as a *mendelian recessive* trait. It is now known that the cystic fibrosis gene is on chromosome 7. There are several different mutations of this gene that result in cystic fibrosis. The most common mutation is the absence of three base pairs in the DNA. This mutation is called *delta F508.*

Presently, about 80% of the gene mutations that cause cystic fibrosis have been identi-

---

*Cystic fibrosis does not exclusively affect the lungs. It also affects the function of exocrine glands in other parts of the body. In addition to the abnormally viscid secretions of the pulmonary system, the disease is clinically manifested by pancreatic deficiency and high NaCl concentrations in sweat.

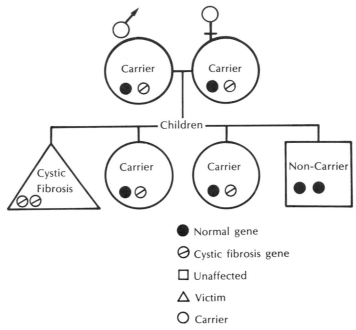

FIG 8-2
Standard mendelian pattern of inheritance of cystic fibrosis.

fied. Diagnostic testing for these abnormal genes is now possible; however, because 100% of the gene mutations responsible for cystic fibrosis are not known, testing is reserved for (1) patients with additional clinical manifestations associated with cystic fibrosis (e.g., excessive bronchial secretions or an elevated sweat chloride) and (2) genetic counseling for individuals that are at high risk for passing the cystic fibrosis gene on to their children.

Other than the fact that the carrier of the cystic fibrosis gene may be identified through genetic testing, the carrier (heterozygotes) does not demonstrate evidence of the disease. If both parents carry the cystic fibrosis gene, the possibility of their children having cystic fibrosis (regardless of their sex) follows the standard mendelian pattern: there is a 25% chance that each child will have cystic fibrosis, a 25% chance that each child will be completely normal (does not carry the gene), and a 50% chance that each child will be a carrier (Fig. 8-2).

Cystic fibrosis is much more common in whites. In the United States, the incidence is estimated to be one in 2,000 live births in Caucasians, one in 17,000 live births in blacks, and one in 90,000 live births in Orientals. About 30,000 white Americans have the disease, and about one in 25 are carriers. The average life expectancy is about 25 years of age, and few patients live past 40 years of age. Death is usually due to pulmonary complications.

OVERVIEW

OF THE CARDIOPULMONARY CLINICAL MANIFESTATIONS ASSOCIATED WITH
CYSTIC FIBROSIS

❏ **INCREASED RESPIRATORY RATE**
    Several pathophysiologic mechanisms operating simultaneously may lead to an increased ventilatory rate. These are (see page 17)
    • Stimulation of peripheral chemoreceptors
    • Anxiety

❏ PULMONARY FUNCTION STUDY FINDINGS

Expiratory Maneuver Findings (see page 41)

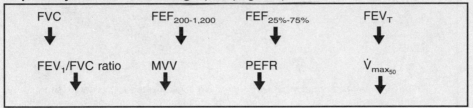

Lung Volume and Capacity Findings (see page 48)

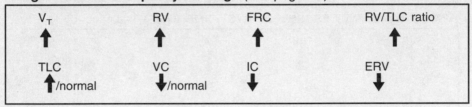

❏ **INCREASED HEART RATE (PULSE), CARDIAC OUTPUT, AND BLOOD PRESSURE** (see page 86)
❏ **INCREASED ANTEROPOSTERIOR CHEST DIAMETER (BARREL CHEST)** (see page 49)
❏ **PURSED-LIP BREATHING** (see page 49)
❏ **USE OF ACCESSORY MUSCLES DURING INSPIRATION** (see page 51)
❏ **USE OF ACCESSORY MUSCLES DURING EXPIRATION** (see page 54)
❏ **ARTERIAL BLOOD GASES**

Mild to Moderate Cystic Fibrosis

Acute Alveolar Hyperventilation with Hypoxemia (see page 57)

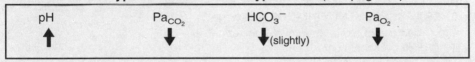

Severe Cystic Fibrosis

Chronic Ventilatory Failure with Hypoxemia (see page 60)

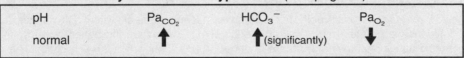

Acute ventilatory changes superimposed on chronic ventilatory failure (see page 65)

Because acute ventilatory changes are frequently seen in patients with chronic ventilatory failure, the respiratory care practitioner must be familiar with and be on alert for (1) acute alveolar hyperventilation superimposed on chronic ventilatory failure and (2) acute ventilatory failure superimposed on chronic ventilatory failure.

□ **CYANOSIS** (see page 68)
□ **OXYGENATION INDICES** (see page 69)

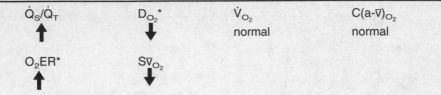

$$\dot{Q}_S/\dot{Q}_T \uparrow \qquad D_{O_2}{}^* \downarrow \qquad \dot{V}_{O_2} \text{ normal} \qquad C(a\text{-}\bar{v})_{O_2} \text{ normal}$$

$$O_2ER^* \uparrow \qquad S\bar{v}_{O_2} \downarrow$$

*The D_{O_2} may be normal in patients who have compensated to the decreased oxygenation status with (1) an increased cardiac output, (2) an increased hemoglobin level, or (3) a combination of both. When the D_{O_2} is normal, the O_2ER is usually normal.

□ **HEMODYNAMIC INDICES (SEVERE CYSTIC FIBROSIS)** (see page 87)

CVP ↑	RAP ↑	$\overline{PA}$ ↑	PCWP normal
CO normal	SV normal	SVI normal	CI normal
RVSWI ↑	LVSWI normal	PVR ↑	SVR normal

□ **POLYCYTHEMIA, COR PULMONALE** (see page 92)
  • Elevated hemoglobin concentration and hematocrit
  • Distended neck veins
  • Enlarged and tender liver
  • Peripheral edema
  • Pitting edema

□ **DIGITAL CLUBBING** (see page 93)
□ **CHEST ASSESSMENT FINDINGS** (see page 6)
  • Decreased tactile and vocal fremitus
  • Hyperresonant percussion note
  • Diminished breath sounds
  • Diminished heart sounds
  • Crackles/rhonchi/wheezing

□ **COUGH, SPUTUM PRODUCTION, AND HEMOPTYSIS** (see page 93)
□ **SPONTANEOUS PNEUMOTHORAX** (see Chapter 18)
    A spontaneous pneumothorax is commonly seen in patients with cystic fibrosis. The incidence is greater than 20% in the adult population. When the patient with cystic fibrosis has a pneumothorax, there is about a 50% chance that it will reoccur. The respiratory care practitioner must be on alert for this complication (e.g., symptoms of pleuritic pain, shoulder pain, and sudden shortness of breath). Precipitating factors include excessive exertion, high altitude, and positive-pressure breathing.
□ **RADIOLOGIC FINDINGS**
  Chest radiograph
    • Translucent (dark) lung fields
    • Depressed or flattened diaphragms

- Right ventricular enlargement
- Areas of atelectasis and fibrosis
- Pneumothorax (spontaneous)
- Abscess formation (occasionally)

During the later stages of cystic fibrosis, the alveoli become hyperinflated, which causes the residual volume and functional residual capacity to increase. This condition decreases the density of the lungs. Consequently, the resistance to x-ray penetration is not as great, and the x-ray film becomes darker in appearance.

Because of the increased residual volume and functional residual capacity, the diaphragm is depressed and appears so on the radiograph (Fig. 8-3). Since right ventricular enlargement and failure often develop as secondary problems during the advanced stages of cystic fibrosis, an enlarged heart may be identified on the radiograph. In some patients, areas of atelectasis, abscess formation, or a pneumothorax may be seen.

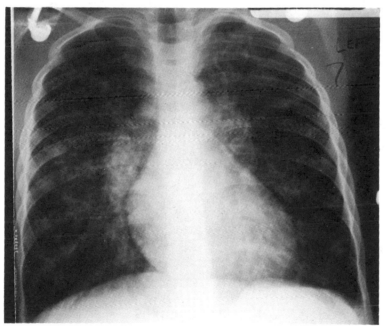

FIG 8-3

Chest x-ray film of a patient with cystic fibrosis.

COMMON NONRESPIRATORY CLINICAL MANIFESTATIONS
Meconium Ileus

Meconium ileus is an obstruction of the small intestine of the newborn that is caused by the impaction of thick, dry, tenacious meconium, usually at or near the ileocecal valve. This results from a deficiency in pancreatic enzymes and is the earliest manifestation of cystic fibrosis. The disease is suspected in newborn infants who demonstrate abdominal distention and fail to pass meconium within 12 hours after birth. Meconium ileus may occur in up to 25% of infants with cystic fibrosis.

Meconium Ileus Equivalent

Meconium ileus equivalent is an intestinal obstruction (similar to meconium ileus in neonates) that occurs in older children and young adults with cystic fibrosis.

Malnutrition and Poor Body Development

In cystic fibrosis, the pancreatic ducts become plugged with mucus, which leads to fibrosis of the pancreas. The pancreatic insufficiency that ensues inhibits the digestion of protein and fat, and this results in vitamin A, D, E, and K deficiencies. Vitamin K deficiency may be the basis of easy bruising and bleeding. Approximately 80% of all patients with cystic fibrosis have the aforementioned vitamin deficiencies and therefore show signs of malnutrition and poor body development throughout life.

Elevated Sweat Chloride Concentration

Although the sweat glands of cystic fibrosis patients are described as microscopically normal, the glands secrete up to four times the normal amount of sodium and chloride. The actual amount of sweat, however, is no greater than that produced by a normal individual. The sweat chloride test is used to measure the electrolyte concentration of the patient's perspiration. This test involves the stimulation of sweat production over the patient's forearm. When about 0.1 ml of sweat is collected under an airtight seal, the electrolyte concentration is measured. In children, a sweat chloride concentration greater than 60 mEq/L is considered to be diagnostic of the disease. In adults, a sweat chloride concentration greater than 80 mEq/L is usually required to confirm the diagnosis.

Nasal Polyps and Sinusitis

About 20% of the patients with cystic fibrosis have nasal polyps and sinusitis. The polyps are usually multiple and may cause nasal obstruction and, in some cases, distortion of normal facial features.

Sterility

Approximately 99% of the men and most women with cystic fibrosis are sterile. The women that do become pregnant are not likely to carry the infant to term. The infant that is carried to term will have cystic fibrosis or will be a carrier.

GENERAL MANAGEMENT OF CYSTIC FIBROSIS

The patient and the patient's family should be instructed as to the disease and how it affects bodily functions. They should be taught home care therapies, the goals of these therapies, and how to administer medications. Patients with severe cystic fibrosis are commonly managed by a pulmonary rehabilitation team. Such teams include a respiratory therapist, physical therapist, respiratory nurse specialist, occupational therapist, dietitian, social worker, and psychologist. A pediatrician or internist trained in respiratory rehabilitation outlines and orchestrates the patient's therapeutic program.

Patients should have regular medical checkups for comparative purposes to determine their general health, weight, height, pulmonary function abilities, and sputum culture. In addition, time-release pancreatic enzymes such as Pancrease are prescribed to patients with cystic fibrosis to aid food digestion. Patients are also encouraged to replace body salts either by heavily salting their food or in pill form. Supplemental multivitamins and minerals are also important.

Mobilization of Bronchial Secretions

Because of the excessive mucus production and accumulation associated with cystic fibrosis, a number of respiratory therapy modalities may be used to enhance the mobilization of bronchial secretions (see Appendix XI). Aggressive and vigorous bronchial hygiene—especially chest physical therapy and postural drainage—should be performed on a regular basis on patients both in the hospital and at home. Although controversial, nightly mist tent therapy is sometimes used for these patients.

Medications

Mucolytic agents.—Mucolytic agents may be used to break down the large amounts of thick tenacious mucus associated with cystic fibrosis. Early results of a new mucolytic agent called rhDNase (Pulmozyme) have been encouraging in patients with cystic fibrosis (see Appendix VI).

Sympathomimetics.—Sympathomimetic drugs are prescribed for patients with cystic fibrosis when bronchial spasm is present (see Appendix II).

Parasympatholytics.—Parasympatholytic agents are also used to offset bronchial smooth muscle constriction (see Appendix III).

Xanthines.—Xanthines are used to enhance bronchial smooth muscle relaxation (see Appendix IV).

Expectorants.—Expectorants are often used when water alone is not sufficient to facilitate expectoration (see Appendix VII).

Antibiotics.—Antibiotics are commonly administered to prevent or combat secondary respiratory tract infections (see Appendix VII).

Other Agents.—The inhalation of amiloride, a potent loop diuretic, is currently being studied as an effective agent to contain water in the lumen of the airway. The long-term benefits of this agent are yet to be determined.

Supplemental Oxygen

Because hypoxemia is often associated with cystic fibrosis, supplemental oxygen may be required. The hypoxemia that develops in cystic fibrosis is caused by the pulmonary shunting associated with the disorder. It should be noted, however, that when the patient demonstrates chronic ventilatory failure during the advanced stages of cystic fibrosis, caution must be taken not to eliminate the patient's hypoxic ventilatory drive.

Continuous Mechanical Ventilation

Because acute ventilatory failure (superimposed on chronic ventilatory failure) is often seen in patients with severe cystic fibrosis, continuous mechanical ventilation may be required to maintain an adequate ventilatory status. Continuous mechanical ventilation is justified when the acute ventilatory failure is thought to be reversible.

Lung or Heart/Lung Transplantation

Several large organ transplant centers are now performing lung or heart/lung transplantations in selected patients with cystic fibrosis.

• • • • **CYSTIC FIBROSIS CASE STUDY** • • • •

ADMITTING HISTORY AND PHYSICAL EXAMINATION

This patient was first seen at the medical center at age 22 months, with a history of cough, fever, and runny nose for seven days. Past history revealed that he had bulky, foul-smelling stools since infancy. His first upper respiratory tract infection was at age 4 months, and he had a chronic cough and intermittent wheezing ever since. He had acute tonsillitis, bronchitis, and otitis media on three separate occasions, always treated with antibiotics. The present illness was diagnosed as "asthmatic bronchitis," and the patient was treated at home with antibiotics and expectorants. Since the "bronchitis" did not improve, the parents were advised to bring the child to the hospital. Family history revealed that the parents were healthy, but that the only other sibling had cystic fibrosis.

Physical examination revealed an active child in no acute distress, but with an almost constant wet-sounding cough. Rectal temperature was 102.3° F. The abdomen was protuberant. The child was in the 40th percentile for height and weight. The tonsils were boggy and edematous. There were coarse crackles and rhonchi over all lung fields. A moderate amount of yellow and opaque sputum was produced with each coughing episode. The chest radiograph revealed atelectasis of the right middle lobe and probable pneumonitis in the same area. Laboratory findings showed a hemoglobin concentration of 17 g%, WBC of 21,000, and Sa_{O_2} of 90% on room air. The patient's sweat chloride concentration was 83 mEq/L (N = <60 mEq/L). A diagnosis of cystic fibrosis was made. At this time, the respiratory therapist recorded this SOAP note:

RESPIRATORY ASSESSMENT AND PLAN

S: Mother reports patient has constant loose cough.

O: Coughing almost constantly. Abdomen protuberant. T 102.3 F. Coarse crackles and rhonchi throughout all lung fields. Moderate amount of yellow and opaque sputum. CXR: RML atelectasis vs. pneumonitis. WBC elevated (21,000). Sa_{O_2} on room air 90%. Sweat chlorides increased (83 mEq/L).

A: • Probable cystic fibrosis (history & sweat chloride level)
      • RML pneumonitis (x-ray & elevated WBC)
      • Airway secretions (moderate amount of sputum)

P: Bronchial hygiene protocol. Aerosolized medication protocol with amiloride. Teach parents postural drainage therapy.

His hospital course was benign. He responded to antibiotics and was discharged on an oral pancreatic enzyme regimen. For the next six years, the family lived in Denver. Apparently, he did well (even at that altitude), taking pancreatic enzyme with each meal. He experienced two bouts of pneumonia, but in both instances the response to therapy was prompt and required no hospitalization; however, he deteriorated rapidly during the next two years. X-rays showed extensive alveolar hyperinflation and depressed diaphragms. His pulmonary functions tests showed a decreased vital capacity and a substantial decrease in flow mechanics. He developed clubbing of the fingers and toes. Six months later, at age 11 years, he developed increased respiratory distress due to bilateral pneumonia and was again admitted to the hospital. The respiratory therapist assigned to assess and treat the patient recorded the following:

RESPIRATORY ASSESSMENT AND PLAN

S: Complains of cough and shortness of breath.

O: Coarse rhonchi throughout all lung fields. BP 160/100, P 125, RR 40/min. Clubbed fingers and toes. CXR: Severe alveolar hyperinflation and bilateral new infiltrates. ABG (room air): pH 7.56, Pa_{CO_2} 67, HCO_3^- 39, Pa_{O_2} 39. Patient appears fatigued.

A: • Bilateral pneumonia (x-ray)
 • Acute alveolar hyperventilation on chronic ventilatory failure with severe hypoxemia in a patient with known cystic fibrosis (severe). (ABG)
 • Impending ventilatory failure (ABG & patient fatigue)
 • Large airway secretions (rhonchi)

P: Family requests no intubation for patient. Vigorous bronchial hygiene. Possible bronchoscopy. Get sputum sample and culture. Increased intensity of aerosolized medication and bronchial hygiene protocols.

His last admission was three months later. At this time, he again had bilateral pneumonia. He improved under vigorous therapy, but on the fifth day of this hospitalization, he suffered a "cardiac arrest." No attempts were made to resuscitate. Postmortem examination was refused by the parents.

DISCUSSION

The long-term prognosis of this hereditary disease seems to be improving with each passing year. Twenty-five years ago, the addition of chest physical therapy to treatment regimens for this condition had a remarkable increase on survival. The impact of genetic therapy on this condition is yet to be assessed, but it promises to be dramatic. Recently, the addition of rhDNase therapy for mucolysis of retained secretions has had a 10% to 15% immediate effect on FVC in most recipients. Cystic fibrosis thus exists as a remarkable testimony to the success of respiratory care modalities and a great challenge for the respiratory care practitioner of the future.

Amiloride, used in this patient, exerts its effect by prohibiting outward migration of fluid from airway secretions, thus reducing their tenacity and improving the ease with which they can be expectorated. Instruction of the patient and his parents in respiratory hygiene modalities through the course of a chronic illness are illustrated here, as is the knowledge, beforehand, that the patient did not wish the use of heroic measures in his last hospitalization. When all was done, the practitioner and the parents could rest easier in the knowledge that they had done all that they could for this unfortunate victim, who enjoyed remarkably good health through the majority of his disease despite the (at that time) "inevitable outcome."

SELF-ASSESSMENT QUESTIONS

Multiple Choice

1. Which of the following is commonly found in the tracheobronchial tree secretions of patients with cystic fibrosis?
   - I. *Staphylococcus*
   - II. *Haemophilus influenzae*
   - III. *Streptococcus*
   - IV. *Pseudomonas aeruginosa*
     - a. I only
     - b. II only
     - c. IV only
     - d. I and IV only
     - e. I, II, and IV

2. When two carriers of cystic fibrosis produce children, there is a
   - I. 75% chance that the baby will be a carrier.
   - II. 25% chance that the baby will be completely normal.
   - III. 50% chance that the baby will have cystic fibrosis.
   - IV. 25% chance that the baby will have cystic fibrosis.
     - a. I only
     - b. III only
     - c. II and IV only
     - d. I and II only
     - e. I, III, and IV only

3. The cystic fibrosis gene is located on chromosome
   - a. 5.
   - b. 6.
   - c. 7.
   - d. 8.
   - e. 9.

4. In cystic fibrosis, the patient commonly demonstrates a(an)
   - I. Increased FEV_T.
   - II. Decreased MVV.
   - III. Increased RV.
   - IV. Decreased FEV_1/FVC ratio.
     - a. I only
     - b. II only
     - c. III only
     - d. III and IV only
     - e. II, III, and IV only

5. During the advanced stages of cystic fibrosis, the patient generally demonstrates
   - I. Bronchial breath sounds.
   - II. Dull percussion notes.
   - III. Diminished breath sounds.
   - IV. Hyperresonant percussion notes.
     - a. I and III only
     - b. II and IV only
     - c. I and IV only
     - d. III and IV only
     - e. II and III only

6. Approximately 80% of all patients with cystic fibrosis demonstrate a deficiency in vitamin(s)
    I. A.
    II. B.
    III. D.
    IV. E.
    V. K.
        a. III and IV only
        b. I, IV, and V only
        c. II, III, and IV only
        d. I, III, IV, and V only
        e. I, II, III, IV, and V

7. In children, which of the following sweat chloride concentration values is diagnostic of cystic fibrosis?
        a. 50 mEq/L
        b. 60 mEq/L
        c. 70 mEq/L
        d. 80 mEq/L
        e. 90 mEq/L

8. Which of the following is/are a mucolytic agent(s)?
    I. N-acetylcysteine
    II. Aristocort
    III. rhDNase
    IV. Aldactone
        a. I only
        b. II only
        c. III only
        d. II and IV only
        e. I and III only

9. In regard to the secretion of sodium and chloride, the sweat glands of patients with cystic fibrosis secrete
        a. 2 times the normal amount.
        b. 4 times the normal amount.
        c. 6 times the normal amount.
        d. 8 times the normal amount.
        e. 10 times the normal amount.

10. Which of the following clinical manifestations are associated with severe cystic fibrosis?
    I. Decreased hemoglobin concentration
    II. Increased central venous pressure
    III. Decreased breath sounds
    IV. Increased pulmonary vascular resistance
        a. I and III only
        b. II and III only
        c. III and IV only
        d. II, III, and IV only
        e. I, II, III, and IV

Answers Appear in Appendix XXI.

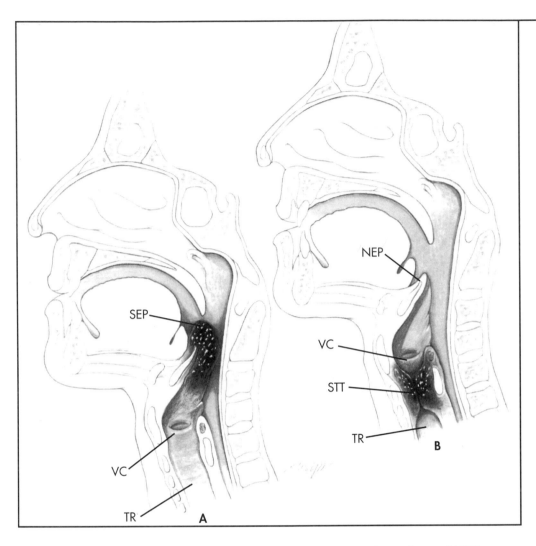

CROUP SYNDROME: LARYNGOTRACHEOBRONCHITIS & ACUTE EPIGLOTTITIS

FIG 9-1

A, acute epiglottitis. *SEP* = swollen epiglottis; *VC* = vocal cords; *TR* = trachea. **B,** laryngo-tracheobronchitis. *NEP* = normal epiglottis; *VC* = vocal cords; *STT* = swollen trachea tissue; *TR* = trachea. (See also Plate 8.)

Croup Syndrome: Laryngotracheobronchitis and Acute Epiglottitis

Croup is a general term used to describe the inspiratory, barking sound associated with the partial upper airway obstruction that develops in the following two disease entities: *laryngotracheobronchitis (subglottic croup)* and *acute epiglottitis (supraglottic croup)* (Fig. 9-1). Clinically, the inspiratory sound heard in croup is also called *inspiratory stridor.*

ANATOMIC ALTERATIONS OF THE UPPER AIRWAY
Laryngotracheobronchitis

Because this disease entity can affect the lower laryngeal area, trachea, and occasionally the bronchi, the term *laryngotracheobronchitis* (LTB) is used as a synonym for "classic" *subglottic croup.* Pathologically, LTB is an inflammatory process that causes edema and swelling of the mucous membranes. Although the laryngeal mucosa and submucosa are vascular, the distribution of the lymphatic capillaries is uneven or absent in this region. Consequently, when edema develops in the upper airway, fluid spreads and accumulates quickly throughout the connective tissues, which causes the mucosa to swell and the airway lumen to narrow. The inflammation also causes the mucous glands to increase their production of mucus and the cilia to lose their effectiveness as a mucociliary transport mechanism.

Because the subglottic area is the narrowest region of the larynx in an infant or small child, even a slight degree of edema can cause a significant reduction in the cross-sectional area. The edema in this area is further aggravated by the rigid, cricoid cartilage, which surrounds the mucous membrane and prevents external swelling as fluid engorges the laryngeal tissues. The edema and swelling in the subglottic region also decreases the ability of the vocal cords to abduct (move apart) during inspiration. This further reduces the cross-sectional area of airway in this region.

Acute Epiglottitis

Acute epiglottitis is a life-threatening emergency. In contrast to LTB, epiglottitis is an inflammation of the supraglottic region. The supraglottic region includes the epiglottis, aryepiglottic folds, and false vocal cords. Epiglottitis does not involve the pharynx, trachea, or other subglottic structures. As the edema in the epiglottis increases, the lateral borders curl, and the tip of the epiglottis protrudes in a posterior and inferior direction. During inspiration, the swollen epiglottis is pulled (or sucked) over the laryngeal inlet. In severe cases, this may completely block the laryngeal opening. Clinically, the classic finding is a swollen, cherry-red epiglottis.

To summarize, the major pathologic or structural changes associated with croup are as follows:

- LTB: airway obstruction due to tissue swelling just below the vocal cords
- Epiglottitis: airway obstruction due to tissue swelling just above the vocal cords

ETIOLOGY
Laryngotracheobronchitis

The most common cause of LTB is a viral infection. The parainfluenza viruses 1, 2, and 3, transmitted via aerosol droplets, are the most frequently identified etiologic agents, with type 1 being the most prevalent. LTB may also be caused by influenza A and B, respiratory syncytial viruses (RSV), rhinovirus, and adenoviruses.

LTB is predominantly seen in children between 3 months and 3 years of age. Males are affected slightly more often than females. The onset of LTB is relatively slow (i.e., symptoms progressively increase over a period of 24 to 48 hours), and it is most often seen during the winter months. A cough is commonly present, and it usually takes on a brassy or barking quality. The child's voice is usually hoarse, and the inspiratory stridor is typically loud and high in pitch. Unlike epiglottitis, the patient usually does not have a fever, drooling, swallowing difficulties, or a toxic appearance.

Acute Epiglottitis

Acute epiglottitis is a bacterial infection almost always caused by *Haemophilus influenzae* B. It is transmitted via aerosol droplets. Although rare, other causative agents such as *Streptococcus pneumoniae, Staphylococcus aureus,* and *Haemophilus parainfluenzae* have been reported. It is estimated that epiglottitis accounts for fewer than 1 per 1,000 pediatric cases. There is no clear-cut geographic or seasonal incidence. Males are affected more than females. Although acute epiglottis may develop in all age groups (neonatal to adulthood), it most of-

---

Table 9-1 General History/Physical Findings of Laryngotracheobronchitis and Epiglottitis

Clinical Finding	LTB	Epiglottitis
Age	3 mo-3 yr	2-4 yr
Onset	Slow (24-48 hr)	Abrupt (2-4 hr)
Fever	Absent	Present
Drooling	Absent	Present
Lateral neck x-ray	Haziness in subglottic area	Haziness in supraglottic area
Inspiratory stridor	High pitched and loud	Low pitched and muffled
Hoarseness	Present	Absent
Swallowing difficulty	Absent	Present
White blood count	Normal (viral)	Elevated (bacterial)

ten occurs in children between two and four years of age. The onset of epiglottis is usually abrupt.

Although the initial clinical manifestations are usually mild, they progress rapidly over a two- to four-hour period. A common scenario includes a sore throat or mild upper respiratory problem that quickly progresses to a high fever, lethargy, and difficulty in swallowing and handling secretions. The child usually appears pale. As the supraglottic area becomes swollen, breathing becomes noisy, the tongue is often thrust forward during inspiration, and the child may drool. Compared with LTB, the inspiratory stridor is usually softer and lower in pitch. The voice and cry are usually muffled rather than hoarse. Older children commonly complain of a sore throat and pain during swallowing. A cough is usually absent in patients with epiglottitis.

The general history and physical findings of LTB and epiglottis are contrasted in Table 9-1.

OVERVIEW

OF THE CARDIOPULMONARY CLINICAL MANIFESTATIONS ASSOCIATED WITH
LARYNGOTRACHEOBRONCHITIS AND EPIGLOTTITIS

❏ **INCREASED RESPIRATORY RATE**
Several pathophysiologic mechanisms operating simultaneously may lead to an increased ventilatory rate. These are (see page 17)
  • Stimulation of peripheral chemoreceptors
  • Anxiety

❏ **INCREASED HEART RATE (PULSE), CARDIAC OUTPUT, AND BLOOD PRESSURE** (see page 86)
❏ **ARTERIAL BLOOD GASES**

Mild to Moderate LTB or Epiglottitis

Acute Alveolar Hyperventilation with Hypoxemia (see page 57)

pH*	Pa_{CO_2}	HCO_3^-*	Pa_{O_2}
↑	↓	↓(slightly)	↓

*When tissue hypoxia is severe enough to produce lactic acid, the pH and HCO_3^- values will be lower than expected for a particular Pa_{CO_2} level.

Severe LTB or Epiglottitis

Acute Ventilatory Failure with Hypoxemia (see page 59)

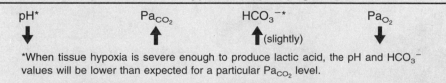

pH*	Pa_{CO_2}	HCO_3^-*	Pa_{O_2}
↓	↑	↑(slightly)	↓

*When tissue hypoxia is severe enough to produce lactic acid, the pH and HCO_3^- values will be lower than expected for a particular Pa_{CO_2} level.

❏ **CYANOSIS** (see page 68)
❏ **USE OF ACCESSORY MUSCLES DURING INSPIRATION** (see page 51)
❏ **SUBSTERNAL/INTERCOSTAL RETRACTION** (see page 98)

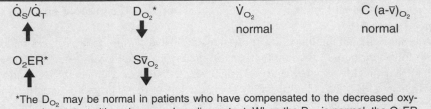

$\dot{Q}_S/\dot{Q}_T$	D_{O_2}*	$\dot{V}_{O_2}$	$C\,(a\text{-}\bar{v})_{O_2}$
↑	↓	normal	normal
O_2ER*	$S\bar{v}_{O_2}$		
↑	↓		

*The D_{O_2} may be normal in patients who have compensated to the decreased oxygenation status with an increased cardiac output. When the D_{O_2} is normal, the O_2ER is usually normal.

□ **CHEST ASSESSMENT FINDING** (see page 6)
- Diminished breath sounds

□ **INSPIRATORY STRIDOR**

Under normal circumstances, the slight narrowing of the upper (extrathoracic) airway that naturally occurs during inspiration is nonsignificant. Because the upper airway is relatively small in infants and children, however, even a slight degree of edema may become significant. Thus, when the cross section of the upper airway is reduced because of the edema, the child will generate stridor during inspiration, when the upper airway naturally becomes smaller. It should also be noted that if the edema becomes severe, the patient may generate both inspiratory and expiratory stridor.

□ **LATERAL NECK X-RAY FILM**
- Haziness in the subglottic area (LTB)
- Haziness in the supraglottic area (epiglottitis)
- Classic thumb sign

Although the diagnosis of epiglottitis or LTB can generally be made on the basis of the patient's clinical history, a lateral neck x-ray film is sometimes used to confirm the diagnosis. When the patient has LTB, a white haziness is demonstrated in the subglottic area. When the patient has acute epiglottitis, there is a white haziness in the supraglottic area. In addition, epiglottitis often appears on a lateral neck x-ray film as the classic "thumb sign." The epiglottis is swollen and rounded, which gives it an appearance of the distal portion of a thumb (Fig 9-2).

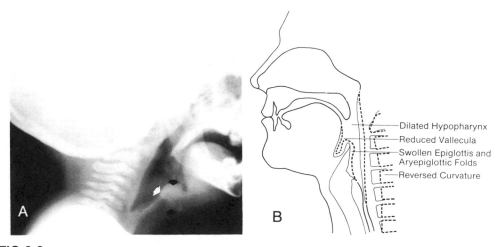

FIG 9-2

The classic "thumb sign" of an edematous epiglottis is evident in this lateral neck film (see *arrows* in **A**). The schematic illustrates the findings to look for in a lateral film in a patient with suspected epiglottitis **(b).** Such films are superfluous in a child with the classic history, signs, and symptoms of epiglottitis; they can be of tremendous help, however, in the diagnosis of mild or questionable cases—particularly when explaining to parents the need for aggressive treatment. (From Ashcraft CK, Steele RW: *J Respir Dis* 1988; 9:48-60. Used by permission.)

GENERAL MANAGEMENT OF LARYNGOTRACHEOBRONCHITIS AND EPIGLOTTITIS

It is important to stress that early recognition of epiglottitis may be lifesaving. A history of upper airway obstruction and a general examination should be secured as soon as possible. But *under no circumstances should the mouth or throat be examined, unless personnel and equipment are readily available to rapidly intubate or tracheostomize the patient. In cases of suspected epiglottitis, examination or inspection of the pharynx and larynx are absolutely contraindicated, except in the operating room with a fully trained team.* This is because the direct examination of the throat (even though depression of the tongue may reveal a bright red epiglottis and confirm the diagnosis) often results in a sudden and complete closure of the upper airway. A lateral neck radiograph may be necessary to differentiate LTB, epiglottitis, or some other upper airway obstruction. Once established, the general management of LTB and acute epiglottitis is as follows:

Supplemental Oxygen

Because hypoxemia is associated with both LTB and epiglottitis, supplemental oxygen is usually required.

Cool Aerosol Mist

Cool aerosol mist therapy (with oxygen) either by face mask or tent is a primary mode of treatment for LTB. It is administered to liquefy thick secretions and to cool and reduce subglottic edema.

Racemic Epinephrine (Micronefrin, Vaponefrin)

Aerosolized racemic epinephrine is usually administered to children with LTB. This α-adrenergic agent is used for its mucosal vasoconstriction and is an effective and safe aerosol decongestant.

Corticosteroids

Corticosteroids have been shown to reduce the severity and duration of LTB. They are generally prescribed when the patient does not respond to cool mist and racemic epinephrine therapy (see Appendix V).

Antibiotic Therapy

Because acute epiglottitis is almost always caused by *Haemophilus influenzae,* appropriate antibiotic therapy should be part of the treatment plan. Ampicillin and chloramphenicol are commonly prescribed to cover the most common organisms that cause acute epiglottitis.

Endotracheal Intubation (Tracheostomy)

In cases of suspected epiglottitis, examination or inspection of the pharynx and larynx are absolutely contraindicated, except in the operating room with a fully trained surgical team in attendance. This is because the epiglottis may obstruct completely in response to even the slightest touch during inspection. The physician, nurse, and respiratory care practitioner should not leave the patient's bedside until successful placement of the endotracheal tube is secured. When the patient is anxious, restless, or uncooperative, restraints may be needed to ensure against accidental extubation.

· · ·   ## LARYNGOTRACHEOBRONCHITIS CASE STUDY   · · ·

ADMITTING HISTORY AND PHYSICAL EXAMINATION

A three-year-old male had a mild viral upper respiratory infection and some hoarseness for three days, when at 10 PM he rapidly developed a brassy cough and high-pitched inspiratory stridor. He became moderately dyspneic. The child was restless and appeared frightened. Rectal temperature was 37° C. The mother claimed that the child was "blue" on two occasions during this episode. She was going to take the child to the emergency room, but the grandmother suggested that she try steam inhalation first. Accordingly, the child was taken to the bathroom, where the shower was turned on full force. The child was also comforted by the grandmother and urged to breathe slowly and deeply. As the bathroom became filled with steam, the respiratory distress abated and within a few minutes the child was free of stridor, breathing essentially normally. The next day, the same symptoms recurred, and the patient was taken to the emergency department. The respiratory therapist documented this assessment and plan:

RESPIRATORY ASSESSMENT AND PLAN

S: Mother reports patients had cough, inspiratory stridor.

O: Confirms above. Lungs clear except for stridor and tracheal breath sounds. RR 50/min. Circumoral pallor noted. O_2 sat. 92% on room air. CXR and soft tissue x-ray of neck suggest laryngotracheobronchitis.

A: Croup, moderate (history & inspiratory stridor)

P: Cool mist aerosol treatment. Med. neb. treatment with racemic epinephrine per protocol. Will obtain throat culture.

The patient did well and, at discharge, the patient's mother was instructed in home treatment of croup, utilizing racemic epinephrine on a prn basis.

DISCUSSION

Home remedies sometimes do work. Any parent who has had a croupy child will recognize himself or herself in the above scenario. What may not be as widely recognized is that sometimes hot, and sometimes cool, aerosols improve this syndrome. Failing this approach, the parents were wise to bring their son to the emergency department for prompt vasoconstrictive therapy accompanied by a cool mist aerosol. This resulted in prompt improvement.

Note again the emphasis on family education, including the use of racemic epinephrine aerosolization for outpatients. These instructions may have resulted in the fact that the patient was never again brought to the emergency department for such an episode.

· · · ·   ## ACUTE EPIGLOTTITIS CASE STUDY   · · · ·

ADMITTING HISTORY AND PHYSICAL EXAMINATION

This 2-year-old female appeared quite well in the evening and was put to bed at the usual time. She woke up two hours later, and the parents were immediately aware that the child was in serious respiratory distress. She was sitting up in bed, drooling, unable to speak or cry and breathing noisily.

The parents wrapped the child in warm blankets and drove her to the emergency room of the nearest hospital. On inspection, the child demonstrated a puffy face, drooling, inspiratory stridor, and cyanotic nail beds. The emergency physician looked at the child and listened to her chest, but did not examine her mouth. Respiratory rate was 42/min, blood pressure was 80/50, and pulse was 140/min. The physician ordered a lateral, soft tissue x-ray of the neck, but while waiting for the x-ray the child became increasingly dyspneic and more cyanotic. At this time, this respiratory SOAP note was charted:

RESPIRATORY ASSESSMENT AND PLAN

S: Mother states patient having severe respiratory distress.

O: RR 42/min, BP 80/50, P 140 regular. Child's face puffy, drooling. Inspiratory stridor (worsening). Nail beds cyanotic. Soft tissue x-ray of neck pending.

A: • Probable acute epiglottitis. No history of foreign body aspiration (general history)
       • Impending acute ventilatory failure (history, vital signs, drooling, inspiratory stridor, & cyanosis)

P: Anesthesiologist & ENT surgeon paged. Mask with 100% oxygen pending their arrival.

The emergency physician placed an emergency page for the anesthesiologist on call and for an ENT surgeon. Immediately, a nonrebreathing oxygen mask was lightly held to the patient's face by the respiratory therapist. As soon as the physicians appeared (about 10 minutes), the child was taken to the operating room. The surgeon stood by to do an emergency cricothyrotomy while the anesthesiologist attempted to intubate the child.

Fortunately, the anesthesiologist was successful, in spite of an enlarged, cherry-red epiglottis partially obstructing the larynx. As soon as the endotracheal tube was in place, the child relaxed and soon went to sleep. She was admitted to the ICU, but was extubated the next day and discharged on the third hospital day. A throat culture taken in the ICU was positive for *H. influenzae*. She was treated orally with amoxicillin.

DISCUSSION

Acute epiglottitis is a life-threatening condition. The key thing to remember here is to avoid examination of the throat until a person qualified in pediatric intubation is nearby. Such manipulation often is unsuccessful and, unless qualified assistance is at hand, the child may asphyxiate.

The treatment suitably selected here was a nonrebreathing oxygen mask while the appropriate team was assembled. Typical of this disease is its abrupt onset and, under appropriate therapy, the rapid manner in which it subsides.

SELF-ASSESSMENT QUESTIONS

True or False

1. LTB is a supraglottic croup.   True _____   False _____
2. Acute epiglottitis is a life-threatening emergency.   True _____   False _____
3. LTB is predominantly seen in children between 2 and 4
   years of age.   True _____   False _____
4. Acute epiglotitis is usually caused by *Haemophilus
   influenzae* B.   True _____   False _____
5. The onset of LTB is relatively slow (24 to 48 hours).   True _____   False _____
6. Drooling is usually present in LTB.   True _____   False _____
7. A fever is associated with acute epiglottitis.   True _____   False _____
8. The inspiratory stridor is usually low pitched and muffled
   in LTB.   True _____   False _____
9. The white blood count is usually elevated in LTB.   True _____   False _____
10. Swallowing is usually difficult in patients with LTB.   True _____   False _____

Answers appear in Appendix XXI.

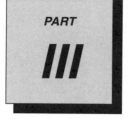

PART

III

INFECTIOUS PULMONARY DISEASES

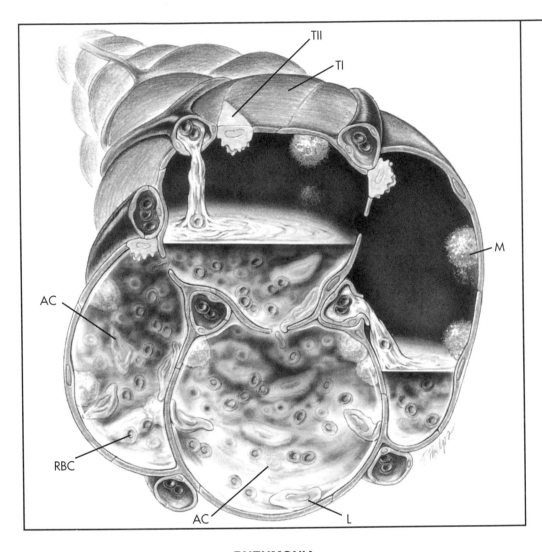

PNEUMONIA

FIG 10-1

Cross-sectional view of alveolar consolidation in pneumonia. *TI* = type I cell; *TII* = type II cell; *M* = macrophage; *AC* = alveolar consolidation; *L* = leukocyte; *RBC* = red blood cell. (See also Plate 9.)

Pneumonia

ANATOMIC ALTERATIONS OF THE LUNGS

Pneumonia, or pneumonitis with consolidation, is an inflammatory process that primarily affects the gas exchange area of the lung. In response to the inflammation, fluid (serum) and some red blood cells (RBCs) from adjacent pulmonary capillaries pour into the alveoli. This fluid transfer is called *effusion*. Polymorphonuclear leukocytes also move into the infected area to engulf and kill invading bacteria on the alveolar walls. This process has been termed "surface phagocytosis." Increased numbers of macrophages also appear in the infected area to remove cellular and bacterial debris. If the infection is overwhelming, the alveoli become completely filled with fluid, RBCs, polymorphonuclear leukocytes, and macrophages. When this occurs, the alveoli are said to be *consolidated* (Fig. 10-1).

To summarize, the major pathologic or structural changes associated with pneumonia are as follows:

- Inflammation of the alveoli
- Alveolar consolidation

ETIOLOGY

In the United States, pneumonia causes more deaths than any other infectious disease. Etiologic agents of pneumonia include bacteria, viruses, fungi, tuberculosis, and anaerobic organisms. Pneumonia can also develop after the aspiration of gastric contents or the inhalation of irritating chemicals, such as chlorine. Involvement of an entire lobe of the lung is called *lobar pneumonia*. When both lungs are involved, it is called *double pneumonia*. The term "walking pneumonia" has no clinical significance, but nevertheless is used to describe a mild case of pneumonia. For example, patients with *Mycoplasma pneumoniae,* who generally have mild symptoms and remain ambulatory, are sometimes told that they have "walking pneumonia."

The major causes of pneumonia are listed in Table 10-1 and are discussed below.

Bacterial Causes

Gram-positive Organisms

Streptococcal pneumonia.—*Streptococcus pneumoniae* (formerly *Diplococcus pneumoniae*) accounts for over 80% of all the bacterial pneumonias. This organism is a gram-positive, nonmotile coccus that is found singly, in pairs, and in short chains (Fig 10-2). The cocci are enclosed in a smooth, thick polysaccharide capsule essential for virulence. There are over 80

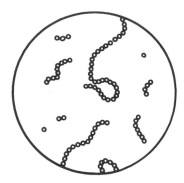

FIG 10-2
The streptococcus organism is a gram-positive, nonmotile coccus that is found singly, in pairs, and in short chains.

Table 10-1 Causes of Pneumonia		
Bacterial Causes	**Viral Causes**	**Other Causes**
Gram-positive organisms	Influenza virus	*Mycoplasma pneumoniae*
Streptococcus	Respiratory syncytial virus	Rickettsial infections
Staphylococcus	Parainfluenza virus	*Chlamydia psittaci*
Gram-negative organisms	Adenovirus	Varicella
Klebsiella		Rubella
Pseudomonas aeruginosa		Aspiration of gastric contents
Haemophilus influenzae		Aspiration of lipids
Legionella pneumophila		*Pneumocystis carinii*
		Cytomegalovirus
		Fungal infections
		Tuberculosis
		Anaerobic organisms

different types of *Streptococcus pneumoniae.* Serotype 3 organisms are the most virulent. Streptococci are generally transmitted by aerosol from a cough or sneeze of an infected individual. Most strains of *Streptococcus pneumoniae* are sensitive to penicillin and its derivatives.

Staphylococcal Pneumonia.—There are two major groups of staphylococci: (1) *Staphylococcus aureus,* which is responsible for most "staph" infections in humans, and (2) *Staphylococcus albus* and/or *epidermidis,* which is part of the normal flora. The staphylococci are gram-positive cocci that are found singly, in pairs, and in irregular clusters (Fig. 10-3). Staphylococcal pneumonia often follows a predisposing virus infection and is seen more commonly in children and immunosuppressed adults. *Staphylococcus aureus* is commonly transmitted by aerosol from a cough or sneeze of an infected individual and indirectly via contact with contaminated floors, bedding, clothes, and the like.

Gram-Negative Organisms

The major gram-negative organisms responsible for pneumonia are rod-shaped microorganisms called *bacilli* (Fig. 10-4).

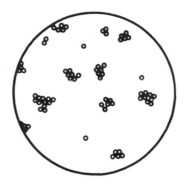

FIG 10-3

The staphylococcus organisms is a gram-positive, nonmotile coccus that is found singly, in pairs, and in irregular clusters.

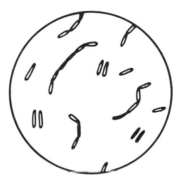

FIG 10-4

The bacilli are rod-shaped microorganisms and are the major gram-negative organisms responsible for pneumonia.

***Klebsiella pneumoniae* (Friedländer's bacillus).**—*Klebsiella pneumoniae* has long been associated with lobar pneumonia, particularly in men over 40 years old and in chronic alcoholics of both sexes. *Klebsiella* is a gram-negative bacillus that is found singly, in pairs, or in chains of varying lengths. It is a normal inhabitant of the human gastrointestinal tract. The organism can be transmitted directly by aerosol or indirectly by contact with freshly contaminated articles. *Klebsiella pneumoniae* is a common nosocomial, or hospital-acquired disease. It is typically transmitted by such routes as clothing, intravenous solutions, foods, and the hands of health care workers. The mortality of patients with *Klebsiella pneumoniae* has been quite high, since septicemia is a frequent complication.

Pseudomonas aeruginosa (Bacillus pyocyaneus).—*Pseudomonas aeruginosa* is a highly motile, gram-negative bacillus. It is found in the human gastrointestinal tract and is a contaminant in many aqueous solutions. It is frequently cultured from the respiratory tract of chronically ill, tracheostomized patients. This makes *Pseudomonas aeruginosa* a particular problem to the respiratory therapy practitioner. Since the *Pseudomonas* organism thrives in dampness, it is frequently cultured from contaminated respiratory therapy equipment. The sputum from patients with *Pseudomonas* infection is frequently green and sweet smelling. The organism is commonly transmitted by aerosol or by direct contact with freshly contaminated articles.

Haemophilus influenzae.—*Haemophilus influenzae* is frequently a cause of a secondary type of pneumonia that follows a primary viral infection. *Haemophilus influenzae* is one of the smallest gram-negative bacilli, measuring about 1.5 μm in length and 0.3 μm in width. There are six types of *Haemophilus influenzae,* designated A to F, but only type B is commonly pathogenic. Pneumonia caused by *Haemophilus influenzae B* is most often seen in children between the ages of 1 month and 6 years. *Haemophilus influenzae B* is almost always the cause of acute epiglottis. The organism is transmitted via aerosol or contact with contaminated objects, but it is sensitive to cold and does not survive long after expectoration.

Legionella pneumophila.—In July 1976, a severe pneumonia-like disease outbreak occurred in an American Legion convention in Philadelphia. The causative agent eluded isolation for many months, despite concerted efforts of the nation's top epidemiologic experts. When the organism was finally recovered from a patient, it was found to be an unusual and fastidious gram-negative bacillus with atypical concentrations of certain branched-chain lipids. The initial isolate was designated as *Legionella pneumophila.* More than 20 *legionella* species have been now been identified.

Most of the species are free-living in soil and water, where they act as decomposer organisms. The organism also multiplies in standing water such as contaminated mud puddles, large air-conditioning systems, and water tanks. The organism is transmitted when it becomes airborne and enters the patient's lungs as an aerosol. There is no convincing evidence that the organism is transmitted from person to person. The organism can be detected in pleural fluid, sputum, or lung tissue by direct fluorescent antibody microscopy. Although it is rarely found outside the lungs, the organism may be found in other tissue. The disease is most commonly seen in middle-aged males who smoke.

Viral Causes

Viruses are minute organisms not visible by ordinary light microscopy. They are parasitic and depend on nutrients inside cells for their metabolic and reproductive needs. About 90% of acute upper respiratory tract infections and 50% of lower respiratory tract infections are due to viruses. The most common viruses that cause respiratory infections are described below.

Influenza virus.—Although there are several subtypes, influenza A and B are the most common causes of viral respiratory tract infections. In the United States, influenza A and B commonly occur in epidemics during the winter months. The virus survives well in conditions with low temperatures and low humidity (winter). Influenza is transmitted from person to person by aerosol droplets. It has also been found in horses, swine, and birds. Influenza viruses have an incubation period of 1 to 3 days, and usually cause upper respiratory tract infections. Young adults in robust health appear to be particularly susceptible. Oftentimes, the first sign of an epidemic is an increase in school absenteeism.

Respiratory syncytial virus (RSV).—The respiratory syncytial virus (RSV) is a member of the paramyxovirus group. Parainfluenza, mumps, and rubella viruses also belong to this group. The RSV is most often seen in children under 6 months of age and in elderly persons with underlying pulmonary disease. Approximately 25% of respiratory illnesses in children less than 1 year old are due to this virus. The infection is rarely fatal in infants. The RSV virus often goes unrecognized but may play an important role as forerunner to bacterial infections. The virus is transmitted by aerosol and by direct contact with infected individuals. RSV infections are most commonly seen in patients during the winter and spring months.

Parainfluenza virus.—The parainfluenza viruses are also members of the paramyxovirus group and, therefore, are related to mumps, rubella, and the respiratory syncytial viruses. There are five types of parainfluenza viruses: types 1, 2, 3, 4A, and 4B. Types 1, 2, and 3 are the major causes of infections in humans. Type 1 is considered a "croup" type of virus. Types 2 and 3 are associated with severe infections. Although type 3 is seen in persons of all ages, it is most commonly seen in infants less than 2 months old; types 1 and 2 are most often seen in children between the ages of 6 months and 5 years. Types 1 and 2 typically occur in the fall, while type 3 infection is most often seen in the late spring and summer. Parainfluenza viruses are transmitted by aerosol droplets and by direct person-to-person contact. The parainfluenza viruses are known for their ability to spread rapidly among members of the same family.

Adenoviruses.—There are over 30 adenovirus subgroups. Serotypes 4, 7, 14, and 21 cause viral infections and pneumonia in all age groups. Serotype 7 has been related to fatal cases of pneumonia in children. Adenoviruses are transmitted by aerosol. Patients with pneumonia caused by adenoviruses are generally seen during the fall, winter, and spring months.

Other Causes

Mycoplasma pneumoniae.—The mycoplasma are small, cell wall-deficient organisms. They are smaller than bacteria but larger than viruses. Their cell walls lack peptidoglycan. The pneumonia caused by the mycoplasmal organism is described as *primary atypical pneumonia,* atypical because the organism escapes isolation by standard bacteriologic tests. *Mycoplasma pneumoniae* infection is not highly communicable. It may take weeks for the organism to spread, even among members of the same family. It is most frequently seen in adolescents and young adults during the late summer and early fall months. The patient with *Mycoplasma pneumoniae* is often said to have "walking pneumonia," since the condition is mild (i.e., slight fever, fatigue, and a characteristic dry, hacking cough) and the patient is usually ambulatory.

Rickettsiae.—Rickettsiae are small, pleomorphic coccobacilli. Most rickettsiae are intracellular parasites possessing both RNA and DNA. There are several pathogenic members of the Rickettsia family: *Rickettsia rickettsii* (Rocky Mountain spotted fever), *Rickettsia akari* (rickettsialpox), *Rickettsia prowazekii* (typhus), and *Rickettsia burnetii,* also called *Coxiella burnetii* (Q fever).

All species of the genus *Rickettsia* are unstable outside of cells except for *Rickettsia burnetii* (Q fever), which is extremely resistant to heat and light. Q fever can cause pneumonia as well as a prolonged febrile illness, an influenza-like illness, and endocarditis. The organism is commonly transmitted by arthropods (lice, fleas, ticks, mites). It may also be transmitted by cattle, sheep, and goats and possibly in raw milk.

Chlamydia psittaci **(Psittacosis).**—Chlamydia psittaci is a small gram-negative bacterium in the respiratory tract and feces in a variety of birds (e.g., parrots, parakeets, lorikeets, cockatoos, chickens, pigeons, ducks, pheasants, and turkeys). *Chlamydia psittaci* is transmitted from birds to humans via aerosol or by direct contact. The clinical manifestations of *Chlamydia psittaci* closely resemble those caused by *Mycoplasma pneumoniae.* A newly named organism, *Chlamydia pneumoniae* (formerly called the TWAR strain of *Chlamydia psittaci*), has recently been identified as the cause of pneumonia in adults.

Varicella (chickenpox).—The varicella virus usually causes a benign disease in children between the ages of 2 and 8 years, and complications of varicella are not common. In some cases, however, varicella has been noted to spread to the lungs and cause a serious secondary pneumonitis.

Rubella (measles).—Measles virus spreads from person to person by the respiratory route. Respiratory complications are often encountered in this disease because of widespread involvement of the mucosa of the respiratory tract.

Aspiration pneumonitis.—Aspiration of gastric juice with a pH of 2.5 or less causes a serious and often fatal pneumonia. Aspiration pneumonitis is commonly missed since acute inflammatory reactions may not begin until several hours after aspiration of the gastric juice. The inflammatory reaction generally increases in severity for 12 to 26 hours and may progress to the adult respiratory distress syndrome (ARDS). In the absence of a secondary bacterial infection, the inflammation usually becomes clinically insignificant in about 72 hours. Mendelson in 1946 first described the clinical manifestations of tachycardia, dyspnea, and cyanosis associated with the aspiration of acid stomach contents. The clinical picture he described is now known as Mendelson's syndrome and is usually confined to aspiration pneumonitis in pregnant females.

Lipoid pneumonitis.—The aspiration of mineral oil, used medically as a lubricant, has also been known to cause pneumonitis. The severity of the pneumonia is dependent on the type of oil aspirated. Oils from animal fats cause the most serious reaction, while oils of vegetable origin are relatively inert. When mineral oil is inhaled in an aerosolized form, an intense pulmonary tissue reaction occurs.

***Pneumocystis carinii* pneumonia.**—*Pneumocystis carinii* is an opportunistic, often fatal, form of pneumonia seen in profoundly immunosuppressed patients. Although the pneumocystic organism has been identified as a protozoa, recent information suggests that it is more closely related to fungi. Currently, pneumocystis pneumonia is the major pulmonary infection seen in patients with AIDS (between 80% and 90% of the cases). In vulnerable hosts, the disease spreads rapidly throughout the lungs.

Cytomegalovirus.—Cytomegalovirus (CMV), a member of the herpesvirus family, is the most common viral pulmonary complication of AIDS. CMV infection commonly coexists with *Pneumocystis carinii* infection.

Fungal infections.—Because most fungi are aerobes, the lung is a prime site for fungal infections. Primary fungal pathogens include *Histoplasma capsulatum, Coccidioides immitis,* and *Blastomyces dermatitidis.*

In addition, the opportunistic yeast pathogens, *Candida albicans, Cryptococcus neoformans,* and *Aspergillus* may also cause pneumonia in certain patients. For example, *Candida albicans,* which occurs as normal flora in the oral cavity, genitalia, and large intestines, is rarely seen in the tracheobronchial tree or lung parenchyma. In patients with AIDS, however, *Candida albicans* commonly causes an infection of the mouth, pharynx, esophagus, vagina, skin, and lungs. A *Candida albicans* infection of the mouth is called thrush, which is characterized by a white, adherent, patchy infection of the membranes of the mouth, gums, cheeks, and throat. *Cryptococcus neoformans* proliferates in the high nitrogen content of pigeon droppings and readily scatters into the air and dust. Today, the highest case rate of cryptococcosis occurs among AIDS patients and persons undergoing steroid therapy. The molds of the genus *Aspergillus* may be the most pervasive of all fungi—especially *A. fumigatus. Aspergillus* is found in soil, vegetation, leaf detritus, food, and compost heaps. Persons that breathe air of graineries, barns, and silos are at the greatest risk. *Aspergillus* infection usually occurs in the lungs. *Aspergillus* is almost always an opportunistic infection and, lately, has posed a serious threat to patients with AIDS. When fungal organisms are inhaled, the initial response of the lung is an inflammatory reaction similar to any acute pneumonia (see Chapter 14).

Tuberculosis.—Tuberculosis (TB) is an infectious disease caused by *Mycobacterium tuberculosis. M. tuberculosis* is a slender, rod-shaped aerobic organism. In the early 1980s, the United States had the lowest TB rate in modern history. Then, in 1985, the TB incidence started rising and has risen ever since. In 1990, Americans were suffering 16 percent more TB than in 1984. The rise in TB is primarily due to the increased incidence and problems associated with homelessness, drug abuse, and AIDS. In fact, TB in AIDS patients is now at epidemic levels. The initial response of the lung is an inflammatory reaction that is similar to any acute pneumonia (see Chapter 13).

Anaerobic organisms.—A lung abscess is most commonly caused by the aspiration of oral and gastrointestinal fluids containing anaerobic organisms such as *Peptococcus, Peptostreptococcus, Bactroides,* and *Fusobacterium.* These anaerobic organisms are normally found throughout the digestive tract and the small grooves and spaces between the teeth and gums. During the early stages of a lung abscess, the pathology is indistinguishable from that of any acute pneumonia (see Chapter 12).

OVERVIEW

OF THE CARDIOPULMONARY CLINICAL MANIFESTATIONS ASSOCIATED WITH
PNEUMONIA

❑ **INCREASED RESPIRATORY RATE**

Several pathophysiologic mechanisms operating simultaneously may lead to an increased ventilatory rate. These are (see page 17)
- Stimulation of peripheral chemoreceptors
- Decreased lung compliance/increased ventilatory rate relationship
- Stimulation of J receptors
- Pain/anxiety/fever

❑ **PULMONARY FUNCTION STUDY FINDINGS**

Expiratory Maneuver Findings (see page 39)

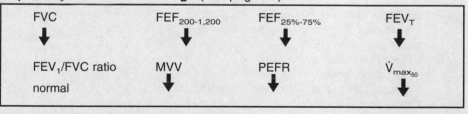

| FVC ↓ | FEF$_{200-1,200}$ ↓ | FEF$_{25\%-75\%}$ ↓ | FEV$_T$ ↓ |
| FEV$_1$/FVC ratio normal | MVV ↓ | PEFR ↓ | $\dot{V}_{max_{50}}$ ↓ |

Lung Volume and Capacity Findings (see page 39)

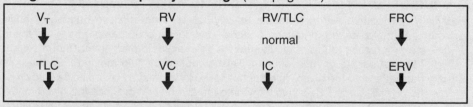

| V$_T$ ↓ | RV ↓ | RV/TLC normal | FRC ↓ |
| TLC ↓ | VC ↓ | IC ↓ | ERV ↓ |

❑ **INCREASED HEART RATE (PULSE), CARDIAC OUTPUT, AND BLOOD PRESSURE** (see page 86)

❏ **ARTERIAL BLOOD GASES**

Mild to Moderate Pneumonia

Acute Alveolar Hyperventilation with Hypoxemia (see page 57)

pH*	Pa_{CO_2}	HCO_3^{-*}	Pa_{O_2}
↑	↓	↓(slightly)	↓

*When tissue hypoxia is severe enough to produce lactic acid, the pH and HCO_3^- values will be lower than expected for a particular Pa_{CO_2} level.

Severe Pneumonia

Acute Ventilatory Failure with Hypoxemia (see page 59)

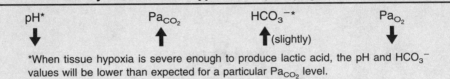

pH*	Pa_{CO_2}	HCO_3^{-*}	Pa_{O_2}
↓	↑	↑(slightly)	↓

*When tissue hypoxia is severe enough to produce lactic acid, the pH and HCO_3^- values will be lower than expected for a particular Pa_{CO_2} level.

❏ **CYANOSIS** (see page 68)
❏ **OXYGENATION INDICES** (see page 69)

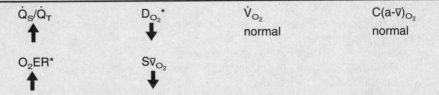

$\dot{Q}_S/\dot{Q}_T$	$D_{O_2}*$	$\dot{V}_{O_2}$	$C(a-\bar{v})_{O_2}$
↑	↓	normal	normal
O_2ER*	$S\bar{v}_{O_2}$		
↑	↓		

*The D_{O_2} may be normal in patients who have compensated to the decreased oxygenation status with an increased cardiac output. When the D_{O_2} is normal, the O_2ER is usually normal.

❏ **CHEST ASSESSMENT FINDINGS** (see page 6)
- Increased tactile and vocal fremitus
- Dull percussion note
- Bronchial breath sounds
- Crackles/rhonchi
- Pleural friction rub (if process extends to pleural surface)
- Whispered pectoriloquy

❏ **PLEURAL EFFUSION** (see Chapter 19)

❏ **COUGH, SPUTUM PRODUCTION, AND HEMOPTYSIS** (see page 93)
Initially, the patient with pneumonia usually has a nonproductive barking or hacking cough. As the disease progresses, however, the cough becomes productive. When the disease progresses to this point, the patient often expectorates small amounts of purulent, blood-streaked, or rusty sputum. This is caused by fluid moving from the pulmonary capillaries into the alveoli in response to the inflammatory process. As fluid crosses into the alveoli, some RBCs also move into the alveoli and produce the blood-streaked or rusty appearance of the fluid (see Fig 10-1). Some of the fluid that moves into the alveoli may also work its way into the bronchioles and bronchi. As the fluid accumulates in the bronchial tree, the subepithelial mechanoreceptors in the trachea, bronchi, and bronchioles are stimulated and initiate a cough reflex. Since the bronchioles and the smaller bronchi are deep in the lung parenchyma, the patient with pneumonia initially has a dry, hacking cough, and fluid cannot be easily expectorated until the process involves the larger bronchi.

❑ **CHEST PAIN/DECREASED CHEST EXPANSION** (see page 98)
❑ **RADIOLOGIC FINDINGS**

Chest radiograph
- Increased density (from consolidation and atelectasis)
- Air bronchograms
- Pleural effusions

Because of the numerous causes of pneumonia, the radiographic signs vary considerably. In general, pneumonia (alveolar consolidation) appears as an area of increased density that may involve a small lung segment, a lobe, or one or both lungs (Fig. 10-5). As the alveolar consolidation intensifies, the alveolar density increases and air bronchograms may be seen (Fig. 10-6). A pleural effusion is easily identified on the chest radiograph (Chapter 19).

CT scan
- Alveolar consolidation and air bronchograms can also be seen on the CT scan (Fig. 10-7).

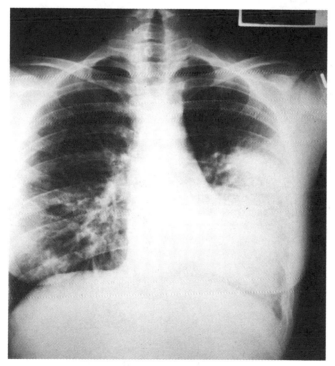

FIG 10-5

Chest x-ray film of a 20-year-old woman with a severe left-lung pneumonia.

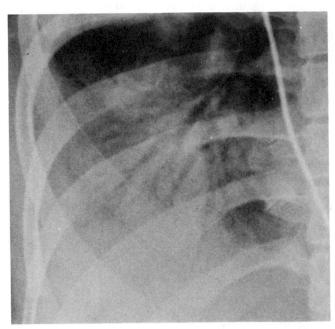

FIG 10-6

Air bronchogram. The branching linear lucencies within the consolidation in the right lower lobe are particularly well demonstrated in this example of staphylococcal pneumonia. (From Armstrong P, Wilson AG, Dee P: *Imaging of Diseases of the Chest,* St. Louis, 1990, Mosby-Year Book. Used by permission.)

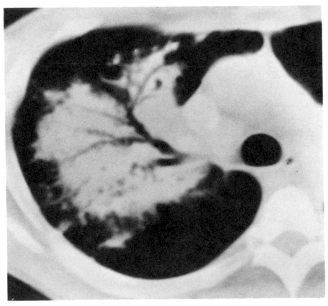

FIG 10-7

Air bronchogram shown by CT in a patient with pneumonia. (From Armstrong P, Wilson AG, Dee P: *Imaging of Diseases of the Chest,* St. Louis, 1990, Mosby-Year Book. Used by permission.)

GENERAL MANAGEMENT OF PNEUMONIA
Hyperinflation Techniques

Hyperinflation techniques are commonly ordered to offset (at least temporarily) the alveolar consolidation associated with pneumonia (see Appendix XII).

Medications

Antibiotic agents.—Where feasible, antibiotics are used to combat the infective agents that cause pneumonia (see Appendix VIII).

Analgesic agents.—Analgesics may be ordered to relieve pleuritic pain. As the pain decreases, the depth of inspiration and cough effort should improve.

Ribavirin aerosol.—Ribavirin (Virazole) has been shown to be effective in treating children with respiratory syncytial virus (RSV) infection. Ribavirin is supplied as 6 g of lyophilized powder in a 100-ml vial, which is reconstituted in 300 ml of sterile water, making a 2% (20 mg/ml) strength solution. The solution is aerosolized and delivered to the patient by means of a device called the *small particle aerosol generator (SPAG)*. The aerosol is administered continuously for 12 to 18 hours per day, for 3 to 7 days, through an oxyhood, face tent, or oxygen tent.

Aerosolized pentamidine.—Pentamidine has been found to be effective against *Pneumocystis carinii* in patients with AIDS. Pentamidine can be administered parenterally or as an inhaled aerosol. When given by inhaled aerosol, pentamidine reaches a much higher concentration in the lungs than when given intravenously.

Supplemental Oxygen

Because of the hypoxemia associated with pneumonia, supplemental oxygen may be required. It should be noted, however, that the hypoxemia that develops in pneumonia is most commonly caused by the alveolar consolidation and capillary shunting associated with the disorder. Hypoxemia caused by capillary shunting is refractory to oxygen therapy.

Thoracentesis

Thoracentesis (also called thoracocentesis) entails the surgical perforation of the chest wall and pleural space with a needle for the aspiration of fluid for diagnostic or therapeutic purposes or for the removal of a specimen for biopsy. The procedure is usually performed using local anesthesia, with the patient in an upright position. Therapeutically, a thoracentesis may be used to treat pleural effusion. Fluid samples may be examined for the following:

- Color
- Odor
- RBC count
- WBC count with differential
- Protein
- Glucose
- Lactic dehydrogenase (LDH)
- Amylase
- pH
- Wright's, Gram's and acid-fast (AFB) stains
- Aerobic, anaerobic, tuberculosis, and fungal cultures
- Cytology

• • • • •   **PNEUMONIA CASE STUDY**   • • • • •

ADMITTING HISTORY AND PHYSICAL EXAMINATION

This 47-year-old male was hunting in northern Michigan with some friends. They spent considerable time out-of-doors in inclement weather and indulged freely in alcoholic beverages during the afternoons and evenings. Previously, the man had been essentially healthy.

Returning home, he felt listless and thought that he was "coming down with a cold." That night he noticed a mild, nonproductive cough. He had a headache and some pain in his right chest on deep inspiration, and he noticed that he was somewhat short of breath when he climbed one flight of stairs. During the night he woke up and felt very chilled then very warm. His wife put her hand on his forehead and was certain that he had a "high fever." Since he felt miserable, they went to the emergency room of the nearest hospital.

On physical examination his vital signs were the following-blood pressure 150/88, pulse 116/min, respirations 28/min, and temperature (oral) 39.9° C. He was in moderate distress. Percussion of the chest revealed dullness on the right lower side, and on inspiration there were fine crackles heard in that area. The breath sounds were described as "bronchial." The chest radiograph showed pneumonic consolidation of the right lower lung field. On room air, his arterial blood gas values were pH 7.53, Pa_{CO_2} 27, HCO_3^- 21, Pa_{O_2} 72. The respiratory therapist assigned to assess and treat the patient charted this SOAP note:

RESPIRATORY ASSESSMENT AND PLAN

S: "I feel miserable!"

O: Alert, cooperative, acutely ill. Temperature 39.9° C, BP 150/88, P 116, RR 28. Dull to percussion over RLL, where crackles are heard. CXR: Pneumonic consolidation RLL. ABG on room air: pH 7.53, Pa_{CO_2} 27, HCO_3^- 21, Pa_{O_2} 72.

A: • RLL consolidation (pneumonia presumed)
   • Acute alveolar hyperventilation with mild hypoxemia (ABG)

P: Oxygen therapy per respiratory care protocol.

The patient was started on oxygen (4 L/min) via a nasal cannula. The physician prescribed intravenous antibiotic therapy. Over the next 72 hours, the patient steadily improved and was discharged on the third hospital day.

DISCUSSION

A history of cold exposure in conjunction with the use of alcoholic beverages prior to the onset of pneumonia is not uncommon.

In cases of pneumonia, the great temptation for the respiratory care practitioner is to want to do too much. Typically, volume expansion therapy, bronchodilator aerosol therapy, and bland aerosol therapy have been ordered for these patients, even in the acute, consolidative stage of their pneumonia. All that was needed for this patient was appropriate selection of antibiotics, rest, fluids, and supplementary oxygen. When the pneumonia "breaks up" (in its resolution stage), excessive airway secretions and even bronchoconstriction may appear. At that time, use of other modalities may be necessary.

SELF-ASSESSMENT QUESTIONS

Multiple Choice

1. Which of the following is known as Friedländer's bacillus?
   a. *Haemophilus influenzae*
   b. *Pseudomonas aeruginosa*
   c. *Legionella pneumophila*
   d. *Klebsiella*
   e. Streptococcus

2. Of the six types of *Haemophilus influenzae*, which type is most frequently pathogenic?
   a. Type A
   b. Type B
   c. Type C
   d. Type D
   e. Type E
   f. Type F

3. Which of the following is associated with Q fever?
   a. *Mycoplasma pneumoniae*
   b. *Rickettsia*
   c. Ornithosis
   d. Varicella
   e. Respiratory syncytial virus

4. Mendelson's syndrome is associated with
   a. Lipoid pneumonitis.
   b. Rubella.
   c. Varicella.
   d. Aspiration pneumonitis.
   e. *Rickettsia.*

5. Which of the following is/are commonly seen in patients with AIDS?
   I. *Aspergillus*
   II. *Cryptococcus*
   III. *Pneumocystis carinii*
   IV. Cytomegalovirus
   a. I only
   b. III only
   c. II and IV only
   d. II, III, and IV only
   e. I, II, III, and IV

6. Ribavirin aerosol has been shown to be effective in treating children with
   a. *Klebsiella.*
   b. *Haemophilus influenzae B.*
   c. Respiratory syncytial virus.
   d. *Pseudomonas aeruginosa.*
   e. *Streptococcus.*

7. Which of the following is almost always the cause of acute epiglottis?
   a. *Haemophilus influenzae B*
   b. *Klebsiella*
   c. *Streptococcus*
   d. *Mycoplasma pneumoniae*
   e. Parainfluenza virus

8. Which of the following is most associated with causing "croup?"
   a. *Streptococcus*
   b. *Parainfluenza*
   c. *Mycoplasma pneumoniae*
   d. Adenovirus
   e. *Chlamydia psittaci*

9. In the absence of a secondary bacterial infection, lung inflammation caused by the aspiration of gastric fluids usually becomes insignificant in about
    a. 2 days.
    b. 3 days.
    c. 5 days.
    d. 7 days.
    e. 10 days.

10. Which of the following is/are associated with pneumonia?
    I. Decreased tactile and vocal fremitus
    II. Increased $C(a-\bar{v})_{O_2}$
    III. Decreased PEFR
    IV. Increased VC
    a. I only
    b. III only
    c. II and IV only
    d. I and III only
    e. II and III only

Answers appear in Appendix XXI.

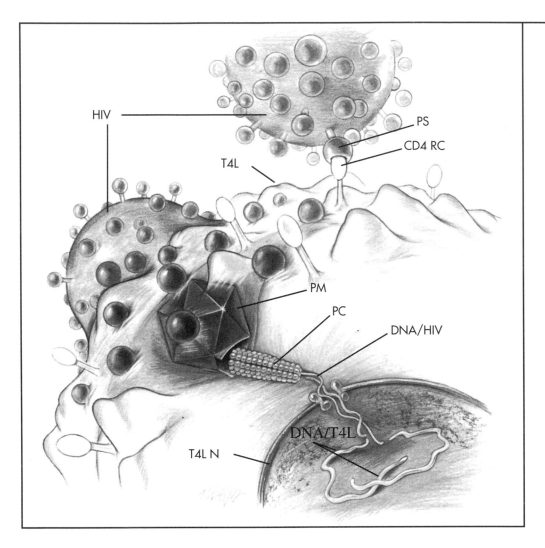

HUMAN IMMUNODEFICIENCY VIRUS ATTACKING T4 LYMPHOCYTE
FIG 11-1

Human immunodeficiency virus attacking T4 lymphocyte. *HIV* = human immunodeficiency virus; *PS* = protein spike (on outer surface of HIV); *CD4 RC* = CD4 receptor site (on outer surface of T4 lymphocyte); *T4L* = T4 lymphocyte; *PM* = protein matrix of HIV (beneath the surface of the T4 lymphocyte); *PC* = protein core of HIV (contains strands of RNA and reverse transcriptase); *DNA/HIV* = DNA of the human immunodeficiency virus; *DNA/T4L* = DNA of the T4 lymphocyte; *T4L N* = nucleus of the T4 lymphocyte. (See also Plate 10.)

CHAPTER 11

Acquired Immunodeficiency Syndrome

Acquired immunodeficiency syndrome (AIDS) was first reported in 1981 in young, previously healthy, homosexual males and in intravenous drug users. These patients presented with a variety of unusual opportunistic infections, including *Pneumocystis carinii* pneumonia (most common), mucosal candidiasis, viral infections, fungal infections, mycobacterial infections, and a relatively rare skin cancer called Kaposi's sarcoma, characterized by purplish blotches or bumps. It was soon discovered that these patients had somehow acquired severe impairment of their immune system, which in turn left them vulnerable to certain types of cancer and to a variety of opportunistic infections.

Since 1981, an enormous amount of research has resulted in (1) the identification of the virus responsible for this devastating illness, (2) a screening system to identify those infected with the AIDS virus, and (3) symptomatic criteria used to identify patients with full-blown AIDS. In 1991, more than 150 countries reported over 300,000 cases of AIDS, and over 8 million people were estimated to be infected with the AIDS virus. It was estimated that 1 million of these cases were in the United States alone.

There still is no known cure or effective means of prevention (short of sexual abstinence and avoidance of nonsterile injectables). What was once thought to be a relatively isolated problem among a specific group of people has since become one of the major worldwide health problems of the twentieth century.

ETIOLOGY

The causative virus of AIDS was isolated in 1983 and is known as the **human immunodeficiency virus (HIV).** There are two major forms of HIV: HIV-1 and HIV-2. Most cases are caused by HIV-1, although the incidence of individuals infected with HIV-2 is increasing in West Africa. HIV is a member of the retrovirus family that must live and reproduce inside human cells. Retroviruses store their genetic information in RNA and contain a unique enzyme, called *reverse transcriptase,* which allows the virus to make DNA from RNA—a reversal of the normal DNA-to-RNA sequence.

Closely related viruses have been discovered in various apes and monkeys, and it is possible that all of these immunodeficiency viruses evolved from one virus type several hundred years ago. It is not known when humans first became infected, but it was probably long before the earliest AIDS cases were reported in 1981.

HIV is a small and fragile virus. Inside the virus are two strands of RNA that contain the genetic information for the virus (most organisms, including humans, store genetic information in DNA). The RNA and various viral enzymes are packed in protein to form a core, which is surrounded by a protein matrix. The matrix, in turn, is covered by a fatty envelope through which protein spikes project.

The protein spikes allow the virus to attach to receptor molecules called *CD4 receptor sites,* which are found on the surface of certain white blood cells and some neural cells. The cells that have the highest concentration of CD4 receptor sites on their surface and, therefore, are the primary target of the HIV are the *T lymphocytes* with *helper* and *inducer* activities. These cells are also called *CD4-positive cells* or *T4 lymphocytes.* The T4 lymphocytes are crucial to immune function, since they stimulate other immune cells—including *killer lymphocytes,* which attack infected cells, and *B lymphocytes,* which produce antibodies. Normally, the T4 lymphocytes comprise about 60% to 70% of the circulating T cells. The T4 lymphocytes progressively decrease in HIV-infected patients.

The T lymphocytes with *cytotoxic* and *suppressor* activities are not directly affected by the virus. These cells are also called CD8-positive cells or T8 lymphocytes. These cells are not reduced in HIV-infected patients and may even increase. The T4 and T8 cells are routinely monitored in known HIV-infected patients. In healthy, noninfected HIV individuals, the T4/T8 ratio is about 2.0. In HIV-infected patients with AIDS, the T4/T8 ratio is usually 0.5 or less.

To a lesser extent, the CD4 receptor sites are also found on the surface of the macrophages. The macrophages are large wandering cells that engulf foreign material and are also vital to the immune response.

As shown in Figure 11-1, the HIV infects an individual's T4 lymphocytes as follows: When the HIV binds to a receptor site of a T4 lymphocyte, the fatty outer layer of the HIV fuses to the membrane of the white blood cell. This action allows the protein matrix (which contains the core of the virus) to enter the white blood cell. Eventually, the protein matrix breaks down, releasing the virus. When this happens, the reverse *transcriptase enzyme,* which is inside the core, converts the RNA to DNA—which, as already mentioned, is the opposite of the normal DNA-to-RNA sequence.

The virus DNA then inserts into the DNA of the white blood cell nucleus. This irreversible joining of the virus DNA with the host DNA is called *integration,* and leaves the white blood cell permanently infected. In this integrated form, the virus can reproduce RNA copies of the HIV, which in turn migrate out of the white blood cell. The new HIV copy is now free to infect other white blood cells. Slowly, the infected white blood cells die.

Although ineffectively, the immune system does mount a response to the invasion of HIV. The B lymphocytes produce antibodies against various components of the virus, and killer lymphocytes attack HIV-infected cells. While these responses may slow the spread of the virus, they fail to clear it from the body and, consequently, the infection remains for life. As the infection advances, the T4-lymphocyte population drops, and the immune system becomes progressively disabled. Eventually, perhaps after many years, the body is left almost totally defenseless against infections.

HIV Transmission

HIV is primarily transmitted through sexual contact with an HIV-infected individual. HIV is easily transferred from one person to another during sexual activities that involve the exchange of body fluids, especially when cuts, scrapes, abrasions, infections, or inflammation are present. In the United States, the largest population of individuals infected with HIV through sexual contact consists of homosexual and bisexual men.

HIV is also transmitted through skin punctures caused by contaminated needles or syringes. In the United States, the second largest group infected with HIV are intravenous drug users. In this group, the virus is primarily transmitted by inserting contaminated needles or syringes into the circulation.

Although it is not as prevalent today (because of new screening tests), HIV can be transmitted to individuals who are recipients of contaminated blood, tissue, or organs. In addition, mothers can transmit the virus to their child before, during, or shortly after the baby is born (e.g., through breast milk). There is a relatively small (but growing) number of persons who have contacted AIDS by heterosexual anal, oral, or vaginal intercourse.

On rare occasions, laboratory and health care workers have been infected during the course of their work. The most common accidents involve use of contaminated sharp instruments (e.g., needles). There also have been very rare incidents where contaminated health care workers (e.g., dentists) have passed the virus on to patients. Although HIV has been detected in tears and saliva, the concentration is said to be too low for effective transmission.

Diagnosis of AIDS

Testing for HIV infection has been available since 1985. There are now several laboratory screening tests available for HIV detection. The screening test most commonly used is a serologic procedure that detects anti-HIV antibodies in the serum. Because a "false positive" for HIV can occur in some patients, each patient with a positive result for the anti-HIV antibody is tested twice. When the second screening test is positive, a third confirmatory test for detecting HIV antibodies is administered. The Western blot assay is the most commonly used confirmatory test. The overall sensitivity and specificity of the Western blot are high.

An important problem with the HIV tests is the delay between the time of HIV infection and the production of anti-HIV antibodies. From the moment an individual acquires the infection, it can take from six weeks to a year before the individual becomes HIV-positive. During this period, an infected person can unknowingly pass the virus on to others.

OVERVIEW

OF THE CLINICAL MANIFESTATIONS ASSOCIATED WITH
HIV INFECTION AND AIDS

The clinical manifestations of individuals with HIV infection are extremely variable, and there is no such thing as a typical course of infection. AIDS is the full-blown, symptomatic phase of the HIV infection, the end stages of the HIV infection when the patient's immune system is critically depressed and unable to fight disease effectively. The time which must elapse between the moment an individual acquires HIV and development of full-blown AIDS is unknown. Evidence suggests, however, that this period may be as short as one year or as long as 10 to 15 years. The general clinical course of HIV infection and AIDS is as follows.

❏ **HIV INFECTION**

During the early stages, most individual infected with HIV demonstrate no signs or symptoms of any health problems. In some cases, however, at the time positive anti-HIV antibodies appear, symptoms similar to influenza or a mononucleosis-like illness develop. Clinical manifestations include fever, generalized aches, lymphadenopathy, rashes of various types, headache, increased temperature, pharyngitis, and joint pains. In addition, some patients manifest a variety of skin disorders such as acne, nonspecific rashes, and oral lesions. Typically, the patient is ill with these symptoms for two to five weeks and then returns to good health.

After the patient's health returns to normal, there is usually a long quiet, or dormant, period that can last for many years in spite of the fact that the HIV continues to replicate. There may be no symptoms, and the person infected may have no idea that anything is wrong. In some cases, however, the patient may have persistent swelling of the lymph nodes, weight loss, fatigue, fever, diarrhea, skin rashes, herpes, thrush (candidiasis of the oral mucosa), or leukoplakia (characterized by white hairlike ridges on the side of the tongue). All of these problems may resolve spontaneously and recur intermittently. This phase may last from less than one year to more than ten years, and ends when the individual's immunity drops so low that full-blown AIDS develops.

❑ AIDS

AIDS is characterized by (1) a number of opportunistic infections that commonly develop in response to a weakened immune system, (2) certain unusual cancers, (3) neurologic disorders, and (4) various constitutional symptoms. These problems result in a wide range of clinical manifestations. The type and severity of clinical manifestations vary from person to person. Some of these conditions can be treated, and some may be present throughout the remainder of the patient's life.

❑ OPPORTUNISTIC INFECTIONS

Although AIDS can lead to serious complications in almost any organ system, the most common problems are infections in the lungs. When pulmonary infections are present, the patient with AIDS will manifest the same clinical findings as any patient with pneumonia. The following are the most common opportunistic infections that affect the respiratory system of patients with AIDS (also see Chapter 10):

Pneumocystis carinii pneumonia

The most common respiratory complication seen in patients with AIDS is *Pneumocystis carinii* pneumonia (between 80% and 90% of the cases). Although the *Pneumocystis* organism has been classified as a protozoan, recent information suggests that it is more closely related to fungi than to protozoa.

Pneumoncystis can normally be found in the lungs of humans, but it does not cause disease in healthy hosts, only in individuals whose immune systems are critically impaired. Before AIDS, *Pneumocystis carinii* pneumonia was seen primarily in patients with malignancy, in organ transplant recipients, or in patients with diseases requiring treatment with large doses of immunosuppressive agents. Today, most cases of *Pneumoncystis carinii* pneumonia are seen in AIDS patients. The early clinical manifestations of *Pneumocystis* in AIDS patients are indistinguishable from any other pneumonia.

Tuberculosis

In individuals with a healthy immune system, infection with *Mycobacterium tuberculosis* generally remains dormant. In patients with AIDS, however, this is not the case. Because the immune system is critically suppressed, reactivation of this latent infection has now emerged as a major respiratory problem, especially in AIDS patients who are intravenous drug users, homeless, or from socially depressed areas.

Atypical mycobacterial infections that frequently cause infections (opportunistic infections) in patients with AIDS include *M. kansasii* and *M. avium-intracellulare (MAI)*. Since the mid-1980s, the incidence of atypical mycobacterial infections has increased dramatically in this group.

Viral pneumonia

Cytomegalovirus (CMV), a member of the herpesvirus family, is the most common viral pulmonary complication of AIDS. CMV also infects other organs, such as the eye, liver, and gastrointestinal tract, and commonly coexists with *Pneumocystis*. Although less common, other herpesviruses, such as herpes simplex and varicella zoster virus, may infect the lungs of patients with AIDS.

Bacterial infection

Patients with AIDS appear to have an increased frequency of bacterial pneumonia as well. *Streptococcus pneumoniae* and *Haemophilus influenzae* are the organisms most commonly found. The increased incidence of bacterial pneumonia in patients with AIDS is presumably related to the depression of the humoral immune system that accompanies the impairment of cellular immunity. It is thought that the loss of T lymphocytes alters the normal relationship between T lymphocytes and the B lymphocytes that produce the antibodies needed to fight bacterial infections.

Fungal diseases

Histoplasmosis and coccidioidomycosis are also seen in AIDS patients, primarily in endemic regions. The criteria for the diagnosis of AIDS are fulfilled when either of these fungal disorders is present in the disseminated form in HIV-positive patients. These two fungal disorders may result from reactivation of dormant spores or from progressive primary infection. Although rarely seen in the tracheobronchial tree or lung parenchyma, the opportunistic yeast pathogens *Candida albicans, Cryptococcus neoformans,* and *Aspergillus* often cause pneumonia in patients with AIDS.

❏ NEOPLASTIC DISEASES

Kaposi's sarcoma is the most common cancer seen in patients with AIDS. Before AIDS, Kaposi's sarcoma was a rare, slow-growing cancer of the skin seen primarily in elderly men. In AIDS, Kaposi's sarcoma is a common clinical manifestation characterized by purplish blotches or bumps on the skin. In AIDS patients, Kaposi's sarcoma spreads much faster than normal.

In AIDS, Kaposi's sarcoma often disseminates to the lungs and gastrointestinal tract. Tumors may be found in the lung parenchyma, bronchi, lymph nodes, and pleura. Tumor nodules are often located on the trunk, neck, and head (especially on the tip of the nose). Pleural involvement commonly leads to pleural effusion. In severe cases, pulmonary hemorrhage may be present. Clinically, pulmonary involvement is difficult to detect. Kaposi's sarcoma is usually suspected when a new, unexplained change suddenly appears on a chest radiograph in patients who already have the skin manifestations of the disease.

The presence of Kaposi's sarcoma alone fulfills the criteria for the diagnosis of AIDS in HIV-infected individuals. Even though treatment for pulmonary Kaposi's sarcoma is generally ineffective, patients with AIDS usually succumb to other coexisting infections or complications of AIDS.

❏ NEUROLOGIC DISEASE

Neurologic complications often develop in patients with AIDS and may involve either the peripheral or central nervous system. Neurologic complications include memory loss, motor problems, poor coordination, and emotional disturbances.

❏ CONSTITUTIONAL SYMPTOMS

Constitutional symptoms involve an unexplained fever and diarrhea, lasting longer than one month, and a weight loss of more than 10%. In full-blown AIDS, weight loss can be extreme. This wasting is particularly common in certain parts of Africa, where AIDS is referred to as the "slim disease."

GENERAL MANAGEMENT OF AIDS

At this time, there is no cure for AIDS. The general management of AIDS consists primarily of (1) supportive care and (2) drugs to control both opportunistic and HIV infections. Agents used to block the HIV infection are actively being investigated. Presently, azidothymidine (AZT or Retrovir or zidovudine) and dedeoxyinosine (DDI or Videx) are approved by the Food and Drug Administration. These agents interrupt and slow the HIV multiplication cycle by merging into the DNA molecule during reverse transcription.

Opportunistic diseases are treated individually. For example, treatment of *Pneumocystis carinii* pneumonia consists of (1) the inhalation of aerosolized pentamidine, (2) oral administration of low doses of trimethoprim sulfamethoxazole, or (3) a combination of both. Penicillins and related agents are used for *Streptococcus* and *Haemophilus influenzae* infections.

The standard pharmacologic agents used to treat tuberculosis consist of multiple drugs for a period of nine months. Isoniazid (INH) and rifampin (Rifadin) are first-line agents prescribed for the entire nine months. Isoniazid is considered to be the most effective first-line antituberculosis agent. Isoniazid is bactericidal and works to prevent the spread of active bacilli. Rifampin is a bactericidal and is most commonly used in combination with isoniazid. During the initial period of two to eight weeks, isoniazid and rifampin are generally supplemented with ethambutol hydrochloride, streptomycin, and/or pyrazinamide. This period is called the *induction phase.* Efforts to reduce the nine-month treatment period to six months have shown some success with the administration of isoniazid, rifampin, pyrazinamide, and either ethambutol hydrochloride or streptomycin for two months, followed by isoniazid and rifampin for four months. For prophylactic use, isoniazid is often given daily for one year to individuals who have been exposed to the tuberculosis bacilli or who have a positive tuberculin reaction (even when the acid-fast stain is negative).

There is no entirely effective treatment for CMV infection, although the antiviral agents ganciclovir and foscarnet sodium may be of some benefit. Amphotericin B is used to treat fungal disorders, and alpha interferon is used to relieve the symptoms associated with Kaposi's sarcoma.

HIV INFECTION/AIDS WITH PNEUMOCYSTIS PNEUMONIA CASE STUDY

ADMITTING HISTORY AND PHYSICAL EXAMINATION

This 37-year-old male has had a long history of numerous homosexual relationships and also developed intravenous drug dependency about two years ago. He had not been feeling well for several weeks and complained of fatigue. He had lost about five pounds and had mild, intermittent diarrhea. For the past 10 days, he had noticed an increasing, nonproductive cough and increasing dyspnea on exertion, and he thought he had a fever. When his respiratory status and malaise did not improve, he decided to go to the emergency room of the local hospital. Two years previously, he had experienced a similar episode and spent three days intubated and on a ventilator.

On physical examination, he was found to be a well-developed, but poorly nourished male who looked somewhat older than his stated age. He was afebrile. Blood pressure was 135/88, pulse 106/min, and respirations 26/min. Percussion and auscultation of the chest were essentially normal. A chest x-ray showed bilateral perihilar infiltrates, consolidation, and atelectasis.

Sputum culture from a bronchoscopic specimen grew *Pneumocystis carinii.* The Western blot test was positive. On room air, his arterial blood gas values were pH 7.56, Pa_{CO_2} 26, HCO_3^- 21, Pa_{O_2} 45. A diagnosis of HIV infection with pneumocystis pneumonia was made, and therapy was started with trimethoprim sulfamethoxazole. At this time, the respiratory care practitioner recorded the following:

RESPIRATORY ASSESSMENT AND PLAN

S: Complains of fatigue, dyspnea, cough, possible fever, 5-pound weight loss.

O: Appears acutely and chronically ill. Afebrile. BP 135/88, P 106 regular, RR 26. Chest exam normal. CXR: Bilateral diffuse infiltrates/consolidation/atelectasis. Sputum silver stain from bronchoscopy: *P. carinii.* Room air ABGs: pH 7.56, Pa_{CO_2} 26, HCO_3^- 21, Pa_{O_2} 45.

A: • HIV infection with *P. carinii* pneumonia (history & sputum culture)
   • Infiltration/consolidation/atelectasis (CXR)
   • Acute alveolar hyperventilation with moderate/severe hypoxemia (ABG)
     • Impending ventilatory failure

P: Admit to ICU per physician's orders. Continuous pulse oximetry. O_2 per protocol. Mask CPAP at +10 cm H_2O for 15 minutes every two hours. ABG in 1 hour and prn. Confer with patient regarding possible need for mechanical ventilation.

Over the next 24 hours, the patient became increasingly dyspneic and anxious. His respiratory rate was 32/min and shallow. On 50% O_2, his arterial blood gases were the following-pH 7.29, Pa_{CO_2} 52, HCO_3^- 22, Pa_{O_2} 39. His chest x-ray was unchanged. He was not coughing productively. A few crackles, but no wheezes or rhonchi could be heard. The patient did not wish to be placed on a ventilator again. The following was documented at this time:

RESPIRATORY ASSESSMENT AND PLAN

S: "I can't seem to get enough air! Please help me!"

O: Extremely dyspneic. Cyanotic on 50% O_2. RR 32 and shallow. pH 7.29, Pa_{CO_2} 52, HCO_3^- 22, Pa_{O_2} 39. CXR unchanged.

A: • Severe pneumocystis pneumonitis (results of bronchoscopy)
   • Infiltration/consolidation/atelectasis (CXR)
   • Acute ventilatory failure with severe hypoxemia (ABG)

P: Patient requests no intubation and no CPR. Discontinue mask CPAP. Titrate O_2 via oxygen therapy protocol. Nasotracheal suction prn. Supportive care as necessary.

DISCUSSION

Recurrent bouts of pneumonia (usually *Pneumocystis carinii* pneumonia) complicating HIV infection are increasingly lethal, as each episode leaves its residual of permanent lung damage. Early determination regarding the wishes of such patients with respect to mechanical ventilation is obviously humane and appropriate.

Hopefully, in the near future, as more specific therapy for the underlying HIV infection becomes available, decisions to forgo ventilator therapy, as occurred in this patient, will become less and less common. The remarkable predilection of such patients to present with pulmonary infections, either *Pneumocystis carinii* pneumonia, multi-drug resistant atypical tuberculosis, or fungal infections, must be kept in mind.

SELF-ASSESSMENT QUESTIONS

Multiple Choice
1. Which of the following white blood cells have a high concentration of CD4 receptor sites on their surface?
   I. Suppressor cells
   II. Helper cells
   III. Inducer cells
   IV. Cytotoxic cells
     a. I only
     b. III only
     c. IV only
     d. II and III only
     e. I and IV only
2. In healthy, noninfected individuals, the T4/T8 ratio is about
     a. 1.
     b. 2.
     c. 3.
     d. 4.
     e. 4.
     f. 5.
3. The most common respiratory complication seen in patients with AIDS is
     a. *Mycobacterium tuberculosis.*
     b. *Pneumocystis carinii.*
     c. Atypical mycobacterium.
     d. Cytomegalovirus.
     e. *Streptococcus pneumoniae.*
4. Which of the following white blood cells is/are the primary target of the HIV?
   I. T4 lymphocytes
   II. Helper cells
   III. CD4-positive cells
   IV. Inducer cells
     a. I only
     b. II only
     c. III and IV only
     d. II and IV only
     e. I, II, III, and IV
5. Normally, the T4 lymphocytes comprise what percent of the circulating T cells?
     a. 20% to 30%
     b. 30% to 40%
     c. 40% to 50%
     d. 50% to 60%
     e. 60% to 70%

Fill in the Blanks
1. The most commonly used HIV confirmatory test is the _____
2. When the HIV enters an individual's T4 lymphocyte, the _____enzyme converts RNA to DNA, which is the reverse of the normal DNA-to-RNA sequence.
3. Treatment of *Pneumocystis carinii* pneumonia consists of the inhalation of aerosolized _____
4. The most common cancer seen in patients with AIDS is _____
5. The irreversible joining of the HIV DNA with the DNA of the white blood cell is called _____

Answers appear in Appendix XXI.

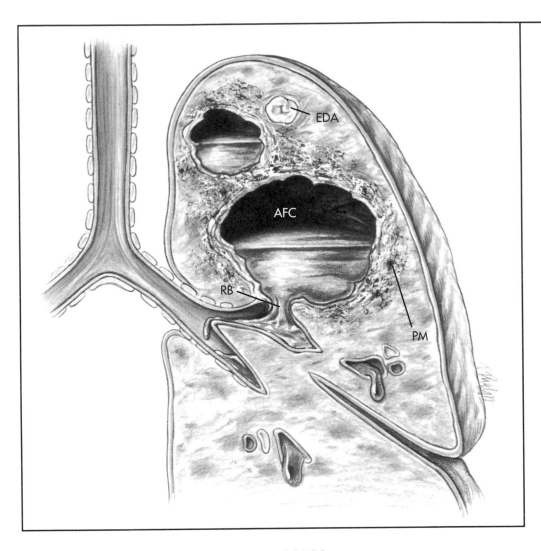

LUNG ABSCESS

FIG 12-1

Cross-sectional view of lung abscess. *AFC* = air-fluid cavity; *RB* = ruptured bronchus (and drainage of the liquified contents of the cavity); *EDA* = early development of abscess; *PM* = pyogenic membrane. (See also Plate 11.)

Lung Abscess

ANATOMIC ALTERATIONS OF THE LUNGS

A lung abscess is defined as a necrosis of lung tissue which, in severe cases, leads to a localized air-fluid cavity. The fluid in the cavity is a collection of purulent exudate that is composed of liquefied white blood cell remains, proteins, and tissue debris. The air-fluid cavity is encapsulated in a so-called pyogenic membrane that consists of a layer of fibrin, inflammatory cells, and granulation tissue.

During the early stages of a lung abscess the pathology is indistinguishable from that of any acute pneumonia. Polymorphonuclear leukocytes and macrophages move into the infected area to engulf any invading organisms. This action causes the pulmonary capillaries to dilate, the interstitium to fill with fluid, and the alveolar epithelium to swell from the edema fluid. In response to this inflammatory reaction, the alveoli in the infected area become consolidated (see Fig 10-1).

As the inflammatory process progresses, tissue necrosis involving all the lung structures occurs. In severe cases, the tissue necrosis will likely rupture into a bronchus and, thus, allow a partial or total drainage of the liquefied contents to the cavity to ensue. An air-fluid cavity may also rupture into the intrapleural space and cause pleural effusion. This may lead to inflammation of the parietal pleura, chest pain, and a decreased chest expansion. After a period of time, fibrosis and calcification of the tissues around the cavity encapsulates the abscess (Fig 12-1).

To summarize, the major pathologic or structural changes associated with a lung abscess are as follows:

- Alveolar consolidation
- Alveolar-capillary and bronchial wall destruction
- Tissue necrosis
- Cavity formation
- Fibrosis and calcification of the lung parenchyma

ETIOLOGY

A lung abscess is most commonly caused by anaerobic organisms. In humans, anaerobic organisms normally inhabit the intestinal tract and are even found in the saliva. Anaerobic organisms often colonize in the small grooves and spaces between the teeth and gums in patients with poor oral hygiene (anaerobic organisms are commonly associated with gingivitis and dead or abscessed teeth). As a general rule, anaerobic organisms enter the lungs when an individual aspirates gastrointestinal fluids that contain the organisms. Anaerobic organisms found in gastrointestinal fluids and saliva include *Peptococcus, Peptostreptococcus, Bactroides,* and *Fusobacterium.* Predisposing factors that frequently lead to the aspiration of gastrointestinal fluids (and anaerobes) are usually related to an altered mental status and include (1) a history of recent alcoholic binge, (2) seizure disorder, (3) a cerebrovascular accident, (4) head trauma, or (5) general anesthesia. The incidence of lung abscesses caused by anaerobic organisms is also high in patients with poor oral hygiene.

Although less frequent, aerobic organisms such as *Staphylococcus aureus, Streptococcus pyogenes, Klebsiella pneumoniae,* and *Escherichia coli* can also cause significant tissue destruction with the formation of a lung abscess. On rare occasions, a lung abscess may also be caused by *Streptococcus pneumoniae, Pseudomonas aeruginosa,* or *Legionella pneumophila.* Typically, more than one type of bacterium is involved, as in an infection with anaerobic organisms mixed with aerobic ones.

Other organisms that may lead to a lung abscess are *Mycobacterium tuberculosis* (including the atypical *Mycobacterium kansasii* and *Mycobacterium avium-intracellulare*) and fungal diseases such as *Histoplasma capsulatum, Coccidioides immitis, Blastomyces,* and *Aspergillus fumigatus.* Some parasites, such as *Paragonimus westermani, Echinococcus,* and *Entamoeba histolytica,* are associated with lung abscess.

Finally, a lung abscess may develop as a result of (1) bronchial obstruction with secondary cavitating infection (e.g., bronchogenic carcinoma or foreign body), (2) vascular obstruction with tissue infarction (e.g., septic embolism or vasculitis), (3) interstitial lung disease with cavity formation (e.g., pneumoconiosis [silicosis], Wegener's granulomatosis, and rheumatoid nodule), (4) cysts that become infected (e.g., congenital or bronchogenic cysts), or (5) a penetrating chest wound that leads to an infection (e.g., bullet wound).

Anatomically, a lung abscess most commonly forms in the superior segments of the lower lobes, and the posterior segments of the upper lobes. The tendency for an abscess to form in these areas is due to the effect of gravity and the dependent position of the tracheobronchial tree at the time of aspiration, which commonly occurs while the patient is in the supine position. The right lung is more commonly involved that the left.

OVERVIEW

OF THE CARDIOPULMONARY CLINICAL MANIFESTATIONS ASSOCIATED WITH
AN ABSCESS OF THE LUNGS

❑ **INCREASED RESPIRATORY RATE**
Several pathophysiologic mechanisms operating simultaneously may lead to an increased ventilatory rate (see page 17):

* Stimulation of peripheral chemoreceptors
* Decreased lung compliance/increased ventilatory rate relationship
* Stimulation of J receptors
* Pain, anxiety/fever

❑ **PULMONARY FUNCTION STUDY FINDINGS (SEVERE AND EXTENSIVE CASES)**

Expiratory Maneuver Findings (see page 39)

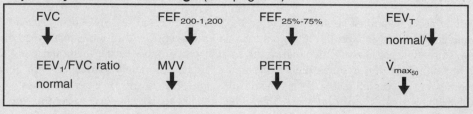

FVC	FEF$_{200-1,200}$	FEF$_{25\%-75\%}$	FEV$_T$
↓	↓	↓	normal/↓
FEV$_1$/FVC ratio normal	MVV ↓	PEFR ↓	$\dot{V}_{max_{50}}$ ↓

Lung Volume and Capacity Findings (see page 39)

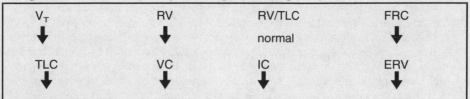

V_T	RV	RV/TLC	FRC
↓	↓	normal	↓
TLC	VC	IC	ERV
↓	↓	↓	↓

❑ **INCREASED HEART RATE (PULSE), CARDIAC OUTPUT, AND BLOOD PRESSURE** (see page 86)
❑ **ARTERIAL BLOOD GASES**

Mild to Moderate Lung Abscess

Acute Alveolar Hyperventilation with Hypoxemia (see page 57)

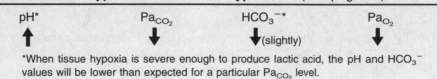

pH*	Pa_{CO_2}	HCO_3^-*	Pa_{O_2}
↑	↓	↓(slightly)	↓

*When tissue hypoxia is severe enough to produce lactic acid, the pH and HCO_3^- values will be lower than expected for a particular Pa_{CO_2} level.

Severe Lung Abscess

Acute Ventilatory Failure with Hypoxemia (see page 59)

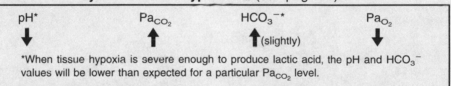

pH*	Pa_{CO_2}	HCO_3^-*	Pa_{O_2}
↓	↑	↑(slightly)	↓

*When tissue hypoxia is severe enough to produce lactic acid, the pH and HCO_3^- values will be lower than expected for a particular Pa_{CO_2} level.

❑ **OXYGENATION INDICES** (see page 69)

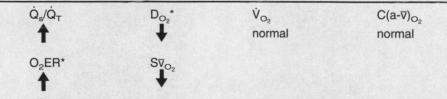

$\dot{Q}_s/\dot{Q}_T$	D_{O_2}*	$\dot{V}_{O_2}$	$C(a-\bar{v})_{O_2}$
↑	↓	normal	normal
O_2ER*	$S\bar{v}_{O_2}$		
↑	↓		

*The D_{O_2} may be normal in patients who have compensated to the decreased oxygenation status with an increased cardiac output. When the D_{O_2} is normal, the O_2ER is usually normal.

❑ **CYANOSIS** (see page 68)
❑ **PLEURAL EFFUSION WITH EMPHYEMA** (see Chapter 19)
❑ **CHEST PAIN/DECREASED CHEST EXPANSION** (see page 98)
❑ **CHEST ASSESSMENT FINDINGS** (see page 6)
- Increased tactile and vocal fremitus
- Crackles/rhonchi
- Directly over the abscess:
  - Dull percussion note
  - Bronchial breath sounds
  - Diminished breath sounds
  - Whispered pectoriloquy
  - Pleural friction rub (if abscess near pleural surface)

❑ **DIGITAL CLUBBING** (see page 93)
❑ **COUGH SPUTUM PRODUCTION AND HEMOPTYSIS** (see page 93)

During the early stages, when the lung abscess is in the inflammatory pneumonia-like phase, the patient generally has a nonproductive barking or hacking cough. If the abscess progresses into an air-fluid cavity and ruptures through a bronchus, the patient may suddenly cough up large amounts of sputum. Foul-smelling brown or gray sputum indicates a putrid infection that is caused by numerous organisms, including anaerobes. An odorless green or yellow sputum indicates a nonputrid infection caused by a single anaerobic organism. Blood-streaked sputum is common in patients with a lung abscess. Occasionally, hemoptysis is seen.

❑ **RADIOLOGIC FINDINGS**
Chest radiograph
  • Increased opacity
  • Cavity formation
  • Fibrosis and calcification
  • Pleural effusion

The chest radiograph typically reveals localized consolidation during the early stages of a lung abscess formation. The characteristic radiograph of a lung abscess appears after (1) the infection ruptures into a bronchus, (2) tissue destruction and necrosis has occurred, and (3) partial evacuation of the purulent contents has occurred. The abcess usually appears on the radiograph as a circular radiolucency that contains an air-fluid level surrounded by a dense wall of lung parenchyma (Fig 12-2).

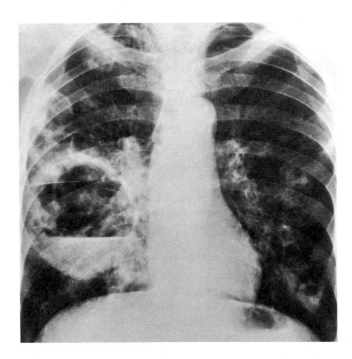

FIG 12-2
Reactivation tuberculosis with a large cavitary lesion containing an air-fluid level in the right lower lobe. Other smaller cavitary lesions are seen in other lobes. (From Armstrong F, Wilson AG, Dee P: *Imaging of diseases of the chest,* St. Louis, 1990, Mosby-Year Book. Used by permission.)

GENERAL MANAGEMENT OF LUNG ABSCESS

When treated properly, most patients with a lung abscess show improvement. In acute cases, the size of the abscess quickly decreases and eventually closes altogether. In severe or chronic cases, the patient's improvement may be slow or insignificant, even under appropriate therapy.

Antibiotic Agents

Antibiotics are the primary treatment for a lung abscess. Penicillin is usually the first drug of choice. For patients who have serious penicillin hypersensitivity, clindamycin, lincomycin, erythromycin, streptomycin, or tetracycline may be used. Methicillin, nafcillin, or vancomycin is commonly used to treat a lung abscess caused by *Staphylococcus aureus*. When *Klebsiella* is the causative agent, kanamycin is commonly administered. For resistant organisms, the antibiotic of choice is based on the results of culture and sensitivity studies.

Mobilization of Bronchial Secretions

Because of the excessive mucus production and accumulation associated with a ruptured abscess, a number of respiratory care modalities (e.g., chest physical therapy and postural drainage) may be used to enhance the mobilization of bronchial secretions (see Appendix XI).

Hyperinflation Techniques

Hyperinflation measures may be used to offset the alveolar consolidation associated with lung abscess (see Appendix XII).

Supplemental Oxygen

Because of the hypoxemia associated with lung abscess, supplemental oxygen may be required. It should be noted, however, that because of the alveolar consolidation produced by a lung abscess, capillary shunting may be present. Hypoxemia caused by capillary shunting is refractory to oxygen therapy.

Surgery

Surgical intervention for drainage or resection of the abcessed lobe or lobes may be helpful in selected, antibiotic-refractory cases.

• • • • **LUNG ABSCESS CASE STUDY** • • • •

ADMITTING HISTORY AND PHYSICAL EXAMINATION

This 64-year-old unemployed male sought medical attention because of an increasingly severe cough that produced moderate amounts of foul-smelling sputum. One year ago, he had undergone splenectomy for removal of a ruptured spleen. He reported that on several occasions recently, he had a slight fever and was anorectic, and he had lost about six pounds. For the past three days, he had noticed some right-sided chest pain, and his cough had become very productive.

Physical examination showed a small and poorly nourished male in moderate distress, coughing throughout the interview. His oral temperature was 100.6° F, and there was brawny discoloration of the legs below the knees. His teeth were in deplorable condition, and he had marked halitosis. Examination of the chest revealed dullness, crackles, rhonchi, and bronchial breath sounds in the right lower lobe.

His frequent cough produced large amounts of foul-smelling brown and gray sputum. The chest x-ray showed a 4-cm diameter density in the right lower lobe with a clear air-fluid level. There was no evidence of empyema. Sputum for a culture and sensitivity study was obtained, but the results were still pending. His arterial blood gas values were the following-pH 7.51, Pa_{CO_2} 29, HCO_3^- 22, Pa_{O_2} 61 on room air. The "Assess and Treat" respiratory care practitioner that was assigned to his case recorded the following:

RESPIRATORY ASSESSMENT AND PLAN

S: "I can't stop coughing." Complains of low-grade fever, loss of appetite, weight loss (6 pounds).

O: Cachectic. T 100.6° orally. Teeth carious. Flat to percussion over RLL Crackles and bronchial breath sounds over RLL CXR: 4-cm-diameter density with fluid level RLL ABGs: pH 7.51, Pa_{CO_2} 29, HCO_3^- 22, Pa_{O_2} 61. Excessive amount of foul-smelling, thick brown and gray sputum.

A: • Malnourished (inspection)
  • Probable lung abscess (CXR & history)
  • Acute alveolar hyperventilation with mild hypoxemia (ABG)
  • Excessive and thick airway secretions (sputum characteristics)

P: Bronchial hygiene with P&D to RLL per protocol. Oxygen therapy per protocol. Spot-check Sa_{O_2}. Encourage deep breathing and coughing. Add mucolytic (acetylcystine) × 5 days. Suggest Social Service and Nutrition Service Comment. Schedule PFT.

Following the results of the sensitivity studies, the physician instituted antibiotic therapy. Over the next 5 days, the patient's general condition improved. His cough and sputum production had decreased remarkably, but not completely. The sputum produced was no longer thick. His Pa_{O_2} increased to 86 mm Hg, and he no longer had acute alveolar hyperventilation. The chest radiograph revealed that his lung abscess was slightly reduced in size when compared with the chest radiograph taken on the day of his admission. His PFT revealed a mild reduction in lung volumes, capacities, and expiratory flow rates. Social service worked with him on two occasions during his hospitalization and scheduled a follow-up appointment at his home four weeks after discharge. The patient was instructed on deep-breathing and coughing techniques and general bronchial hygiene, and was discharged on the morning of the sixth day.

DISCUSSION

The appropriate respiratory care of patients with lung abscess closely resembles that of those with bronchiectasis (see Chapter 6). Identification of this patient's lung abscess in the right lower lobe allowed targeted chest physical therapy to be practiced. The suggestion that the Social Service representative see the patient was entirely appropriate. Extraction of his carious teeth might also improve his outlook.

SELF-ASSESSMENT QUESTIONS

Multiple Choice

1. Which of the following is/are anaerobic organisms?
    I. *Klebsiella*
    II. *Peptococcus*
    III. *Coccidioides immitis*
    IV. *Bacteroides*
        a. I and II only
        b. II and IV only
        c. III and IV only
        d. II, III, and IV only
        e. I, III, and IV only

2. Which of the following is/are predisposing factors to the aspiration of gastrointestinal fluids (and anaerobes)?
    I. Seizure disorders
    II. Head trauma
    III. Alcoholic binges
    IV. General anesthesia
        a. I and III only
        b. II and IV only
        c. II and III only
        d. II, III, and IV only
        e. I, II, III, and IV

3. Which of the following aerobic organisms is/are associated with the formation of a lung abscess?
    I. *Fusobacterium*
    II. *Staphylococcus aureus*
    III. *Klebsiella*
    IV. *Streptococcus pyogenes*
        a. I only
        b. III only
        c. II and IV only
        d. II, III, and IV only
        e. I, II, III, and IV

4. Anatomically, a lung abscess most commonly forms in the
    I. Posterior segment of the upper lobe.
    II. Lateral basal segment of the lower lobe.
    III. Anterior segment of the upper lobe.
    IV. Superior segment of the lower lobe.
        a. I only
        b. III only
        c. I and IV only
        d. II and III only
        e. II, III, and IV only

5. Which of the following pulmonary function findings are associated with a severe and extensive lung abscess?
    I. Decreased FVC
    II. Increased PEFR
    III. Decreased RV
    IV. Increased FRC
        a. I only
        b. III only
        c. II and IV only
        d. III and IV only
        e. I and III only

True or False

1. Penicillin is usually the first drug of choice in treating a lung abscess.

   True _____   False _____

2. An odorless green or yellow sputum indicates a putrid infection that is caused by numerous organisms.

   True _____   False _____

3. In humans, anaerobic organisms normally inhabit the intestines and are found in the saliva.

   True _____   False _____

4. Some parasites, such as *Echinococcus,* are associated with lung abscess.

   True _____   False _____

5. A lung abscess is more commonly found in the left lung rather than the right lung.

   True _____   False _____

Answers appear in Appendix XXI.

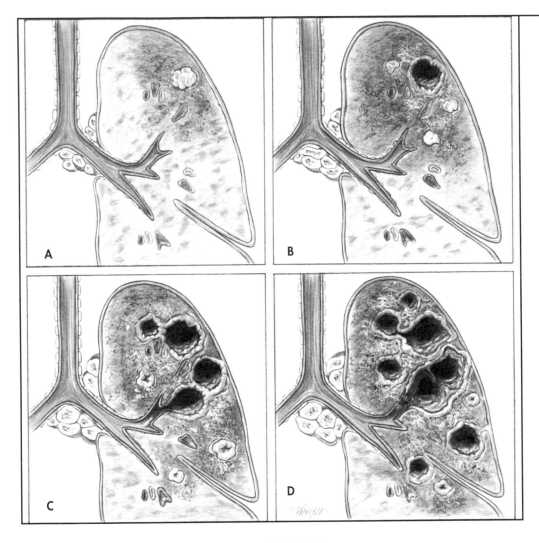

TUBERCULOSIS

FIG 13-1

Tuberculosis. **A,** early primary infection. **B,** cavitation of a caseous tubercle and new primary lesions developing. **C,** further progression and development of cavitations and new primary infections. **D,** severe lung destruction caused by tuberculosis. (See also Plate 12.)

Tuberculosis

ANATOMIC ALTERATIONS OF THE LUNGS

Tuberculosis (TB) is a chronic, bacterial infection that primarily affects the lungs, although it may occur in almost any part of the body. Clinically, tuberculosis is separated into the following three categories: **primary tuberculosis, postprimary tuberculosis,** and **disseminated tuberculosis.**

Primary Tuberculosis

Primary tuberculosis (also called the primary infection stage) entails the patient's first exposure to the pathogen. Primary tuberculosis begins when inhaled bacilli implant in the alveoli. As the bacilli multiply over a three- to four-week period, the initial response of the lungs is an inflammatory reaction that is similar to any acute pneumonia (see Fig 10-1). In other words, there is a large influx of polymorphonuclear leukocytes and macrophages that move into the infected area to engulf (but not fully kill) the bacilli. This action also causes the pulmonary capillaries to dilate, the interstitium to fill with fluid, and the alveolar epithelium to swell from the edema fluid. Eventually, the alveoli become consolidated (i.e., filled with fluid, polymorphonuclear leukocytes, and macrophages). Clinically, this phase of tuberculosis coincides with a *positive tuberculin reaction.*

Unlike pneumonia, however, the lung tissue that surrounds the infected area slowly produces a protective cell wall called a *tubercle,* or *granuloma,* that surrounds and encases the bacilli. A tubercle consists of a central core containing TB bacilli and enlarged macrophages and an outer wall composed of fibroblasts, lymphocytes, and neutrophils. It takes about 2 to 10 weeks for a tubercle to form. Although the formation of a tubercle works to prevent further spread of infection, it also carries the potential for more damage. For example, the center of the tubercle frequently breaks down and fills with necrotic tissue that resembles dry cottage cheese. When this occurs, the tubercle is called a *caseous lesion* or *caseous granuloma.*

If the bacilli are controlled (either by the patient's immunologic defense system or by antituberculous drugs), fibrosis and calcification of the lung parenchyma ultimately replace the tubercle during the healing process. As a result of the fibrosis and calcification, the lung tissue retracts and becomes rigid. Because of the destruction, calcification, and fibrosis, distortion and dilation of the bronchi (bronchiectasis) are commonly seen.

Postprimary Tuberculosis

Postprimary tuberculosis (also called secondary or reinfection tuberculosis) is used to describe the reactivation of the tuberculosis months or even years after the initial infection has been controlled. Even though most of the patients with primary tuberculosis recover completely, it is important to note that live tubercle bacilli can remain dormant for decades. This is why a positive tuberculin reaction generally persists even after the primary infection stage has been controlled. At any time, the bacilli encased in a tubercle may become reactivated, especially in patients with weakened immunity. If uncontrolled, cavitation of the caseous tubercle develops. In severe cases, a deep tuberculous cavity may rupture and allow air and infected material to flow into the pleural space or into the tracheobronchial tree. Pleural complications are common in tuberculosis (Fig 13-1).

Disseminated Tuberculosis

Disseminated tuberculosis (also called extrapulmonary tuberculosis) refers to bacilli that escape from a tubercle and rapidly disseminate to sites other than the lungs by means of the pulmonary lymphatic system or bloodstream. In general, the bacilli that gain entrance into the bloodstream usually gather and multiply in portions of the body that have a high tissue oxygen tension. The most common location is the apex of the lungs. Other oxygen-rich areas in the body include the regional lymph nodes, kidneys, the ends of long bones, genital tract, brain, and meninges. When a large number of bacilli are freed into the bloodstream, they can produce a condition called *miliary tuberculosis,* i.e., the presence of numerous small tubercles (about the size of a pinhead) scattered throughout the body.

To summarize, the major pathologic or structural changes of the lungs associated with tuberculosis (mainly postprimary tuberculosis) are as follows:

* Alveolar consolidation
* Alveolar-capillary destruction
* Caseous tubercles or granulomas
* Cavity formation
* Fibrosis and calcification of the lung parenchyma
* Distortion and dilation of the bronchi

ETIOLOGY

TB is one of the oldest diseases known to man and remains one of the most widespread diseases in the world. The remains of ancient skeletons from 4000 B.C. have been found with characteristic tuberculous changes. TB was a common disease in Egypt around 1000 B.C. In early writings, the disease was commonly called **"consumption," "Captain of the Men of Death,"** and **"white plague."** In the 19th century, the disease was named **tuberculosis,** which arose mainly from the tubercle formation described during postmortem examinations.

In the early 1980s, the incidence of TB in the United States was at its lowest level in modern history. Then, in 1985, the rate of TB started rising and has risen ever since. In 1990, the incidence of TB had risen 16% since 1984. The increased incidence of TB has primarily been due to the higher rate of infection among homeless people, AIDS patients, and drug addicts.

In humans, tuberculosis is primarily caused by *Mycobacterium tuberculosis.* The mycobacteria are long, slender, straight, or curved rods. There are about 50 different mycobacteria species, and several can cause tuberculosis in humans (e.g., *M. povis, M. ulcerans, M. kansasii, M. avium,* and *M. intracellulare* complex). Mycobacterial infections caused by species other than *M. tuberculosis* are called **MOTT** (Mycobacteria other than tuberculosis), or **atypi-**

cal mycobacterial infections. In immunosuppressed patients (e.g., AIDS), the incidence of tuberculous disease associated with atypical mycobacterial infections is rapidly increasing—especially those caused by *M. kansasii* and *M. avium-intracellulare (MAI)* complex.

The mycobacteria are highly aerobic organisms and thrive best in areas of the body with high oxygen tension (e.g., the apex of the lung). When stained, the hard outer layer of the tubercle bacilli resists decolorization by acid or alcohol and, hence, are called *acid-fast* bacilli. In addition, the hard, outer coat of the tubercle bacillus also protects the organism against killing and digestion by phagocytes and renders the bacilli more resistant to antituberculous drugs.

The tubercle bacillus is almost exclusively transmitted within aerosol droplets produced by the coughing, sneezing, or laughing of an individual with active tuberculosis. In fact, in fine dried aerosol droplets, the tubercle bacillus can remain suspended in air for several hours after a cough or sneeze. When inhaled, some of the tubercle bacilli may be trapped in the mucus of the nasal passages and removed. The smaller bacilli, however, can easily be inhaled into the bronchioles and alveoli. People living in closed, small rooms with limited access to sunlight and fresh air are especially at risk. The bacillus may also gain entrance into the body through skin lesions, laboratory accidents (e.g., needle puncture from an infected site), or ingestion (e.g., drinking unpasteurized milk that is infected with *M. bovis*).

Although the factors responsible for postprimary tuberculosis are not fully understood, conditions that weaken the local and systemic body defenses seem to play a major role. Such conditions include AIDS, diabetes mellitus, surgery, childbirth, puberty, treatment with immunosuppressive drugs, alcoholism, nutritional deficiency, chronic debilitating disorders, and old age. TB in patients with AIDS is now at epidemic levels.

DIAGNOSIS

The most frequently used diagnostic methods for tuberculosis are the tuberculin skin test, acid-fast stain and sputum cultures, and chest radiographs.

Tuberculin Skin Testing

The tuberculin skin test measures the delayed hypersensitivity (cell mediated, type IV) that follows exposure to tuberculoproteins. The most commonly used tuberculin test is the *Mantoux test,* which consists of an intradermal injection of a small amount of a purified protein derivative (PPD) of the tuberculin bacillus. In the Mantoux test, 0.1 ml of PPD is injected into the forearm to produce an immediate small bleb. The skin is then observed for induration (wheal) after 48 hours and 72 hours. An induration less than 5 mm is negative. An induration between 5 mm and 9 mm is considered suspicious, and retesting is required. An induration of 10 mm or greater is considered positive. A positive reaction is fairly sound evidence of recent or past infection or disease. It should be stressed, however, that a positive reaction does not necessarily confirm that a patient has active tuberculosis, only that there has been exposure to the bacillus and that cell-mediated immunity to the bacillus has developed.

Acid-Fast Stain and Sputum Culture

An acid-fast stain of sputum is commonly used to confirm the diagnosis of *M. tuberculosis.* There are several variations of the acid-fast stain currently in use. The Ziehl-Neelsen stain reveals bright red acid-fast bacilli (AFB) against a blue background. Another technique involves a fluorescent acid-fast stain that reveals luminescent yellow-green bacilli against a dark brown background. The fluorescent acid-fast stain is becoming the acid-fast test of choice because it is easier to read and provides a striking contrast.

A positive acid-fast stain should be followed by a sputum culture. A culture is necessary to differentiate *M. tuberculosis* from other acid-fast organisms. Culture results can take up to six to eight weeks to obtain. Culturing also identifies drug-resistant bacilli and their sensitivity to antibiotic therapy. The sputum specimen should be obtained from deep in the lungs early in the morning. Saliva or nasal secretions are not acceptable.

OVERVIEW

OF THE CARDIOPULMONARY CLINICAL MANIFESTATIONS ASSOCIATED WITH
TUBERCULOSIS

❏ **INCREASED RESPIRATORY RATE**

Several pathophysiologic mechanisms operating simulatenously may lead to an increased ventilatory rate. These are (see page 17)
- Stimulation of peripheral chemoreceptors
- Decreased lung compliance/increased ventilatory rate relationship
- Stimulation of J receptors
- Pain/anxiety/fever

❏ **PULMONARY FUNCTION STUDY FINDINGS**

Expiratory Maneuver Findings (see page 39)

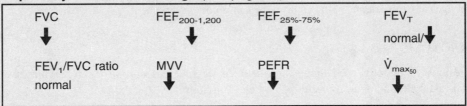

FVC	FEF$_{200-1,200}$	FEF$_{25\%-75\%}$	FEV$_T$
↓	↓	↓	normal/↓
FEV$_1$/FVC ratio normal	MVV ↓	PEFR ↓	$\dot{V}_{max_{50}}$ ↓

Lung Volume and Capacity Findings (see page 39)

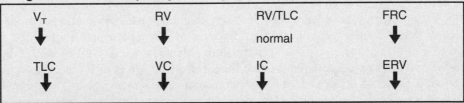

V$_T$	RV	RV/TLC	FRC
↓	↓	normal	↓
TLC ↓	VC ↓	IC ↓	ERV ↓

❏ **INCREASED HEART RATE (PULSE), CARDIAC OUTPUT, AND BLOOD PRESSURE** (see page 86)

❏ **ARTERIAL BLOOD GASES**

Mild to Moderate Tuberculosis

Acute Alveolar Hyperventilation with Hypoxemia (see page 57)

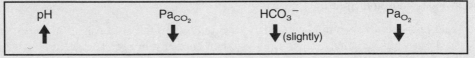

| pH | Pa$_{CO_2}$ | HCO$_3^-$ | Pa$_{O_2}$ |
| ↑ | ↓ | ↓ (slightly) | ↓ |

Severe Tuberculosis

Chronic Ventilatory Failure with Hypoxemia (see page 60)

pH	Pa_{CO_2}	HCO_3^-	Pa_{O_2}
normal	↑	↑ (significantly)	↓

Acute ventilatory changes superimposed on chronic ventilatory failure (see page 65)

Because acute ventilatory changes are frequently seen in patients with chronic ventilatory failure, the respiratory care practitioner must be familiar with and be on the alert for (1) *acute alveolar hyperventilation superimposed on chronic ventilatory failure,* and (2) *acute ventilatory failure superimposed on chronic ventilatory failure.*

❑ **OXYGENATION INDICES** (see page 69)

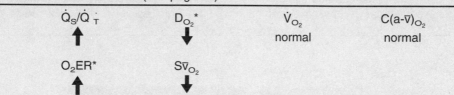

$\dot{Q}_S/\dot{Q}_T$	D_{O_2}*	$\dot{V}_{O_2}$	$C(a-\bar{v})_{O_2}$
↑	↓	normal	normal

O_2ER*	$S\bar{v}_{O_2}$		
↑	↓		

*The D_{O_2} may be normal in patients who have compensated for the decreased oxygenation status with an increased cardiac output, an increased hemoglobin level, or a combination of both. When the D_{O_2} is normal, the O_2ER is usually normal.

❑ **CYANOSIS** (see page 68)
❑ **HEMODYNAMIC INDICES (SEVERE TUBERCULOSIS)** (see page 87)

CVP	RAP	$\overline{PA}$	PCWP
↑	↑	↑	normal
CO	SV	SVI	CI
normal	normal	normal	normal
RVSWI	LVSWI	PVR	SVR
↑	normal	↑	normal

❑ **POLYCYTHEMIA, COR PULMONALE** (see page 92)
 • Elevated hemoglobin concentration and hematocrit
 • Distended neck veins
 • Enlarged and tender liver
 • Pitting edema

❑ **CHEST ASSESSMENT FINDINGS** (see page 6)
 • Increased tactile and vocal fremitus
 • Dull percussion note
 • Bronchial breath sounds
 • Crackles/rhonchi/wheezing
 • Pleural friction rub (if process extends to pleural surface)
 • Whispered pectoriloquy

❑ **PLEURAL EFFUSION** (see Chapter 19)
❑ **COUGH, SPUTUM PRODUCTION, AND HEMOPTYSIS** (see page 93)

❑ **CHEST PAIN/DECREASED CHEST EXPANSION** (see page 98)
❑ **RADIOLOGIC FINDINGS**
  Chest radiograph
  • Increased opacity
  • Ghon complex
  • Cavity formation
  • Pleural effusion
  • Calcification and fibrosis
  • Retraction of lung segments or lobe
  • Right ventricular enlargement

Chest radiography is most valuable in the diagnosis of pulmonary tuberculosis. During the initial primary infection stage, peripheral inflammation can be identified. As the disease progresses, the combination of tubercles and the involvement of the lymph nodes in the hilar region (the Ghon complex) can be seen. In severe cases, cavity formation and pleural effusion can readily be seen (Fig 13-2). Healed lesions appear fibrotic or calcified. Retraction of the healed lesions or segments will also be revealed on chest radiographs. In patients with postprimary tuberculosis of the lungs, lesions involving the apical and posterior segments of the upper lobes are often seen. Finally, because right-sided heart failure may develop as a secondary problem during the advanced stages of tuberculosis, an enlarged heart may be seen on the chest radiograph.

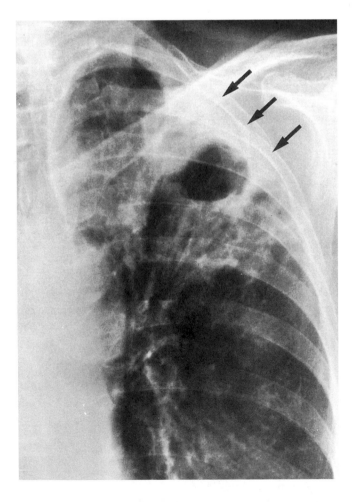

FIG 13-2
Cavitary reactivation tuberculosis showing localized pleural thickening (arrows). (From Armstrong P, Wilson AG, Dee P: *Imaging of diseases of the chest,* St. Louis, 1990, Mosby-Year Book. Used by permission.)

GENERAL MANAGEMENT OF TUBERCULOSIS

Because the tubercle bacillus can exist in open cavitary lesions, in closed lesions, and within the cytoplasm of macrophages, a drug that may be effective in one of these environments may be ineffective in another. In addition, some of the tuberculosis bacilli are often drug-resistant. Because of this problem, several drugs are usually prescribed concurrently. Since there is toxicity associated with antituberculosis drugs, frequent examinations are performed to identify toxicity manifested in the kidneys, liver, eyes, and ears. When the disease is identified, the patient is typically hospitalized for the first week of therapy to ensure proper compliance with the prescribed drug regimen, to monitor the patient for adverse effects, and to encourage rest and good nutrition.

Pharmacologic Agents Used to Treat Tuberculosis

The standard pharmacologic agents used to treat tuberculosis consist of multiple drugs for nine months. Isoniazid (INH) and rifampin (Rifadin) are first-line agents prescribed for the entire nine months. Isoniazid is considered to be the most effective first-line antituberculosis agent. Isoniazid is bactericidal and works to prevent the spread of active bacilli. Rifampin is bactericidal and is most commonly used in combination with isoniazid.

During the initial period of two to nine weeks, isoniazid and rifampin are generally supplemented with ethambutol, streptomycin, or pyrazinamide. This period is called the *induction phase*. Efforts to reduce the nine-month treatment period to six months have shown some success with the administration of the following four drugs: isoniazid, rifampin, pyrazinamide, and either ethambutol or streptomycin for two months, followed by isoniazid and rifampin for four months.

Finally, it should be noted that the prophylactic use of isoniazid is often prescribed as a daily dose for one year in individuals who have been exposed to the tuberculosis bacilli, or who have a positive tuberculin reaction (even when acid-fast stain is negative).

Supplemental Oxygen

Because of the hypoxemia associated with tuberculosis, supplemental oxygen may be required. It should be noted, however, that because of the alveolar consolidation and destruction caused by tuberculosis, capillary shunting is present. Hypoxemia caused by capillary shunting is refractory to oxygen therapy. In addition, when the patient demonstrates chronic ventilatory failure during the advanced stages of tuberculosis, caution must be taken not to eliminate the patient's hypoxic drive to breathe.

• • • • TUBERCULOSIS CASE STUDY • • • •

ADMITTING HISTORY AND PHYSICAL EXAMINATION

A 60-year-old male had been in good health until about four months prior to admission, when he first noticed the onset of night sweats, occasionally accompanied by chills. Three months ago, he noticed that his appetite was decreasing, and he had lost about 25 pounds since that time.

Three weeks ago, he noticed that his "smoker's cough" of long standing had become more productive. For the past two weeks, his daily sputum production had increased to about a cup of thick yellow sputum with an occasional fleck or two of blood. There was a concomitant increase in dyspnea. About 10 days ago, he had the gradual onset of moderately sharp, left-sided chest pain. It was aggravated by deep breathing, but did not radiate.

The past history gave little useful information. The last time the patient sought medical assistance was 33 years ago when he suffered a broken arm in an industrial accident. At that time, he was told that he had a positive tuberculin reaction, but that he had no specific pulmonary problems. He has had several chest x-rays in mobile chest x-ray units since then, once for an insurance application. The last one was five years ago.

For the past 35 years, he was employed in a foundry as a "cone maker" and "shaker." He volunteered the information that he worked in a "dusty" environment and was wearing a protective mask only for the past few months. His family history was noncontributory.

Physical examination revealed a thin elderly man who appeared chronically and acutely ill. Temperature was 102.4° F orally, pulse 116, blood pressure 132/90, and respirations 32/min. There was marked dullness to percussion in both apical areas. There were diffuse inspiratory crackles and expiratory rhonchi in the right upper and middle lobes. A chest x-ray demonstrated extensive bilateral apical calcification with cavity formation in the right upper lobe, and a diffuse infiltrate in the right middle lobe. He was admitted to the hospital. This initial respiratory assessment and plan was entered into the patient's chart:

RESPIRATORY ASSESSMENT AND PLAN

S: Productive cough, slight hemoptysis, moderate dyspnea. History of left-sided chest pain for 10 days.

O: Febrile to 102.4° F, RR 32, P 116, BP 132/90. Crackles and rhonchi in right upper and right middle lobes. CXR: Apical calcification; RUL cavity; RML infiltrate.

A: • Probable tuberculosis (patient possibly infectious).
       • Large airway secretion in RUL and RML (rhonchi)

P: Flag chart: Respiratory isolation pending smear results. Obtain sputum for routine, anaerobic and acid-fast cultures and cytology—induce if necessary. Obtain baseline ABG on room air. Based on ABG results, titrate oxygen therapy per protocol. Discuss need for bedside spirogram with physician.

DISCUSSION

Currently, there is a near epidemic of tuberculosis in the United States. In almost every hospital of any size, the number of acute tuberculosis cases being admitted per year is increased. Much of this epidemic is associated with multiple-drug resistant organisms in patients who have not completed initial courses of chemotherapy. Another large proportion of these cases are in patients with HIV disease, or other immune system disorders. Elderly patients who live in crowded quarters, such as those in nursing homes and convalescent hospitals are also at risk. This diagnosis is first made on the basis of a strong clinical suspicion, particularly in these settings.

The history of a positive tuberculin reaction, fever, cough, hemoptysis, and an apical infiltrate with abscess formation strongly suggests a diagnosis of tuberculosis.

The inpatient respiratory care of such patients is made slightly more complex by the recent OSHA requirements regarding at least six room air changes an hour, particulate scrubbers, and protective masks that must be worn by all health care workers. The decision by the respiratory care practitioner (who was the first person on the ward to see the patient) to place him in isolation pending smear results was entirely appropriate. Had there been difficulty obtaining a sputum specimen, sputum induction, postural drainage, induction with hypertonic saline, or even bronchoscopy may have been necessary.

The patient indeed did produce sputum containing acid-fast organisms. The attending physician prescribed isoniazid, rifampin, and streptomycin for two months followed by a course of isoniazid and rifampin as an outpatient for four months. The patient did well through follow-up.

SELF-ASSESSMENT QUESTIONS

Multiple Choice

1. The first stage of tuberculosis is known as
    I. Reinfection tuberculosis.
    II. Primary tuberculosis.
    III. Secondary tuberculosis.
    IV. Primary infection stage.
        a. I only
        b. II only
        c. III only
        d. I and III only
        e. II and IV only

2. What is the protective cell wall called that surrounds and encases lung tissue infected with tuberculosis?
    I. Miliary tuberculosis
    II. Reinfection tuberculosis
    III. Granuloma
    IV. Tubercle
        a. I only
        b. III only
        c. IV only
        d. III and IV only
        e. II and III only

3. The tubercle bacillus is
    I. Highly aerobic.
    II. Acid-fast.
    III. Capable of surviving for months.
    IV. Rod-shaped.
        a. I only
        b. II only
        c. IV only
        d. II and III only
        e. I, II, III, and IV

4. At which size wheal is a tuberculin skin test considered to be positive?
        a. greater than 4 mm
        b. greater than 6 mm
        c. greater than 8 mm
        d. greater than 10 mm
        e. greater than 12 mm

5. Which of the following is often prescribed as a daily dose for one year in individuals who have been exposed to the tuberculosis bacilli?
        a. Streptomycin
        b. Ethambutol
        c. Isoniazid
        d. Rifampin
        e. Pyrazinamide

True or False

1. Pleural space complications are common in patients with tuberculosis.   True _____   False _____
2. A positive reaction to the tuberculin skin test confirms that a patient has active tuberculosis.   True _____   False _____
3. Tuberculosis commonly develops in the apex of the lungs.   True _____   False _____
4. The tuberculin skin test measures the delayed hypersensitivity that follows exposure to the tubercle bacillus.   True _____   False _____
5. Miliary tuberculosis is a small, isolated tubercle lesion.   True _____   False _____

Answers appear in Appendix XXI.

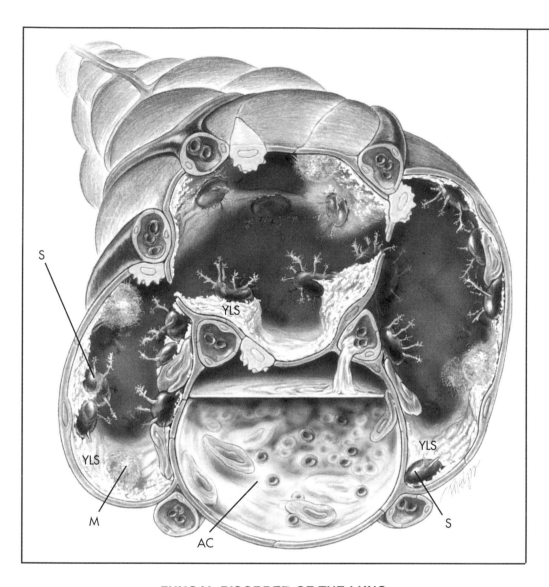

FUNGAL DISORDER OF THE LUNG

FIG 14-1

Cross-sectional view of alveoli infected with *Histoplasma capsulatum. S* = spore; *YLS* = yeastlike substance; *AC* = alveolar consolidation; *M* = macrophage. (See also Plate 13.)

Fungal Diseases
of the Lungs

ANATOMIC ALTERATIONS OF THE LUNGS

When fungal spores are inhaled, they may reach the lungs and germinate. When this happens, the spores produce a frothy, yeastlike substance that leads to an inflammatory response. Polymorphonuclear leukocytes and macrophages move into the infected area and engulf the fungal spores. The pulmonary capillaries dilate, the interstitium fills with fluid, and the alveolar epithelium swells with edema fluid. Regional lymph node involvement commonly occurs during this period. Because of the inflammatory reaction, the alveoli in the infected area eventually become consolidated (Fig 14-1).

In severe cases, tissue necrosis, granulomas, and cavity formation may be seen. During the healing process, fibrosis and calcification of the lung parenchyma ultimately replace the granulomas. In response to the fibrosis and calcification, the lung tissue retracts and becomes rigid. The apical and posterior segments of the upper lobes are most commonly involved. The anatomic changes of the lungs caused by fungal diseases are similar to those seen in tuberculosis.

To summarize, the major pathologic or structural changes of the lungs associated with fungal diseases of the lungs are as follows:

- Alveolar consolidation
- Alveolar-capillary destruction
- Granuloma formation
- Cavity formation
- Fibrosis and calcification of the lung parenchyma

ETIOLOGY

Fungal spores are widely distributed throughout the air, soil, dust, fomites, animals, and even among the normal flora of humans. It is estimated that as many as 300 fungal species may be linked to disease in animals. Among plants, fungal disease is the most common cause of destruction. In humans, most exposures to fungal pathogens do not lead to overt infection. This is because humans have a relatively high resistance to fungal pathogens. Human fungal disease (also called *mycotic disease* or *mycosis*) can be caused, however, by "primary" or "true" fungal pathogens that exhibit some degree of virulence, or with "opportunistic" or "secondary" pathogens that take advantage of a weakened defense system (e.g., AIDS).

PRIMARY PATHOGENS
Histoplasmosis

Histoplasmosis is the most common fungal infection in the United States. It is caused by the dimorphic fungus *Histoplasma capsulatum*. In the United States, it is estimated that the incidence of histoplasmosis is about 500,000 cases per year, with several thousand cases requiring hospitalization. A small number of cases result in death. The prevalence of histoplasmosis is especially high along the major river valleys of the Midwest (e.g., Ohio, Michigan, Illinois, Mississippi, Missouri, Kentucky, Tennessee, Georgia, and Arkansas). In fact, on the basis of skin test surveys it is estimated that 80% to 90% of the population throughout these areas show signs of prior infection—hence, histoplasmosis is often called *Ohio Valley fever*.

Histoplasma capsulatum is commonly found in soils enriched with bird excreta such as the soil near chicken houses, pigeon lofts, barns, and trees where starlings and blackbirds roost. The birds themselves, however, do not carry the organism, although the *Histoplasma capsulatum* spore may be carried by bats. Generally, an individual acquires the infection by inhaling the fungal spores that are released when the soil from an infected area is disturbed (e.g., children playing in dirt).

When the *H. capsulatum* organism reaches the alveoli, at body temperature it converts from its mycelial form (mold) to a parasitic yeast form. The clinical manifestations of histoplasmosis are strikingly similar to those seen in tuberculosis. Depending on the individual's immune system, the disease may take on one of four forms: latent asymptomatic disease, primary pulmonary histoplasmosis, chronic histoplasmosis, or disseminated infection. The incubation period for the infection is about 14 days. Only about 40% of those infected demonstrate symptoms, and only about 10% of these patients are ill enough to consult a physician.

Latent asymptomatic histoplasmosis is characterized by healed lesions in the lungs or hilar lymph nodes as well as a positive histoplasmin skin test.

Primary pulmonary histoplasmosis appears as a mild, self-limiting, febrile, respiratory infection. Early clinical manifestations include muscle and joint pains and a dry, hacking cough. Hivelike lesions (erythema multiforme) and subcutaneous nodules (erythema nodosum) may appear. During this phase of the disease, the patient's chest radiograph generally shows single- or multiple-infection sites.

Chronic histoplasmosis is characterized by infiltration and cavity formation in the upper lobes of one or both lungs. Clinically, this stage of the disease is similar to postprimary tuberculosis and is more commonly seen in middle-aged men who smoke. The patient often has a productive cough, fever, night sweats, and weight loss. Oftentimes, the infection is self-limiting. In some patients, however, there may be progressive destruction of lung tissue and dissemination of the infection.

Disseminated histoplasmosis may follow either self-limited histoplasmosis or chronic histoplasmosis. It is most often seen in the very old or very young or in patients with abnormal immune systems (e.g., patients with AIDS). Even though the macrophages can remove the fungi from the bloodstream, they are unable to kill them. The clinical manifestations of disseminated histoplasmosis include high-grade fever, generalized lymph node enlargement, hepatosplenomegaly, muscle wasting, anemia, leukopenia, and thrombocytopenia. The patient may be hoarse and have ulcerations of the mouth and tongue, nausea, vomiting, diarrhea, and abdominal pain.

The *histoplasmosis skin test,* which entails the injection of a fungal extract called *histoplasmin* into the skin, is used to determine the presence of the organism. The presence of *H. capsulatum* causes a delayed hypersensitivity immune response. A positive finding does not reveal whether the disease is recent or old. Confirmation of histoplasmosis requires culture and identification of the organism.

When the histoplasmosis organism is present, the infection causes a delayed hypersensitivity immune response and, therefore, the production of antibodies. Even though these antibodies are not protective, they serve as excellent evidence for the presence of the disease.

The complement fixation (CF) test is used to show the presence of these antibodies. The presence of antibodies can also be shown with the immunodiffusion (ID) test. Both CF and ID tests become positive two weeks after the clinical manifestions of the disease appear.

Coccidioidomycosis

Coccidioidomycosis is caused by inhaling the spores of *Coccidioides immitis,* which are spherical fungi carried by wind-borne dust particles. The disease is endemic in hot, dry regions. It is estimated that about 100,000 new cases occur annually. In the United States, coccidioidomycosis is especially prevalent in California, Arizona, Nevada, New Mexico, Texas, and Utah. About 80% of the people in the San Joaquin Valley are coccidioidin skin test positive. Because the prevalence of coccidioidomycosis is high in these regions, the disease is also known as *California disease, desert fever, San Joaquin Valley disease,* or *valley fever.* The fungus has been isolated in these regions from soils, plants, and a large number of vertebrates (e.g., mammals, birds, reptiles, and amphibians).

When *Coccidioides immitis* spores are inhaled, they settle in the lungs, begin to germinate, and form round, thin-walled cells called *spherules.* The spherules, in turn, produce endospores that make more spherules (the spherule-endospore phase). The disease usually takes the form of an acute, primary self-limiting pulmonary infection with or without systemic involvement. Some cases, however, progress to a disseminated disease.

Clinical manifestations are absent in about 60% of the people who have a positive skin test. In the remaining 40%, most of the patients demonstrate coldlike symptoms such as fever, chest pain, cough, headaches, and malaise. In uncomplicated cases, the patient generally has complete recovery and lifelong immunity. In about one out of 200 cases, however, the primary infection does not resolve, and progresses with varied clinical manifestations. Chronic progressive pulmonary disease is characterized by nodular growths called *fungomas* and cavity formation in the lungs. Disseminated coccidioidomycosis occurs in about one out of 6,000 exposed persons. When this condition exists, there may be involvement of the lymph nodes, meninges, spleen, liver, kidney, skin, and adrenals. The skin lesions (e.g., bumps on the face and chest) are commonly accompanied by arthralgia or arthritis, especially in the ankles and knees. This condition is commonly called *desert bumps, desert arthritis,* or *desert rheumatism.* Death is most commonly caused by meningitis.

The diagnosis of coccidioidomycosis can be made by the direct visualization of distinctive spherules in microscopy of the patient's sputum, tissue exudates, biopsies, or spinal fluid. This finding can be further supported when the spores are isolated and cultured. Two antigen tests, the *immunodiffusion test* and the *latex agglutination test,* are also useful in the diagnosis of coccidioidomycosis. Two skin tests, the *coccidioidin skin test* or the *spherulin skin test* can also be used to determine whether the disease is present. Neither test, however, indicates whether the disease is recent or old.

Blastomycosis

Blastomycosis (also called Chicago disease) is caused by *Blastomyces dermatitidis. Blastomycosis* is most common in North America. In general, blastomycosis is seen from southern Canada to southern Louisiana and from Minnesota to the Carolinas and Georgia. Cases have also been reported in Central America, South America, Africa, and the Middle East. *Blastomyces dermatitidis* inhabits areas high in organic matter such as forest soil, decaying wood, animal manure, and abandoned buildings. Blastomycosis is most common among pregnant women and middle-aged black males. The disease is also found in dogs, cats, and horses.

The primary portal of entry of *B. dermatitidis* is the lungs. The acute clinical manifestations resemble those of acute histoplasmosis, including fever, cough, hoarseness, aching of the joints and muscles, and in some cases, pleuritic pain. Unlike histoplasmosis, however, the cough is frequently productive, and the sputum is purulent. Acute pulmonary infections may be self-limiting or progressive. When progressive, nodules and abscesses develop in the lungs. Extrapulmonary lesions commonly involve the skin, bones, reproductive tract, spleen, liver, kidney, or prostate gland. The skin lesions may, in fact, be the first signs of the disease. It often begins on the face, hand, wrist, or leg as a subcutaneous nodule that erodes to skin surface. Dissemination of the yeast may also cause arthritis and osteomyelitis, and involvement of the central nervous system causes headache, convulsions, coma, and mental confusion. The diagnosis of blastomycosis can be made from direct visualization of the yeast in sputum smears. Culture of the fungus can also be performed. An accurate blastomycin skin test is not available.

Opportunistic Pathogens

Opportunistic yeast pathogens such as *Candida albicans, Cryptococcus neoformans,* and *Aspergillus* are also associated with lung infections in certain patients. For example, under normal circumstances, *Candida albicans* occurs as a normal flora in the oral cavity, genitalia, and large intestines. In patients with AIDS, however, *Candida albicans* often becomes excessive and causes an infection of the mouth, pharynx, vagina, skin, and lungs. A *Candida albicans* infection of the mouth is called *thrush* and is characterized by a white, adherent, patchy infection of the membranes of the mouth, gums, cheeks, and throat. *Cryptococcus neoformans* proliferates in the high nitrogen content of pigeon droppings and are readily scattered into the air and dust. Today, the highest incidence of *Cryptococcus* is seen among patients with AIDS and persons undergoing steroid therapy. The molds of *Aspergillus* may be the most pervasive of all fungi—especially *A. fumigatus. Aspergillus* is found in soil, vegetation, leaf detritus, food, and compost heaps. Persons breathing air of graineries, barns, and silos are at the greatest risk. *Aspergillus* infection usually occurs in the lungs. *Aspergillus* is almost always an opportunistic infection, and poses a serious threat to patients with AIDS.

OVERVIEW
OF THE CARDIOPULMONARY CLINICAL MANIFESTATIONS ASSOCIATED WITH
FUNGAL DISEASES OF THE LUNGS

❑ **INCREASED RESPIRATORY RATE**

Several pathophysiologic mechanisms operating simultaneously may lead to an increased ventilatory rate. These are (see page 17)

- Stimulation of peripheral chemoreceptors
- Decreased lung compliance/increased ventilatory rate relationship
- Stimulation of J receptors
- Pain/anxiety/fever

❑ **PULMONARY FUNCTION STUDY FINDINGS**

Expiratory Maneuver Findings (see page 39)

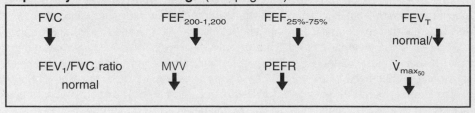

FVC	FEF$_{200-1,200}$	FEF$_{25\%-75\%}$	FEV$_T$
↓	↓	↓	normal/↓
FEV$_1$/FVC ratio	MVV	PEFR	$\dot{V}_{max_{50}}$
normal	↓	↓	↓

Lung Volume and Capacity Findings (see page 39)

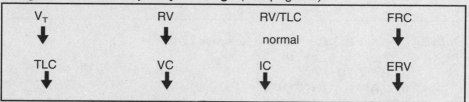

V_T	RV	RV/TLC	FRC
↓	↓	normal	↓
TLC	VC	IC	ERV
↓	↓	↓	↓

❑ **INCREASED HEART RATE (PULSE), CARDIAC OUTPUT, AND BLOOD PRESSURE** (see page 86)
❑ **ARTERIAL BLOOD GASES**

Mild to Moderate Fungal Disease

Acute Alveolar Hyperventilation with Hypoxemia (see page 57)

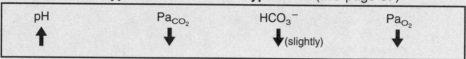

pH	Pa_{CO_2}	HCO_3^-	Pa_{O_2}
↑	↓	↓(slightly)	↓

Severe Fungal Disease

Chronic Ventilatory Failure with Hypoxemia (see page 60)

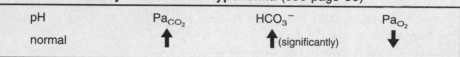

pH	Pa_{CO_2}	HCO_3^-	Pa_{O_2}
normal	↑	↑(significantly)	↓

Acute ventilatory changes superimposed on chronic ventilatory failure (see page 65)

Because acute ventilatory changes are frequently seen in patients with chronic ventilatory failure, the respiratory care practitioner must be familiar with and on the alert for (1) *acute alveolar hyperventilation superimposed on chronic ventilatory failure*, and (2) *acute ventilatory failure superimposed on chronic ventilatory failure*.

❑ **OXYGENATION INDICES** (see page 69)

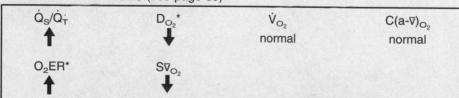

$\dot{Q}_S/\dot{Q}_T$	D_{O_2}*	$\dot{V}_{O_2}$	$C(a-\bar{v})_{O_2}$
↑	↓	normal	normal
O_2ER*	$S\bar{v}_{O_2}$		
↑	↓		

*The D_{O_2} may be normal in patients who have compensated for the decreased oxygenation status with an increased cardiac output, an increased hemoglobin level, or a combination of both. When the D_{O_2} is normal, the O_2ER is usually normal.

❑ **CYANOSIS** (see page 68)
❑ **HEMODYNAMIC INDICES (SEVERE FUNGAL DISEASE)** (see page 87)

CVP	RAP	$\overline{PA}$	PCWP
↑	↑	↑	normal
CO	SV	SVI	CI
normal	normal	normal	normal
RVSWI	LVSWI	PVR	SVR
↑	normal	↑	normal

❏ **CHEST ASSESSMENT FINDINGS** (see page 6)
  • Increased tactile and vocal fremitus
  • Dull percussion note
  • Bronchial breath sounds
  • Crackles/rhonchi/wheezing
  • Pleural friction rub (if process extends to pleural surface)
  • Whispered pectoriloquy

❏ **PLEURAL EFFUSION** (see Chapter 19)
❏ **COUGH, SPUTUM PRODUCTION, AND HEMOPTYSIS** (see page 93)
❏ **CHEST PAIN/DECREASED CHEST EXPANSION** (see page 98)
❏ **RADIOLOGIC FINDINGS**
  Chest radiograph
    • Increased opacity
    • Cavity formation
    • Pleural effusion
    • Calcification and fibrosis

During the early stages, localized infiltration and consolidation with or without lymph node involvement are commonly seen (Fig 14-2). Single or multiple spherical nodules may be seen (Fig 14-3). During the advanced stages, bilateral cavities in the apical and posterior segments of the upper lobes are often seen (Fig 14-4). In disseminated disease, a diffuse bilateral micronodular pattern and pleural effusion may be seen. Fibrosis and calcification of healed lesions can be identified.

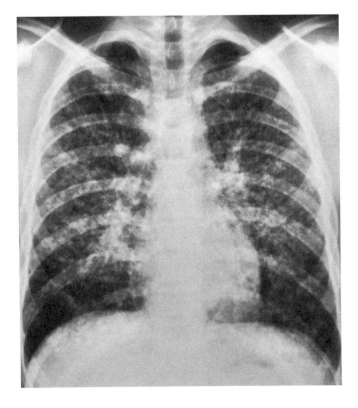

FIG 14-2
Acute inhalational histoplasmosis in an otherwise healthy patient. This young man developed fever and cough after tearing down an old barn. The study shows bilateral hilar adenopathy. (From Armstrong P, Wilson AG, Dee P: *Imaging of diseases of the chest,* St. Louis, 1990, Mosby-Year Book. Used by permission.)

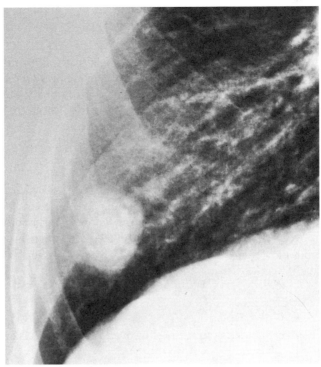

FIG 14-3
Histoplasmoma, showing a well-defined spherical nodule. The central portion of the nodule shows calcification. (From Armstrong P, Wilson AG, Dee P: *Imaging of diseases of the chest,* St. Louis, 1990, Mosby-Year Book. Used by permission.)

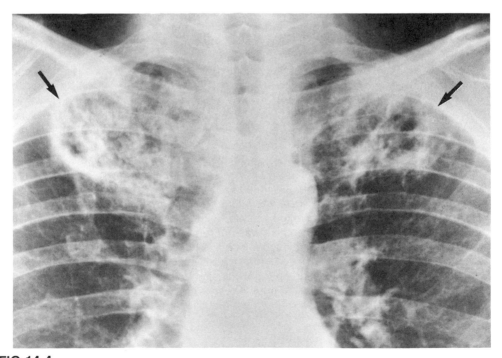

FIG 14-4
Chronic cavitary histoplasmosis. Note the striking upper zone predominance of the shadows. Multiple large cavities are present. (From Armstrong P, Wilson AG, Dee P: *Imaging of diseases of the chest,* St. Louis, 1990, Mosby-Year Book. Used by permission.)

GENERAL MANAGEMENT OF FUNGAL DISEASES
Medications

Antifungal agents.—Drugs commonly used to treat fungal diseases of the lungs are amphotericin B, ketoconazole, or miconazole. Amphotericin B is administered intravenously (IV) and is the drug of choice in severe cases. Ketoconazole is given orally and takes up to three weeks to produce its effect. Ketoconazole is also used to treat progressive or disseminated fungal diseases of the lung.

Supplemental Oxygen

Because of the hypoxemia associated with fungal disorders, supplemental oxygen may be required. It should be noted, however, that because of the alveolar consolidation produced by a fungal disorder, capillary shunting may be present. Hypoxemia caused by capillary shunting is refractory to oxygen therapy. In addition, when the patient demonstrates chronic ventilatory failure during the advanced stages of a fungal disorder, caution must be taken not to eliminate the patient's hypoxic drive.

Surgery

Surgery to remove affected masses in the lungs or other organs may also be helpful.

• • • **FUNGAL DISEASE OF THE LUNG CASE STUDY** • • •

ADMITTING HISTORY AND PHYSICAL EXAMINATION

This patient is a 29-year-old housewife and graduate student who was born and raised in Germany. She had been living in New Mexico for eight months, when two months ago she developed myalgia in both shoulders and a cough occasionally productive of yellow sputum. She had a transient, raised erythematous rash over her extremities, which disappeared after three days. She sought no medical help at that time and attributed the symptoms to "flu."

She was quite well for the past two months, but in the past week she developed pain and swelling over the right sternoclavicular joint. Two days ago, she developed swelling, pain, warmth, and erythema over the left ankle, which became steadily worse over the next 24 hours. She also noticed the appearance of several scattered, nodular skin lesions. Her cough reappeared and became slightly more productive. She did not feel well and finally decided to seek medical assistance.

On admission, the patient was a well-developed, well-nourished young female in moderate distress. Her temperature was 37.6° C orally, pulse 82/min, blood pressure 130/80 mm Hg. There was a small ulcerated lesion under her left nipple and three small nodular areas on her left calf. There was slight swelling and tenderness over the right sternoclavicular junction and marked warmth, tenderness, erythema, and swelling of the left ankle. Auscultation of the chest was not remarkable. The chest x-ray revealed a single nodular density in the right upper lobe and some irregular hilar adenopathy on the right. Laboratory studies revealed a highly positive complement fixation test for coccidioides. Latex agglutination and agar gel diffusion tests were also positive. Both the sputum and biopsy specimen taken from the ulcer on her breast contained spherules of *Coccidioides immitis*. The respiratory care practitioner recorded this in the patient's chart:

RESPIRATORY ASSESSMENT AND PLAN

S: Complains of cough. No dyspnea.

O: Afebrile. Lungs clear to auscultation. CXR: 1.0 cm nodule in RUL. Lab tests:

Coccidioidin skin test positive; serologies positive for *C. immitis;* sputum contains coccidioides spherules. Nodular skin lesions on legs.

A: • Coccidioidomycosis (history & lab tests)
       • Possibly disseminated (skin lesions)

P: No reason for respiratory care treatment. Will see prn as requested.

She was treated with amphotericin B and recovered completely.

DISCUSSION

The most common diseases which together constitute a category of "fungal disease of the lungs" include coccidioidomycosis (in the southwest) and histoplasmosis (in the Ohio and Mississippi River Valleys). There are several other less common ones (e.g., *Candida albicans,* aspergillosis), but they rarely come to the attention of respiratory care practitioners.

Exotic as these cases may be, the therapist had enough information in his assessment note to suspect that his services were not necessary. Specifically, the patient was not particularly dyspneic or cyanotic, and her sputum was not particularly tenacious. Thus, once his assessment was completed, he "signed off" the case. It is in precisely this manner that therapist-driven protocols save the patient, the hospital, and society much expense.

SELF-ASSESSMENT QUESTIONS

Multiple Choice
1. Which of the following is the most common fungal infection in the United States?
       a. Coccidioidomycosis
       b. Histoplasmosis
       c. San Joaquin Valley disease
       d. Blastomycosis
       e. Desert fever
2. Incidence of histoplasmosis is especially high in which of the following areas?
     I. Arizona
     II. Mississippi
    III. Nevada
    IV. Texas
       a. II only
       b. IV only
       c. II and IV only
       d. II and III only
       e. I, III, and IV only
3. The condition called desert bumps, desert arthritis, or desert rheumatism is associated with which fungal disorder?
       a. Ohio Valley fever
       b. Blastomycosis
       c. Coccidioidomycosis
       d. *Aspergillus*
       e. *Candida albicans*
4. Which of the following is/are used to treat fungal diseases?
     I. Streptomycin
     II. Amphotericin B
    III. Penicillin G
    IV. Ketoconazole
       a. I only
       b. II only
       c. IV only
       d. II and IV only
       e. I, II, and III only
5. Which of the following forms of histoplasmosis are characterized by healed lesions in the hilar lymph nodes as well as a positive histoplasmin skin test response?
       a. Disseminated infection
       b. Latent asymptomatic disease
       c. Chronic histoplasmosis
       d. Self-limiting primary disease
       e. None of the above

True or False
1. *Histoplasma capsulatum* is commonly found in soils near chicken houses and pigeon lofts.   True _____ False _____
2. It is estimated that about 50,000 new cases of coccidioidomycosis occur annually.   True _____ False _____
3. Blastomycosis is also known as valley or desert fever.   True _____ False _____
4. Two skin tests, the coccidioidin skin test and the spherulin skin test may be used in the diagnosis of coccidioidomycosis.   True _____ False _____
5. Blastomycosis is most common in young men living in North America.   True _____ False _____

Answers appear in Appendix XXI.

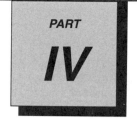
PULMONARY
VASCULAR DISEASES

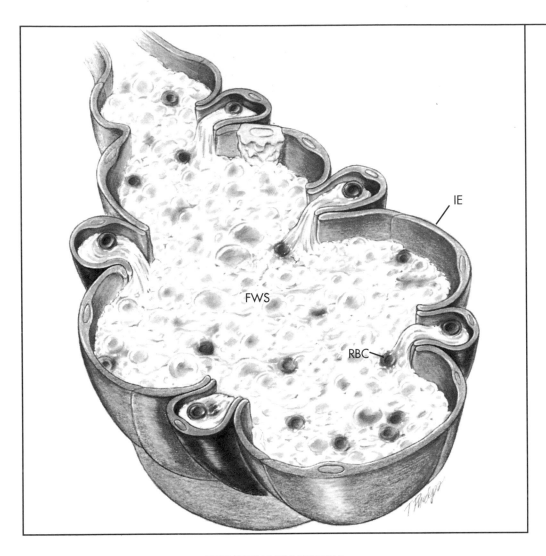

PULMONARY EDEMA

FIG 15-1

Cross-sectional view of alveoli and alveolar duct with pulmonary edema. *FWS* = frothy white secretions; *IE* = interstitial edema; *RBC* = red blood cell. (See also Plate 14.)

Pulmonary Edema

ANATOMIC ALTERATIONS OF THE LUNGS

Pulmonary edema is an excessive movement of fluid from the pulmonary vascular system to the extravascular system and air spaces of the lungs. Fluid first seeps into the perivascular and peribronchial interstitial spaces and, depending on the degree of severity, progressively moves into the alveoli, bronchioles, and bronchi.

As a consequence of this fluid movement, the alveolar walls and interstitial spaces swell. As this condition intensifies, the alveolar surface tension increases and causes alveolar skrinkage and atelectasis. Moreover, much of the fluid that accumulates in the tracheobronchial tree is churned into a frothy, white (sometimes blood-tinged or pink) sputum as a result of air moving in and out of the lungs. The abundance of fluid in the interstitial spaces causes the lymphatic vessels to widen and the lymph flow to increase (Fig 15-1).

To summarize, the major pathologic or structural changes associated with pulmonary edema are as follows:

- Interstitial edema, including fluid engorgement of the perivascular and peribronchial spaces and the alveolar wall interstitium
- Increased surface tension
- Alveolar shrinkage and atelectasis
- Frothy white (or pink) secretions throughout the tracheobronchial tree

ETIOLOGY

The etiology of pulmonary edema can be divided into two major categories: cardiogenic and noncardiogenic.

Cardiogenic Pulmonary Edema

Ordinarily, hydrostatic pressure of about 10 to 15 mm Hg tends to move fluid out of the pulmonary capillaries into the interstitial space. This force is normally offset by colloid osmotic forces of about 25 to 30 mm Hg that tend to keep fluid in the pulmonary capillaries. The colloid osmotic pressure is referred to as *oncotic pressure* and is produced by the albumin and globulin particles in the blood. The stability of fluid within the pulmonary capillaries is therefore determined by the balance between *hydrostatic* and *oncotic* pressure. This hydrostatic and oncotic relationship also maintains fluid stability in the interstitial compartments.

Movement of fluid in and out of the capillaries is expressed by Starling's equation:

$$J = K (Pc - Pi) - (\pi c - \pi i)$$

where *J* is the net fluid movement out of the capillary, *K* is the capillary permeability factor, *Pc* and *Pi* are the hydrostatic pressures in the capillary and interstitial space, and πc and πi are the oncotic pressures in the capillary and interstitial space.

Though conceptually valuable, this equation has limited practical use. Of the four pressures, only the oncotic and hydrostatic pressures of the pulmonary capillaries can be identified with any certainty. The oncotic and hydrostatic pressures within the interstitial compartments cannot be readily determined.

When the hydrostatic pressure within the pulmonary vascular system rises to more than 25 to 30 mm Hg, the oncotic pressure loses its holding force over the fluid within the pulmonary capillaries. Consequently, fluid will start to spill into the interstitial and air spaces of the lungs.

Increased pulmonary capillary hydrostatic pressure is considered the most common cause of pulmonary edema. In alphabetical order, some causes of cardiogenic pulmonary edema follow:

- Arrhythmias (e.g., Premature Ventricular Contractions, bradycardia)
- Congenital heart defects
- Excessive fluid administration
- Left ventricular failure
- Mitral or aortic valve disease
- Myocardial infarction
- Pulmonary embolus
- Renal failure
- Rheumatic heart disease (myocarditis)
- Systemic hypertension

Noncardiogenic Pulmonary Edema

Increased capillary permeability.—Pulmonary edema may develop due to increased capillary permeability as a result of infectious, inflammatory, and other processes. The following are some causes of increased capillary permeability:

- Alveolar hypoxia
- Adult respiratory distress syndrome
- Inhalation of toxic agents such as chlorine, sulfur dioxide, nitrogen oxides, ammonia, and phosgene
- Pneumonia
- Therapeutic radiation of the lungs

Lymphatic insufficiency.—Should the lungs' normal lymphatic drainage be decreased, intravascular and extravascular fluid begins to pool, and pulmonary edema ensues. Lymphatic drainage may be slowed because of obliteration or distortion of lymphatic vessels. The lymphatic vessels may be obstructed by tumor cells in lymphangitic carcinomatosis. Because the lymphatic vessels empty into systemic veins, increased systemic venous pressure may slow lymphatic drainage. Lymphatic insufficiency has also been observed following lung transplantation.

Decreased intrapleural pressure.—Reduced intrapleural pressure may cause pulmonary edema. During severe airway obstruction, for example, the negative pressure exerted by the patient during inspiration may create a suction effect on the pulmonary capillaries and cause fluid to move into the alveoli. Furthermore, the increased negative intrapleural pressure promotes filling of the right side of the heart and hinders blood flow in the left side of the heart. This condition may cause pooling of the blood in the lungs and, subsequently, an elevated hydrostatic pressure and pulmonary edema. Another related kind of pulmonary edema is caused by the sudden removal of a pleural effusion. Clinically, this condition is called "decompression pulmonary edema."

Decreased oncotic pressure.—Although this condition is rare, if the oncotic pressure is reduced from its normal 25 to 30 mm Hg and falls below the patient's normal hydrostatic pressure of 10 to 15 mm Hg, fluid may begin to seep into the interstitial and air spaces of the lungs. Decreased oncotic pressure may be caused by the following:

- Overtransfusion and/or rapid transfusion of intravenous fluids
- Uremia
- Hypoproteinemia (e.g., severe malnutrition)
- Acute nephritis
- Polyarteritis nodosa

Other Causes

Although the exact mechanisms are not known, pulmonary edema is also associated with the following:

- Allergic reaction to drugs
- Chronic alcohol ingestion
- Aspiration (e.g., near drowning)
- Central nervous system (CNS) stimulation
- Cerebral hemorrhage
- Encephalitis
- Excessive sodium consumption
- Drug-induced (e.g., heroin, amphetamines, cocaine, antituberculosis agents, and cancer chemotherapy agents)
- Metal poisoning (e.g., cobalt, iron, and lead)
- Skull trauma
- Cardiac tamponade

OVERVIEW

OF THE CARDIOPULMONARY CLINICAL MANIFESTATIONS ASSOCIATED WITH
PULMONARY EDEMA

❏ **INCREASED RESPIRATORY RATE**

Several pathophysiologic mechanisms operating simultaneously may lead to an increased ventilatory rate. These are (see page 17)
- Stimulation of peripheral chemoreceptors
- Decreased lung compliance/increased ventilatory rate relationship
- Stimulation of J receptors
- Anxiety

□ CHEYNE-STOKES RESPIRATION (see page 18)

Cheyne-Stokes respiration may be seen in patients with severe left-sided heart failure and pulmonary edema. It is suggested that the cause of Cheyne-Stokes respiration in these patients may be related to the prolonged circulation time between the lungs and the central chemoreceptors.

□ PULMONARY FUNCTION STUDY FINDINGS

Expiratory Maneuver Findings (see page 39)

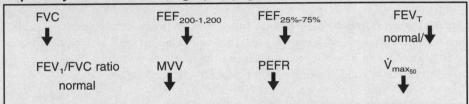

FVC	FEF$_{200-1,200}$	FEF$_{25\%-75\%}$	FEV$_T$
↓	↓	↓	normal/↓
FEV$_1$/FVC ratio normal	MVV ↓	PEFR ↓	$\dot{V}_{max_{50}}$ ↓

Lung Volume and Capacity Findings (see page 39)

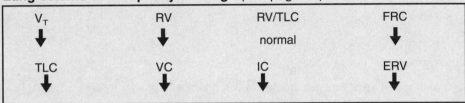

V$_T$	RV	RV/TLC	FRC
↓	↓	normal	↓
TLC ↓	VC ↓	IC ↓	ERV ↓

□ DECREASED DIFFUSION CAPACITY (see page 48)

□ ARTERIAL BLOOD GASES

Mild to Moderate Pulmonary Edema

Acute Alveolar Hyperventilation with Hypoxemia (see page 57)

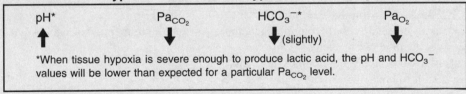

pH*	Pa$_{CO_2}$	HCO$_3^-$*	Pa$_{O_2}$
↑	↓	↓ (slightly)	↓

*When tissue hypoxia is severe enough to produce lactic acid, the pH and HCO$_3^-$ values will be lower than expected for a particular Pa$_{CO_2}$ level.

Severe Pulmonary Edema

Acute Ventilatory Failure with Hypoxemia (see page 59)

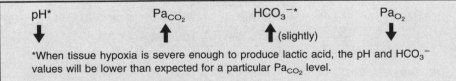

pH*	Pa$_{CO_2}$	HCO$_3^-$*	Pa$_{O_2}$
↓	↑	↑ (slightly)	↓

*When tissue hypoxia is severe enough to produce lactic acid, the pH and HCO$_3^-$ values will be lower than expected for a particular Pa$_{CO_2}$ level.

□ OXYGENATION INDICES (see page 69)

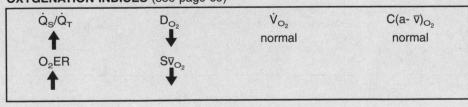

$\dot{Q}_S/\dot{Q}_T$	D$_{O_2}$	$\dot{V}_{O_2}$	C(a-$\bar{v}$)$_{O_2}$
↑	↓	normal	normal
O$_2$ER ↑	S$\bar{v}_{O_2}$ ↓		

❑ **CYANOSIS** (see page 68)
❑ **HEMODYNAMIC INDICES (CARDIOGENIC PULMONARY EDEMA)** (see page 87)

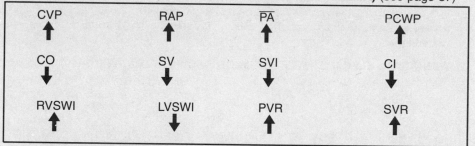

❑ **COUGH AND SPUTUM (FROTHY AND PINK IN APPEARANCE)** (see page 93)
❑ **CHEST ASSESSMENT FINDINGS** (see page 6)
  • Increased tactile and vocal fremitus
  • Crackles/rhonchi/wheezing

❑ **PLEURAL EFFUSION** (see Chapter 19)
❑ **PAROXYSMAL NOCTURNAL DYSPNEA AND ORTHOPNEA**

Patients with pulmonary edema often awaken with severe dyspnea after several hours of sleep. This condition is called *paroxysmal nocturnal dyspnea*. This is particularly true of patients with cardiogenic pulmonary edema. While the patient is awake, more time is spent in the erect position and, as a result, excess fluids tend to accumulate in the dependent portions of the body. When the patient lies down, however, the excess fluids from the dependent parts of the body move into the bloodstream and cause an increase in venous return to the lungs. This action raises the pulmonary capillary pressure and promotes pulmonary edema. The pulmonary edema in turn promotes pulmonary shunting, venous admixture, and hypoxemia. When the hypoxemia becomes severe, the peripheral chemoreceptors are stimulated and initiate an increased ventilatory rate (see Fig 1-26). The decreased lung compliance, J receptor stimulation, and anxiety may also contribute to the paroxysmal nocturnal dyspnea commonly seen in this disorder at night. A patient is said to have **orthopnea** when dyspnea increases while the patient is in a recumbent position.

❑ **RADIOLOGIC FINDINGS**
Chest radiograph
  • Fluffy opacities
  • Left ventricular hypertrophy
  • Kerley's A and B lines
  • Pleural effusion

Cardiogenic pulmonary edema
Since x-ray densities primarily reflect alveolar filling and not interstitial edema, by the time abnormal findings are encountered the pathologic changes associated with pulmonary edema are advanced. Chest radiography typically reveals dense, fluffy opacities that spread outward from the hilar areas to the peripheral borders of the lungs (Fig. 15-2). The peripheral portion of the lungs often remains clear, and this produces what is described as a "butterfly" or "batwing" distribution. Left ventricular hypertrophy and enlarged pulmonary vessels are commonly seen. Pleural effusions may be seen. Kerley's A and B lines may appear earlier in the radiograph. Kerley's A lines are 1- to 2-cm lines of interstitial edema extending out from the hilum. Kerley's B lines are short, thin lines of interstitial edema that extend inward from the pleural surface of the lower regions of the lungs. Kerley's B lines originate from the septa that separate the lung lobules. When thickened by pulmonary edema, these septa form the so-called septal lines or Kerley's B lines.

Noncardiogenic pulmonary edema
In noncardiogenic pulmonary edema, the chest radiograph commonly shows areas of fluffy densities that are usually more dense near the hilum. The density may be unilateral or bilateral. Pleural effusion is usually not present, and the cardiac silhouette is not enlarged.

❏ **ABNORMAL ELECTROLYTES (CARDIOGENIC PULMONARY EDEMA)** (see page 100)
  • Hypokalemia
  • Hyponatremia

Hypokalemia and hyponatremia are often seen in patients with left-sided heart failure and may result from diuretic therapy or excessive fluid retention.

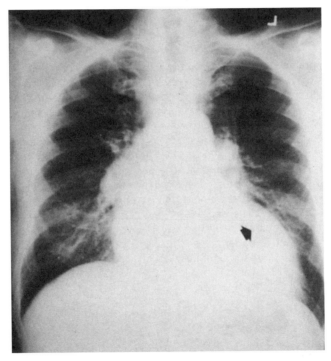

FIG 15-2
Left-sided heart failure (arrow) with accompanying edema.

GENERAL MANAGEMENT OF PULMONARY EDEMA

The treatment of pulmonary edema is based on the underlying etiology. Common therapeutic interventions include the following:

Medications

Positive inotropic agents.—When left-sided heart failure is present, positive inotropic drugs (e.g., digitalis, dobutamine, and amrinone) are commonly administered to increase cardiac output (see Appendix IX).

Afterload reduction agents.—The work of the heart can be reduced and contractility improved with afterload reduction agents. Systemic hypertension (elevated afterload) is most often reduced with direct-acting vasodilators such as nitroglycerin, nitroprusside, hydralazine, and minoxidil.

Morphine sulfate.—This agent is also used to reduce afterload by inducing venodilation and venous pooling, and for sedation and relief of anxiety.

Diuretic agents.—Diuretic agents are prescribed to promote fluid excretion (see Appendix X).

Sympathomimetic agents.—Sympathomimetic drugs are prescribed to patients with pulmonary edema when there is accompanying bronchospasm (see Appendix II).

Alcohol (ethanol, ethyl alcohol).—Because alcohol is a specific surface-active agent, it may be aerosolized into the patient's lungs to lower the surface tension of the frothy secretions. This action enhances the mobilization of secretions. Between 5 and 15 ml of 30% to 50% alcohol solution is generally administered. This is rarely used today.

Albumin and mannitol.—Albumin or mannitol is sometimes administered to increase the patient's oncotic pressure in an effort to offset the increased hydrostatic forces of cardiogenic pulmonary edema if the patient's osmotic pressure is low.

Hyperinflation Techniques

Hyperinflation therapy is commonly prescribed to offset the fluid accumulation and alveolar shrinkage associated with pulmonary edema (see Appendix XII). For example, high-flow mask continuous positive airway pressure (CPAP) has been shown to produce a significant and rapid improvement in the oxygenation and ventilatory status in patients with pulmonary edema. It is believed that mask CPAP improves lung compliance, decreases the work of breathing, enhances gas exchange, and decreases vascular congestion in patients with pulmonary edema. In fact, mask CPAP is frequently prescribed (at least for a trial period) for patients with pulmonary edema who have arterial blood gas values that reveal impending, or acute, ventilatory failure—the hallmark clinical manifestations for mechanical ventilation. Oftentimes, mask CPAP dramatically improves the oxygenation and ventilatory status in these patients and eliminates the need for mechanical ventilation.

Supplemental Oxygen

Because of the hypoxemia associated with pulmonary edema, supplemental oxygen is usually required. It should be noted, however, that the hypoxemia that develops in pulmonary edema is most commonly caused by the alveolar fluid, atelectasis, and capillary shunting associated with the disorder. Hypoxemia caused by capillary shunting is refractory to oxygen therapy.

Methods of Decreasing Hydrostatic Pressure

In an effort to lower the elevated hydrostatic pressure, the physician may order the following:

- Positioning the patient in the Fowler's position (sitting up)
- Rotating tourniquets (rarely used)
- Phlebotomy (rarely used)

• • • •　**PULMONARY EDEMA CASE STUDY**　• • • •

ADMITTING HISTORY AND PHYSICAL EXAMINATION

A 76-year-old male was admitted to the emergency room in obvious respiratory distress. His wife reported that her husband had gone to bed feeling well. He woke up about 0230, very short of breath. She became concerned and called an ambulance. Neither the patient or his wife were good historians, but they did report that the patient had been under a physician's care for some time for "heart trouble" and that he was taking "little white pills" on a daily basis. For the past three days he had not taken any medications.

On admission to the emergency room the patient was mildly disoriented and slightly cyanotic, and he repeatedly tried to take the oxygen mask from his face. He complained of a feeling of suffocation. His neck veins were distended and the skin of his extremities was mottled. On auscultation, there were coarse rhonchi and crackles in both lower lung fields, and some crackles in the middle and upper lung fields.

Cough was productive of pinkish, frothy sputum. Heart rate was 124 bpm, respiratory rate was 29/min, and blood pressure was 105/50. ECG showed evidence of an old infarct, a sinus tachycardia, and an occasional premature ventricular contraction. X-rays taken in the emergency room with the patient in a sitting position revealed bilateral fluffy infiltrates, more marked in the lower lung fields. The heart was enlarged. Laboratory findings were within normal limits. Blood gases on $F_{I_{O_2}}$ of 0.30 were pH 7.11, Pa_{CO_2} 72, HCO_3^- 25, and Pa_{O_2} 68.

RESPIRATORY ASSESSMENT AND PLAN

S: Patient has "a feeling of suffocation."

O: Cyanosis; disorientation; HR 124; RR 29; BP 105/50; ECG, sinus tachycardia and occasional premature ventricular contractions. Distended neck veins; mottled extremities; coarse rhonchi and crackles bilaterally; frothy pink sputum; X-ray: bilateral fluffy infiltrates and an enlarged heart; ABG: pH 7.11, Pa_{CO_2} 72, HCO_3^- 25, and Pa_{O_2} 68 ($F_{I_{O_2}}$: 0.30).

A: • Acute pulmonary edema
　　• Acute ventilatory failure with mild hypoxemia (ABG)
　　• Large and small airway secretions (rhonchi & crackles)
　　• Bilateral alveolar infiltrate (X-ray)

P: Increase $F_{I_{O_2}}$ to 0.80, mask CPAP at 25 cm H_2O, 50% ethanol aerosol every 60 minutes, be on standby for emergency endotracheal intubation and ventilator support, continue ECG and oximetric monitoring, and repeat ABG in 30 minutes.

The patient was admitted to the cardiology service with the admission diagnosis of pulmonary edema—congestive heart failure. ECG monitoring and continuous oximetry were followed. Treatment consisted of intravenous administration of furosemide, dopamine, and nitroprusside, and mask CPAP at 25 cm H_2O pressure with an $F_{I_{O_2}}$ of 0.8. A Foley catheter was placed.

Two hours later, the patient's condition was much improved. Heart rate was 96 bpm, respiratory rate was 18/min, and blood pressure was 126/70. ECG revealed mild sinus tachycardia and no ectopic beats. Auscultation revealed considerable improvement. There were still some basilar crackles, but the upper lung fields were clear. Cough was much reduced and no longer productive. Repeat chest x-ray (also at bedside) showed considerable improvement. Urine output was in excess of 600 ml/hr. The patient was calm and rational. Repeat arterial blood gases revealed a pH of 7.35, a Pa_{CO_2} of 46, HCO_3^- of 23, and a Pa_{O_2} of 120.

RESPIRATORY ASSESSMENT AND PLAN

S: Patient is "less short of breath. No pain."

O: No longer cyanotic. HR 96; RR 18; BP 126/70; ECG, mild sinus tachycardia without ectopic beat; breath sounds, less crackles; no sputum production; x-ray, improved; ABG: pH 7.35, Pa_{CO_2} 46, HCO_3^- 23, Pa_{O_2} 120 (FI_{O_2}: 0.8).

A: • Decreased pulmonary edema (overall impression from above data)
     • No longer in ventilatory failure (ABG)
     • Excessively corrected hypoxemia (ABG)
     • Secretions controlled (no sputum & less crackles)

P: Discontinue CPAP at 25 cm H_2O and 50% ethanol. Place on oxygen mask (FI_{O_2}: 0.40 to 0.60). Continue ECG and oximetric monitoring. Repeat ABG in 60 minutes.

DISCUSSION

Acute pulmonary edema is a classic finding in left-sided heart failure. The management consists of improving myocardial efficiency, decreasing the cardiovascular afterload, decreasing the hypervolemia, and improving oxygenation. Furosemide is a potent loop diuretic, dopamine has direct inotropic effects, and nitroprusside is a potent peripheral vasodilator. The combination of these drugs with CPAP resulted in a marked improvement of myocardial activity and in a rapid change in the clinical picture.

This patient had an acute respiratory problem, but the basic cause was cardiac. Once the cardiac efficiency was increased, the respiratory symptoms disappeared. CPAP and an increased oxygen fraction were adequate, and this patient was spared the trauma and risk associated with intubation and mechanical ventilation. No evidence of acute myocardial infarction was found. Ethanol aerosol was given to decrease the surface tension of his airway secretions. He was discharged after 48 hours, his condition much improved. He was instructed to take his cardiac medication and his diuretics without fail and to return to his family physician in three days.

SELF-ASSESSMENT QUESTIONS

Multiple Choice

1. In pulmonary edema, fluid first moves into the
    I. Alveoli.
    II. Perivascular interstitial space.
    III. Bronchioles.
    IV. Peribronchial interstitial space.
        a. I only
        b. II only
        c. III only
        d. I and III only
        e. II and IV only

2. What is the normal hydrostatic pressure in the pulmonary capillaries?
        a. 5 to 10 mm Hg
        b. 10 to 15 mm Hg
        c. 15 to 20 mm Hg
        d. 20 to 25 mm Hg
        e. 25 to 30 mm Hg

3. What is the normal oncotic pressure of the blood?
        a. 5 to 10 mm Hg
        b. 10 to 15 mm Hg
        c. 15 to 20 mm Hg
        d. 20 to 25 mm Hg
        e. 25 to 30 mm Hg

4. Causes of cardiogenic pulmonary edema include
    I. Excessive fluid administration.
    II. Right ventricular failure.
    III. Mitral valve disease.
    IV. Pulmonary embolus.
        a. III and IV only
        b. I and II only
        c. I, II, and III only
        d. II, III, and IV only
        e. I, III, and IV

5. As a result of pulmonary edema, the patient's
    I. RV is decreased.
    II. FRC is increased.
    III. VC is increased.
    IV. TLC is increased.
        a. I only
        b. I and IV only
        c. II and III only
        d. III and IV only
        e. II, III, and IV only

True or False

1. Morphine sulfate induces venodilation.   True _____   False _____
2. Patients with pulmonary edema frequently receive 30% to
   50% aerosolized alcohol.   True _____   False _____
3. A patient is said to have orthopnea if dyspnea increases
   when the patient is in the upright position.   True _____   False _____
4. Kerley's B lines on chest x-ray films are believed to
   originate from edematous interlobular septa.   True _____   False _____
5. Hyperproteinemia reduces oncotic pressure.   True _____   False _____

Fill in the Blank

1. An agent used to increase the patient's oncotic pressure to counteract the increased hydrostatic forces associated with cardiogenic pulmonary edema is _____ .

Answers appear in Appendix XXI.

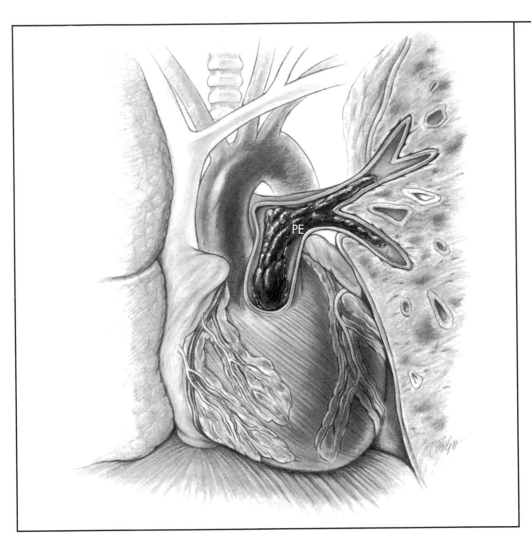

PULMONARY EMBOLISM

FIG 16-1
Pulmonary embolism (PE). (See also Plate 15.)

Pulmonary Embolism and Infarction

ANATOMIC ALTERATIONS OF THE LUNGS

A pulmonary embolism is a blood clot (thrombus) or obstruction from other particulate matter that has become dislodged elsewhere in the body and has impacted in the natural filter system of the pulmonary vasculature. If the embolism significantly disrupts pulmonary blood flow, pulmonary infarction develops and causes alveolar atelectasis, consolidation, and tissue necrosis. In addition, bronchial smooth muscle constriction typically accompanies pulmonary embolism. Although the precise mechanism is not known, it is believed that the embolism causes the release of cellular mediators such as serotonin, histamine, and prostaglandins from platelets, which in turn leads to bronchoconstriction. Local areas of alveolar hypocapnia and hypoxemia may also contribute to the bronchoconstriction associated with pulmonary embolism.

Embolism may occur as one large thrombus or as a shower of small thrombi that may or may not interfere with the right heart's ability to perfuse the lungs adequately. When a large embolus detaches from a thrombus and passes through the right heart, it commonly lodges in the bifurcation of the pulmonary artery where it forms what is known as a *saddle embolus* (Fig 16-1). This is often fatal.

To summarize, the major pathologic or structural changes associated with pulmonary embolism are as follows:

- Blockage of the pulmonary vascular system
- Pulmonary infarction
- Alveolar atelectasis
- Alveolar consolidation
- Pulmonary tissue necrosis
- Bronchial smooth muscle constriction (bronchospasm)

ETIOLOGY

Although there are many possible sources of pulmonary emboli (e.g., fat, air, amniotic fluid, bone marrow, or tumor fragments), blood clots are by far the most common source.

Most pulmonary emboli originate from deep veins in the lower part of the body, i.e., the leg and pelvic veins and the inferior vena cava. When a thrombus or a piece of a thrombus breaks loose in a deep vein, the clot is carried through the venous system to the right chambers of the heart and ultimately lodges in the pulmonary arteries or arterioles. The following are some of the factors predisposing to pulmonary embolism:

Venous Stasis

- Prolonged bed rest and/or immobilization
- Prolonged sitting (e.g., car or plane travel)
- Congestive heart failure
- Varicose veins
- Thrombophlebitis

Trauma

- Bone fractures (especially of the pelvis and the long bones of the lower extremities)
- Extensive injury to soft tissue

Postoperative or Postpartum States

- Extensive hip or abdominal operations
- Phlegmasia alba dolens puerperarum (milk-leg)

Hypercoagulation Disorders

- Oral contraceptives
- Polycythemia
- Multiple myeloma

Others

- Obesity
- Malignant neoplasms
- Pregnancy
- Burns

OVERVIEW

OF THE CARDIOPULMONARY CLINICAL MANIFESTATIONS ASSOCIATED WITH
PULMONARY EMBOLISM

❏ **INCREASED RESPIRATORY RATE**

There are probably several unique mechanisms working simultaneously to increase the rate of breathing in patients with pulmonary embolism, the major of which follow:

Stimulation of peripheral chemoreceptors

When an embolus lodges in the pulmonary vascular system, blood flow is reduced or completely absent distal to the obstruction. Consequently, the alveolar ventilation beyond the obstruction is wasted, or dead space, ventilation. That is, there is no carbon dioxide-oxygen exchange. The $\dot{V}/\dot{Q}$ ratio distal to the pulmonary embolus is high and may even be infinite if there is no perfusion at all (Fig 16-2).

Although portions of the lungs have a high $\dot{V}/\dot{Q}$ ratio at the onset of a pulmonary embolism, this condition is quickly reversed, and there is a decrease in the $\dot{V}/\dot{Q}$ ratio. The pathophysiologic mechanisms responsible for the decreased $\dot{V}/\dot{Q}$ ratio are as follows: In response to the pulmonary embolus, pulmonary infarction develops and causes alveolar atelectasis, consolidation, and parenchymal necrosis. In addition the embolus is believed to activate the release of humoral agents such as serotonin, histamine, and prostaglandins into the pulmonary circulation, which cause bronchial constriction. Collectively, the alveolar atelectasis, consolidation, tissue necrosis, and bronchial constriction lead to a decreased alveolar ventilation relative to the alveolar perfusion (decreased $\dot{V}/\dot{Q}$ ratio). As a result of the decreased $\dot{V}/\dot{Q}$ ratio, pulmonary shunting and venous admixture ensue.

The end result of the venous admixture is a decrease in the patient's Pa_{O_2} and Ca_{O_2} (Fig 16-3). It should be emphasized that *it is not the pulmonary embolism but rather the decreased $\dot{V}/\dot{Q}$ ratio that develops from the pulmonary infarction (atelectasis and consolidation) and bronchial constriction (release of cellular mediators) that actually causes the reduction of the patient's arterial oxygen level.* As this condition intensifies, the patient's oxygen level may decline to a point low enough to stimulate the peripheral chemoreceptors, which in turn initiates an increased ventilatory rate.

Reflexes from the aortic and carotid sinus baroreceptors

The normal function of the aortic and carotid sinus baroreceptors, located near the aortic and carotid peripheral chemoreceptors, is to initiate reflexes that cause decreased heart and ventilatory rates in response to an elevated systemic blood pressure and increased heart and ventilatory rates in response to a reduced systemic blood pressure.

If obstruction of the pulmonary vascular system is severe, left ventricular output will diminish and cause the systemic blood pressure to drop. The decreased systemic blood pressure reduces the tension of the walls of the aorta and carotid artery, which activates the baroreceptors. Activation of the baroreceptors in turn initiates an increased heart rate and ventilatory rate.

Other pathophysiologic mechanisms that may increase the patient's ventilatory rate include the following (see page 17):

- Stimulation of the J receptors
- Anxiety/pain/fever

❑ ARTERIAL BLOOD GASES

Minimal Pulmonary Embolism

Acute Alveolar Hyperventilation with Hypoxemia (see page 57)

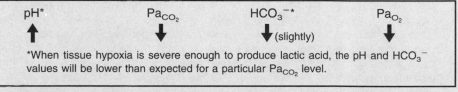

| pH* | Pa_{CO_2} | HCO_3^-* | Pa_{O_2} |
| ↑ | ↓ | ↓ (slightly) | ↓ |

*When tissue hypoxia is severe enough to produce lactic acid, the pH and HCO_3^- values will be lower than expected for a particular Pa_{CO_2} level.

Extensive Pulmonary Embolism and Infarction

Acute Ventilatory Failure with Hypoxemia (see page 59)

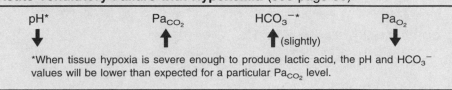

| pH* | Pa_{CO_2} | HCO_3^-* | Pa_{O_2} |
| ↓ | ↑ | ↑ (slightly) | ↓ |

*When tissue hypoxia is severe enough to produce lactic acid, the pH and HCO_3^- values will be lower than expected for a particular Pa_{CO_2} level.

❑ **CYANOSIS** (see page 68)
❑ **OXYGENATION INDICES** (see page 69)

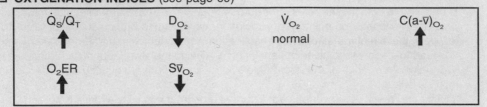

❑ **HEMODYNAMIC INDICES (EXTENSIVE PULMONARY EMBOLISM)** (see page 87)

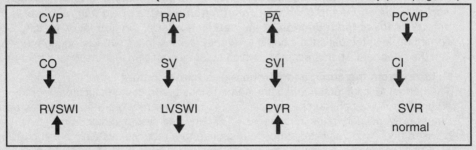

Normally, the pulmonary artery pressure is 25/10 mm Hg, with a mean pulmonary artery pressure of around 15 mm Hg. Most patients with pulmonary embolism, however, have a mean pulmonary artery pressure in excess of 20 mm Hg. Three major mechanisms may contribute to the pulmonary hypertension: (1) decreased cross-sectional area of the pulmonary vascular system due to the emboli, (2) vasoconstriction induced by humoral agents, and (3) vasoconstriction induced by alveolar hypoxia.

Decreased Cross-Sectional Area of the Pulmonary Vascular System Due to the Embolus.— The cross-sectional area of the pulmonary vascular system may decrease significantly if a large embolus becomes lodged in a major artery or if many small emboli become lodged in numerous small pulmonary vessels.

Vasoconstriction Induced by Humoral Agents.—One of the consequences of pulmonary embolism is the release of certain humoral agents, primarily serotonin and prostaglandin. These agents induce smooth muscle constriction of both the tracheobronchial tree and the pulmonary vascular system. Such smooth muscle constriction may further reduce the total cross-sectional area of the pulmonary vascular system and cause the pulmonary artery pressure to rise.

Vasoconstriction Induced by Alveolar Hypoxia.—In response to the humoral agents liberated in pulmonary embolism, the smooth muscles of the tracheobronchial tree constrict and cause the $\dot{V}/\dot{Q}$ ratio to decrease and the $P_{A_{O_2}}$ to decline. Although the precise mechanism is unclear, when the $P_{A_{O_2}}$ decreases, pulmonary vasoconstriction ensues. This action appears to be a normal compensatory mechanism to offset the shunt produced by the underventilated alveoli. When the number of hypoxic areas becomes significant, however, generalized pulmonary vasoconstriction may develop and further contribute to the increase in pulmonary blood pressure. When the pulmonary embolism is severe, right-heart strain and cor pulmonale may ensue. Cor pulmonale leads to an increased CVP, distended neck veins, and a swollen and tender liver.

❑ **COR PULMONALE** (see page 92)
   • Distended neck veins
   • Swollen and tender liver

❑ **PLEURAL EFFUSION** (see Chapter 19)

❑ **CHEST ASSESSMENT FINDINGS** (see page 6)
  * Crackles/wheezing
  * Pleural friction rub (especially when pulmonary infarction involves the pleura)

❑ **SYSTEMIC HYPOTENSION**

When significant pulmonary hypertension develops, systemic hypotension is nearly always present. This is due to the decrease in the cross-sectional area of the pulmonary vascular system, which reduces blood flow to the left heart and causes a decrease in left ventricular output and systemic hypotension.

❑ **SYNCOPE, LIGHT-HEADEDNESS, AND CONFUSION**

If the left ventricular output and systemic blood pressure decrease substantially, blood flow to the brain may also diminish significantly. This may cause periods of light-headedness, confusion, and even syncope.

❑ **INCREASED HEART RATE**

The two major mechanisms responsible for the increased heart rate associated with pulmonary embolism are (1) reflexes from the aortic and carotid sinus baroreceptors and (2) stimulation of the pulmonary reflex mechanism.

For a discussion of reflexes from the aortic and carotid sinus baroreceptors, see the previous section on increased respiratory rate in this chapter. The increased heart rate may also reflect an indirect response of the heart to hypoxic stimulation of the peripheral chemoreceptors, mainly the carotid bodies. When the carotid bodies are so stimulated, the patient's ventilatory rate increases. As a result of the increased rate of lung inflation, the pulmonary reflex mechanism is activated; this mechanism triggers tachycardia.

❑ **ABNORMAL ELECTROCARDIOGRAPHIC PATTERNS**
  * Sinus tachycardia
  * Atrial arrhythmias
      Atrial tachycardia
      Atrial flutter
      Atrial fibrillation
  * Acute right ventricular strain pattern and right bundle branch block

In some cases, the obstruction of pulmonary blood flow produced by pulmonary emboli leads to abnormal electrocardiographic (ECG) patterns. However, there is no ECG pattern diagnostic of pulmonary embolism. Abnormal patterns merely suggest the possibility. Sinus tachycardia is the most common arrhythmia seen. The sinus tachycardia and atrial arrhythmias sometimes noted are also thought to be indirectly related to the increased right-heart strain and cor pulmonale.

❑ **ABNORMAL HEART SOUNDS**
  * Increased second heart sound (S_2)
  * Increased splitting of the second heart sound (S_2)
  * Third heart sound (or ventricular gallop)

Increased Second Heart Sound (S_2).—Following pulmonary embolization, abnormally high blood pressure develops in the pulmonary artery. This condition causes the pulmonic valve to close more forcefully. As a result, the sound produced by the pulmonic valve (P_2) is often louder than the aortic sound (A_2), which causes a louder second heart sound, or S_2.

Increased Splitting of the Second Heart Sound (S_2).—Two major mechanisms either individually or together may contribute to the increased splitting of S_2 sometimes noted in pulmonary embolism: (1) increased pulmonary hypertension and (2) incomplete right bundle branch block.

In response to the increased pulmonary hypertension, the blood pressure in the pulmonic valve area is frequently higher than normal during ventricular contraction. This delays closure of the pulmonic valve and therefore abnormally widens the S_2 split.

The incomplete right bundle branch block that sometimes accompanies pulmonary embolism may also contribute to the increased splitting of S_2. In an incomplete block, the electrical activity through the right heart is delayed; this delayed activity in turn slows right ventricular contraction. The blood pressure in the pulmonic valve area remains higher than normal and for a longer period of time during right ventricular contraction. As a result, there is delayed closure of the pulmonic valve, which may further widen the S_2 split.

Third Heart Sound (Ventricular Gallop).—A third heart sound (S_3), or ventricular gallop, is sometimes heard in patients with pulmonary embolism. It occurs early in diastole, about 0.12 to 0.16 seconds after S_3. Although its precise origin is unknown, it is thought that S_3 is created by vibrations during diastole when the rush of blood into the ventricles is abruptly stopped by ventricular walls that have lost some of their elasticity because of hypertrophy.

Thus, when pulmonary embolism causes right-heart strain, or hypertrophy, an S_3, or ventricular gallop, may be noted. An S_3 generated in the right ventricle usually is best heard to the right of the apex close to the lower sternal border and during inspiration.

❑ OTHER CARDIAC MANIFESTATIONS

Right Ventricular Heave or Lift.—As a consequence of the elevated pulmonary blood pressure, right ventricular strain and/or right ventricular hypertrophy often develops. When this occurs, a sustained lift of the chest wall can be felt at the lower left side of the sternum during systole (Fig 16-4). This is because the right ventricle lies directly beneath the sternum.

❑ COUGH/HEMOPTYSIS (SEE PAGE 93)

As a result of the pulmonary hypertension, the pulmonary hydrostatic pressure, normally about 15 mm Hg, often becomes higher than the pulmonary oncotic pressure (normally about 25 mm Hg). This permits plasma and red blood cells to move across the alveolar-capillary membrane and into alveolar spaces. If this process continues, the subepithelial mechanoreceptors located in the bronchioles, bronchi, and trachea will be stimulated. Such stimulation initiates a cough reflex and the expectoration of blood-tinged sputum.

❑ CHEST PAIN/DECREASED CHEST EXPANSION (see page 98)

Chest pain is frequently noted in patients with pulmonary embolism. The origin of the pain is obscure. It may be cardiac or pleural, but it is one of the common, early findings in all forms of pulmonary embolism, even in the absence of obvious cor pulmonale or pleural involvement.

❑ RADIOLOGIC FINDINGS

Chest radiograph
* Increased density (in infarcted areas)
* Hyperradiolucency distal to the embolus (in noninfarcted areas)
* Dilatation of the pulmonary artery
* Pulmonary edema
* Cor pulmonale
* Pleural effusion

Although there are often no radiographic signs seen in patients with a pulmonary embolus, a density with a diffuse border similar to pneumonia may be seen if infarction has occurred. There may also be hyperradiolucency distal to the embolus that is caused by decreased vascularity. Dilatation of the pulmonary artery on the affected side, pulmonary edema (common after a fat embolus), cor pulmonale, and pleural effusion may also be seen.

Abnormal perfusion lung scan vs. normal ventilation scan findings

Ventilation lung scanning can provide additional information on perfusion defects. The patient breathes a gas mixture containing a small amount of radioactive gas, usually xenon 133. The presence of the xenon is detected by an external scintillation camera during a wash-in or wash-out breathing maneuver. Patients with pulmonary embolism often demonstrate normal ventilation in the region of their perfusion defect (Fig 16-5, (*A*).

An intravenous injection of radiolabeled particles 20 to 50 μm in diameter is used in determining the presence of pulmonary embolism. Particles labeled with a γ-emitting isotope, usually iodine or technetium, are injected into venous blood. The isotope accompanies the venous blood through the right-heart chambers and on into the pulmonary vascular system. Because blood flow is decreased or absent distal to a pulmonary embolus, fewer radioactive particles are present in this area. This is recorded by an external scintillation camera (Fig 16-5, *B*).

Abnormal pulmonary angiographic findings

Pulmonary angiography is the "gold standard" used to confirm the presence of pulmonary embolism in patients with "borderline" or "indeterminant" ventilation-perfusion lung scans. A catheter is advanced through the right heart and into the pulmonary artery. A radiopaque dye is then rapidly injected into the pulmonary artery while serial roentgenograms are taken. Pulmonary embolism is confirmed by abnormal filling within the artery or a cutoff of the artery. A dark area appears on the angiogram distal to the embolization since the radiopaque material is prevented from flowing past the obstruction (Fig 16-6). The procedure generally poses no risk to the patient unless there is severe pulmonary hypertension (mean pulmonary artery pressure >45 mm Hg) or the patient is in shock or allergic to the contrast medium. The pulmonary angiogram is rarely positive if the ventilation-perfusion lung scan is normal.

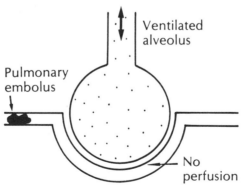

FIG 16-2
Dead-space ventilation in pulmonary embolism.

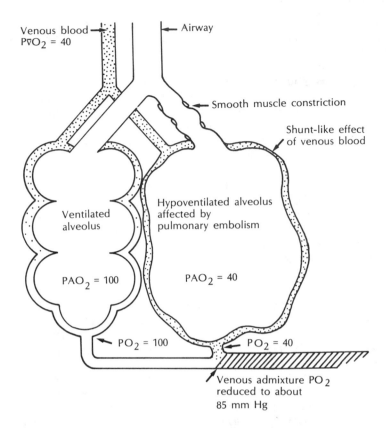

Venous blood
$P\bar{v}O_2 = 40$

Airway

Smooth muscle constriction

Shunt-like effect
of venous blood

Ventilated
alveolus

Hypoventilated alveolus
affected by
pulmonary embolism

$PAO_2 = 100$

$PAO_2 = 40$

$PO_2 = 100$

$PO_2 = 40$

Venous admixture PO_2
reduced to about
85 mm Hg

FIG 16-3

Venous admixture develops in pulmonary embolism as a result of bronchial smooth muscle constriction (shuntlike effect). Venous admixture may also occur when an embolus leads to pulmonary infarction and causes alveolar atelectasis and consolidation (true capillary shunt). Alveolar atelectasis and consolidation are not shown in this illustration.

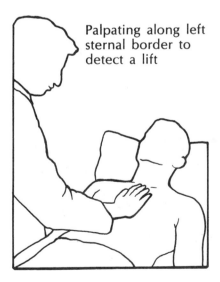

Palpating along left
sternal border to
detect a lift

FIG 16-4

A right ventricular lift can sometimes be detected in patients with a pulmonary embolism.

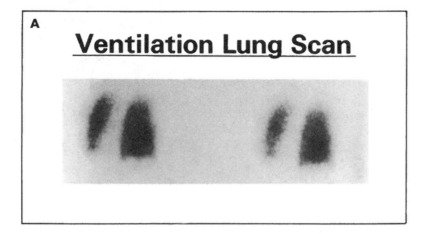

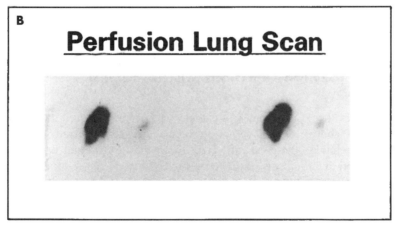

FIG 16-5

A normal ventilation lung scan and an abnormal perfusion lung scan are commonly seen in patients with severe pulmonary embolism. **A,** A normal ventilation scan shows a uniform distribution of gas, with the dark areas reflecting the presence of the radioactive gas and, therefore, good ventilation (right lung is on viewer's left). **B,** An abnormal perfusion scan. The dark area shown in the right lung represents good blood flow. The white or light areas shown in the left lung represent a decreased or complete absence of blood flow (right lung is on viewer's left).

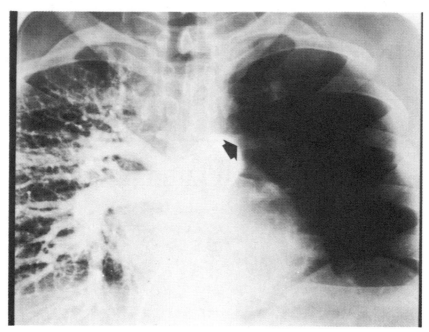

FIG 16-6
Abnormal pulmonary angiogram. Radiopaque material injected into the blood is prevented from flowing past the pulmonary embolism *(arrow).* This causes the angiogram to appear dark distal to the obstruction.

GENERAL MANAGEMENT OF PULMONARY EMBOLISM
Preventive Measures

Preventive measures should be initiated in patients who are predisposed to pulmonary embolism *(see* Etiology, above). Low doses of subcutaneously administered heparin have been proved extremely helpful in these patients. Tight-fitting elastic stockings have also been helpful in patients prone to thrombosis of the leg veins.

Management of Pulmonary Embolism

Heparin, administered intravenously, is the primary anticoagulant used to treat patients with acute pulmonary embolism. Warfarin (Coumadin) and dicumarol are the most commonly used oral anticoagulants. These latter agents are used primarily for the prevention of any additional or recurrent pulmonary emboli. They do nothing to eliminate existing pulmonary emboli. Supplemental oxygen is given to offset hypoxemia. Cardiotonic drugs are sometimes employed to reduce right-heart strain, and ECG monitoring is used to detect arrhythmias.

Thrombolytic Agents

Urokinase and streptokinase, two fibrinolytic agents, have been proved beneficial in treating pulmonary embolism. These thrombolytic agents are sometimes used along with heparin. Because of the excessive risk of bleeding, however, the use of fibrinolytic agents in treating pulmonary embolism has been limited.

Pulmonary Embolectomy

Surgical removal of blood clots from the pulmonary circulation is generally a last resort in treating pulmonary embolism because of the mortality associated with the procedure and because of the availability of fibrinolytic agents to adequately treat pulmonary embolism.

· **PULMONARY EMBOLISM AND INFARCTION CASE STUDY** ·

ADMITTING HISTORY AND PHYSICAL EXAMINATION

A 59-year-old white male slipped while shoveling snow and suffered a trimalleolar fracture of his right ankle. He was taken to the emergency room of the medical center. After appropriate workup, he was taken to the operating room where, under spinal anesthesia, the ankle fracture was reduced and a full-length cast was applied. He was discharged the next morning.

At home, he was doing well for about ten days when at about 3 PM he suddenly developed a nonproductive cough and severe dyspnea. He was taken by ambulance to the emergency room, and on arrival he was found to be unconscious and mildly cyanotic. At this time, his vital signs were blood pressure 90/40, pulse 126/min, and respiratory rate 36/min. Chest auscultation was unremarkable. P_2 was loud. On O_2 at 2 lpm, his arterial blood gas values were pH 7.51, Pa_{CO_2} 28, HCO_3^- 21, and Pa_{O_2} 39. A portable chest x-ray was reported as normal.

At this time, a nonrebreathing oxygen mask was placed on the patient. The cyanosis disappeared. He was taken to the radiology department where a ventilation-perfusion lung scan was performed. The scan showed a large perfusion defect in the left lower lung. At this point, the physician elected to transfer the patient to the ICU, intubate, and ventilate with 100% oxygen. After ten minutes on the mechanical ventilator, the patient's vital signs were blood pressure 90/40, pulse 126/min with frequent premature ventricular contractions, and respiratory rate of 12/min (12 mechanical ventilation breaths). Auscultation revealed mild bilateral wheezing. Blood gases on an $F_{I_{O_2}}$ of 1.0 were the following: pH 7.44, Pa_{CO_2} 32, HCO_3^- 23, and Pa_{O_2} 126. At this time, the respiratory therapist working with the patient recorded this:

RESPIRATORY ASSESSMENT AND PLAN

S: N/A (patient unconscious, intubated)

O: BP 90/40; P 126/min with frequent PVCs. Bilateral wheezing; loud P_2; On 100% O_2 and mechanical ventilation: pH 7.44, Pa_{CO_2} 32, HCO_3^- 23, Pa_{O_2} 126; Perfusion deficit left lung.

A: · Acute pulmonary embolism, left lung, probably secondary to immobilization of right leg ($\dot{V}/\dot{Q}$ scan)
   · Ventilatory and oxygenation status adequate on present ventilator settings (mildly over-oxygenated) (ABG)
   · Bronchospasm (wheezing)

P: Start continuous pulse oximetry. Reduce $F_{I_{O_2}}$ per oxygen therapy protocol. Wean from ventilator support per mechanical ventilation protocol. Bronchodilator therapy per protocol.

Serious consideration was given to surgical embolectomy, but the patient was stable at this time and began to respond. The decision, therefore, was to manage the pulmonary embolus conservatively, and the patient was anticoagulated intravenously with heparin. He was extubated without difficulty on the third hospital day.

The patient stated that he was feeling much better and did not feel short of breath or any pain. His cough was productive of rusty sputum. His vital signs were blood pressure 138/82, pulse 90 (regular), and respiratory rate 20/min. Crackles were heard over the left lower lobe. A chest x-ray showed a small left pleural effusion, and some "plate-like" atelectasis in the left lower lobe. On 2 lpm oxygen, his Sa_{O_2} was greater than 92%. The respiratory care practitioner charted the following at this time:

RESPIRATORY ASSESSMENT AND PLAN

S: Patient says he is feeling much better. Not dyspneic. No chest pain.

O: BP 138/82, P 90 & regular, RR 20. Crackles left base. CXR: small left pleural effusion, some atelectasis. Pulse oximetry 92% on 2 lpm.

A: • Pulmonary embolism
- Now, probably has infarcted LLL (crackles & CXR)
- Small pleural effusion & atelectasis (CXR)
- Good oxygenation on 2 lpm (oximetry)

P: Titrate O_2 per protocol. Lung hyperinflation (volume expansion protocol). Monitor pleural effusion with CXR in two to three days.

The physician monitored the patient's SGOT, LDH, and enzyme fractions as the patient improved steadily and recovered within the next seven days.

DISCUSSION

Unless acute ventilatory failure occurs, the role of the respiratory practitioner in the care of the patient with pulmonary embolism is somewhat limited. As we see here, oxygenation status must be monitored and appropriate oxygen given. If necessary, ventilatory support may be required.

Once infarction of the embolized segment has occurred, atelectasis in the area (often complicated by a pleural effusion) frequently occurs. At this point, volume expansion therapy such as incentive spirometry may be helpful. Through this period, oxygenation must be assured.

There is some debate as to whether the bronchospasm (as seen in this patient) deserves treatment. Some investigators feel this problem results from release of bronchoconstrictors from the vascular clot itself. Whether or not this patient benefited from bronchodilator therapy was not clear from our examination of the records. Such therapy was certainly not contraindicated in his case. Ventilator management of such patients is complicated by the large amount of wasted ventilation that they demonstrate.

SELF-ASSESSMENT QUESTIONS

Multiple Choice

1. Most pulmonary emboli originate from thrombi in the
   a. Lungs.
   b. Right heart.
   c. Leg and pelvic veins.
   d. Left heart.
   e. Pulmonary veins.

2. The aortic and carotid sinus baroreceptors initiate the following in response to a decreased systemic blood pressure:
   I. Increased heart rate
   II. Increased ventilatory rate
   III. Decreased heart rate
   IV. Decreased ventilatory rate
   V. Ventilatory rate is not affected by the aortic and carotid sinus baroreceptors
   a. I and IV only
   b. II and III only
   c. III and IV only
   d. I and II only
   e. V only

3. What is the normal mean pulmonary artery pressure?
   a. 5 mm Hg
   b. 10 mm Hg
   c. 15 mm Hg
   d. 20 mm Hg
   e. 25 mm Hg

4. Pulmonary hypertension develops in pulmonary embolism because of
   I. Increased cross-sectional area of the pulmonary vascular system.
   II. Vasoconstriction due to humoral agent release.
   III. Vasoconstriction induced by decreased arterial oxygen pressure (Pa_{O_2}).
   IV. Vasoconstriction induced by decreased alveolar oxygen pressure (PA_{O_2}).
   a. I and III only
   b. II and III only
   c. I, II, and III only
   d. II, III, and IV only
   e. II and IV only

5. In severe pulmonary embolism, common hemodynamic indices seen is/are:
   I. Decreased PVR
   II. Increased $\overline{PA}$
   III. Decreased CVP
   IV. Increased PCWP
   a. II only
   b. III only
   c. IV only
   d. I and II only
   e. II, III, and IV only

6. S_2 is sometimes louder in pulmonary embolism because of a more forceful closure of the
   a. Tricuspid valve.
   b. Pulmonic valve.
   c. Mitral valve.
   d. Bicuspid valve.

7. When humoral agents such as serotonin are released into the pulmonary circulation
    I. The bronchial smooth muscles dilate.
    II. The $\dot{V}/\dot{Q}$ ratio decreases.
    III. The bronchial smooth muscles constrict.
    IV. The $\dot{V}/\dot{Q}$ ratio increases.
        a. I only
        b. II only
        c. IV only
        d. II and III only
        e. I and IV only

8. Which of the following is a thrombolytic agent?
    I. Urokinase
    II. Heparin
    III. Warfarin
    IV. Streptokinase
        a. I only
        b. IV only
        c. II and III only
        d. I and IV only
        e. I, II, III, and IV

9. Which of the following is the most prominent source of pulmonary emboli?
        a. Fat
        b. Blood clots
        c. Bone marrow
        d. Air
        e. Malignant neoplasms

10. Which of the following is the most common arrhythmia seen in pulmonary embolism?
        a. Sinus tachycardia
        b. Atrial flutter
        c. Left bundle-branch block
        d. Incomplete right bundle-branch block
        e. Complete right bundle-branch block

Answers appear in Appendix XXI.

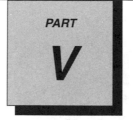
CHEST AND PLEURAL TRAUMA

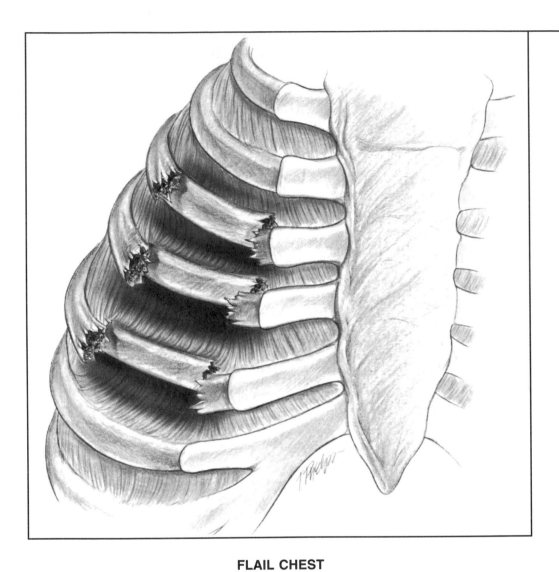

FLAIL CHEST

FIG 17-1

Flail chest. Double fractures of at least three or more adjacent ribs. (See also Plate 16.)

Flail Chest

ANATOMIC ALTERATIONS OF THE LUNGS

A flail chest is the result of double fractures (i.e., two fractures along the length of the same rib) of at least three or more adjacent ribs, which causes the thoracic cage to become unstable (Fig 17-1). The affected ribs cave in (flail) during inspiration as a result of the subatmospheric intrapleural pressure. This compresses and restricts the underlying lung area and promotes atelectasis and lung collapse. In severe cases there may also be contusion of the lung under the fractured ribs.

To summarize, the major pathologic or structural changes associated with flail chest are as follows:

- Double fracture of multiple adjacent ribs
- Rib instability
- Lung restriction
- Atelectasis
- Lung collapse
- Lung contusion

ETIOLOGY

A crushing injury to the chest is usually the cause of a flail chest. Such trauma may result from the following:

- Direct compression by a heavy object
- Automobile accident
- Industrial accident

OVERVIEW

OF THE CARDIOPULMONARY CLINICAL MANIFESTATIONS ASSOCIATED WITH
FLAIL CHEST

❏ **INCREASED RESPIRATORY RATE**

Several pathophysiologic mechanisms operating simultaneously may lead to an increased ventilatory rate. These are (see page 17)

Stimulation of peripheral chemoreceptors

As a result of the paradoxical movement of the chest wall, the lung area directly beneath the broken ribs is compressed during inspiration and is pushed outward through the flail area during expiration. This abnormal chest and lung movement causes air to be shunted from one lung to another during a ventilatory cycle.

When the lung on the affected side is compressed during inspiration, gas moves into the lung on the unaffected side. During expiration, however, air from the unaffected lung moves into the affected lung. The shunting of air from one lung to another is known as *pendelluft* (Fig 17-2). In consequence of the pendelluft, the patient rebreathes dead-space gas and hypoventilates. In addition to the hypoventilation produced by the pendelluft, alveolar ventilation may also be decreased by the lung compression and atelectasis associated with an unstable chest.

As a result of the pendelluft, lung compression, and atelectasis, the $\dot{V}/\dot{Q}$ ratio decreases. This leads to intrapulmonary shunting and venous admixture (Fig 17-3). Because of the venous admixture, the patient's Pa_{O_2} and Ca_{O_2} decrease. As this condition intensifies, the patient's oxygen level may decline to a point low enough to stimulate the peripheral chemoreceptors which, in turn, initiate an increased ventilatory rate.

Other possible mechanisms
- Decreased lung compliance/increased ventilatory rate relationship
- Activation of the deflation receptors
- Activation of the irritant receptors
- Stimulation of the J receptors
- Pain/anxiety

❏ **PULMONARY FUNCTION STUDY FINDINGS**

Lung Volume and Capacity Findings (see page 39)

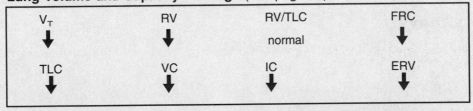

V_T	RV	RV/TLC	FRC
↓	↓	normal	↓
TLC	VC	IC	ERV
↓	↓	↓	↓

❏ **INCREASED HEART RATE (PULSE), CARDIAC OUTPUT, AND BLOOD PRESSURE** (see page 86)

❏ **ARTERIAL BLOOD GASES**

Mild Flail Chest

Acute Alveolar Hyperventilation with Hypoxemia (see page 57)

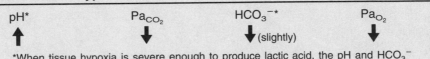

pH*	Pa_{CO_2}	HCO_3^-*	Pa_{O_2}
↑	↓	↓ (slightly)	↓

*When tissue hypoxia is severe enough to produce lactic acid, the pH and HCO_3^- values will be lower than expected for a particular Pa_{CO_2} level.

Severe Flail Chest

Acute Ventilatory Failure with Hypoxemia (see page 59)

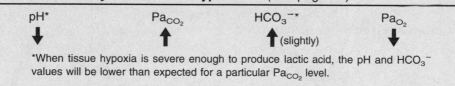

*When tissue hypoxia is severe enough to produce lactic acid, the pH and HCO_3^- values will be lower than expected for a particular Pa_{CO_2} level.

❏ **CYANOSIS** (see page 68)
❏ **OXYGENATION INDICES** (see page 69)

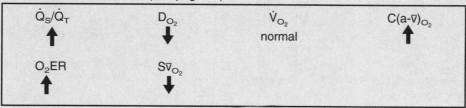

❏ **HEMODYNAMIC INDICES (SEVERE FLAIL CHEST)** (see page 87)

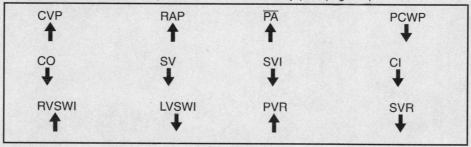

❏ **PARADOXICAL MOVEMENT OF THE CHEST WALL**

When double fractures exist in at least three or more adjacent ribs, a paradoxical movement of the chest wall is seen. During inspiration, the fractured ribs are pushed inward by the atmospheric pressure surrounding the chest. During expiration, the flail area bulges outward when the intrapleural pressure becomes greater than the atmospheric pressure.

❏ **RADIOLOGIC FINDINGS**
Chest Radiograph
   • Increased capacity (in atelectatic areas)
   • Rib fractures (may need special films—rib series—to demonstrate)

Because of the lung compression and atelectasis associated with a flail chest, the density of the lungs increases. The increase in lung density is revealed on the chest radiograph as an increased opacity (i.e., whiter in appearance). The chest radiograph will also show the rib fractures (Fig 17-4).

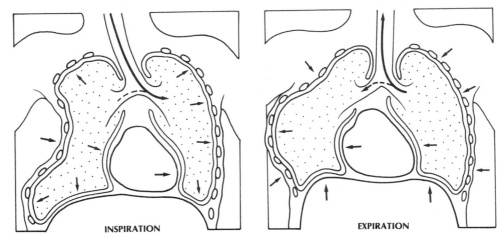

FIG 17-2
Lateral flail chest with accompanying pendelluft.

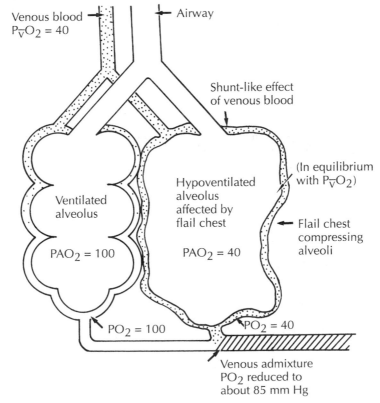

FIG 17-3
Venous admixture in flail chest.

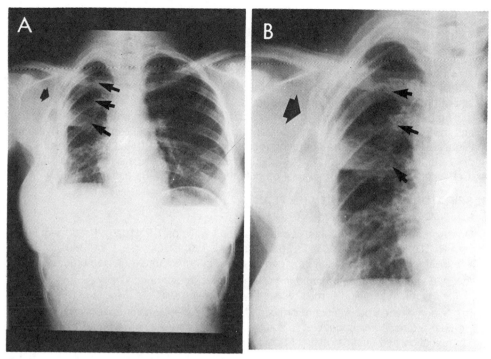

FIG 17-4

A, chest x-ray film of a 20-year-old female with a severe right-sided flail chest. **B,** close-up of the same x-ray film.

GENERAL MANAGEMENT OF FLAIL CHEST

In mild cases, medication for pain and routine bronchial hygiene may be all that is needed. In more severe cases, however, stabilization of the chest is usually required to allow bone healing and to prevent atelectasis. Today, controlled volume ventilation, sometimes accompanied by positive end-expiratory pressure (PEEP), is commonly used to stabilize a flail chest. Generally, mechanical ventilation for 5 to 10 days is an adequate time for adequate bone healing to occur.

Supplemental Oxygen

Because of the hypoxemia associated with a flail chest, supplemental oxygen may be required. It should be noted, however, that the hypoxemia that develops in a flail chest is most commonly caused by the aleveolar atelectasis and capillary shunting associated with the disorder. Hypoxemia caused by capillary shunting is often refractory to oxygen therapy.

• • • • • **FLAIL CHEST CASE STUDY** • • • • • •

ADMITTING HISTORY AND PHYSICAL EXAMINATION

A 40-year-old truck driver was involved in a serious, four-vehicle automobile accident and was taken to the emergency room of a nearby medical center where he was found to be markedly agitated, obese, and uncooperative. He was concious, and in obvious respiratory distress. His vital signs were blood pressure 80/62, pulse 90/min, respirations 42/min and shallow. There was bilateral paradoxical movement of the chest wall.

There was a laceration of the right eye, and deep lacerations of the right thigh with rupture of the patellar tendon. There was pain and tenderness on palpation of the right posterior chest wall. The AP diameter of the chest was increased. Breath sounds were decreased bilaterally, and expiration was prolonged.

X-ray examination revealed posterolateral fractures of ribs 2 through 10 on the right and of the necks of ribs 11 and 12 on the left. He had a 4^+ hematuria, but his other laboratory findings were within normal limits.

The patient was intubated in the emergency department. An arterial line was placed, and the patient was taken to the operating room where surgical repair of the eye and thigh was performed. In the operating room, with an $F_{I_{O_2}}$ of 1.0, his blood gases were pH 7.48, Pa_{CO_2} 30, HCO_3^- 23, Pa_{O_2} 360. The patient was transferred to the surgical ICU, where the respiratory therapist on duty made the following assessment:

RESPIRATORY ASSESSMENT AND PLAN

S: N/A—intubated, sedated.

O: No paradoxical movement of chest wall on ventilator. BP 110/70, P 100 regular, RR 12 on vent. On 100% O_2, pH 7.48, Pa_{CO_2} 30, HCO_3^- 23, Pa_{O_2} 360. CXR: bilateral rib fractures, left lung contused, no pneumothorax, no hemothorax.

A: • Bilateral flail chest (history, paradoxical chest movement, CXR)
• Hyperoxygenation & mild respiratory alkalemia (ABG)

P: Wean oxygen per ventilator protocol. Maintain patient on controlled ventilation per protocol until chest wall is stable. Physician and/or charge nurse to increase sedation and muscle relaxant should patient begin to inhale between preset mechanical ventilation rate. Continuous Sa_{O_2} monitoring. Careful chest assessment and auscultation to watch for significant pneumothorax.

The patient was kept intubated and ventilated with an $F_{I_{O_2}}$ of 0.3 and a mechanical ventilation rate of 12/min. His hospital course was stormy. On the second day, a right pneumothorax was demonstrated and a chest tube was inserted. The next day his pulse rose to 160/min, and the PA catheter showed evidence of left ventricular failure. He was rapidly digitalized and diuresed, and his cardiac function improved dramatically. His Swan-Ganz catheter failed to "wedge." Over the next few days, the chest x-ray showed dense infiltrates in both lungs, and it was difficult to maintain adequate oxygenation, even with high inspired oxygen concentrations. It was noted that whenever his arterial saturation dropped below 90%, he became restless and agitated. At this time, the respiratory assessment was as follows:

RESPIRATORY ASSESSMENT AND PLAN

S: N/A—intubated, sedated.

O: Afebrile. P 140 regular, BP 142/82, RR 12 (on vent). Right chest tube shows air leak. Crackles bilaterally. CXR: fractures appear in line; bilateral dense infiltrates. ABG: pH 7.37, Pa_{CO_2} 38, HCO_3^- 23, Pa_{O_2} 58 on $F_{I_{O_2}}$ of 0.7. Sputum thick, yellow.

A: • Persistent flail chest bilaterally (CXR)
• Bilateral dense infiltrates suggest pulmonary edema/ARDS (CXR)
• Adequate ventilatory status with moderate hypoxemia on present ventilatory settings. Oxygenation continues to worsen (ABG)
• Thick, yellow bronchial secretions (sputum)
• Bronchopleural fistula on right side (chest tube bubbles)

P: Mechanical ventilation and PEEP per protocol. Continue oxygen therapy per protocol. Instill acetylcysteine and suction prn. Closely monitor patient's fluid intake and output. Assist physician in the replacement of the Swan-Ganz catheter to optimize fluid therapy. Continue Sa_{O_2} monitoring. Obtain sputum for Gram's stain and culture.

During the first week of his hospitalization, his BUN increased to 60 mg% and his creatinine to 1.9 mg%. Liver function tests remained within normal limits. The abnormal BUN and creatinine gradually returned to normal during the second week. The patient was slowly but successfully weaned off the ventilator over the next two weeks. His total hospital stay was 40 days. Over 120 respiratory (SOAP) assessments were documented in the patient's chart at discharge.

DISCUSSION

This complicated case demonstrates the care of the traumatized patient with multi-organ failure. In this case, the second organ effected was the cardiovascular system, probably secondary to fluid overload. Initial therapy included chest wall rest and internal fixation with mechanical ventilation. One could argue that PEEP could have been added to his management at this point.

Later (when what appears to be ARDS supervened), PEEP was added, both for its effect on the ARDS and secondarily to stabilize the chest wall. Although these problems were dramatic enough, the therapist alertly noted the thick, yellow bronchial secretions and added acetylcysteine and vigorous suctioning to deal with this problem. The ordering of a sputum Gram's stain and culture was appropriate.

Clearly, a patient this ill should be assessed at least once—possibly more—per shift. As this patient was hospitalized for 40 days, more than 120 such assessments were found in his chart! As we reviewed his case, this certainly did not seem to be excessive.

SELF-ASSESSMENT QUESTIONS

Multiple Choice

1. When the deflation reflex is activated,
   I. The lungs deflate.
   II. The expiratory time increases.
   III. The ventilatory rate increases.
   IV. The Hering-Breuer inflation reflex is activated.
      a. I only
      b. II only
      c. III only
      d. III and IV only
      e. I, III, and IV only

2. When a patient has a severe flail chest,
   I. Venous return increases.
   II. Cardiac output decreases.
   III. Systemic blood pressure increases.
   IV. Central venous pressure increases.
      a. I only
      b. III only
      c. III and IV only
      d. II and IV only
      e. I, III, and IV only

3. A flail chest consists of a double fracture of at least
      a. Two adjacent ribs.
      b. Three adjacent ribs.
      c. Four adjacent ribs.
      d. Five adjacent ribs.
      e. Six adjacent ribs.

4. As a consequence of a severe flail chest, the
   I. RV increases.
   II. V_T decreases.
   III. VC increases.
   IV. FRC decreases.
      a. IV only
      b. I and III only
      c. II and IV only
      d. II, III, and IV only
      e. I, II, III, and IV

5. When mechanical ventilation is used to stabilize a flail chest, how much time is generally needed for bone healing to occur?
      a. 5 to 10 days
      b. 10 to 15 days
      c. 15 to 20 days
      d. 20 to 25 days
      e. 25 to 30 days

True or False

1. The shunting of air from one lung to another is known as pendelluft.   True _____   False _____

2. The fractured ribs of a severe flail chest commonly move outward during expiration.   True _____   False _____

3. In pendelluft, lung compression and atelectasis cause the $\dot{V}/\dot{Q}$ ratio to increase.   True _____   False _____

4. The irritant receptors may be stimulated in a flail chest.   True _____   False _____

5. During the advanced stages of a severe flail chest, the increased HCO_3^- level in the arterial blood gases is secondary to the increased Pa_{CO_2}.   True _____   False _____

Answers appear in Appendix XXI.

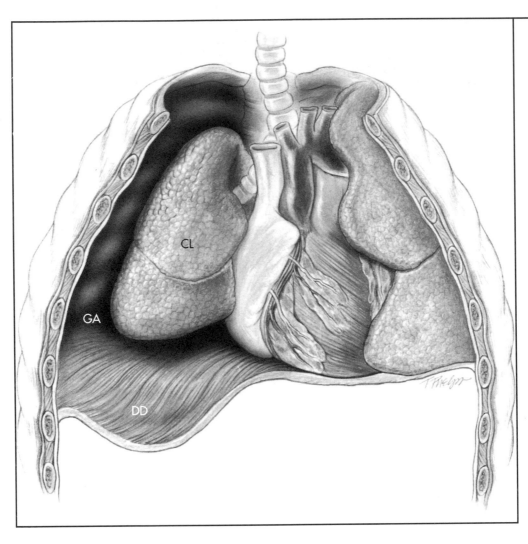

PNEUMOTHORAX

FIG 18-1

Right-sided pneumothorax. *GA* = gas accumulation; *DD* = depressed diaphragm; *CL* = collapsed lung. (See also Plate 17.)

CHAPTER 18

Pneumothorax

ANATOMIC ALTERATIONS OF THE LUNGS

A pneumothorax exists when gas accumulates in the pleural space (Fig 18-1). When gas enters the pleural space, the visceral and parietal pleura separate. This enhances the natural tendency of the lungs to recoil, or collapse, and the natural tendency of the chest wall to move outward, or expand. As the lung collapses the alveoli are compressed, and atelectasis ensues. In severe cases, the great veins may be compressed and cause the venous return to the heart to diminish.

To summarize, the major pathologic or structural changes associated with a pneumothorax are as follows:

- Lung collapse
- Atelectasis
- Chest wall expansion
- Compression of the great veins and decreased cardiac venous return

ETIOLOGY

There are three ways in which gas can gain entrance to the pleural space:

- From the lungs through a perforation of the visceral pleura
- From the surrounding atmosphere through a perforation of the chest wall and parietal pleura or, rarely, through an esophageal fistula or from a perforated abdominal viscus
- From gas-forming microorganisms in an empyema in the pleural space

A pneumothorax may be classified as either closed or open according to how gas gains entrance to the pleural space. In a *closed pneumothorax,* gas in the pleural space is not in direct contact with the atmosphere. An *open pneumothorax,* on the other hand, implies that the pleural space is in direct contact with the atmosphere and that gas can move freely in and out. A pneumothorax in which the intrapleural pressure exceeds the intra-alveolar (or atmospheric) pressure is known as a *tension pneumothorax.* Some etiologic forms of pneumothorax are as follows:

- Traumatic pneumothorax
- Spontaneous pneumothorax
- Iatrogenic pneumothorax

Traumatic Pneumothorax

Penetrating wounds to the chest wall from a knife, bullet, or an impaling object in an automobile or industrial accident are common causes of a traumatic pneumothorax. When this type of trauma occurs, the pleural space is in direct contact with the atmosphere, and gas can move in and out of the pleural cavity. This condition is known as a *sucking chest wound* and is classified as an *open pneumothorax* (Fig 18-2).

A piercing chest wound may also result in a *closed (valvular) pneumothorax* through a one-way valve-like action of the ruptured parietal pleura. In this form of pneumothorax, gas enters the pleural space during inspiration but cannot leave during expiration because the parietal pleura (or more remotely, the chest wall itself) acts as a check valve. This condition may cause the intrapleural pressure to exceed the atmospheric pressure in the affected area. Technically, this form of pneumothorax is classified as a *tension pneumothorax* (Fig 18-3).

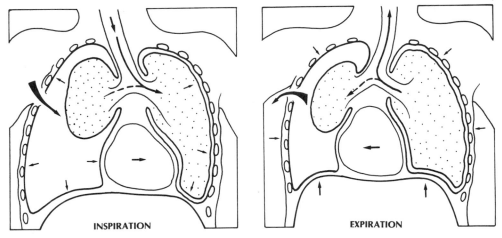

FIG 18-2
Sucking chest wound with accompanying pendelluft.

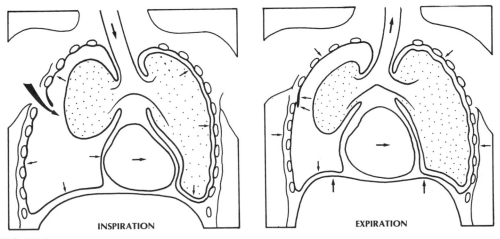

FIG 18-3
Closed (valvular) pneumothorax produced by a chest wall wound.

When a crushing chest injury occurs, the pleural space may not be in direct contact with the atmosphere, but the sharp end of a fractured rib may pierce or tear the visceral pleura. This may permit gas to leak into the pleural space from the lungs. Technically, this form of pneumothorax is classified as a *closed pneumothorax.*

Spontaneous Pneumothorax

When pneumothorax occurs suddenly and without any obvious underlying cause, it is referred to as a spontaneous pneumothorax. Spontaneous pneumothorax is secondary to certain underlying pathologic processes such as pneumonia, tuberculosis, and chronic obstructive pulmonary disease. A spontaneous pneumothorax is sometimes caused by the rupture of a small bleb or bulla on the surface of the lung. This type of pneumothorax often occurs in tall persons between the ages of 15 and 35 years. It may be due to the high negative intrathoracic pressure and mechanical stresses that take place in the upper zone of the upright lung.

A spontaneous pneumothorax may also behave as a valvular pneumothorax. Air from the lung parenchyma may enter the pleural space via a tear in the visceral pleura during inspiration but is unable to leave during expiration since the visceral tear functions as a check valve (Fig 18-4). This condition may cause the intrapleural pressure to exceed the intra-alveolar pressure. This form of pneumothorax is classified as both a *closed* and a *tension pneumothorax.*

Iatrogenic Pneumothorax

An *iatrogenic pneumothorax* sometimes occurs during specific diagnostic or therapeutic procedures. For example, a pleural or liver biopsy may cause a pneumothorax. Thoracentesis, intercostal nerve block, cannulation of a subclavian vein, and tracheostomy are possible causes of an iatrogenic pneumothorax. *An iatrogenic pneumothorax is always a hazard during positive-pressure mechanical ventilation.*

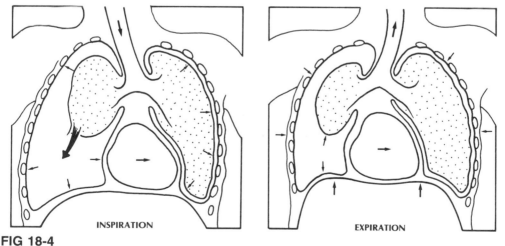

INSPIRATION   EXPIRATION

FIG 18-4
Valvular pneumothorax produced by a rupture in the visceral pleura.

OVERVIEW
OF THE CARDIOPULMONARY CLINICAL MANIFESTATIONS ASSOCIATED WITH
PNEUMOTHORAX

❑ **INCREASED RESPIRATORY RATE**

Several pathophysiologic mechanisms operating simultaneously may lead to an increased ventilatory rate. These are the following:

Stimulation of peripheral chemoreceptors

As gas moves into the pleural space, the visceral and parietal pleura separate, and the lung on the affected side begins to collapse. As the lung collapses, atelectasis develops, and alveolar ventilation decreases.

If the patient has a pneumothorax due to a sucking chest wound, an additional mechanism may also promote hypoventilation. That is, when a patient with this type of pneumothorax inhales, the intrapleural pressure on the unaffected side decreases. As a result, the mediastinum often moves to the unaffected side, where the pressure is lower, and compresses the normal lung. The intrapleural pressure on the affected side may also decrease, and some air may enter through the chest wound and further shift the mediastinum toward the normal lung. During expiration, the intrapleural pressure on the affected side rises above atmospheric pressure, and gas escapes from the pleural space through the chest wound. As gas leaves the pleural space, the mediastinum moves back toward the affected side. Because of this back-and-forth movement of the mediastinum, some gas from the normal lung may enter the collapsed lung during expiration and cause it to expand slightly. During inspiration, however, some of this "rebreathed dead-space gas" may move back into the normal lung. This paradoxical movement of gas within the lungs is known as *pendelluft*. As a result of the pendelluft, the patient hypoventilates (see Fig 18-2).

Thus, when a patient has a pneumothorax, alveolar ventilation is reduced because of lung collapse and atelectasis. Should the pneumothorax be accompanied by a sucking chest wound, alveolar ventilation may be further decreased by pendelluft.

As a result of the reduced alveolar ventilation the patient's $\dot{V}/\dot{Q}$ ratio decreases. This leads to intrapulmonary shunting and venous admixture (Fig 18-5). Because of the venous admixture, the Pa_{O_2} and Ca_{O_2} decrease. As this condition intensifies, the patient's oxygen level may decline to a point low enough to stimulate the peripheral chemoreceptors. Stimulation of the peripheral chemoreceptors in turn initiates an increased ventilatory rate.

Other possible mechanisms (see page 17)
- Decreased lung compliance/increased ventilatory rate relationship
- Activation of the deflation receptors
- Activation of the irritant receptors
- Stimulation of the J receptors
- Pain/anxiety

❑ **PULMONARY FUNCTION STUDY FINDINGS**

Lung Volume and Capacity Findings (see page 39)

V_T	RV	RV/TLC	FRC
↓	↓	normal	↓
TLC	VC	IC	ERV
↓	↓	↓	↓

❑ **INCREASED HEART RATE (PULSE), CARDIAC OUTPUT, AND BLOOD PRESSURE (SMALL PNEUMOTHORAX)** (see page 86)
❑ **ARTERIAL BLOOD GASES**

Small Pneumothorax

Acute Alveolar Hyperventilation with Hypoxemia (see page 57)

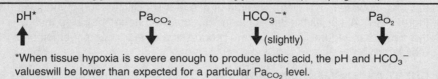

pH*	Pa_{CO_2}	HCO_3^-*	Pa_{O_2}
↑	↓	↓ (slightly)	↓

*When tissue hypoxia is severe enough to produce lactic acid, the pH and HCO_3^- valueswill be lower than expected for a particular Pa_{CO_2} level.

Large Pneumothorax

Acute Ventilatory Failure with Hypoxemia (see page 59)

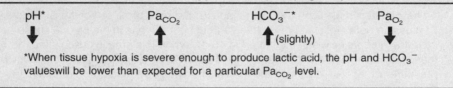

pH*	Pa_{CO_2}	HCO_3^-*	Pa_{O_2}
↓	↑	↑ (slightly)	↓

*When tissue hypoxia is severe enough to produce lactic acid, the pH and HCO_3^- valueswill be lower than expected for a particular Pa_{CO_2} level.

❑ **CYANOSIS** (see page 68)
❑ **OXYGENATION INDICES** (see page 69)

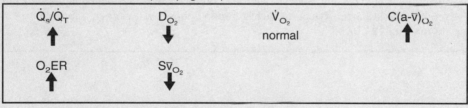

$\dot{Q}_s/\dot{Q}_T$	D_{O_2}	$\dot{V}_{O_2}$	$C(a\text{-}\bar{v})_{O_2}$
↑	↓	normal	↑
O_2ER	$S\bar{v}_{O_2}$		
↑	↓		

❑ **HEMODYNAMIC INDICES (LARGE PNEUMOTHORAX)** (see page 87)

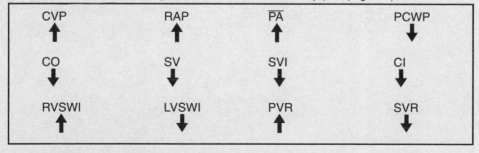

CVP	RAP	$\overline{PA}$	PCWP
↑	↑	↑	↓
CO	SV	SVI	CI
↓	↓	↓	↓
RVSWI	LVSWI	PVR	SVR
↑	↓	↑	↓

❑ **RADIOLOGIC FINDINGS**
Chest radiograph
- Increased translucency (darker area) on the side of pneumothorax
- Mediastinal shift to unaffected side in tension pneumothorax
- Depressed diaphragm
- Lung collapse
- Atelectasis

Ordinarily, the presence of a pneumothorax is easily identified on the chest radiograph in the upright posteroanterior view (Fig 18-6). A small collection of air is often visible if the exposure is made at the end of maximal expiration because the translucency of the pneumothorax is more obvious when contrasted to the density of a partially deflated lung. The pneumothorax is usually seen in the upper part of the pleural cavity when the film is exposed while the patient is in the upright position. Severe adhesions, however, may limit a volume of gas to a specific portion of the pleural space. Figure 18-7, *A,* shows the development of a tension pneumothorax in the lower part of the right lung. Figure 18-7, *B,* shows progression of the same pneumothorax 30 minutes later.

❏ CHEST ASSESSMENT FINDINGS

- Hyperresonant percussion note
- Diminished breath sounds
- Tracheal shift
- Displaced heart sounds
- Increased diameter on the affected side

As gas accumulates in the pleural space, the ratio of air to solid tissue increases. Percussion notes resonate more freely throughout the gas in the pleural space as well as in the air spaces within the lung (Fig 18-8). When this area is auscultated, however, the breath sounds are diminished (Fig 18-9). When intrapleural gas accumulation and pressure are excessively high, the mediastinum may be forced to the unaffected side. If this is the case, there will be a tracheal shift and the heart sounds will be displaced during auscultation. Finally, the gas that accumulates in the pleural space enhances not only the natural tendency of the lungs to collapse but also the natural tendency of the chest wall to expand. Thus, in a large pneumothorax, the chest often appears larger on the affected side. This is especially true in patients with a severe tension pneumothorax (Fig 18-10).

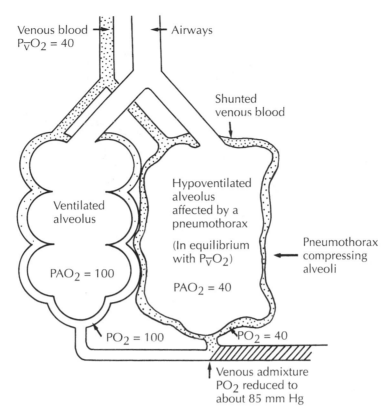

FIG 18-5
Venous admixture in pneumothorax.

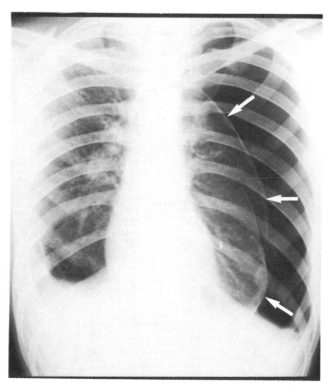

FIG 18-6
Left-sided pneumothorax *(arrows)*. Notice the shift of the heart and mediastinum to the right, away from the tension pneumothorax.

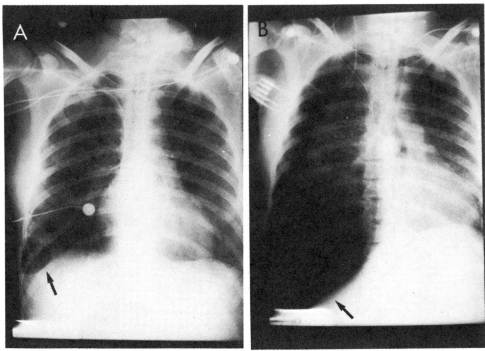

FIG 18-7

A, development of a small tension pneumothorax in lower part of the right lung *(arrow).* **B,** the same pneumothorax 30 minutes later. Notice the shift of the heart and mediastinum to the left, away from the tension pneumothorax. Also notice the depression of the right hemidiaphragm (*arrow*).

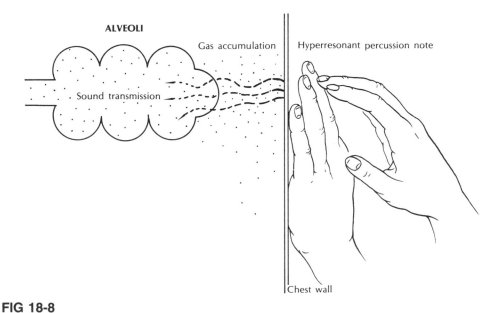

FIG 18-8

Because the ratio of air to solid tissue increases in a pneumothorax, hyperresonant percussion notes are produced over the affected area.

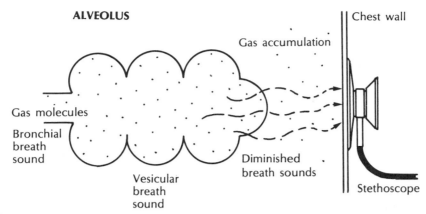

FIG 18-9
Breath sounds diminish as gas accumulates in the intrapleural space.

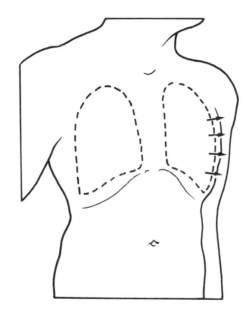

FIG 18-10
As gas accumulates in the intrapleural space, the chest diameter increases on the affected side in a tension pneumothorax.

GENERAL MANAGEMENT OF PNEUMOTHORAX

The management of pneumothorax depends on the degree of lung collapse. When the pneumothorax is relatively small (15% to 20%), the patient may need only bed rest or limited physical activity. In such cases, resorption of intrapleural gas usually occurs within 30 days.

When the pneumothorax is greater than 20%, the gas should be evacuated. In less severe cases when the pneumothorax is confined to a relatively small area, air may simply be withdrawn from the pleural cavity by needle aspiration. In more serious cases, however, a chest tube attached to an underwater seal is inserted into the patient's pleural cavity. Such a tube permits evacuation of air and enhances the reexpansion and pleural adherence of the affected lung. The chest tube may or may not be attached to gentle negative suction. When suction is used, the negative pressure usually does not exceed -12 cm H_2O, and -5 cm H_2O is generally all that is needed. After the lung has reexpanded, the chest tube is left in place for another 24 to 48 hours.

Supplemental Oxygen

Because of the hypoxemia associated with a pneumothorax, supplemental oxygen may be required. It should be noted, however, that the hypoxemia that develops in a pneumothorax is most commonly caused by the alveolar atelectasis and capillary shunting associated with the disorder. Hypoxemia caused by capillary shunting is refractory to oxygen therapy.

• • **SPONTANEOUS PNEUMOTHORAX CASE STUDY** • •

ADMITTING HISTORY AND PHYSICAL EXAMINATION

This patient was a 20-year-old male university student who was in excellent health until five hours prior to admission. He was sitting quietly in his dorm room studying for an examination, when he suddenly developed a sharp pain in his left lower thoracic region. It was most acute in the anterior axillary line. The pain was exacerbated by deep inspiration and radiated anteriorly, almost to the midline. It did not radiate into the shoulder or neck. The patient became mildly dyspneic and had episodes of nonproductive cough, which seemed to increase the chest pain. These symptoms worsened, and at 1 AM, his roommate drove him to the university hospital emergency room.

On examination, the patient was a well-nourished, well-developed young male in moderately acute distress. His trachea was shifted to the right of the midline. His blood pressure was 150/82, pulse 96, respirations 28 and shallow. The left chest was tympanitic to percussion, and the breath sounds were described as "distant." The patient was not cyanotic. The emergency department physician was momentarily busy with another patient and asked the respiratory therapist on duty to assess the patient's respiratory status. The respiratory therapist assigned to the emergency room during the night shift made the following assessments and plans:

RESPIRATORY ASSESSMENT AND PLAN

S: Left chest pain worsened by cough; shortness of breath.

O: Normal vital signs. Left chest hyperresonant. Trachea shifted to the right. Breath sounds on left "distant."

A: Probable left pneumothorax (history & objective indicators)

P: Notify physician (who is in the next room). Stat CXR & ABG. Oxygen therapy via partial rebreathing mask ($F_{I_{O_2}}$ 0.6 to 0.8). Obtain supplies for tube thoracotomy and place at patient's bedside.

The chest radiograph confirmed the diagnosis of left-sided pneumothorax with mediastinal shift to the right. The arterial blood gas values on the partial rebreathing mask were pH 7.53, Pa_{CO_2} 29, HCO_3^- 21, Pa_{O_2} 56. The physician was still busy with the patient in the next room. With this new information the respiratory therapist charted the following:

RESPIRATORY ASSESSMENT AND PLAN

S: "This oxygen mask helps a little."

O: Persistent symptoms as in SOAP-1 above. CXR: 50% left *tension pneumothorax.* Mediastinum shifted to right. Nonrebreathing mask ABGs: pH 7.53, Pa_{CO_2} 29, HCO_3^- 21, Pa_{O_2} 56.

A: • 50% left pneumothorax with mediastinal shift (CXR)

   • Acute alveolar hyperventilation with mild hypoxemia (ABG)

P: Inform physician of above assessment. Increase $F_{I_{O_2}}$ to 0.8 to 1.0 via a nonrebreathing mask. Stay at patient's bedside until physician arrives. Will assist in placement of chest tube.

Fifteen minutes later, the attending physician entered the room and quickly reviewed the clinical data and assessments. Moments later, he introduced a thoracostomy tube and began underwater drainage. The lung expanded well, and the tube was removed after 48 hours. Follow-up examination after two weeks revealed full expansion of the left lung. There was no evidence of blebs or bullae. A tuberculin skin test was negative.

DISCUSSION

Few respiratory conditions persist with a "crisis" onset, and this is one of them. Other instances include foreign body aspiration, pulmonary embolism, anaphylactic shock, and some cases of asthma.

Though the respiratory care administered in this case (oxygen therapy) was fairly pedestrian, the therapist's assistance in assessment of this patient and his presence at bedside made a great difference in the ease with which the patient was treated. The value of an assessing/treating therapist in this situation cannot be underestimated.

SELF-ASSESSMENT QUESTIONS

Multiple Choice

1. When gas moves between the pleural space and the atmosphere during a ventilatory cycle, the patient is said to have a/an
   I. Closed pneumothorax.
   II. Open pneumothorax.
   III. Valvular pneumothorax.
   IV. Sucking chest wound.
      a. I only
      b. II only
      c. III only
      d. I and III only
      e. II and IV only

2. When gas enters the pleural space during inspiration but is unable to leave during expiration, the patient is said to have a/an
   I. Iatrogenic pneumothorax.
   II. Valvular pneumothorax.
   III. Tension pneumothorax.
   IV. Open pneumothorax.
      a. I only
      b. III only
      c. II and III only
      d. III and IV only
      e. II, III, and IV only

3. A pneumothorax may be caused by
   I. Pneumonia.
   II. Tuberculosis.
   III. Chronic obstructive pulmonary disease.
   IV. Blebs.
      a. IV only
      b. I and II only
      c. II and III only
      d. II, III, and IV only
      e. I, II, III, and IV

4. When a patient has a pneumothorax due to a sucking chest wound,
   I. Intrapleural pressure on the unaffected side increases during inspiration.
   II. The mediastinum often moves to the unaffected side during inspiration.
   III. Intrapleural pressure on the affected side often rises above the atmospheric pressure during expiration.
   IV. The mediastinum often moves to the affected side during expiration.
      a. I and IV only
      b. I and III only
      c. II and III only
      d. II, III, and IV only
      e. I, II, III, and IV

5. The increased ventilatory rate commonly manifested in patients with pneumothorax may be due to
   I. Stimulation of the J receptors.
   II. Increased lung compliance.
   III. Increased stimulation of the Hering-Breuer reflex.
   IV. Stimulation of the irritant reflex.
      a. I and IV only
      b. II and III only
      c. III and IV only
      d. II, III, and IV only
      e. I, II, III, and IV

6. The physician usually elects to evacuate the intrathoracic gas when the pneumothorax is greater than
     a. 5%.
     b. 10%.
     c. 15%.
     d. 20%.
     e. 25%.

7. When treating a pneumothorax with a chest tube and suction, the negative (suction) pressure usually does not exceed
     a. 4 cm H_2O.
     b. 6 cm H_2O.
     c. 8 cm H_2O.
     d. 10 cm H_2O.
     e. 12 cm H_2O.

8. A patient with a severe tension pneumothorax demonstrates
   I. Diminished breath sounds.
   II. Hyperresonant percussion note.
   III. Dull percussion notes.
   IV. Whispered pectoriloquy.
     a. II only
     b. I and II only
     c. III and IV only
     d. I, II, and IV only
     e. I, II, III, and IV

9. When a patient has a large tension pneumothorax, the
   I. Pa_{CO_2} decreases.
   II. pH increases.
   III. HCO_3^- decreases.
   IV. Pa_{CO_2} increases.
     a. I only
     b. IV only
     c. III and IV only
     d. II and III only
     e. I, II, and III only

10. When a patient has a large tension pneumothorax, the
   I. PVR decreases.
   II. $\overline{PA}$ increases.
   III. CVP decreases.
   IV. CO increases.
     a. I only
     b. II only
     c. III only
     d. I and III only
     e. II and IV only

Answers appear in Appendix XXI.

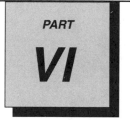
DISORDERS OF THE PLEURA AND OF THE CHEST WALL

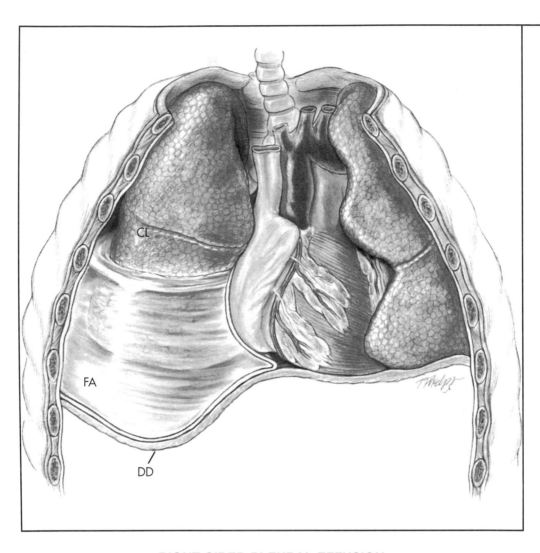

RIGHT-SIDED PLEURAL EFFUSION

FIG 19-1

Right-sided pleural effusion. *FA* = fluid accumulation; *DD* = depressed diaphragm; *CL* = collapsed lung (partially collapsed). (See also Plate 18.)

19

Pleural Diseases

ANATOMIC ALTERATIONS OF THE LUNGS

A number of pleural diseases can cause fluid to accumulate in the pleural space, and this fluid is called a *pleural effusion* (Fig 19-1). Similar to gas in the pleural space, fluid accumulation will separate the visceral and parietal pleura and compress the lungs. In severe cases, atelectasis will develop, the great veins may be compressed, and cardiac venous return may be diminished. Pleural effusion produces a restrictive lung disorder.

To summarize, the major pathologic or structural changes associated with significant pleural effusion are as follows:

* Lung compression
* Atelectasis
* Compression of the great veins and decreased cardiac venous return

ETIOLOGY

A pleural effusion may be transudative or exudative. Transudate develops when fluid from the pulmonary capillaries moves into the pleural space. The fluid produced is thin and watery and it contains a few blood cells and little protein. The pleural surfaces are not involved in producing the transudate.

In contrast, an exudate develops when the pleural surfaces are diseased. The fluid has a high protein content and a great deal of cellular debris. Exudate is usually caused by inflammation.

Major Causes of a Transudate Pleural Effusion

Congestive Heart Failure.—Congestive heart failure is probably the most common cause of a pleural effusion. Both right- and left-sided heart failure can result in pleural effusion. In right-sided heart failure, an increase in the hydrostatic pressure in the systemic circulation can (1) increase the rate of pleural fluid formation and (2) decrease lymphatic drainage from the pleural space because of the elevated systemic venous pressure. In left-sided heart failure, an increase in the hydrostatic pressures in the pulmonary circulation can (1) decrease the rate of pleural fluid absorption through the visceral pleura and (2) cause fluid movement through the visceral pleura into the pleural space. In general, left-sided heart failure is more likely to produce pleural effusion than right-sided heart failure.

Hepatic Hydrothorax.—Occasionally, pleural effusions can develop as a complication of hepatic cirrhosis, particularly when ascitic fluid is present. The pleural effusion in these patients is generally right-sided.

Peritoneal Dialysis.—As in the pleural effusion that occurs as a result of ascites, pleural fluid may also develop as a complication of peritoneal dialysis. When the peritoneal dialysis is stopped, the pleural effusion usually disappears rapidly.

Nephrotic Syndrome.—Pleural effusion is commonly seen in patients with nephrotic syndrome. It is generally bilateral. The effusion is a result of the decreased plasma oncotic pressure that develops in this disorder.

Pulmonary Embolus.—It is estimated that between 30% and 50% of patients with pulmonary emboli develop pleural effusion. Two distinct mechanisms are responsible. First, obstruction of the pulmonary vasculature can lead to right-sided heart failure, which in turn can lead to pleural effusion. The second mechanism involves the increased permeability of the capillaries in the visceral pleura that develops in response to the ischemia caused by the pulmonary emboli.

Major Causes of an Exudate Pleural Effusion

Malignant Pleural Effusions.—Metastatic disease of the pleura or of the mediastinal lymph nodes is the most common cause of exudative pleural effusions. Carcinoma of the lung and breast and lymphomas account for about 75% of malignant pleural effusions.

Malignant Mesotheliomas.—Malignant mesotheliomas arise from the mesothelial cells that line the pleural cavities. Individuals with chronic asbestos exposure have a much greater risk of developing this neoplasm. The pleural fluid is exudative and generally contains a mixture of normal mesothelial cells, differentiated and undifferentiated malignant mesothelial cells, and a varying number of lymphocytes and polymorphonuclear leukocytes.

Pneumonias.—As many as 40% of patients with bacterial pneumonia have an accompanying pleural effusion. Most pleural effusions associated with pneumonia resolve without any specific therapy. About 10%, however, will need some sort of therapeutic intervention. If appropriate antibiotic therapy is not instituted, bacteria invade the pleural fluid from the lung parenchyma. Eventually, pus will accumulate in the pleural cavity (*empyema*). Pleural effusion can also be produced by viruses, *Mycoplasma pneumoniae,* and rickettsiae, although the pleural effusions are usually small.

Tuberculosis.—Pleural effusion may develop from a rupture of a caseous tubercle into the pleural cavity. It is also possible that the inflammatory reaction that develops in tuberculosis obstructs the lymphatic pores in the parietal pleural. This in turn leads to an accumulation of protein and fluid in the pleural space. Pleural effusion due to tuberculosis is generally unilateral and small to moderate in size.

Fungal Diseases.—Patients with fungal diseases occasionally have secondary pleural effusions. Common fungal diseases that may produce a pleural effusion are histoplasmosis, coccidioidomycosis, and blastomycosis.

Pleural Effusion Due to Diseases of the Gastrointestinal Tract.—Pleural effusion is sometimes associated with diseases of the gastrointestinal tract such as pancreatic disease, subphrenic abscess, intrahepatic abscess, esophageal perforation, abdominal operations, and diaphragmatic hernia.

Pleural Effusion Due to Collagen Vascular Diseases.—Pleural effusion occasionally develops as a complication of collagen vascular diseases. Such diseases include rheumatoid pleuritis, systemic lupus erythematosus, Sjögren's syndrome, familial Mediterranean fever, and Wegener's granulomatosis.

Other Pathologic Fluids That Separate the Parietal From the Visceral Pleura

In addition to transudate and exudate, there are other pathologic fluids that can separate the parietal pleura from the visceral pleura.

Empyema.—The accumulation of \pus in the pleural cavity is called empyema. Empyema commonly develops as a result of inflammation. Thoracentesis may confirm the diagnosis and determine the specific causative organism. The pus is usually removed by chest tube drainage.

Chylothorax.—Chylothorax (also called chylopleura) is the presence of chyle in the pleural cavity. Chyle is a milky liquid produced from the food in the small intestine during digestion. It consists mainly of fat particles in a stable emulsion. Chyle is taken up by fingerlike, intestinal lymphatics, called lacteals, and transported by the thoracic duct to the neck. From the thoracic duct, the chyle moves into the venous circulation and mixes with blood.

The presence of chyle in the pleural cavity is usually due to trauma to the neck or thorax or to a tumor occluding the thoracic duct.

Hemothorax.—The presence of blood in the pleural space is known as a hemothorax. Most of these are caused by penetrating or blunt chest trauma. An iatrogenic hemothorax may develop from trauma caused by the insertion of a central venous catheter.

Blood can gain entrance into the pleural space from trauma to the chest wall, diaphragm, lung, or mediastinum. Hemothorax may also be caused by the rupture of small blood vessels. A hematocrit should always be obtained if the pleural fluid looks like blood. A hemothorax is said to be present only when the hematocrit of the pleural fluid is at least 50% that of the peripheral blood.

OVERVIEW

OF THE CARDIOPULMONARY CLINICAL MANIFESTATIONS ASSOCIATED WITH
PLEURAL EFFUSION

❏ **INCREASED RESPIRATORY RATE**
  Several pathophysiologic mechanisms operating simultaneously may lead to an increased ventilatory rate. These are (see page 17)
  • Stimulation of peripheral chemoreceptors
  • Decreased lung compliance/increased ventilatory rate relationship
  • Activation of the deflation receptors
  • Activation of the irritant receptors
  • Stimulation of the J receptors
  • Pain/anxiety

❏ **PULMONARY FUNCTION STUDY FINDINGS**

Lung Volume and Capacity Findings (see page 39)

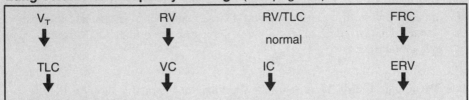

❏ **INCREASED HEART RATE (PULSE), CARDIAC OUTPUT, AND BLOOD PRESSURE (SMALL PLEURAL EFFUSION)** (see page 86)
❏ **ARTERIAL BLOOD GASES**

Small Pleural Effusion

Acute Alveolar Hyperventilation with Hypoxemia (see page 57)

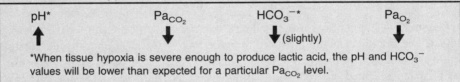

*When tissue hypoxia is severe enough to produce lactic acid, the pH and HCO_3^- values will be lower than expected for a particular Pa_{CO_2} level.

Large Pleural Effusion

Acute Ventilatory Failure with Hypoxemia (see page 59)

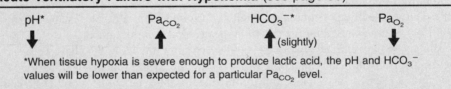

*When tissue hypoxia is severe enough to produce lactic acid, the pH and HCO_3^- values will be lower than expected for a particular Pa_{CO_2} level.

❏ **CYANOSIS** (see page 68)
❏ **OXYGENATION INDICES** (see page 69)

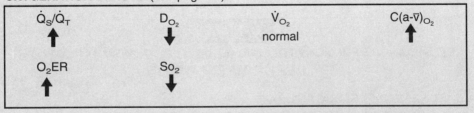

❏ **HEMODYNAMIC INDICES (LARGE PLEURAL EFFUSION)** (see page 87)

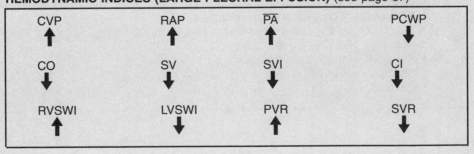

❏ **CHEST PAIN/DECREASED CHEST EXPANSION** (see page 98)
❏ **COUGH (DRY, NONPRODUCTIVE)** (see page 93)
❏ **CHEST ASSESSMENT FINDINGS** (see page 6)
   • Tracheal shift
   • Decreased tactile and vocal fremitus
   • Dull percussion note
   • Diminished breath sounds
   • Displaced heart sounds

❏ **RADIOLOGIC FINDINGS**
Chest radiograph
   • Blunting of the costophrenic angle
   • Depressed diaphragm
   • Mediastinal shift (possibly) to unaffected side
   • Atelectasis

   The diagnosis of a pleural effusion is generally based on the chest x-ray film. A pleural effusion of less than 300 ml usually cannot be seen on an upright chest x-ray film. In moderate pleural effusion (1,000 ml) in the upright position, an increased density usually appears at the costophrenic angle. The fluid first accumulates posteriorly in the most dependent part of the thoracic cavity, between the inferior surface of the lower lobe and the diaphragm. As the fluid volume increases, it extends upward around the anterior, lateral, and posterior thoracic walls. Interlobar fissures are sometimes highlighted as a result of fluid filling. On the typical radiograph the lateral costophrenic angle is obliterated, and the outline of the diaphragm on the affected side is lost (Figs 19-2 and 19-3).

   In severe cases, the weight of the fluid may cause the diaphragm to become inverted (concave). Clinically, this inversion is only seen in left-sided pleural effusions; the gastric air bubble is pushed downward and the superior border of the left diaphragmatic leaf is concave. In addition, the mediastinum may be shifted to the unaffected side, and the intercostal spaces may appear widened.

   Pleural effusion, atelectasis, and parenchymal infiltrates can obliterate one or both diaphragms. Thus, when a posteroanterior or lateral chest radiograph suggests pleural effusion, additional radiographic studies are generally needed to document the presence of pleural fluid or other pathology present. The lateral decubitus radiograph is recommended since free fluid gravitates to the most dependent part of the pleural space (Fig 19-4).

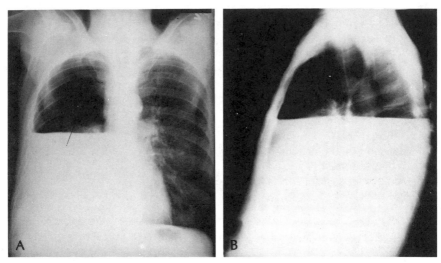

FIG 19-2

Posteroanterior **(A)** and lateral **(B)** radiographs of a patient with a hydropneumothorax. Note that the fluid level extends throughout the length and width of the hemithorax. This hydropneumothorax followed an attempted thoracentesis in this patient with a massive right pleural effusion. (From Light RL: *Pleural diseases,* Philadelphia, Lea & Febiger, 1983. Used by permission.)

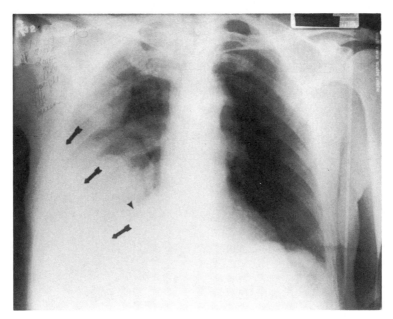

FIG 19-3

Chest radiograph of a patient with a pulmonary abscess in the right lung, extrapleural bleed *(arrows),* and pleural effusion. (From Rau JL Jr, Pearce DJ: *Understanding chest radiographs.* Denver, Multi-Media Publishing Co, 1984. Used by permission.)

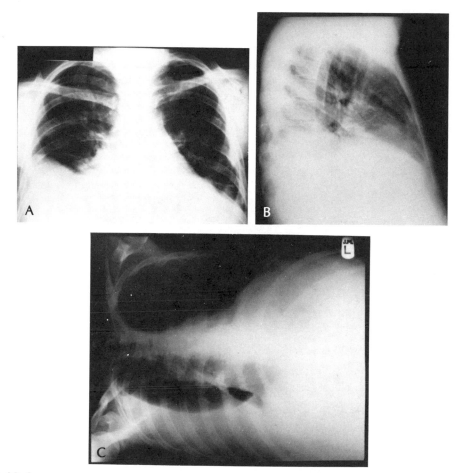

FIG 19-4
Subpulmonic pleural effusion. **A,** posteroanterior chest radiograph demonstrating clear lateral costophrenic angles but apparent elevation of the right diaphragm. **B,** lateral chest radiograph of the same patient demonstrates a blunted posterior costophrenic angle. **C,** lateral decubitus film of this patient demonstrates a large amount of free pleural fluid. (From Light RL: *Pleural diseases.* Philadelphia, Lea & Febiger, 1983. Used by permission.)

GENERAL MANAGEMENT OF PLEURAL EFFUSION

The management of each patient with a pleural effusion must be individualized. Questions to be asked include the following: What is the appropriate antibiotic? Should a thoracentesis be performed? Should a chest tube be inserted? Can the underlying cause be treated?

An etiologic diagnosis is necessary to appropriately treat a patient with pleural effusion. Examination of the effusion may reveal blood following trauma or surgery, pus in empyema, or milky fluid in chylothorax. The presence of blood in the pleural fluid in the absence of trauma or surgery suggests a malignant disease or pulmonary embolization.

When the cause of the pleural effusion is not readily evident, microscopic and chemical examination of pleural fluid may determine whether the effusion is a transudate or an exudate. If the fluid is a transudate, treatment is directed to the underlying problem (e.g., congestive heart failure, cirrhosis, or nephrosis). When an exudate is present, a cytologic examination may identify a malignancy. The fluid may also be examined for its biochemical makeup (e.g., protein, sugar, and various enzymes) and for the presence of bacteria.

Thoracentesis

Thoracentesis (also called thoracocentesis) entails the perforation of the chest wall and pleural space with a needle for the aspiration of fluid for diagnostic or therapeutic purposes or for the removal of a specimen for biopsy. The procedure is usually performed using local anesthesia, with the patient in an upright position. Therapeutically, a thoracentesis may be used to treat pleural effusion. Fluid samples may be examined for the following:

- Color
- Odor
- RBC count
- WBC count with differential
- Protein
- Glucose
- Lactic dehydrogenase (LDH)
- Amylase
- pH
- Wright's, Gram's and acid-fast (AFB) stains
- Aerobic, anaerobic, tuberculosis, and fungal cultures
- Cytology

Hyperinflation Techniques

Hyperinflation measures are commonly ordered to offset the alveolar consolidation and atelectasis associated with pleural effusion (see Appendix XII).

Supplemental Oxygen

Because of the hypoxemia associated with a pleural effusion, supplemental oxygen may be required. It should be noted, however, that the hypoxemia that develops in a pleural effusion is most commonly caused by the alveolar atelectasis and capillary shunting associated with the disorder. Hypoxemia caused by capillary shunting is refractory to oxygen therapy.

• • • • ▐ **PLEURAL DISEASE CASE STUDY** ▌ • • • •

ADMITTING HISTORY AND PHYSICAL EXAMINATION

A 55-year-old male came to the emergency department because of dull, right-sided chest pain of about two weeks' duration, dry, nonproductive cough, and increasing dyspnea. He had a history of having worked with asbestos insulating materials for about one month, almost 30 years previously. The patient had never smoked.

On physical examination, the patient appeared older than his stated age and was in obvious, moderately severe respiratory distress. His oral temperature was 98.6° F; blood pressure was 150/86, pulse 100/min, and respirations 32/min. Examination of the chest showed decreased respiratory excursion on the right side, with dullness to percussion and diminished breath sounds in this area. No wheezes or rhonchi were heard.

Bedside spirometry revealed an FVC that was 50% of predicted. The chest radiograph revealed a large pleural effusion with pleural thickening in the lower right lung area. Room air blood gases were pH 7.52, Pa_{CO_2} 29, HCO_3^- 22, Pa_{O_2} 55. His WBC was 10,400.

While the physician prepared the patient for a thoracentesis, the respiratory care practitioner recorded this assessment and plan:

RESPIRATORY ASSESSMENT AND PLAN

S: "This cough is driving me crazy!" Also complains of right-sided pleuritic chest pain.

O: Afebrile. BP 150/86, P 100, RR 32. Decreased lung expansion on right, with dullness to percussion and decreased breath sounds at right base. FVC 50% of predicted. CXR: large right pleural effusion with pleural thickening. ABG on room air: pH 7.52, Pa_{CO_2} 29, HCO_3^- 22, Pa_{O_2} 55.

A: • Large right pleural effusion with pleural thickening (CXR)
• Acute alveolar hyperventilation with moderate hypoxemia (ABG)

P: Oxygen therapy (O_2 mask) per oxygen therapy protocol. Remain on standby to assist physician with thoracentesis. Reassess after thoracentesis.

The thoracentesis yielded 850 ml of grossly bloody fluid, which was high in protein (4.5 g/dl) and lactic dehydrogenase (300 IU/L). On cytologic examination of the fluid, a diagnosis of malignant mesothelioma was made. The patient's acute alveolar hyperventilation rapidly returned to normal after the thoracentesis, although continuous oxygen therapy was still needed to correct the hypoxemia. His cough diminished significantly, and his vital signs returned to normal. Hyperinflation directed by volume expansion protocol was prescribed for the next 24 hours. At discharge, arrangements were made for home oxygen.

DISCUSSION

Here again, the respiratory care practitioner's involvement in care of patients with pleural disease/pleural effusion is somewhat limited. Oxygen therapy per protocol was certainly indicated because of the patient's hypoxemia, despite the alveolar hyperventilation. The respiratory care practitioner shows, in this case, that he is "on top of the situation" by his intention to reassess the patient after thoracentesis. At that time, several less-than-optimum results might occur, e.g. insufficient removal of the pleural effusion or the development of a post-thoracentesis pneumothorax.

This case well illustrates the fact that the respiratory care practitioner needs to be cautious in even the simplest of respiratory care situations. The fact that the respiratory care practitioner is not directly involved in the thoracentesis does not relieve him of the responsibility for continual assessment of the patient after the procedure is completed.

SELF-ASSESSMENT QUESTIONS

Multiple Choice

1. Which of the following is/are associated with exudative effusion?
   - I. Few blood cells
   - II. Inflammation
   - III. Thin and watery fluid
   - IV. Disease of the pleural surfaces
       - a. I only
       - b. II only
       - c. IV only
       - d. I and III only
       - e. II and IV only
2. Which of the following is probably the most common cause of a transudative pleural effusion?
       - a. Pulmonary embolus
       - b. Congestive heart failure
       - c. Hepatic hydrothorax
       - d. Nephrotic syndrome
       - e. Peritoneal dialysis
3. A hemothorax is said to be present when the hematocrit of the pleural fluid is at least what percentage of the peripheral blood?
       - a. 20
       - b. 30
       - c. 40
       - d. 50
       - e. 60
4. Approximately what percentage of patients with pulmonary emboli develop pleural effusion?
       - a. 0 to 20
       - b. 20 to 30
       - c. 30 to 50
       - d. 50 to 60
       - e. 60 to 80
5. Which of the following is/are associated with pleural effusion?
   - I. Increased RV
   - II. Decreased FRC
   - III. Increased V_T
   - IV. Decreased VC
       - a. I only
       - b. III only
       - c. I and III only
       - d. II and IV only
       - e. II, III, and IV only

True or False

1. Chyle in the pleural cavity is commonly caused by trauma to the neck.   True _____ False _____
2. A hyperresonant percussion note is associated with a pleural effusion.   True _____ False _____
3. Left-sided heart failure is more likely to cause a pleural effusion than right-sided heart failure.   True _____ False _____
4. The accumulation of pus in the pleural cavity is called empyema.   True _____ False _____
5. Pleural effusion may be caused by a gastrointestinal disorder.   True _____ False _____

Answers appear in Appendix XXI.

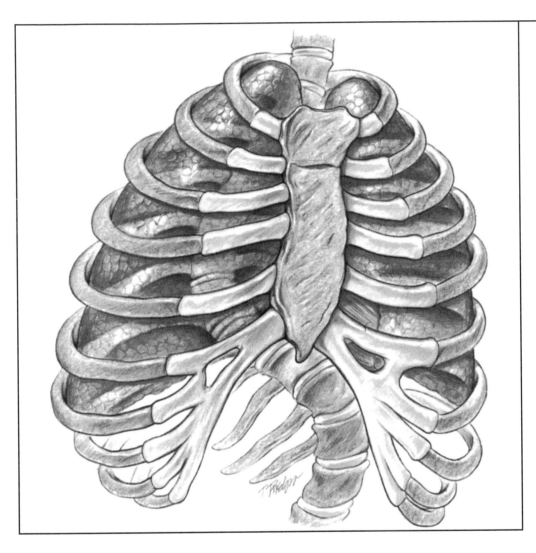

KYPHOSCOLIOSIS

FIG 20-1

Kyphoscoliosis. Posterior and lateral curvature of the spine, causing lung compression and atelectasis. (See also Plate 19.)

Kyphoscoliosis

ANATOMIC ALTERATIONS OF THE LUNGS

Kyphoscoliosis is a combination of two thoracic deformities that commonly appear together. *Kyphosis* is a posterior curvature of the spine (humpback), and *scoliosis* is a lateral curvature of the spine.

In severe kyphoscoliosis, the deformity of the thorax compresses the lungs and restricts alveolar expansion, which in turn causes alveolar hypoventilation and atelectasis. In addition, the patient's ability to cough and mobilize secretions may also be impaired, further causing atelectasis as secretions accumulate throughout the tracheobronchial tree. Because kyphoscoliosis involves both a posterior and lateral curvature of the spine, the thoracic contents generally twist in such a way as to cause a mediastinal shift in the same direction as the lateral curvature of the spine. Kyphoscoliosis causes a restrictive lung disorder (Fig 20-1) and difficulty clearing airway secretions.

To summarize, the major pathologic or structural changes of the lungs associated with kyphoscoliosis are as follows:

* Lung restriction and compression as a result of the thoracic deformity
* Mediastinal shift
* Mucus accumulation throughout the tracheobronchial tree
* Atelectasis

ETIOLOGY

Kyphoscoliosis affects approximately 10% of the U.S. population. Of this group, only about 1% have a notable deformity. The precise cause of kyphoscoliosis is unknown in about 80% to 85% of the cases. When kyphoscoliosis arises without a known cause, it is called idiopathic kyphoscoliosis. There are, however, a number of pathologic conditions known to cause kyphoscoliosis. These include congenital vertebral defects, neuromuscular disease (e.g., paralytic poliomyelitis, cerebral palsy, spinal muscular atrophy or injury), and vertebral disease.

OVERVIEW

OF THE CARDIOPULMONARY CLINICAL MANIFESTATIONS ASSOCIATED WITH
KYPHOSCOLIOSIS

❑ **INCREASED RESPIRATORY RATE**

Several pathophysiologic mechanisms operating simultaneously may lead to an increased ventilatory rate. These are (see page 17)
- Stimulation of peripheral chemoreceptors
- Decreased lung compliance/increased ventilatory rate relationship
- Activation of the deflation receptors
- Activation of the irritant receptors
- Stimulation of the J receptors
- Pain/anxiety

❑ **PULMONARY FUNCTION STUDY FINDINGS**

Expiratory Maneuver Findings (see page 39)

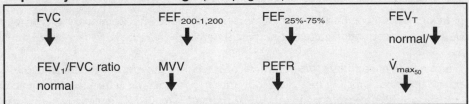

FVC	$FEF_{200-1,200}$	$FEF_{25\%-75\%}$	FEV_T
↓	↓	↓	normal/↓
FEV_1/FVC ratio	MVV	PEFR	$\dot{V}_{max_{50}}$
normal	↓	↓	↓

Lung Volume and Capacity Findings (see page 39)

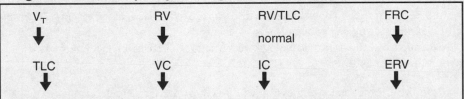

V_T	RV	RV/TLC	FRC
↓	↓	normal	↓
TLC	VC	IC	ERV
↓	↓	↓	↓

❑ **INCREASED HEART RATE (PULSE), CARDIAC OUTPUT, AND BLOOD PRESSURE** (see page 86)

❑ **ARTERIAL BLOOD GASES**

Moderate Kyphoscoliosis

Acute Alveolar Hyperventilation with Hypoxemia (see page 57)

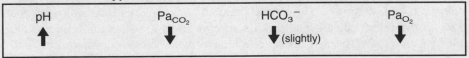

pH	Pa_{CO_2}	HCO_3^-	Pa_{O_2}
↑	↓	↓ (slightly)	↓

Severe Kyphoscoliosis

Chronic Ventilatory Failure with Hypoxemia (see page 60)

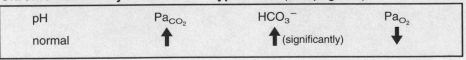

pH	Pa_{CO_2}	HCO_3^-	Pa_{O_2}
normal	↑	↑ (significantly)	↓

Acute Ventilatory Changes Superimposed on Chronic Ventilatory Failure
(see page 65)

Because acute ventilatory changes are frequently seen in patients with chronic ventilatory failure, the respiratory care practitioner must be familiar with and be on alert for (1) *acute alveolar hyperventilation superimposed on chronic ventilatory failure,* and (2) *acute ventilatory failure superimposed on chronic ventilatory failure.*

❏ **CYANOSIS** (see page 68)
❏ **OXYGENATION INDICES** (see page 69)

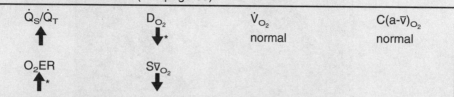

$\dot{Q}_S/\dot{Q}_T$	D_{O_2}	$\dot{V}_{O_2}$	$C(a-\bar{v})_{O_2}$
↑	↓*	normal	normal
O_2ER	$S\bar{v}_{O_2}$		
↑*	↓		

*The D_{O_2} may be normal in patients who have compensated for the decreased oxygenation status with an increased cardiac output, an increased hemoglobin level, or a combination of both. When the D_{O_2} is normal, the O_2ER is usually normal.

❏ **HEMODYNAMIC INDICES** (see page 87)

CVP	RAP	$\overline{PA}$	PCWP
↑	↑	↑	normal
CO	SV	SVI	CI
normal	normal	normal	normal
RVSWI	LVSWI	PVR	SVR
↑	normal	↑	normal

❏ **POLYCYTHEMIA, COR PULMONALE** (see page 92)
 • Distended neck veins
 • Enlarged and tender liver
 • Peripheral edema
 • Pitting edema

❏ **COUGH AND SPUTUM PRODUCTION** (see page 93)
❏ **CHEST ASSESSMENT FINDINGS** (see page 6)
 • Obvious thoracic deformity
 • Tracheal shift
 • Increased tactile and vocal fremitus
 • Dull percussion note
 • Bronchial breath sounds
 • Crackles/rhonchi/wheezing

❏ **RADIOLOGIC FINDINGS**
 Chest radiograph
 • Thoracic deformity
 • Mediastinal shift
 • Increased lung opacity
 • Atelectasis
 • Enlarged heart (cor pulmonale)

The extent of the thoracic deformity in kyphoscoliosis is demonstrated in anteroposterior and lateral radiographs. When present, a mediastinal shift is best shown on an anteroposterior chest radiograph. As the alveoli collapse, the density of the lung increases and is revealed on the chest radiograph as increased opacity. In severe cases, cor pulmonale may be seen (Fig 20-2).

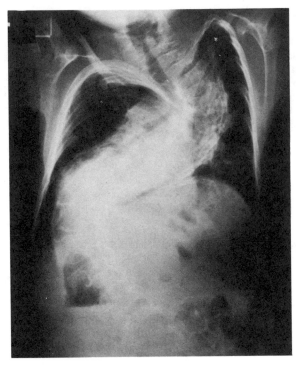

FIG 20-2
Severe kyphoscoliosis in a 14-year-old male.

GENERAL MANAGEMENT OF KYPHOSCOLIOSIS
Bracing

When signs of kyphoscoliosis are identified early in life, a body brace may prevent progression of the deformity as the thoracic skeleton matures.

Electrical Stimulation

Electrical stimulation is an alternative to the body brace. Two methods are in use: the implantable stimulator, which is popular in Europe, and the surface electrode system. Both methods are used to strengthen the muscles that surround the spine.

Surgery

Surgery may entail fusion of the involved vertebrae or insertion of a metal brace to provide correction and stability, including the Harrington and Luque rods.

Mobilization of Bronchial Secretions

Because of the excessive mucus accumulation associated with kyphoscoliosis, a number of respiratory therapy modalities may be used to enhance the mobilization of bronchial secretions (see Appendix XI).

Hyperinflation Techniques

Hyperinflation measures are commonly ordered to offset the atelectasis associated with kyphoscoliosis (see Appendix XII).

Supplemental Oxygen

Because of the hypoxemia associated with a kyphoscoliosis, supplemental oxygen may be required. It should be noted, however, that the hypoxemia that develops in kyphoscoliosis is most commonly caused by the atelectasis and capillary shunting associated with the disorder. Hypoxemia caused by capillary shunting is often refractory to oxygen therapy.

In addition, when the patient demonstrates chronic ventilatory failure during the advanced stages of kyphoscoliosis, caution must be taken not to eliminate the patient's hypoxic drive to breathe.

• • • • **KYPHOSCOLIOSIS CASE STUDY** • • • •

ADMITTING HISTORY AND PHYSICAL EXAMINATION

A 62-year-old male had poliomyelitis 52 years ago, after which he developed increasing anteroposterior and lateral curvature of the spine as a consequence of unilateral muscle weakness. He was able to function quite well in spite of his severe physical handicap, and had a distinguished career as a writer. His exercise tolerance was reasonably good, and he became dyspneic only after climbing two flights of stairs. He had smoked cigarettes for about 20 years but stopped smoking 15 years ago. He sought medical attention because of a three-day long history of cough that became productive of yellow, tenacious sputum. He was now mildly dyspneic at rest.

In the chest clinic, physical examination revealed severe kyphoscoliosis. The patient was in obvious respiratory distress. He was pale, and the lips and nail beds were "dusky." The patient frequently coughed throughout the examination, producing large amounts of thick, tenacious, yellow sputum. His oral temperature was 103.2°; blood pressure 150/92; pulse 100/min and regular; respirations 36/min and shallow. Auscultation revealed crackles and rhonchi over the left base posteriorly. The chest x-ray revealed an infiltrate that caused consolidation in the left lower lung field, and increased vascular markings throughout the left lung. Laboratory examination showed a WBC count of 15,000, with 10% bands and 60% segmented forms. On room air, the patient's arterial blood gas values were the following: pH 7.54; Pa_{CO_2} 65, HCO_3^- 31, Pa_{O_2} 57. At this time, the respiratory therapist documented this assessment and plan:

RESPIRATORY ASSESSMENT AND PLAN

S: Complains of severe productive cough and shortness of breath.

O: Acutely ill. Temp. 103.2° F; BP 150/92; P 100; RR 36. Cyanotic. Productive cough: large amount of thick tenacious yellow sputum. Crackles and rhonchi at left base. WBC 15,000 (10B, 60S). Blood cultures pending. CXR: LLL infiltrate and consolidation. Room air ABGs: pH 7.54; Pa_{CO_2} 65, HCO_3^- 31, Pa_{O_2} 57.

A: • Severe kyphoscoliosis aggravated by LLL infiltrate and consolidation (history & CXR)
  • Acute alveolar hyperventilation superimposed on chronic ventilatory failure with moderate hypoxemia (ABG)
    • Possibly impending ventilatory failure
  • Thick and tenacious yellow sputum accumulation (sputum production)

P: Discuss with physician the possibility of impending ventilatory failure and need for mechanical ventilation. Obtain stat sputum Gram's stain, culture, and cytology. Continuous pulse oximetry. Oxygenate per oxygen therapy protocol. Med. nebs: mucolytic agent per protocol. Institute LLL postural drainage per bronchial hygiene protocol.

While intubation and assisted or controlled ventilation were seriously considered, it was decided to treat him conservatively, at least initially. He was started on massive antibiotic therapy and was monitored closely in the respiratory intensive care unit. He responded well to therapy. Within 48 hours, his Pa_{O_2} increased to 68 mm Hg, and his acute alveolar hyperventilation (superimposed on chronic ventilatory failure) returned to baseline values.

He was able to cough and clear secretions well. His cough and respiratory rate diminished. His chest radiograph revealed significant improvement in the right lower lung lobe pneumonia. Prior to discharge, a pulmonary function test showed a significant decrease in lung volumes and capacities. The discharge diagnosis was severe restrictive pulmonary disease secondary to kyphoscoliosis, complicated by acute pneumococcal pneumonia.

DISCUSSION

The respiratory care practitioner here is faced with a clinical situation in which two restrictive processes (kyphoscoliosis and complicating pneumonia) tend to be more than additive in their impact on the patient's oxygenation and acid-base homeostasis.

With the increasing popularity of negative pressure (curaiss) ventilation, pressure support, and PEP therapy, the respiratory care practitioner's options in this setting tend to increase. Appropriately, the respiratory care practitioner's first attention is directed, however, to bronchial hygiene and control of the patient's hypoxemia, followed closely by attention to the secretion problem. The therapist infers (in the assessment portion of the SOAP note) that subsequent blood gas data may suggest the need (or lack of it) for assisted ventilation.

SELF-ASSESSMENT QUESTIONS

Multiple Choice

1. What kind of curvature of the spine is manifested in kyphosis?
   - a. Posterior
   - b. Anterior
   - c. Lateral
   - d. Medial
   - e. Posterior and lateral

2. Kyphoscoliosis affects approximately what percentage of the U.S. population?
   - a. 2
   - b. 5
   - c. 10
   - d. 15
   - e. 20

3. Which of the following is/are associated with kyphoscoliosis?
   - I. Increased FRC
   - II. Decreased V_T
   - III. Increased TLC
   - IV. Decreased RV
     - a. I only
     - b. IV only
     - c. II and IV only
     - d. III and IV only
     - e. II, III, and IV only

4. Which of the following is/are associated with kyphoscoliosis?
   - I. Bronchial breath sounds
   - II. Hyperresonant percussion note
   - III. Whispered pectoriloquy
   - IV. Diminished breath sounds
     - a. I and III only
     - b. II and IV only
     - c. III and IV only
     - d. II, III, and IV only
     - e. I, II, and III only

5. During the advanced stages of kyphoscoliosis, the patient commonly demonstrates which of the following arterial blood gas values?
   - I. Increased HCO_3^-
   - II. Decreased pH
   - III. Increased Pa_{CO_2}
   - IV. Normal pH
   - V. Decreased HCO_3^-
     - a. I only
     - b. II only
     - c. III and IV only
     - d. II and V only
     - e. I, III, and IV only

True or False

1. When kyphoscoliosis arises without a known cause, it is called idiopathic kyphoscoliosis. True _____ False _____
2. Kyphoscoliosis is classified as an obstructive lung disorder. True _____ False _____
3. The precise cause of kyphoscoliosis is unknown in about 80% to 85% of cases. True _____ False _____
4. The anatomic alterations of the lungs associated with kyphoscoliosis cause a shuntlike effect. True _____ False _____
5. Kyphoscoliosis causes the patient's PEFR to increase. True _____ False _____

Answers appear in Appendix XXI.

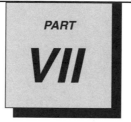
ENVIRONMENTAL
LUNG DISEASE

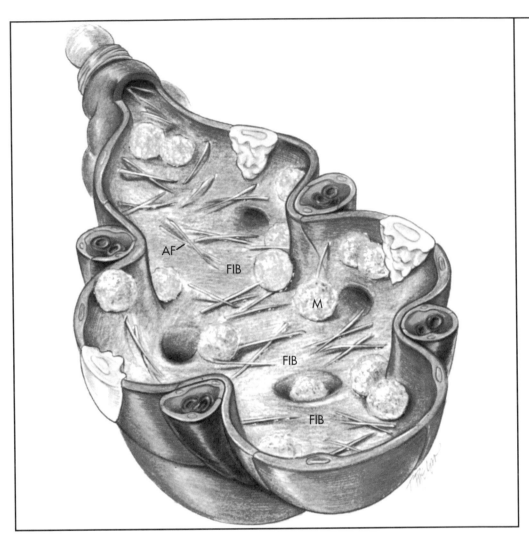

PNEUMOCONIOSIS

FIG 21-1

Asbestosis (close-up of one alveolar unit). *AF* = asbestos fiber; *FIB* = fibrosis; *M* = macrophage. (See also Plate 20.)

CHAPTER 21

Pneumoconiosis

ANATOMIC ALTERATIONS OF THE LUNGS

Pneumoconiosis is a general term used to describe diseases of the lungs that are caused by the chronic inhalation of inorganic dusts and particulate matter, usually of occupational or environmental origin (e.g., coal dust, asbestos, silica). When inorganic dusts or particulate matter are inhaled, the smaller particles stick to the moist surfaces of the respiratory bronchioles, alveolar ducts, and alveoli.

The initial lung response is inflammation and phagocytosis by alveolar macrophages. The macrophages engulf and carry the particles to the terminal bronchioles from where they are then propelled out of the lungs by the mucociliary escalator. Some particles are carried to the lymphatic vessels and then to the lymph nodes, primarily the nodes around the hilum. During excessive exposure, however, the mucociliary system becomes overwhelmed, which results in the accumulation of particles. When this happens, the dust particles become enmeshed in a network of collagen and fibrin, and the lungs stiffen (lung compliance decreases). Characteristic of pneumoconioses is the fact that the pulmonary fibrosis may continue despite the cessation of dust exposure.

Some dust particles (e.g., silica) have a toxic effect on the macrophages that ingest them. The macrophages disintegrate and release chemicals that activate successive waves of macrophages. When the newly recruited macrophages engulf the liberated dust particles, they in turn disintegrate. Some particles have the ability to penetrate the interstitial space (e.g., asbestos, coal dust, silica). As the disease progresses, the alveoli and adjacent pulmonary capillaries are destroyed and replaced by fibrous, cystlike structures. The cysts are commonly about 1.0 cm in diameter and produce a honeycomb appearance on gross examination. In severe cases, and particularly in asbestosis, fibrotic thickening and calcification of the pleura often produce fibrocalcific pleural plaques. This pathologic process frequently extends into—or involves—the diaphragm. Some environmental irritants may also be carcinogenic.

In general, the pneumoconioses produce a restrictive pulmonary disease. However, because the inorganic dusts and particular matter can also accumulate in the small airways, chronic inflammation, swelling, and bronchial obstruction frequently develop. When this condition is present, clinical manifestations of airway obstruction are seen. Thus, the patient with pneumoconiosis may demonstrate a restrictive disorder, an obstructive disorder, or a combination of both.

To summarize, the major pathologic or structural changes associated with the pneumoconioses are as follows:

- Destruction of the alveoli and adjacent pulmonary capillaries
- Fibrotic thickening of the respiratory bronchioles, alveolar ducts, and alveoli

- Cystlike structures (honeycomb appearance)
- Fibrocalcific pleural plaques
- Airway obstruction caused by inflammation and bronchial constriction
- Bronchogenic carcinoma

ETIOLOGY

The etiologic determinants include (1) the size of the dust particle (only those particles between 0.3 and 0.5 μm are likely to reach the alveoli), (2) its chemical nature, (3) its concentration, (4) the length of exposure, and (5) the individual's susceptibility to specific inorganic dusts or particulate matter. Clinically, the diagnosis of a specific cause of a pneumoconiosis may be difficult. In general, the diagnosis is based on the work history of the individual, x-ray films, and pulmonary function studies.

Some of the major causes of the pneumoconioses are covered in the subsequent sections.

Asbestosis

Exposure to asbestos causes asbestosis. Asbestos fibers are a mixture of fibrous minerals composed of hydrous silicates of magnesium, sodium, and iron in various proportions. There are two primary types: the *amphiboles* (crocidolite, amosite, and anthophyllite) and *chrysotile* (most commonly used in industry). Asbestos fibers typically range between 50 and 100 mm in length and are about 0.5 mm in diameter. The chyrsotiles are characterized by having the longest and strongest fibers.

Industrial areas and commercial products associated with asbestos fibers include the following:

- Acoustic products
- Automobile undercoating
- Brake lining
- Cements
- Clutch casing
- Floor tiles
- Fire-fighting suits
- Fireproof paints
- Insulation
- Mill work
- Roofing materials
- Ropes
- Ship construction
- Steam pipe material

Asbestos fibers can often be seen within the thickened septa as brown or orange baton-like structures. The fibers characteristically stain for iron with Perl's stain. Uniform involvement of the lungs is rare. The pathologic process may only affect one lung, a lobe, or a segment of a lobe. The lower lobes are most commonly affected (Fig 21-1).

Coal Worker's Pneumoconiosis

The deposition and accumulation of large amounts of coal dust causes what is known as coal worker's pneumoconiosis (CWP). CWP is also known as *coal miner's lung, black lung, black phthisis,* and *miner's phthisis.* Miners who use cutting machines at the coal face have the greatest exposure.

Simple CWP is characterized by pinpoint nodules throughout the lungs called *coal mac-*

ules (black spots). The coal macules often develop around the first- and second-generation respiratory bronchioles and cause the adjacent alveoli to retract. This condition is called *focal emphysema.*

Complicated CWP or progressive massive fibrosis (PMF) is characterized by massive areas of fibrotic nodules greater than 1 cm. The fibrotic nodules generally appear in the peripheral regions of upper lobes and extend toward the hilum with growth. The nodules are composed of dense collagenous tissue with black pigmentation. Finally, it should be noted that coal dust by itself is chemically inert. The fibrotic changes in CWP are usually due to silica.

Silicosis

Silicosis (also called grinder's disease and quartz silicosis) is caused by the chronic inhalation of crystalline, free silica or silicon dioxide particles. Silica is the main component of more than 95% of the rocks of the earth. It is found in sandstone, quartz (beach sand is mostly quartz), flint, granite, many hard rocks, and some clays.

Simple silicosis is characterized by small rounded nodules scattered throughout the lungs. No single nodule is greater than 9 mm. Patients with simple silicosis are usually symptom free.

Complicated silicosis is characterized by nodules that coalesce and form large masses of fibrous tissues, usually in the upper lobes and perihilar regions. In severe cases, the fibrotic regions may undergo tissue necrosis and cavitate.

Occupations that may expose an individual to silica include the following:

- Tunneling
- Hard-rock mining
- Sandblasting
- Quarrying
- Stonecutting
- Grinding of pottery materials
- Foundry work
- Ceramics work
- Abrasives work
- Brick making
- Paint making
- Polishing
- Stone drilling
- Well drilling

Berylliosis

Beryllium is a steel-gray, lightweight metal found in certain plastics and ceramics, rocket fuels, and x-ray tubes. As a raw ore, beryllium is not hazardous. When it is processed into the pure metal or one of its salts, however, it may cause a tissue reaction when inhaled or implanted into the skin. The acute inhalation of beryllium fumes or particles may cause a toxic or allergic pneumonitis sometimes accompanied by rhinitis, pharyngitis, and tracheo-bronchitis. The more complex form of berylliosis is characterized by the development of granulomas and a diffuse interstitial inflammatory reaction. Additional causes of pneumoconiosis include the following:

Aluminum

- Ammunition workers

Baritosis (barium)

- Barite millers and miners
- Ceramics workers

Kaolinosis (clay)

- Brick makers
- Ceramics workers
- Potters

Siderosis (iron)

- Welders

Talcosis (certain talcs)

- Ceramics workers
- Papermakers
- Plastics workers
- Rubber workers

OVERVIEW

OF THE CARDIOPULMONARY CLINICAL MANIFESTATIONS ASSOCIATED WITH
PNEUMOCONIOSES

❑ **INCREASED RESPIRATORY RATE**

Several pathophysiologic mechanisms operating simultaneously may lead to an increased ventilatory rate. These are (see page 17)

- Stimulation of peripheral chemoreceptors
- Decreased lung compliance/increased ventilatory rate relationship
- Stimulation of the J receptors
- Pain/anxiety

❑ **PULMONARY FUNCTION STUDY FINDINGS**

Expiratory Maneuver Findings (see page 41)

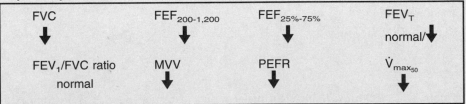

Lung Volume and Capacity Findings (see page 39)

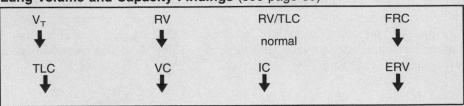

❑ **DECREASED DIFFUSION CAPACITY** (see page 48)

❑ **INCREASED HEART RATE (PULSE), CARDIAC OUTPUT, AND BLOOD PRESSURE** (see page 86)
❑ **ARTERIAL BLOOD GASES**

Moderate Pneumoconiosis

Acute Alveolar Hyperventilation with Hypoxemia (see page 57)

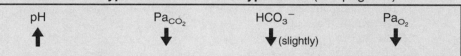

pH	Pa_{CO_2}	HCO_3^-	Pa_{O_2}
↑	↓	↓ (slightly)	↓

Severe Pneumoconiosis

Chronic Ventilatory Failure with Hypoxemia (see page 60)

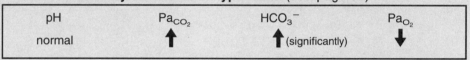

pH	Pa_{CO_2}	HCO_3^-	Pa_{O_2}
normal	↑	↑ (significantly)	↓

Acute Ventilatory Changes Superimposed on Chronic Ventilatory Failure (see page 65)

Because acute ventilatory changes are frequently seen in patients with chronic ventilatory failure, the respiratory care practitioner must be familiar with and on alert for (1) *acute alveolar hyperventilation superimposed on chronic ventilatory failure,* and (2) *acute ventilatory failure superimposed on chronic ventilatory failure.*

❑ **CYANOSIS** (see page 68)
❑ **OXYGENATION INDICES** (see page 69)

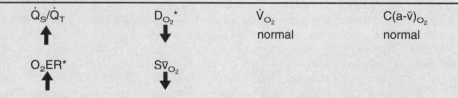

$\dot{Q}_S/\dot{Q}_T$	D_{O_2}*	$\dot{V}_{O_2}$	$C(a-\bar{v})_{O_2}$
↑	↓	normal	normal
O_2ER*	$S\bar{v}_{O_2}$		
↑	↓		

*The D_{O_2} may be normal in patients who have compensated for the decreased oxygenation status with an increased cardiac output, an increased hemoglobin level, or a combination of both. When the D_{O_2} is normal, the O_2ER is usually normal.

❑ **HEMODYNAMIC INDICES (SEVERE)** (see page 87)

CVP	RAP	$\overline{PA}$	PCWP
↑	↑	↑	normal
CO	SV	SVI	CI
normal	normal	normal	normal
RVSWI	LVSWI	PVR	SVR
↑	normal	↑	normal

❑ **POLYCYTHEMIA, COR PULMONALE** (see page 92)
  • Distended neck veins
  • Enlarged and tender liver
  • Peripheral edema
  • Pitting edema

❑ **DIGITAL CLUBBING** (see page 93)
❑ **COUGH AND SPUTUM PRODUCTION** (see page 93)
❑ **PLEURAL EFFUSION** (associated with abestosis) (see Chapter 19)
❑ **CHEST ASSESSMENT FINDINGS** (see page 6)
   • Increased tactile and vocal fremitus
   • Dull percussion note
   • Bronchial breath sounds
   • Crackles/rhonchi/wheezing
   • Pleural friction rub
   • Whispered pectoriloquy

❑ **RADIOLOGIC FINDINGS**
   Chest radiograph
   • Small rounded opacities scattered throughout the lung
   • Irregularly shaped opacities
   • Irregular cardiac and diaphragmatic borders
   • Pleural plaques
   • Honeycomb appearance

Because of the inflammation, tissue thickening, fibrosis, calcification, and pleural plaques, the density of the lungs progressively increases. This increased lung density resists x-ray penetration and is revealed on x-ray films as increased opacity (i.e., whiter in appearance).

Patients with simple silicosis often show small rounded opacities scattered throughout the lungs. In complicated silicosis, huge densities are often seen in the upper lung fields. The hilar region may be elevated, and the lower lobes may show emphysematous changes. Another characteristic feature in a small percentage of patients with silicosis is the appearance of eggshell-like calcifications around the hilar region.

In patients with coal worker's pneumoconiosis, the rounded opacities scattered throughout the lung are smaller and less well defined than are those seen in silicosis. In general, however, the radiographic appearance of silicosis and coal worker's pneumoconiosis is very similar. When large opacities are present (greater than 1 cm), complicated coal worker's pneumoconiosis is indicated. Cavity formation may also be revealed on chest x-ray films.

In patients with asbestosis, the opacity is frequently described as a clouding or "ground-glass" appearance and is particularly noticed in the lower lung lobes (Fig 21–2). When there are substantial calcifications and pleural plaques in the pleural space, irregularly shaped opacities are often seen. Calcified pleural plaques may also be seen on the superior border of the diaphragm (Fig 21–3). The inflammatory response elicited by the asbestos fibers may also produce a fuzziness and irregularity in the cardiac and diaphragmatic borders. Pleural effusion may be present in patients with asbestosis.

Finally, because several of the pneumoconioses are capable of causing cavity formation and cystlike structures, a honeycomb pattern may be seen.

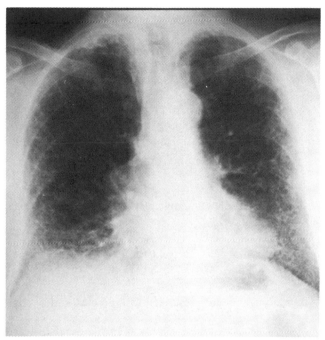

FIG. 21-2
Chest x-ray film of a patient with asbestosis.

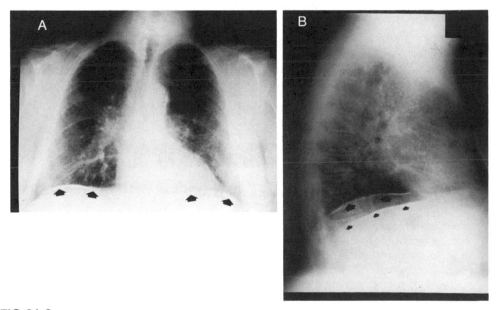

FIG 21-3
Calcified pleural plaques on the superior border of the diaphragm *(arrows)* in a patient with asbestosis. **A,** anteroposterior view. **B,** lateral view.

GENERAL MANAGEMENT OF PNEUMOCONIOSIS

Control and prevention of occupational diseases is the responsibility of the individual worker, management, the community health service, and the state and federal governments. As in all occupational diseases, prevention is the key. It involves education in protective measures, management's cooperation in supplying proper equipment and conditions, inspection and testing services provided by management and by the government, adequate medical and first-aid services at the work site, adequate hospitalization insurance and compensation, and research to provide better methods of safety.

Once the disease is established, there is no effective cure. Individuals who demonstrate suspicious clinical manifestations should be removed from any environment in which they are exposed to inorganic dusts and particulate matter. The long-term prognosis of workers who develop pneumoconiosis is poor. Treatment is directed toward symptoms of the disease.

Medications

Sympathomimetics.—Sympathomimetic drugs may be prescribed to offset bronchial smooth muscle constriction (see Appendix II).

Parasympatholytics.—Parasympatholytic agents are also used to offset bronchial smooth muscle constriction (see Appendix III).

Diuretic agents.—Diuretic agents are prescribed to promote fluid excretion (see Appendix X).

Supplemental Oxygen

Because of the hypoxemia associated with a pneumoconiosis disorder, supplemental oxygen may be required. It should be noted, however, that the hypoxemia that develops in pneumoconiosis is most commonly caused by the alveolar thickening, fibrosis, and capillary shunting associated with the disorder. Hypoxemia caused by capillary shunting is refractory to oxygen therapy.

In addition, when the patient demonstrates chronic ventilatory failure during the advanced states of a pneumoconiosis disorder, caution must be taken not to eliminate the patient's hypoxic drive to breathe.

●　　●　　●　　● **PNEUMOCONIOSIS CASE STUDY** ●　　●　　●　　●

ADMITTING HISTORY AND PHYSICAL EXAMINATION

A 60-year-old male with respiratory distress presented in the emergency department. He reported respiratory difficulties of several years' duration and was currently on total disability because of his pulmonary problems. He had worked on the mine face in a Kentucky coal mine for 35 years. About 15 years ago, he was told that he had "black lung" disease. At that time he quit smoking—a habit he had had for 30 years. He had a mild, nonproductive cough for many years.

On examination, there was severe digital clubbing, distended neck veins, and +2 pitting edema over his ankles. His respiratory rate was 33/min, heart rate 105 bpm, blood pressure 146/100. Breath sounds were "distant," and there were wheezes and rhonchi bilaterally. X-ray examination showed 1- to 3-mm rounded opacities scattered throughout all lung fields and a moderately enlarged right heart. Arterial blood gases on room air were pH 7.39, Pa_{CO_2} 68, HCO_3^- 34, and Pa_{O_2} 54. His bedside FVC was

50% of predicted. His SVC was 70% of predicted. At this time, the following respiratory assessment and plan was entered into the patient's chart:

RESPIRATORY ASSESSMENT AND PLAN

S: Complains of severe shortness of breath

O: Dyspneic. HR 105, BP 146/100, RR 33. Fingers clubbed, distended neck veins, and +3 pitting edema. Distant breath sounds with bilateral wheezes and rhonchi. No sputum production. CXR: 1- to 3-mm opacities throughout both lungs, and moderately enlarged right heart. Room air ABGs: pH 7.39, Pa_{CO_2} 68, HCO_3^- 34, Pa_{O_2} 54. FVC and SVC 50% of predicted.

A: • Chronic pneumoconiosis (history of silica exposure)
• Possible combined restrictive and obstructive lung disorder (FVC, SVC)
• Cor pulmonale (CXR, distended neck veins & pitting edema)
• Chronic ventilatory failure with moderate hypoxemia (ABG)
• Bronchospasm and large airway secretions (wheezes & rhonchi)

P: Continuous pulse oximetry. O_2 per oxygen protocol—per N.C. at 3 lpm. Bronchial hygiene protocol. Trial of bronchodilator therapy with albuterol 0.5 ml in 2.0 ml normal saline every 6 hours.

Over the next hour, the patient was started on a digitalis preparation, oxygen therapy, bronchial hygiene therapy, and bronchodilator therapy. The patient's Sa_{O_2} increased from 88% to 96%. He became increasingly somnolent. Breath sounds were unchanged. Purulent sputum was expectorated. His respiratory rate decreased to 10/min. A STAT ABG on 3 lpm showed pH 7.26, Pa_{CO_2} 92, HCO_3^- 36, and Pa_{O_2} 90. At this point, the respiratory care practitioner wrote the following note:

RESPIRATORY ASSESSMENT AND PLAN

S: Patient incoherent, rambling.

O: Semicomatose. RR 10/min. On 3 lpm: pH 7.26, Pa_{CO_2} 92, HCO_3^- 36, Pa_{O_2} 90, Sa_{O_2} 96%. Wheezes and rhonchi persist.

A: • Acute ventilatory failure on top of chronic ventilatory failure (secondary to hyperoxygenation) (history & ABG)
• Bronchospasm (wheezes)
• Large airway secretions (rhonchi)

P: Emergency intubation. Place on SIMV/PSV per mechanical ventilation protocol. Continuous pulse oximetry. Continue bronchodilator and bronchial hygiene therapy per protocol. Obtain sputum for Gram's stain and culture.

After several days of assisted ventilation, with the ventilator settings at a rate of 4 (IMV), with pressure support of 8 mm Hg, CPAP of +5 cm H_2O, and an $F_{I_{O_2}}$ of 0.30 the arterial blood gases were pH 7.23, Pa_{CO_2} 80, HCO_3^- 35, and Pa_{O_2} 62. His NIF was −10 cm H_2O. He was alert and oriented. His spontaneous respiratory rate off the ventilator was 34/min, average non-IMV V_T was 280 ml, heart rate 110 bpm. His lungs were clear to auscultation. X-ray showed a normal heart size and unchanged lung markings. He no longer had distended neck veins or pitting edema. At this time, this assessment and plan was written in the patient's chart:

RESPIRATORY ASSESSMENT AND PLAN

S: Patient cannot communicate verbally. Indicates he wants ET tube out.

O: Afebrile. Lungs clear. NIF, −10 cm H_2O. On IMV of 4/min, spontaneous V_T 280 ml. ABGs: pH 7.23, Pa_{CO_2} 80, HCO_3^- 35, Pa_{O_2} 62. CXR: enlarged right heart back to normal size, no acute infiltrate, otherwise unchanged.

A: Persistent acute ventilatory failure on chronic ventilatory failure when ventilator weaning attempted. Patient not ready to be extubated. (NIF & ABG)

P: Increase IMV to 12/min and let patient rest for the night. Continue pressure support ventilation. Suggest nutrition assessment. Reactivate ventilator weaning protocol tomorrow morning.

DISCUSSION

The care of uncomplicated pneumoconiosis is often only supportive (including oxygen therapy). When acute bronchitis, pneumonia, or other respiratory insults complicate the case, however, clearly more care is required.

This patient's initial history does not suggest an acute exacerbation. After the initiation of bronchial hygiene therapy (on the basis of wheezes and rhonchi), it became clear that the patient had an infectious exacerbation of his underlying restrictive pulmonary disease process. By then, he was slipping into worsening respiratory failure and intubation was required. Once an airway had been established, and good bronchial hygiene begun, he improved rapidly, although his weaning process was prolonged.

After approximately two weeks, the patient was successfully extubated. He was discharged after four weeks of hospitalization on supplemental oxygen therapy. Pneumococcal vaccine and flu prophylaxis were given. He was urged to promptly report any infectious symptoms to his physician.

SELF-ASSESSMENT QUESTIONS

Multiple Choice

1. The length of asbestos fibers commonly ranges between
    - a. 5 and 10 mm.
    - b. 10 and 20 mm.
    - c. 15 and 25 mm.
    - d. 25 and 50 mm.
    - e. 50 and 100 mm.

2. Which of the following expiratory maneuver findings is/are associated with the pneumoconioses?
    - I. Increased MVV
    - II. Decreased FEV_T
    - III. Increased PEFR
    - IV. Decreased FVC
    - a. II only
    - b. III only
    - c. I and III only
    - d. II and IV only
    - e. I, III, and IV only

3. Which of the following oxgenation indices is/are associated with the pneumoconioses?
    - I. Decreased $C(a-\bar{v})_{O_2}$
    - II. Increased O_2ER
    - III. Decreased $S\bar{v}_{O_2}$
    - IV. Increased $\dot{V}_{O_2}$
    - a. I only
    - b. III only
    - c. II and III only
    - d. I and IV only
    - e. II, III, and IV only

4. The fibrotic changes that develop in coal worker's pneumoconiosis are usually due to
    - a. Barium.
    - b. Silica.
    - c. Iron.
    - d. Coal dust.
    - e. Clay.

5. Which of the following is/are associated with the pneumoconioses?
    - I. Pleural friction rub
    - II. Dull percussion note
    - III. Cor pulmonale
    - IV. Elevated $\overline{PA}$
    - a. I and II only
    - b. II and IV only
    - c. III and IV only
    - d. II, II, and IV only
    - e. I, II, III, and IV

Fill in the Blanks

The five major etiologic determinants of the pneumoconioses are the following:

1. _____
2. _____
3. _____
4. _____
5. _____

Answers appear in Appendix XXI.

PART

VIII

NEOPLASTIC DISEASE

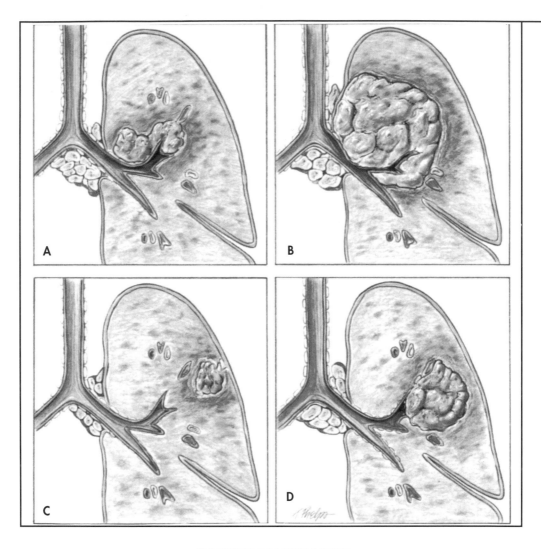

CANCER OF THE LUNG

FIG 22-1

A, squamous (epidermoid) cell carcinoma. **B,** small-cell (oat cell) carcinoma. **C,** adenocarcinoma. **D,** large-cell carcinoma. (See also Plate 21.)

CHAPTER 22

Cancer of the Lung

ANATOMIC ALTERATIONS OF THE LUNGS

Cancer is a general term that refers to abnormal new tissue growth characterized by the progressive, uncontrolled multiplication of cells. Clinically, this abnormal growth of new cells is called a *neoplasm* or *tumor*. A tumor may be localized or invasive, benign or malignant.

Benign tumors do not endanger life unless they interfere with the normal functions of other organs or affect a vital organ. They grow slowly, push aside normal tissue, but do not invade it. They are usually encapsulated, well-demarcated growths. They are not invasive or metastatic, i.e., tumor cells do not travel via the bloodstream and invade or form secondary tumors in other organs.

Malignant tumors are composed of embryonic, primitive, or poorly differentiated cells. They grow in a disorganized manner and so rapidly that nutrition of the cells becomes a problem. For this reason, necrosis, ulceration, and cavity formation are commonly associated with malignant tumors. They also invade surrounding tissues and are metastatic.

Although malignant changes may develop in any portion of the lung, they most commonly originate in the mucosa of the tracheobronchial tree. A tumor that originates in the bronchial mucosa is called *bronchogenic carcinoma*. The terms *lung cancer* and *bronchogenic carcinoma* are used interchangeably.

As a tumor enlarges, the surrounding bronchial airways and alveoli become irritated, inflamed, and swollen. The adjacent alveoli may fill with fluid and become consolidated or collapse. In addition, as the tumor protrudes into the tracheobronchial tree, excessive mucus production and airway obstruction develop. As the surrounding blood vessels erode, blood enters the tracheobronchial tree. Peripheral tumors may also invade the pleural space and impinge on the mediastinum, chest wall, ribs, or diaphragm. A secondary pleural effusion is often seen in lung cancer. A pleural effusion further compresses the lung and causes atelectasis.

To summarize, the major pathologic or structural changes associated with bronchogenic carcinoma are as follows:

- Inflammation, swelling, and destruction of the bronchial airways and alveoli
- Excessive mucus production
- Tracheobronchial mucus accumulation and plugging
- Airway obstruction (either from mucus accumulation or from a tumor projecting into a bronchus)
- Atelectasis
- Alveolar consolidation

- Cavity formation
- Pleural effusion (when a tumor invades the parietal pleura and mediastinum)

ETIOLOGY

There are four major types of bronchogenic tumors: (1) squamous (epidermoid) cell carcinoma, (2) small-cell (oat-cell) carcinoma, (3) adenocarcinoma, and (4) large-cell carcinoma.

Squamous (Epidermoid) Cell Carcinoma

This is the most common form of bronchogenic carcinoma (about 30% to 50% of the cases). The tumor originates from the basal cells of the bronchial epithelium and grows through the epithelium before invading the surrounding tissues. The tumor has a late metastatic tendency and a doubling time of about 100 days. It is commonly located in the large bronchi near the hilar region. Squamous cell tumors may be seen to project into the bronchi during bronchoscopy. In about one third of the cases, squamous cell carcinoma originates in the periphery. Cavity formation with or without an air-fluid interface is seen in 10% to 20% of the cases (Fig 22-1, *A*).

Small-Cell (Oat-Cell) Carcinoma

This form of bronchogenic carcinoma arises from the Kulchitsky's (or K-type) cells in the bronchial epithelium and is commonly found near the hilar region. The tumor grows very rapidly, metastasizes early, and has a doubling time of about 30 days. Because the tumor cells are often compressed into an oval shape, this form of cancer is commonly referred to as oat-cell carcinoma. Small-cell carcinoma accounts for about 20% to 25% of bronchogenic cancer (Fig 22-1, *B*).

Adenocarcinoma

This type of bronchogenic carcinoma arises from the mucus glands of the tracheobronchial tree. In fact, the glandular configuration and the mucus production caused by this type of cancer are the pathologic features that distinguish adenocarcinoma from the other types of bronchogenic carcinoma. The growth rate and metastatic tendency of adenocarcinoma is moderate. The tumor has a doubling time of about 180 days. Adenocarcinoma is most commonly found in the peripheral portions of the lung parenchyma. Cavity formation is common, although less so than with squamous or large-cell carcinoma. Adenocarcinoma accounts for about 15% to 35% of bronchogenic carcinoma cases (Fig 22-1, *C*).

Large-Cell Carcinoma

Large-cell carcinoma may be found in either the peripheral or central regions of the lungs. Its growth rate is rapid, with an early metastatic tendency, and the tumor has a doubling time of about 100 days. Cavity formation is common. Large-cell carcinoma is seen in about 15% to 35% of bronchogenic carcinoma cases (Fig 22-1, *D*).

Bronchogenic carcinoma represents 90% to 95% percent of all the lung cancer types. In the United States, lung cancer is a leading cause of death among men, and it is steadily increasing in women. In fact, during the mid-1980s, the incidence of lung cancer surpassed breast cancer in women. Presently, lung cancer strikes about 130,000 persons every year. It is most commonly seen in persons between 40 and 70 years of age.

Over the past 50 years, a massive amount of evidence strongly correlates cigarette smoking with lung cancer. It is estimated that about 85% of lung cancer cases are due to cigarette smoking. Studies have shown that the risk of developing lung cancer increases directly with the number of cigarettes smoked per day. Squamous and small-cell carcinoma are strongly associated with cigarette smoking. The average male smoker is ten times more likely to develop lung cancer than is a nonsmoker. Various industrial hazards can also cause lung cancer. For example, exposure to asbestos has been recognized for years as a cause of lung cancer.

OVERVIEW
OF THE CARDIOPULMONARY CLINICAL MANIFESTATIONS ASSOCIATED WITH
CANCER OF THE LUNG

❏ **INCREASED RESPIRATORY RATE**

Several pathophysiologic mechanisms operating simultaneously may lead to an increased ventilatory rate. These are (see page 17)
* Stimulation of peripheral chemoreceptors
* Decreased lung compliance/increased ventilatory rate relationship
* Stimulation of the J receptors
* Pain/anxiety

❏ **PULMONARY FUNCTION STUDY FINDINGS**
Expiratory Maneuver Findings (When Tumor Obstructs the Airway)
(see page 39)

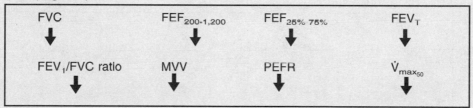

Lung Volume and Capacity Findings (see page 39)

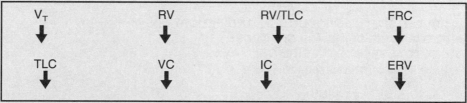

❏ **INCREASED HEART RATE (PULSE), CARDIAC OUTPUT, AND BLOOD PRESSURE** (see page 86)

❏ **ARTERIAL BLOOD GASES**

Localized (e.g., Lobar) Lung Cancer

Acute Alveolar Hyperventilation with Hypoxemia (see page 57)

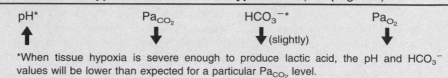

*When tissue hypoxia is severe enough to produce lactic acid, the pH and HCO_3^- values will be lower than expected for a particular Pa_{CO_2} level.

Acute Ventilatory Failure with Hypoxemia (see page 59)

pH^* ↓ Pa_{CO_2} ↑ HCO_3^{-*} ↑ (slightly) Pa_{O_2} ↓

*When tissue hypoxia is severe enough to produce lactic acid, the pH and HCO_3^- values will be lower than expected for a particular Pa_{CO_2} level.

☐ **CYANOSIS** (see page 68)
☐ **OXYGENATION INDICES** (see page 69)

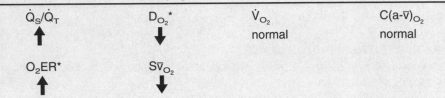

$\dot{Q}_S/\dot{Q}_T$ ↑ $D_{O_2}^*$ ↓ $\dot{V}_{O_2}$ normal $C(a-\bar{v})_{O_2}$ normal

O_2ER^* ↑ $S\bar{v}_{O_2}$ ↓

*The D_{O_2} may be normal in patients who have compensated for the decreased oxygenation status with an increased cardiac output. When the D_{O_2} is normal, the O_2ER is usually normal.

☐ **HEMODYNAMIC INDICES (WHEN HYPOXEMIA AND ACIDEMIA ARE PRESENT, OR WHEN A TUMOR INVADES THE MEDIASTINUM AND COMPRESSES THE SUPERIOR VENA CAVA)** (see page 87)

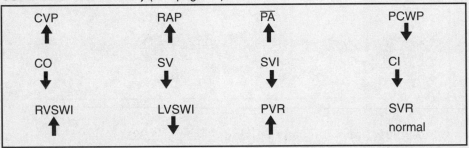

CVP ↑   RAP ↑ $\overline{PA}$ ↑   PCWP ↓

CO ↓   SV ↓   SVI ↓   CI ↓

RVSWI ↑   LVSWI ↓   PVR ↑   SVR normal

☐ **COUGH, SPUTUM PRODUCTION, AND HEMOPTYSIS** (see page 93)
☐ **PLEURAL EFFUSION** (see Chapter 19)
☐ **CHEST ASSESSMENT FINDINGS** (see page 6)
   • Crackles/rhonchi/wheezing

☐ **RADIOLOGIC FINDINGS**
Chest radiograph
   • Small oval or coin lesion
   • Large irregular mass
   • Alveolar consolidation
   • Atelectasis
   • Pleural effusion
   • Involvement of the mediastinum or the diaphragm

A routine chest x-ray often provides the first indication or suspicion of lung cancer. Depending on how long the tumor has been growing, the chest x-ray may show a small white nodule (called a coin lesion) or a large irregular white mass. Unfortunately, by the time a tumor is identified radiographically, regardless of its size, it is usually in the invasive stage and thus difficult to treat. The most common x-ray presentation of lung cancer is that of volume loss involving a single lobe or an individual segment within a lobe.

Because there are four major forms of lung cancer, chest x-ray film findings are variable. In general, squamous and small-cell carcinomas usually appear as a white mass near the hilar region, adenocarcinoma appears in the peripheral portions of the lung, and large-cell carcinoma may appear in either the peripheral or central portion of the lung. Figure 22-2 is a representative example of a bronchogenic carcinoma in the right upper lobe and a coin lesion in the left lung field. Common secondary chest x-ray findings caused by bronchial obstruction include alveolar consolidation, atelectasis, pleural effusion, and mediastinal or diaphragm involvement. The x-ray appearance of cavity formation within a bronchogenic carcinoma is similar regardless of the type of cancer.

❑ **BRONCHOSCOPY FINDINGS** (see page 105)
  * Bronchial tumor or mass lesion

The fiberoptic bronchoscope is commonly used for direct visualization of a bronchial tumor for further inspection and assessment of the extent of the disease (Fig. 22-3).

❑ **COMMON NONRESPIRATORY CLINICAL MANIFESTATIONS**
  * Hoarseness
  * Difficulty in swallowing
  * Superior vena cava syndrome
  * Weakness
  * Electrolyte abnormalities

When a bronchogenic tumor invades the mediastinum, it may involve the left recurrent laryngeal nerve, the esophagus, or the superior vena cava. When the tumor involves the left recurrent laryngeal nerve, the patient's voice becomes hoarse. When the tumor compresses the esophagus, swallowing may become difficult. When a tumor invades the mediastinum and compresses the superior vena cava, blood flow to the heart from the head and upper part of the body may be interrupted. When obstruction occurs, the symptoms include an increased ventilatory rate and cough, which is greatly aggravated by recumbency. Clinically, this condition is called *superior vena cava syndrome*.

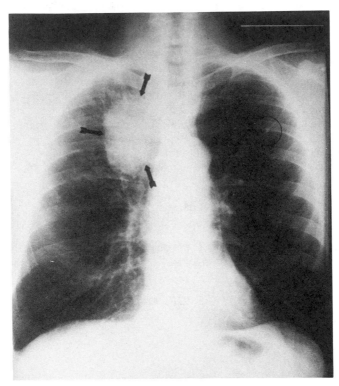

FIG 22-2
Posteroanterior chest radiograph showing a large mass in the right upper lobe *(arrows)*. Note the nodular density in the left lung field *(circle)*. (From Rau JL Jr, Pearce DJ: *Understanding chest radiographs.* Denver, Multi-Media Publishing Inc, 1984. Used by permission.)

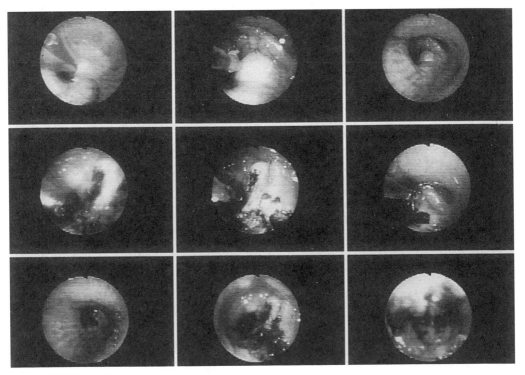

FIG 22-3
Bronchoscopic views of obstructed airways.

GENERAL MANAGEMENT OF CANCER OF THE LUNG

The treatment of lung cancer falls into three major categories: curative, palliative, and adjunctive. The most commonly used treatment modalities for lung cancer are surgery, radiation, and chemotherapy. Recently, immunotherapy and interferon therapy have also been incorporated in the treatment of cancer on an experimental basis.

Surgery

Surgery is used in the diagnosis of the disease, in removal of the tumor, and for the relief of symptoms (palliative) when a cure is not possible. Small tumors can often be completely removed. When the tumor is large or involves vital organs, surgical removal may not be possible.

Radiation Therapy

Radiation therapy is used in about 50% of the cancer cases, either alone or in combination with other forms of treatment. Radiation therapy involves the use of sophisticated equipment that generates high-voltage x-ray and electronic beams that deliver radiation to the tumor without causing lethal damage to the surrounding tissues. Radioactive particles kill tumor cells by causing chemical bonds to break, by disrupting DNA, and by interfering with cellular mitosis.

Chemotherapy

Chemotherapy has evolved as a major treatment for cancer. Drugs may be used as the only treatment modality or in combination with other treatments. Drugs used for chemotherapy act at the cellular level in several ways, including disrupting enzyme production; inhibiting DNA, RNA, and protein synthesis; and interfering with cell mitosis.

Immunotherapy and Interferon

At present, immunotherapy and interferon are used only experimentally in combination with other forms of treatment.

Respiratory Care

Mobilization of bronchial secretions.—Because of the excessive mucus production and accumulation associated with lung cancer, a number of respiratory therapy modalities may be used to enhance the mobilization of bronchial secretions (see Appendix XI).

Hyperinflation techniques.—Hyperinflation techniques may be ordered to (at least temporarily) offset the alveolar compression and consolidation associated with lung cancer (see Appendix XII).

Supplemental oxygen.—Because of the hypoxemia associated with lung cancer, supplemental oxygen may be required. It should be noted, however, that because of the alveolar compression and consolidation produced by lung cancer, capillary shunting may be present. Hypoxemia caused by capillary shunting is refractory to oxygen therapy.

• • •   **BRONCHOGENIC CARCINOMA CASE STUDY**   • • •

ADMITTING HISTORY AND PHYSICAL EXAMINATION

This 52-year-old male factory worker was apparently in good health until about two months prior to admission, when he developed a cough productive of moderate amounts of yellowish sputum. The cough was most severe in the morning, but persisted throughout the day. He also complained of general malaise and reported a recent weight loss of five pounds. He had no night sweats and was afebrile.

He was seen by his private physician and was treated with antibiotics. No x-rays were taken, but the physical exam was described as being within normal limits. On a follow-up telephone call one week later, the patient reported some improvement. Over the next two weeks, the patient developed moderate shortness of breath and marked hoarseness. There was no history of exposure to industrial irritants, but the patient admitted to a moderately heavy intake of alcohol and had a smoking history of 50 pack-years. As his symptoms persisted, he presented to the chest clinic for evaluation.

On physical examination, he was a well-developed, mildly obese middle-aged male who appeared slightly older than his stated age. He was in obvious but not severe respiratory distress. His vital signs were heart rate 125/min, blood pressure 155/95, and respiratory rate 28/min. It was believed by one examiner that there was cyanosis of the lips, fingers, and toenails, although this was questioned by another health care practitioner. The patient's voice was distinctly husky. The trachea was slightly deviated to the left side, and indirect laryngoscopy revealed paralysis of the left vocal cord.

The left lung fields were dull to percussion, and there were markedly diminished breath sounds on this side. A chest x-ray showed a large mass greater than 2 cm in diameter at the left hilum, and loss of lung volume on the left. The physician asked the respiratory therapist to document this information as he prepared the patient for bronchoscopy and biopsy. He also indicated that he planned to obtain secretions for cytology and routine cultures during the bronchoscopy. The following was documented in the patient's chart:

RESPIRATORY ASSESSMENT AND PLAN

S: Cough, hoarseness, moderate shortness of breath.

O: Cyanotic (?), hoarse voice; trachea deviated to the left. HR 125, BP 155/95, RR 28. Laryngoscopy: paralyzed left vocal cord. Decreased breath sounds on left. CXR: large (> 2.0 cm) left hilar mass, mild loss of volume on the left.

A: Probable bronchogenic carcinoma with atelectasis (deviated trachea and CXR).

P: Obtain ABG. Respiratory therapist to remain on standby to assist the physician with the bronchoscopy/biopsy of left lung lesion. Reassess when arterial blood gas results are received from the lab.

DISCUSSION

The role of the respiratory care practitioner in the outpatient care of patients with carcinoma of the lung is often exactly the same as illustrated here—assistance at a diagnostic procedure.

The notes that the practitioner has made in this case are entirely appropriate. Note that in the press of the outpatient situation, the physician may be working at the same pace as the respiratory care practitioner in the assessment and treatment of the patient.

The therapist's role here is that of an active participant in preparing the patient for bronchoscopy, assisting the physician during the procedure, making sure that the obtained specimens are appropriately labeled and handled, and monitoring the patient at the close of the procedure.

SELF-ASSESSMENT QUESTIONS

Multiple Choice
1. Which of the following is the most common form of bronchogenic carcinoma?
    a. Squamous cell carcinoma
    b. Oat-cell carcinoma
    c. Large-cell carcinoma
    d. Adenocarcinoma
    e. Small-cell carcinoma.
2. Which of the following arises from the mucus glands of the tracheobronchial tree?
    a. Small-cell carcinoma
    b. Adenocarcinoma
    c. Squamous cell carcinoma
    d. Oat-cell carcinoma
    e. Large-cell carcinoma
3. Which of the following is/are strongly associated with cigarette smoking?
    I. Adenocarcinoma
    II. Small-cell carcinoma
    III. Large-cell carcinoma
    IV. Squamous cell carcinoma
    a. I only
    b. III only
    c. II and IV only
    d. I and III only
    e. II, III, and IV only
4. Which of the following has the fastest growth rate?
    a. Large-cell carcinoma
    b. Small-cell carcinoma
    c. Adenocarcinoma
    d. Squamous cell carcinoma
    e. Epidermoid carcinoma
5. Which of the following is associated with bronchogenic carcinoma?
    I. Alveolar consolidation
    II. Pleural effusion
    III. Alveolar hyperinflation
    IV. Atelectasis
    a. III only
    b. II and III only
    c. I and IV only
    d. II and III only
    e. I, II, and IV only

True or False
1. Necrosis, ulceration, and cavitation are commonly associated with malignant tumors. True _____ False _____
2. It is estimated that about 85% of lung cancer cases are due to cigarette smoking. True _____ False _____
3. Small-cell carcinoma arises from the Kulchitsky's cells in the bronchial epithelium True _____ False _____
4. Benign tumors are metastatic. True _____ False _____
5. Adenocarcinoma is most commonly found in the peripheral portion of the lung parenchyma. True _____ False _____

Answers appear in Appendix XXI.

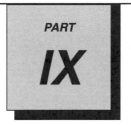

PART

IX

DIFFUSE ALVEOLAR DISEASES

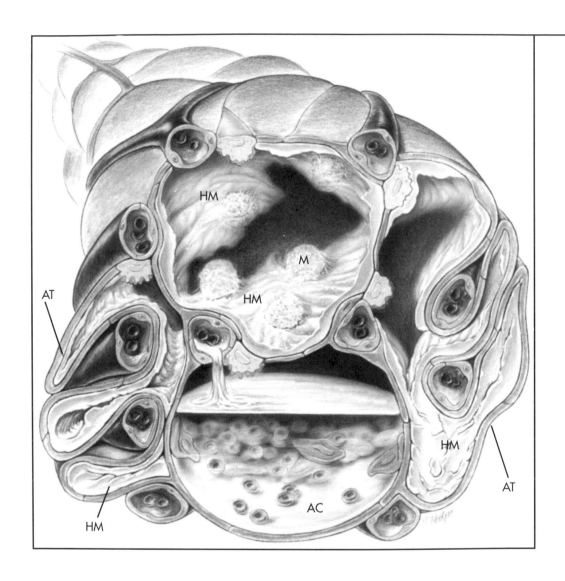

ADULT RESPIRATORY DISTRESS SYNDROME

FIG 23-1

Cross-sectional view of alveoli in adult respiratory distress syndrome. *HM* = hyaline membrane; *AT* = atelectasis; *AC* = alveolar consolidation; *M* = macrophage. (See also Plate 22.)

Adult Respiratory
Distress Syndrome

ANATOMIC ALTERATIONS OF THE LUNGS

The lungs of patients affected by adult respiratory distress syndrome (ARDS) undergo similar anatomic changes, regardless of the etiology of the disease. In response to injury, the pulmonary capillaries become engorged, and the permeability of the alveolar-capillary membrane increases. Interstitial and intra-alveolar edema and hemorrhage ensue, as well as scattered areas of hemorrhagic alveolar consolidation. These processes result in a decrease in alveolar surfactant and in alveolar collapse, or atelectasis.

As the disease progresses, the intra-alveolar walls become lined with a thick, rippled hyaline membrane identical to the hyaline membrane seen in newborns with infant respiratory distress syndrome (hyaline membrane disease). The membrane contains fibrin and cellular debris. In prolonged cases there is hyperplasia and swelling of the type II cells. Fibrin and exudate develop and lead to intra-alveolar fibrosis.

In gross appearance, the lungs of ARDS victims are heavy and "red," "beefy," or "liver-like" in appearance. The anatomic alterations that develop in ARDS create a restrictive lung disorder (Fig 23-1).

To summarize, the major pathologic or structural changes associated with ARDS are as follows:

- Interstitial and intra-alveolar edema and hemorrhage
- Alveolar consolidation
- Intra-alveolar hyaline membrane
- Pulmonary surfactant deficiency or abnormality
- Atelectasis

Historically, ARDS was referred to as "shock lung syndrome" when the disease was first identified in combat casualties during World War II. Since that time, the disease has appeared in the medical literature under many different names, all based on the etiology believed to be responsible for the disease. In 1967, the disease was first described as a specific entity, and the term *adult respiratory distress syndrome* was suggested. This term is predominantly used today. In alphabetical order, some of the names that have appeared in the medical journals to identify ARDS are as follows:

- Acute alveolar failure
- Adult hyaline membrane disease
- Capillary leak syndrome

- Congestion atelectasis
- Da Nang lung (because of the high incidence of ARDS associated with casualties in the Viet Nam War)
- Hemorrhagic pulmonary edema
- Noncardiac pulmonary edema
- Oxygen pneumonitis
- Oxygen toxicity
- Postnontraumatic pulmonary insufficiency
- Postperfusion lung
- Postpump lung
- Posttraumatic pulmonary insufficiency
- Shock lung syndrome
- Stiff lung syndrome
- Wet lung
- White lung syndrome

ETIOLOGY

There appears to be a multitude of etiologic factors that may produce ARDS. In alphabetical order, some of the better-known causes follow:

- Aspiration (e.g., of gastric contents or of water in near-drowning episodes)
- Central nervous system (CNS) disease (particularly when complicated by increased intracranial pressure)
- Cardiopulmonary bypass (especially when the bypass is prolonged)
- Congestive heart failure (leads to increased alveolar fluid leakage)
- Disseminated intravascular coagulation (seen in patients with shock and is a paradox of simultaneous clotting and bleeding, which produces microthrombi in the lungs)
- Drug overdose (e.g., heroin, barbiturates, morphine, methadone)
- Fat or air emboli (the fat emboli act as a source of harmful vasoactive material such as fatty acids and serotonin)
- Fluid overload (promotes alveolar fluid leakage)
- Infections (bacterial, viral, fungal, parasitic, mycoplasmal)
- Inhalation of toxins and irritants (e.g., chlorine gas, nitrogen dioxide, smoke, ozone; oxygen may also be included in this section)
- Immunologic reaction (e.g., allergic alveolar reaction to inhaled material or Goodpasture's syndrome)
- Massive blood transfusion (in stored blood, the quantity of aggregated white blood cells [WBCs], red blood cells [RBCs], platelets, and fibrin increases; these blood components in turn may occlude or damage small blood vessels)
- Nonthoracic trauma
- Oxygen toxicity (e.g., when patients are treated with an excessive oxygen concentration—usually over 60%—for a prolonged period of time)
- Pulmonary ischemia (due to shock and hypoperfusion; may cause tissue necrosis, vascular damage, and capillary leak)
- Radiation-induced lung injury
- Shock (e.g., hypovolemia)
- Systemic reactions to processes initiated outside the lungs (e.g., reactions caused by hemorrhagic pancreatitis, burns, complicated abdominal surgery, septicemia)
- Thoracic trauma (i.e., direct contusion to the lungs)
- Uremia

OVERVIEW

OF THE CARDIOPULMONARY CLINICAL MANIFESTATIONS ASSOCIATED WITH
ADULT RESPIRATORY DISTRESS SYNDROME

❑ **INCREASED RESPIRATORY RATE**

Several pathophysiologic mechanisms operating simultaneously may lead to an increased ventilatory rate. These are (see page 17)
- Stimulation of peripheral chemoreceptors
- Decreased lung compliance/increased ventilatory rate relationship
- Stimulation of the J receptors
- Anxiety

❑ **PULMONARY FUNCTION STUDY FINDINGS**

Lung Volume and Capacity Findings (see page 39)

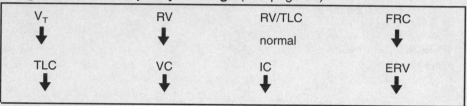

V_T	RV	RV/TLC	FRC
↓	↓	normal	↓
TLC	VC	IC	ERV
↓	↓	↓	↓

❑ **INCREASED HEART RATE (PULSE), CARDIAC OUTPUT, AND BLOOD PRESSURE** (see page 86)
❑ **ARTERIAL BLOOD GASES**

Early Stage ARDS

Acute Alveolar Hyperventilation with Hypoxemia (see page 57)

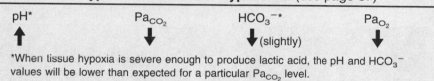

| pH* | Pa_{CO_2} | HCO_3^-* | Pa_{O_2} |
| ↑ | ↓ | ↓ (slightly) | ↓ |

*When tissue hypoxia is severe enough to produce lactic acid, the pH and HCO_3^- values will be lower than expected for a particular Pa_{CO_2} level.

End-Stage ARDS

Acute Ventilatory Failure with Hypoxemia (see page 59)

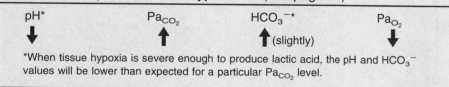

| pH* | Pa_{CO_2} | HCO_3^-* | Pa_{O_2} |
| ↓ | ↑ | ↑ (slightly) | ↓ |

*When tissue hypoxia is severe enough to produce lactic acid, the pH and HCO_3^- values will be lower than expected for a particular Pa_{CO_2} level.

❑ **CYANOSIS** (see page 68)
❑ **OXYGENATION INDICES** (see page 69)

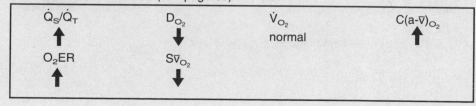

$\dot{Q}_S/\dot{Q}_T$	D_{O_2}	$\dot{V}_{O_2}$	$C(a-\bar{v})_{O_2}$
↑	↓	normal	↑
O_2ER	$S\bar{v}_{O_2}$		
↑	↓		

❏ **HEMODYNAMIC INDICES (END-STAGE ARDS)** (See page 87)

CVP ↑	RAP ↑	PA̅ ↑	PCWP normal
CO normal	SV normal	SVI normal	CI normal
RVSWI ↑	LVSWI normal	PVR ↑	SVR normal

❏ **SUBSTERNAL/INTERCOSTAL RETRACTION** (see page 98)
❏ **CHEST ASSESSMENT FINDINGS** (see page 6)
* Dull percussion note
* Bronchial breath sounds
* Crackles

❏ **RADIOLOGIC FINDINGS**
Chest radiograph
* Increased opacity

The structural changes that develop in ARDS increase the radiodensity of the lungs. The increased lung density resists x-ray penetration and is revealed on the radiograph as increased opacity (i.e., whiter in appearance). Thus, the more severe the ARDS, the denser the lungs become, and the whiter the radiograph (Fig 23-2).

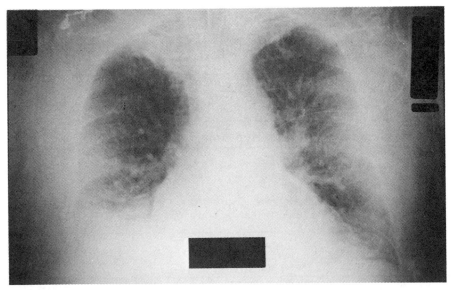

FIG 23-2
Chest x-ray of patient with moderately severe ARDS.

GENERAL MANAGEMENT OF ARDS
Hyperinflation Techniques

Hyperinflation measures are commonly ordered to offset the alveolar consolidation and atelectasis associated with ARDS (see Appendix XII).

Medications

Diuretic agents.—Diuretic agents are frequently ordered for patients with ARDS to attempt to reduce interstitial edema (see Appendix X).

Corticosteroids.—Although the exact mode of action of corticosteroids is not known, they have been shown to be somewhat effective in treating patients with ARDS. The corticosteroids are used to suppress inflammation and edema (see Appendix V).

Antibiotic agents.—Antibiotics are frequently administered in an effort to prevent or treat secondary bacterial infection (see Appendix VIII).

Supplemental Oxygen

Because of the hypoxemia associated with ARDS, supplemental oxygen is always required. It should be noted, however, that the hypoxemia that develops in ARDS is most commonly caused by the alveolar consolidation, atelectasis, and capillary shunting associated with the disorder. Hypoxemia caused by capillary shunting is refractory to oxygen therapy.

• • • • • • **ARDS CASE STUDY** • • • • • •

ADMITTING HISTORY AND PHYSICAL EXAMINATION

This comatose 47-year-old female was admitted to the emergency room of a small community hospital. She had been found by her husband, lying in bed with an empty bottle of "sleeping pills" on the bedside table and a "good-bye note" on the desk blaming her husband's infidelity for her suicide attempt.

In the emergency department she was found to be in moderately deep coma, responding to deep painful stimulation but otherwise nonresponsive. She was of average size and, according to the husband, had previously been in good health. She did not smoke or drink and was taking no other medication. Her blood pressure and pulse were within normal limits, but her respirations were shallow and noisy.

The emergency room physician decided to lavage her stomach. During the introduction of the nasogastric tube, the patient vomited and aspirated liquid gastric contents. At this time it was decided to transfer her by ambulance to a tertiary care medical center about 30 miles away. The pH of the gastric contents was not determined.

On arrival at the medical center the patient was still comatose, but responded to mild painful stimulation. Her weight was 60 kg. Her blood pressure was 100/60, pulse 114 bpm, and respirations were 28/min. On auscultation, there were scattered crackles on the right. A chest x-ray showed bilateral moderate fluffy infiltrates, mostly on the right side. Blood gases on room air were pH 7.51, Pa_{CO_2} 29, HCO_3^- 22, and Pa_{O_2} 52. At this time, the respiratory assessor recorded this SOAP note:

RESPIRATORY ASSESSMENT AND PLAN

S: N/A.

O: Patient is comatose. BP 100/60; P 114; RR 28; bilateral crackles; CXR: bilateral infiltrates, worse on right side; ABG on room air: pH 7.51, Pa_{CO_2} 29, HCO_3^- 22, Pa_{O_2} 52.

A: • Sedative drug overdose with coma (history)
   • Acute alveolar hyperventilation with moderate hypoxemia (ABG)
     • Possibly impending failure
   • Aspiration pneumonitis without prior history of pulmonary disease (history & x-ray)

P: Confer with physician. Plan intubation and ventilatory support according to protocol. Arterial line placement. Continuous oximetry. Repeat ABG one hour following intubation, or prn.

She was admitted to the intensive care unit, intubated and mechanically ventilated with these settings: V_T 750 ml, IMV 12 bpm, F_{IO_2} .4, and +10 cm H_2O of PEEP. An arterial line was placed in her left radial artery, and an intravenous infusion was started with lactated Ringer's solution. An hour later, blood gases were pH 7.43, Pa_{CO_2} 36, HCO_3^- 23, and Pa_{O_2} 40.

Over the next 72 hours, the patient's oxygenation status continued to deteriorate in spite of an increased F_{IO_2}, PEEP, and mechanical ventilatory rate. When the arterial oxygen tension did not improve appreciably on an F_{IO_2} of 0.75 and a PEEP of 20 cm H_2O, a Swan-Ganz catheter was placed in the pulmonary artery. In view of the PEEP, the results were difficult to interpret. A mean pulmonary artery pressure of 27 mm Hg, however, did suggest increased pulmonary vascular resistance.

A chest x-ray confirmed good position of the endotracheal tube and revealed ARDS with extensive, diffuse infiltrates and atelectasis, worse on the right side. Arterial blood gases on an F_{IO_2} of 1.0, + 25 cm H_2O of PEEP, V_T of 1000, and IMV of 16 were pH 7.41, Pa_{CO_2} 41, HCO_3^- 24, and Pa_{O_2} 38. Her respiratory rate was 40 per minute (in between the mechanically ventilated breaths), and there were crackles, wheezes and rhonchi in all lung fields. Moderate to large amounts of purulent sputum was frequently suctioned from the endotracheal tube. Her blood pressure was 90/60, and her pulse was 130 bpm. At this time, the respiratory care practitioner charted this SOAP note:

RESPIRATORY ASSESSMENT AND PLAN

S: N/A.

O: Patient remains comatose. BP 90/60, HR 130, RR 40. Bilateral crackles, rhonchi & wheezes. ABGs on F_{IO_2} 1.0 and + 25 PEEP: pH 7.41, Pa_{CO_2} 41, HCO_3^- 24, Pa_{O_2} 38. CXR: ARDS with bilateral infiltrates and atelectasis, worse on the right side. Purulent sputum. PA pressure (mean) 27 mm Hg.

A: • Severe and worsening hypoxemia (ABG)
   • Persistent coma (physical exam)
   • Aspiration pneumonitis progressing to ARDS with bilateral infiltrates and atelectasis (x-ray)
   • Increasing airway secretions with infection (crackle, rhonchi & purulent sputum)

P: Call physician: Discuss neuromuscular paralysis, inverse I:E ratio ventilation, and ECMO. Gram's stain and culture sputum. Add 2 ml acetylcysteine and 0.5 ml albuterol aerosol Q2°. Suction PRN.

Since it was apparent that current management was not going to be successful, it was decided to alert the ECMO team and place the patient on extracorporeal membrane oxygenation. This was done, and the patient was maintained on ECMO for 13 hours when she developed ventricular tachycardia followed by ventricular fibrillation. Attempts to reestablish normal cardiac function were not successful, and the patient was pronounced dead 45 minutes later.

DISCUSSION

This was a preventable death. Gastric lavage should *NEVER* be performed on an unconscious patient without first protecting the airway with a cuffed endotracheal tube. This is one of the very few categorical imperatives in medicine. The following three etiologic factors known to produce ARDS may have been operative in this patient: drug overdose, aspiration of gastric contents, and breathing an excessive $F_{I_{O_2}}$ for a long period of time (less probable). As time progressed, the patient's lungs became stiffer and physiologically nonfunctional as a result of the anatomic alterations associated with ARDS. Increasing the $F_{I_{O_2}}$ and PEEP, adding bronchodilator and mucolytic aerosols and, finally, going to ECMO to manage this case, while clearly indicated and appropriate, were not enough in the final analysis.

SELF-ASSESSMENT QUESTIONS

Multiple Choice

1. In response to injury, the lungs of an ARDS patient undergo these changes:
   - I. Atelectasis
   - II. Decreased alveolar-capillary membrane permeability
   - III. Interstitial and intra-alveolar edema
   - IV. Hemorrhagic alveolar consolidation
     - a. I and III only
     - b. II and IV only
     - c. I, II, and IV only
     - d. I, III, and IV only
     - e. I, II, III, and IV

2. Historically, ARDS was first referred to as
   - a. Oxygen toxicity.
   - b. Shock lung syndrome.
   - c. Adult hyaline membrane disease.
   - d. Congestion atelectasis.
   - e. White lung.

3. The generic name of Lasix is
   - a. Furosemide.
   - b. Spironolactone.
   - c. Aldactone.
   - d. Thiazide.
   - e. Hydrochlorothiazide.

4. During the early stages of ARDS, the patient commonly demonstrates which arterial blood gas values?
   - I. Decreased pH
   - II. Increased Pa_{CO_2}
   - III. Decreased HCO_3^-
   - IV. Normal Pa_{O_2}
     - a. II only
     - b. III only
     - c. II and III only
     - d. III and IV only
     - e. I and II only

5. Which of the following oxygenation indices is/are associated with ARDS?
   - I. Increased $\dot{V}_{O_2}$
   - II. Decreased D_{O_2}
   - III. Increased $S\bar{v}_{O_2}$
   - IV. Decreased $\dot{Q}_S/\dot{Q}_T$
     - a. I only
     - b. II only
     - c. III only
     - d. II and III only
     - e. I, III, and IV only

True or False

1. The hyaline membrane that develops in ARDS is identical to the hyaline membrane seen in newborns with infant respiratory distress syndrome.   True _____ False _____
2. The lung compliance of patients with ARDS is very high.   True _____ False _____
3. Bronchial breath sounds are associated with ARDS.   True _____ False _____
4. The RV is increased in patients with ARDS.   True _____ False _____
5. Chest x-ray findings in ARDS reveal a decreased opacity.   True _____ False _____

Answers appear in Appendix XXI.

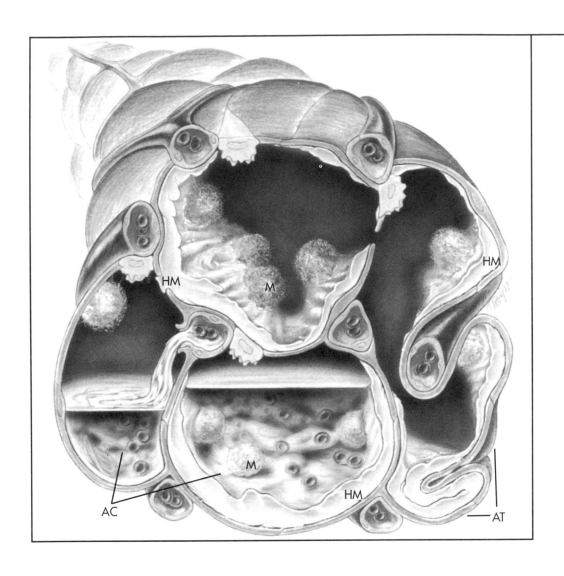

IDIOPATHIC (INFANT) RESPIRATORY DISTRESS SYNDROME

FIG 24-1

Cross sectional view of alveoli in idiopathic (infant) respiratory distress syndrome. *HM* = hyaline membrane; *AT* = atelectasis; *AC* = alveolar consolidation; *M* = macrophage. (See also Plate 23.)

Idiopathic (Infant) Respiratory Distress Syndrome

ANATOMIC ALTERATIONS OF THE LUNGS

On gross examination the lungs are dark red and liverlike. Under the microscope the lungs appear solid because of countless areas of alveolar collapse. The pulmonary capillaries are congested, and the lymphatic vessels are distended. There are extensive interstitial and intra-alveolar edema and hemorrhage.

In what appears to be an effort to offset alveolar collapse, the respiratory bronchioles, alveolar ducts, and some alveoli are dilated. As the disease intensifies, the intra-alveolar walls become lined with a dense, rippled hyaline membrane identical to the hyaline membrane that develops in the adult respiratory distress syndrome (ARDS). The membrane contains fibrin and cellular debris.

During the later stages of the disease, leukocytes are present, and the hyaline membrane is often fragmented and partially ingested by macrophages. Type II cells begin to proliferate, and secretions begin to accumulate in the tracheobronchial tree. The anatomic alterations in infant respiratory distress syndrome (IRDS) produce a restrictive type of lung disorder (Fig 24-1).

To summarize, the major pathologic or structural changes associated with IRDS are as follows:

- Interstitial and intra-alveolar edema and hemorrhage
- Alveolar consolidation
- Intra-alveolar hyaline membrane
- Pulmonary surfactant deficiency or abnormality
- Atelectasis

In alphabetical order, the following are some of the terms that have been used as synonyms for IRDS:

- Asphyxial membrane
- Congenital alveolar dysplasia
- Hyaline atelectasis
- Hyaline-like membrane
- Hyaline membrane disease (perhaps the most popular although an incorrect term)
- Myelin formation in the lungs
- Neonatal atelectasis
- Neonatal pulmonary ischemia

- Pulmonary hypoperfusion syndrome
- Surfactant deficiency syndrome
- Vernix membrane

ETIOLOGY

Although the exact cause of IRDS is controversial, the most popular theory suggests that the disorder develops as a result of (1) a pulmonary surfactant abnormality or deficiency and (2) pulmonary hypoperfusion evoked by hypoxia.

Some of the known factors that predispose an infant to a pulmonary surfactant abnormality or deficiency are as follows:

- Cesarean birth
- Diabetic mother
- Maternal bleeding
- Premature birth (birth weight less than 2.5 kg)
- Prenatal asphyxia
- Prolonged labor
- Second-born twin

The pulmonary hypoperfusion evoked by hypoxia is probably a secondary response to the surfactant abnormality. The probable steps in the development of IRDS are as follows:

1. Because of the pulmonary surfactant abnormality, alveolar compliance decreases, and this results in alveolar collapse.
2. The pulmonary atelectasis causes the infant's work of breathing to increase.
3. Alveolar ventilation decreases in response to the decreased lung compliance, as well as infant fatigue, and causes the alveolar oxygen tension ($P_{A_{O_2}}$) to decrease.
4. The decreased $P_{A_{O_2}}$ (alveolar hypoxia) stimulates a reflex pulmonary vasoconstriction.
5. Because of the pulmonary vasoconstriction, blood bypasses the infant's lungs through fetal pathways—the patient ductus and the foramen ovale.
6. The lung hypoperfusion in turn causes lung ischemia and decreased lung metabolism.
7. Because of the decreased lung metabolism, the production of pulmonary surfactant is reduced even further, and a vicious cycle develops (Fig 24-2).

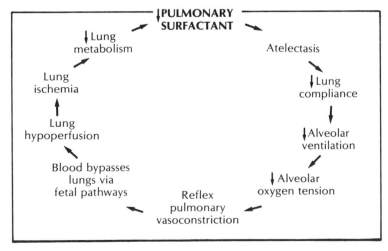

FIG 24-2
Probable etiologic steps in the development of IRDS.

OVERVIEW

OF THE CARDIOPULMONARY CLINICAL MANIFESTATIONS ASSOCIATED WITH
INFANT RESPIRATORY DISTRESS SYNDROME

❏ **INCREASED RESPIRATORY RATE**

Normally, a newborn infant's respiratory rate is about 40 to 60 breaths per minute. In IRDS, the respiratory rate is generally well over 60 breaths per minute. On the basis of anatomic alterations of the lung associated with IRDS, there may be several pathophysiologic mechanisms operating simultaneously that lead to an increased ventilatory rate. The possible mechanisms are as follows (see page 17):

- Stimulation of peripheral chemoreceptors
- Decreased lung compliance/increased ventilatory rate relationship
- Stimulation of the central chemoreceptors

❏ **INCREASED HEART RATE (PULSE), CARDIAC OUTPUT, AND BLOOD PRESSURE** (see page 86)

❏ **PULMONARY FUNCTION STUDY FINDINGS**

Lung Volume and Capacity Findings (see page 39)

V_T	RV	RV/TLC	FRC
↓	↓	normal	↓
TLC	VC	IC	ERV
↓	↓	↓	↓

❏ **CLINICAL MANIFESTATIONS ASSOCIATED WITH INCREASED NEGATIVE INTRAPLEURAL PRESSURES DURING INSPIRATION**
- Intercostal retractions
- Substernal retraction/abdominal distention ("seesaw" movement)
- Cyanosis of the dependent portion of the thoracic/abdominal area

The thorax of the newborn infant is very flexible, i.e., the compliance of the infant's thorax is high. This is due to the large amount of cartilage found in the skeletal structure of newborns. Because of the structural alterations associated with IRDS, however, the compliance of the infant's lungs is low.

In an effort to offset the decreased lung compliance, the infant must generate increased negative intrapleural pressure during inspiration. This causes the following:

- The soft tissues between the ribs retract during inspiration.
- The substernal area retracts, and the abdominal area protrudes in a seesaw fashion during inspiration. The substernal retraction is due to increased negative intrapleural pressure, and the abdominal distention is due to the increased contraction—or depression—of the diaphragm during inspiration.
- The blood vessels in the more dependent portions of the thoracic/abdominal area dilate and pool blood. This causes these areas to appear cyanotic (Fig 24-3).

❏ **FLARING NOSTRILS**

Flaring nostrils are frequently observed in infants in respiratory distress. This is probably a facial reflex to facilitate the movement of gas into the tracheobronchial tree. The *dilator naris,* which originates from the maxilla and inserts into the ala of the nose, is the muscle responsible for this clinical manifestation. When activated, the dilator naris pulls the alae laterally and widens the nasal aperture. This provides a larger orifice for gas to enter during inspiration.

❑ EXPIRATORY GRUNTING

An audible expiratory grunt is frequently heard in infants with IRDS. Depending on the auditory perception of the listener, the expiratory grunt may sound like an expiratory sign or cry. It is often first detected on auscultation.

The expiratory grunt is a natural physiologic mechanism that generates greater positive pressures in the alveoli. This counteracts the hypoventilation associated with the disorder, that is, as the gas pressure in the alveoli increases, the infant's $P_{A_{O_2}}$ increases. During exhalation the infant's epiglottis covers the glottis, which causes the intrapulmonary air pressure to increase. When the epiglottis abruptly opens, gas rushes past the infant's vocal cords and produces an expiratory grunt or cry.

❑ RADIOLOGIC FINDINGS

Chest radiograph
Increased opacity (ground-glass appearance)

On chest x-ray films of infants with IRDS, the air-filled tracheobronchial tree typically stands out against a dense opaque (or white) lung. This white density is often described as having a fine ground-glass appearance throughout the lung fields.

Because of the pathologic processes the density of the lungs is increased. Increased lung density resists x-ray penetration and is revealed on x-ray films as increased opacity. Thus, the more severe the IRDS, the whiter the x-ray film will be (Fig 24-4).

❑ ARTERIAL BLOOD GASES

Advanced Stages of IRDS

Acute Ventilatory Failure with Hypoxemia (see page 59)

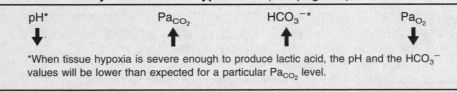

pH*	Pa_{CO_2}	HCO_3^-*	Pa_{O_2}
↓	↑	↑	↓

*When tissue hypoxia is severe enough to produce lactic acid, the pH and the HCO_3^- values will be lower than expected for a particular Pa_{CO_2} level.

Decreased Pa_{O_2}

There are three major mechanisms responsible for the decreased Pa_{O_2} observed in IRDS: (1) pulmonary shunting and venous admixture, (2) persistent pulmonary hypertension of the neonate (PPHN), and (3) infant fatigue.

The infant's Pa_{O_2} decreases in IRDS because of the reduced V̇/Q̇ ratio, intrapulmonary shunting, and venous admixture associated with the disorder.

As the infant's Pa_{O_2} declines, a reflex pulmonary vasoconstriction may be stimulated. Because of the pulmonary vasoconstriction, nonreoxygenated blood begins to bypass the infant's lungs through fetal pathways—the patient ductus and foramen ovale. This is known as *persistent pulmonary hypertension of the neonate,* previously known as *persistent fetal circulation* (Fig 24-5).

If the pathologic processes persist for a long period of time, the infant becomes *fatigued* (because of the increased work of breathing) and begins to hypoventilate. This causes a further reduction of the Pa_{O_2}.

Increased Pa_{CO_2}

There are two major mechanisms responsible for the increased Pa_{CO_2} noted in IRDS: (1) decreased lung compliance and (2) infant fatigue.

Due to the pulmonary surfactant abnormality, alveolar compliance decreases, and alveolar hypoventilation ensues. This in turn causes the Pa_{CO_2} to increase.

Because of the increased work of breathing required, the infant may become fatigued and hypoventilate even more. When this occurs, alveolar ventilation slowly decreases and causes the Pa_{O_2} to decrease and the Pa_{CO_2} to increase (Fig 24-6).

Increased HCO$_3^-$
Decreased pH

When acute ventilatory failure and a progressive increase in Pa$_{CO_2}$ develop during the advanced stages of IRDS, a secondary increase in the HCO$_3^-$ level and a decreased pH will be present. The decreased pH may also be due to the decreased Pa$_{O_2}$ and the metabolic acidosis that result from anaerobic metabolism and lactic acid accumulation. If this is the case, the calculated HCO$_3^-$ reading and pH will be lower than expected for a particular Pa$_{CO_2}$ level.

❑ **CYANOSIS** (see page 68)
❑ **CHEST ASSESSMENT FINDINGS** (see page 6)
- Bronchial (or harsh) breath sounds
- Fine crackles

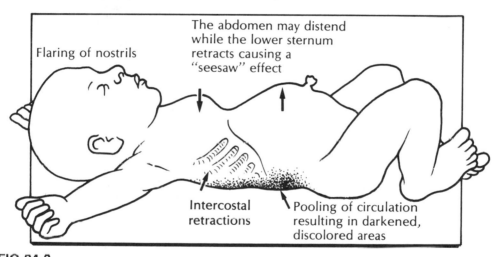

FIG 24-3

Clinical manifestations associated with an increased negative intrapleural pressure during inspiration in infants with IRDS.

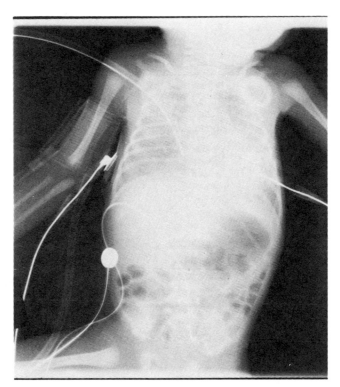

FIG 24-4
Chest x-ray film of an infant with IRDS.

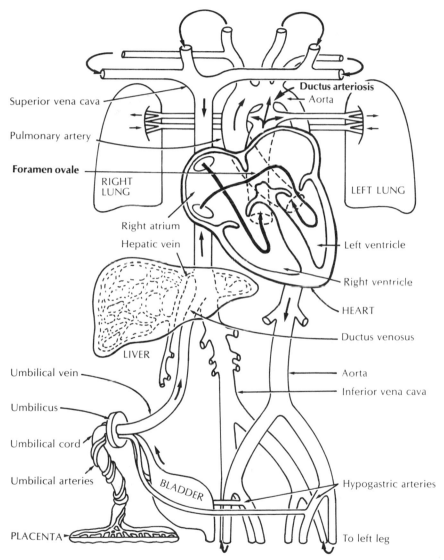

FIG 24-5
Fetal circulation.

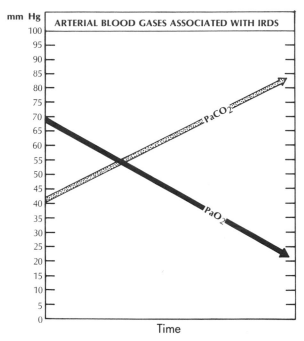

FIG 24-6

Pa$_{O_2}$ and Pa$_{CO_2}$ trends associated with IRDS.

GENERAL MANAGEMENT OF IRDS

During the early stages of IRDS, continuous positive-airway pressure (CPAP) is the treatment of choice. Mechanical ventilation is usually avoided as long as possible. CPAP generally works well with these patients since it (1) increases the functional residual capacity, (2) decreases the work of breathing, and (3) works to increase the Pa$_{O_2}$ while the infant is receiving a lower inspired concentration of oxygen. A Pa$_{O_2}$ between 40 and 70 mm Hg is normal for newborn infants. No effort should be made to get an infant's Pa$_{O_2}$ within the normal adult range (80 to 100 mm Hg). Special attention should be given to the thermal environment of the infant with IRDS, since the infant's oxygenation could be further compromised if the body temperature is above or below normal.

Finally, because of the decreased pulmonary surfactant associated with IRDS, the administration of exogenous surfactant preparations such as Survanta or Exosurf is helpful. The calculated dose of Survanta (Beractant) is administered to the infant in quarters, one fourth at a time. Each quarter dose is instilled directly into the trachea through a 5-F catheter placed into the endotracheal tube. The catheter is taken out after each administration, and the infant is manually ventilated or returned to the ventilator for 30 seconds or until the infant is stable.

Exosurf (composed of Colfosceril palmitate, cetyl alcohol, and tyloxapol) is instilled directly into the endotracheal tube through a side-port adapter that attaches to the endotracheal tube. Exosurf is administered in two stages. The first half of the dose is given in short bursts, timed to correlate with each inspiration. This first half of the dose is administered with the infant in supine position. After the first half of the dose has been given, the infant is rotated to the right and ventilated for about 30 seconds. The second half of the dose is then administered with the patient in the supine position, again in short bursts that coincide with each inspiration. After the second half of the dose has been given, the infant is rotated to the left and ventilated for about 30 seconds.

IDIOPATHIC (INFANT) RESPIRATORY DISTRESS SYNDROME CASE STUDY

ADMITTING HISTORY AND PHYSICAL EXAMINATION

This premature male infant was delivered after 34 weeks of gestation. The mother was a 19-year-old, unmarried primigravida who claimed to be in good health during the entire pregnancy until six hours prior to admission. At that time she noticed the onset of painless vaginal bleeding. She called her obstetrician, who told her he would meet her in the emergency department of the medical center.

On examination she was found to be a healthy young female, approximately 34 weeks pregnant, in early labor, and bleeding slightly from the vagina. Her vital signs were stable and within normal limits. A diagnosis of premature separation of the placenta was made. Since bleeding was minimal and both mother and fetus seemed to be doing well, it was decided to deliver her vaginally. She was monitored very closely, and labor progressed satisfactorily for about eight hours, at which time she was delivered under epidural anesthesia without any obstetrical complications. The baby weighed 2100 grams. The Apgar scores were 7 after one minute and 9 after five minutes. Physical examination was entirely normal for an infant of this size.

On admission to the newborn nursery 30 minutes after delivery, the infant was noted to have some moderate respiratory distress. His respiratory rate was 40/min. There was flaring of the nostrils. A chest x-ray obtained at this time suggested the presence of left upper lobe atelectasis, but no other pulmonary abnormality was noted.

During the next five hours, the infant deteriorated rapidly, and the respiratory distress became markedly accentuated. The baby was cyanotic, retracting, and using the accessory muscles of respiration. The respiratory rate was 64/min, and respirations were described as "grunting" in nature. His heart rate was 165/minute. Crackles were heard bilaterally. A chest x-ray taken at this time revealed generalized haziness that one radiologist described as "ground glass." Arterial blood gases on an $F_{I_{O_2}}$ of 0.30 were pH 7.25, Pa_{CO_2} 52, HCO_3^- 22, Pa_{O_2} 35. The Sa_{O_2} was 60%. At this time, the respiratory therapist working with the baby recorded this assessment and plan:

RESPIRATORY ASSESSMENT AND PLAN

S: N/A (newborn).

O: Dyspneic and cyanotic. Retracting and using accessory muscles. Flaring of nostrils. RR 64 with "grunting." HR 165. Bilateral crackles. CXR: bilateral "ground glass" haziness. ABGs: pH 7.25, Pa_{CO_2} 52, HCO_3^- 22, Pa_{O_2} 35, Sa_{O_2} 60%.

A: • Infant respiratory distress syndrome (history)
• Alveolar hyaline membrane/consolidation/atelectasis (CXR)
• Acute ventilatory failure with hypoxemia (ABG)

P: Intubate/ventilate/PEEP per NICU Protocol. Continuous transcutaneous oximetry. Exosurf per protocol.

The baby was intubated and put on a ventilator with PEEP ranging from +4 to +10 cm H_2O. Artificial surfactant (Exosurf) therapy was begun. The inspired oxygen concentration varied from 30% to 50%. Adjustments were made on the basis of numerous arterial blood gas and electrolyte determinations. Fluid and electrolyte balance was maintained within normal levels. ECMO was considered, but since the baby was doing well on a more conservative regimen, it was decided not to use it at the time. On this management, the baby was weaned from PEEP in 72 hours and from artificial ventilation in 96 hours. Chest x-ray examination on the seventh day showed no residual pathology. The baby was discharged on the 15th day and has been healthy ever since.

DISCUSSION

Most respiratory therapy students greatly look forward to and enjoy their rotation through neonatal intensive care units. In these units, respiratory care practitioners' expertise is core to the functioning of the unit, since the majority of patients there have respiratory disorders. Indeed, many of the first reports of therapist-driven protocols came from just this setting.

Idiopathic respiratory distress syndrome is a fascinating disorder in which meticulous respiratory care of the small infant is crucial. The recent availability of artificial surfactant (Exosurf) has markedly improved the outlook for these infants. Most such units are staffed by an in-house neonatologist, who can guide the therapist through the intricacies of therapy. As in adults with ARDS (in which the pathology is very similar), constant surveillance must be given to the possibility of nosocomial infection, fluid overload, and cardiovascular instability.

SELF-ASSESSMENT QUESTIONS

Multiple Choice

1. When persistent fetal circulation exists in IRDS, blood bypasses the infant's lungs through the
   I. Ductus venosus.
   II. Umbilical vein.
   III. Ductus arteriosus.
   IV. Foramen ovale.
      a. I only
      b. I and II only
      c. I and III only
      d. II and III only
      e. III and IV only

2. It is suggested that IRDS is a result of a
   I. Vernix membrane.
   II. Decreased perfusion of the lungs.
   III. Pulmonary surfactant abnormality.
   IV. Congenital alveolar dysplasia.
      a. I and III only
      b. II and III only
      c. I and IV only
      d. II, III, and IV only
      e. I, II, III, and IV

3. When an infant with IRDS creates a greater-than-normal negative intrapleural pressure during inspiration, the
   I. Soft tissue between the ribs bulges outward.
   II. Substernal area protrudes outward.
   III. Abdominal area retracts inward.
   IV. Dependent blood vessels dilate and pool blood.
      a. II only
      b. IV only
      c. II and III only
      d. I, III, and IV only
      e. II, III, and IV only

4. Infants with severe IRDS often have
   I. Diminished breath sounds.
   II. Bronchial breath sounds.
   III. Hyperresonate percussion notes.
   IV. Fine crackles.
      a. I only
      b. I and IV only
      c. III and IV only
      d. II and III only
      e. II and IV only

5. Continuous positive-airway pressure (CPAP) is often administered to infants with IRDS in an effort to
   I. Increase the infant's FRC.
   II. Decrease the infant's work of breathing.
   III. Increase the infant's Pa_{O_2}.
   IV. Decrease the $F_{I_{O_2}}$ necessary to oxygenate the infant.
      a. I and III only
      b. II and III only
      c. III and IV only
      d. II, III, and IV only
      e. I, II, III, and IV

True or False

1. The intra-alveolar hyaline membrane seen in IRDS is identical to the hyaline membrane seen in adult respiratory distress syndrome (ARDS).   True _____   False _____
2. Alveolar consolidation develops in IRDS.   True _____   False _____
3. When activated, the dilator naris muscle widens the glottis.   True _____   False _____
4. Chest x-ray films of infants with severe IRDS appear more translucent.   True _____   False _____
5. The Pa_{O_2} of infants with IRDS should be maintained between 80 and 100 mm Hg.   True _____   False _____

Fill in the Blank

1. A premature birth is when the infant's weight is less than _____ .

Answers appear in Appendix XXI.

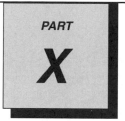

PART

X

CHRONIC NONINFECTIOUS PARENCHYMAL DISEASES

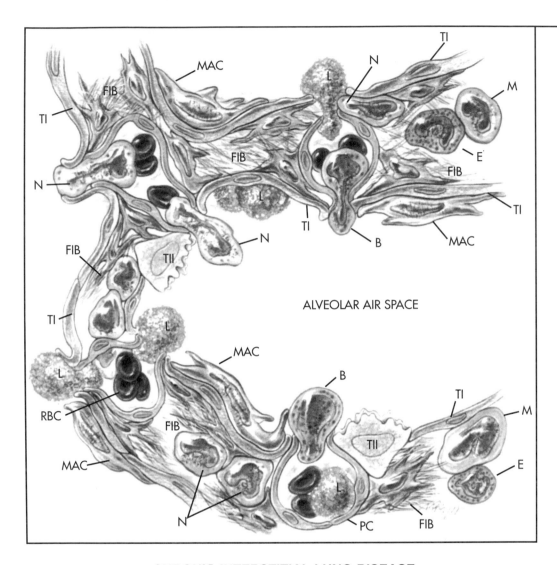

CHRONIC INTERSTITIAL LUNG DISEASE

FIG 25-1

Chronic interstitial lung disease. Cross-sectional, microscopic view of alveolar-capillary unit. N = neutrophil; E = eosinophil; B = basophil; M = monocyte; MAC = macrophage; L = lymphocyte; FIB = fibroblasts (fibrosis); TI = type I alveolar cell; TII = type II alveolar cell; RBC = red blood cell; PC = pulmonary capillary. (See also Plate 24.)

Chronic Interstitial Lung Diseases

ANATOMIC ALTERATIONS OF THE LUNGS

Interstitial lung diseases comprise a large group of pulmonary disorders that are all associated with pulmonary inflammatory changes. Often times, the term interstitial lung disorder is made more specific by using a name closely related to the etiology, or specific pathology, associated with the disease. For example, *farmer's lung* (caused by inhalation of moldy hay) and pulmonary *alveolar proteinosis* (so named because of the protein like material that fills the alveoli) are both considered interstitial lung disorders, and both manifest the same basic pulmonary pathophysiology. The anatomic alterations may involve the bronchi, alveolar walls, and adjacent alveolar spaces. In severe cases, the extensive inflammation will lead to fibrosis, granulomas, honeycombing, and cavitation.

During the *acute stage* of any interstitial lung disease, the general inflammatory condition is characterized by edema and by the infiltration of a variety of white blood cells (e.g., neutrophils, eosinophils, basophils, monocytes, macrophages, and lymphocytes) in the alveolar walls and interstitial spaces (Fig. 25-1). Bronchial inflammation and bronchial smooth muscle constriction may also be present.

During the *chronic stage,* the general inflammatory response is characterized by the infiltration of numerous white blood cells (especially monocytes, macrophages, and lymphocytes) and some fibroblasts in the alveolar walls and interstitial spaces. Airway hyperactivity may be present. This stage may be followed by further interstitial thickening, fibrosis, granulomas, and, in some cases, honeycombing and cavity formation. Pleural effusion may also be present. In the chronic stages, the basic pathologic features of interstitial fibrosis are identical in any interstitial lung disorder.

In general, the interstitial lung disorders produce a restrictive pattern in pulmonary function testing. However, because inflammation and smooth muscle constriction can also develop in the small airways, the clinical manifestations associated with an obstructive disorder may also be seen. Thus, the patient with interstitial lung disease may demonstrate a restrictive disorder, an obstructive disorder, or a combination of both.

Although a fully satisfactory classification system is not available, the interstitial lung disorders are commonly divided into two broad groups based on whether the alveolar inflammation and fibrosis are associated with the presence or absence of *granuloma*. The term granuloma is an imprecise description applied to (1) any small nodular, delimited aggregation of mononuclear inflammatory cells, or (2) a similar collection of modified macrophages resembling epithelial cells, usually surrounded by a rim of lymphocytes. Granuloma formation represents a chronic inflammatory response initiated by various infective and noninfective agents.

To summarize, the major pathologic or structural changes associated with chronic interstitial lung diseases are as follows:

* Fibrotic thickening of the respiratory bronchioles, alveolar ducts, and alveoli
* Granulomas
* Destruction of the alveoli and adjacent pulmonary capillaries
* Honeycombing and cavity formation
* Airway obstruction caused by inflammation and bronchial constriction

ETIOLOGY

Over 140 distinctly different disease processes are known to produce an interstitial lung disorder, and the list continues to grow. In this group of disease entities, however, no specific etiologic agent can be identified in more than 65% of the cases, in spite of the fact that a specific name may be attached to a particular disease entity. Table 25-1 lists some of the more common interstitial lung disorders. A discussion of the more common interstitial lung diseases follows.

Interstitial Inflammation with Granuloma Formation
Extrinsic Allergic Alveolitis

Extrinsic allergic alveolitis (also called hypersensitivity pneumonitis) is an immunologically mediated inflammation of the lungs caused by the inhalation of a variety of offending agents (antigens) such as pollen, animal dander, organic dusts, and spores of certain molds. Table 25-2 lists a variety of offending agents known to cause extrinsic allergic alveolitis. The term *extrinsic allergic alveolitis* is often renamed according to the specific causative agent known to cause the disorder. For example, extrinsic allergic alveolitis caused by inhalation of moldy hay is called *farmer's lung* (see Table 25-2).

Table 25-1 Common Interstitial Lung Disorders

Interstitial Inflammation With Granuloma Formation	Interstitial Inflammation Without Granuloma Formation	Miscellaneous Diffuse Interstitial Lung Diseases
Extrinsic allergic alveolitis (Hypersensitivity pneumonitis)	Idiopathic pulmonary fibrosis	Goodpasture's syndrome
Sarcoidosis	Drug-induced interstitial lung disease	Idiopathic pulmonary hemosiderosis
Eosinophilic granuloma (Histiocystosis X)	Radiation-induced interstitial lung disease	Chronic eosinophilic pneumonia
Pulmonary vasculitides	Irritant gases	Bronchiolitis obliterans with organizing pneumonia
Wegener's granulomatosis	Collagen vascular diseases	Lymphangioleiomyomatosis
Churg-Strauss syndrome	Rheumatoid arthritis	Alveolar proteinosis
Lymphomatoid granulomatosis	Systemic lupus erythematosus	
	Polymyositis-dermatomyositis	
	Progressive systemic sclerosis	
	Sjögren's syndrome	

To understand the clinical and pathophysiologic features of extrinsic allergic alveolitis, a basic understanding of hypersensitivity reaction is required (Table 25-3). There are four types of allergic or hypersensitivity reactions; three are mediated by humoral antibodies, and one is mediated by T cells. It appears that the Type III hypersensitivity reaction is the underlying cause for most of the pathologic changes associated with extrinsic allergic alveolitis. The diagnosis of extrinsic allergic alveolitis generally depends on an occupational history and, subsequently, is confirmed with blood tests (antibody measurements) or skin testing.

Sarcoidosis

Sarcoidosis is a multisystem granulomatous disease of unknown etiology. It may affect any part of the body, but most frequently involves the lung, lymph nodes, liver, spleen, skin, eyes, and small bones of the hands and feet. The lung is the most frequently affected organ, with manifestations generally including interstitial lung disease, enlargement of the mediastinal lymph nodes, or a combination of both. One of the clinical hallmarks of sarcoidosis is an increase in all three major immunologins (IgM, IgG, and IgA).

The incidence of sarcoidosis is variable from one country to another and even in different regions of the same country. For example, Sweden, North Ireland, Denmark, and Germany have a high prevalence, whereas neighboring countries, such as Finland, have a relatively low prevalance. In the United States, the incidence is about 10 cases per 100,000. The disease is more common among blacks and appears most frequently in patients between 10 and 40 years of age, with the highest incidence between 20 and 30 years of age. Women are affected more than men, especially among blacks.

Table 25-2 Antigens, Their Source, and the Disease Entities that can Produce Hypersensitivity Pneumonitis

Disease	Source of Antigen	Antigens
Air-conditioning and humidifier lung	Fungi in air conditioners and humidifiers	Thermophilic actinomycetes
Aspergillosis	Ubiquitous	*Aspergillus fumigatus, A. flavus, A. niger, A. nidulans*
Bagassosis (sugar cane workers)	Moldy bagasse	*Thermoactinomyces vulgaris*
Bird breeder's lung	Pigeon, parrot, hen droppings	Avian proteins
Byssinosis	Cotton, flex, hemp workers	Unknown
Farmer's lung	Moldy hay	*Micropolyspora faeni, T. vulgaris*
Malt worker's lung	Moldy barley, malt dust	*A. clavatus, A. fumigatus*
Maple-bark pneumonitis	Moldy maple bark	*Coniosporium corticale*
Mushroom worker's lung	Mushroom compost	*M. faeni, T. vulgaris*
"New Guinea" lung	Moldy thatch dust	Thatch of huts
Pituitary snuff-taker's lung	Heterologous pituitary powder	Heterologous antigen of pituitary snuff
Sisal worker's lung	Unknown	Unknown
Small pox handler's lung	Not yet demonstrated	Not yet demonstrated
Suberosis	Moldy oak bark, cork dust	*Pencillium*
Wheat weevil disease	Infested wheat flour	*Sitophilus granarius*

Table 25-3 Hypersensitivity or Allergic Reaction

Group	Reaction	Pulmonary Pathology	Example
TYPE I: Anaphylaxis	When first exposed to a certain antigen, the lymphoid cells form specific IgE antibodies which, in turn, bond to the surface of the mast cells. Subsequent exposure to the same antigen creates an antigen-antibody reaction on the surface of the mast cell, which causes the mast cell to degranulate and release chemical mediators such as histamine, leukotrienes [formerly called slow-reacting substance of anaphylaxis (SRS-A)], eosinophilic chemotactic factor of anaphylaxis (ECFA), neutrophil chemotactic factor (NCF), prostaglandins, and platelet-activating factor (PAF).	The release of chemical mediators causes smooth muscle constriction of the bronchi, dilation of blood vessels, increased capillary permeability, infiltration of eosinophils, and tissue edema.	Bronchial asthma, allergic rhinitis, and eczema
TYPE II: Cytotoxic	When certain antigens are introduced into the body, they may bond to the surface of red blood cells, leukocytes, or platelets. When this happens, antibodies are formed to destroy the antigens attached to the cells. Which disease develops depends on which blood cell the antigen is attached to. For example, when antibodies attack the antigen attached to red blood cells, hemolysis, jaundice, and anemia develop. When antibodies attack the leukocytes, increased susceptibility to infection ensues. When antiplatelets antibodies are formed, the results may be thrombocytopenia and hemorrhagic manifestations. Unlike the Type I reaction, only one exposure to the antigen is necessary in the Type II reaction.	Cellular and tissue inflammation	Goodpasture's syndrome, blood transfusion, penicillin therapy (occasionally)
TYPE III: Immune ComplexMediated Hypersensitivity	When an offending soluble or particulate antigen is introduced into the body (e.g., inhaled into the lungs) antibodies are formed. The antibodies, in turn, attach themselves to the capillaries at the spot where the antigen entered the body. The next exposure to the offending antigen elicits immune complexes that lead to the destruction of endothelial cells by the individual's own immunologic defense system.	Damage to the endothelial lining, deposition of fibrin in the wall of the blood vessel, microthrombosis, local ischemia, necrosis of the vessel walls, and granuloma formation	Extrinsic allergic alveolitis (hypersensitivity pneumonitis)
TYPE IV: Cell-Mediated Reactions	The Type IV reaction is mediated by T lymphocytes and involves the same basic mechanism related to the protective response to the T cells. The reaction takes 24 to 48 hours to develop, and is therefore called "delayed hypersensitivity."	Infiltration of macrophages and lymphocytes with possible granuloma formation, caseation, and necrosis	Tuberculosis, poison ivy, poison oak, contact dermatitis, and eczema; possibly sarcoidosis and Wegener's granulomatosis

The initial diagnosis of sarcoidosis is usually based on the clinical presentation, followed by confirmation with chest radiograph and histologic evidence obtained by biopsy.

Eosinophilic Granuloma

Eosinophilic granuloma (also called histiocytosis X) is characterized by numerous small interstitial granulomas scattered throughout the lungs. Often their location is just below the visceral pleura of the lungs. The interstitial granulomas are composed of moderately large, pale *histiocytes* (also called histiocytosis X cells), which are the hallmark of this disorder. Histiocytic cells are a particular type of macrophage having unique rodlike structures called *X bodies* within their cytoplasm that can be seen with electron microscopy. In addition to histiocytes, there is an infiltration by eosinophils, lymphocytes, and alveolar macrophages. Eosinophilic granuloma is a disorder of unknown etiology. It most commonly appears in smokers and ex-smokers between 20 and 40 years of age, and males are slightly more often affected than females.

The Pulmonary Vasculitides

The pulmonary vaculitides (also called granulomatous vasculitides) consist of a heterogeneous group of pulmonary disorders characterized by inflammation and destruction of the pulmonary vessels. The major disorders in this category include Wegener's granulomatosis, Churg-Strauss syndrome, and lymphomatoid granulomatosis.

Wegener's granulomatosis.—Wegener's granulomatosis is a multisystem disorder characterized by (1) a necrotizing, granulomatous vasculitis, (2) focal and segmental glomerulonephritis, and (3) variable degrees of systemic vasculitis of the small veins and arteries. In the lungs, multiple 1- to 9-cm-diameter nodules are commonly seen in the upper lobes, and cavity formation is often associated with the larger lesions.

Wegener's granulomatosis is considered an aggressive and fatal disorder, although the prognosis has significantly improved with the recent availability of cytotoxic agents (e.g., cyclophosphamide). This disorder is most commonly seen in males over 50 years of age. Diagnosis is confirmed by an open lung biopsy. Histologic examination reveals lesions with a marked central necrosis. The area surrounding the necrotizing lesion consists of inflammatory WBCs with some fibroblasts. Inflammatory cell infiltrate and necrotizing vasculitis are seen in the adjacent blood vessels.

Churg-Strauss syndrome.—Churg-Strauss syndrome is a necrotizing vasculitis that predominately involves the small vessels of the lungs. The granulomatous lesions are characterized by a heavy infiltrate of eosinophils, central necrosis, and peripheral eosinophilia. Cavity formation is rare in this disorder. Clinically, symptoms of asthma usually precede the onset of vasculitis. Neurologic disorders such as mononeuritis multiplex, a simultaneous disease of several peripheral nerves, are frequently associated with this disorder. Diagnosis is usually confirmed with an open lung biopsy, and the disease is often rapidly fatal.

Lymphomatoid granulomatosis.—Lymphomatoid granulomatosis is a rare necrotizing vasculitis that primarily involves the lungs, although neurologic and cutaneous lesions are sometimes seen. The lesions are usually in the lower lobes, and cavities develop in more than one third of the cases. Pleural effusion is common.

Although the clinical presentation is similar to that of Wegener's granulomatosis, there are some distinct differences. For example, more mature lymphoreticular cells are involved in the formation of the granulomatous lesions and no glomerulonephritis is seen. Histologically, the lesions simulate malignant lymphoma. This disorder is most commonly seen in males between 50 and 70 years of age. Diagnosis is confirmed by means of an open lung biopsy.

Interstitial Inflammation Without Granuloma Formation
Idiopathic Pulmonary Fibrosis

Idiopathic pulmonary fibrosis (IPF) is a progressive inflammatory disease with varying degrees of fibrosis and, in severe cases, honeycombing. The precise etiology is unknown. Although IPF is the most frequent term used for this disorder, numerous other names appear in the literature, such as acute interstitial fibrosis of the lung, cryptogenic fibrosing alveolitis, Hamman-Rich syndrome, honeycomb lung, interstitial fibrosis, and interstitial pneumonitis.

IPF is commonly separated into the following two major disease entities according to the predominant histologic appearance: *desquamative interstitial pneumonita* (DIP) and *usual interstitial pneumonita* (UIP). In DIP, the most prominent features are hyperplasia and desquamation of the alveolar type II cells, the alveolar spaces are packed with macrophages, and there is an even distribution of the interstitial mononuclear infiltrate.

In UIP, the most prominent features are interstitial and alveolar wall thickening caused by chronic inflammatory cells and fibrosis. In severe cases, fibrotic connective tissue replaces the alveolar walls, the alveolar architecture becomes distorted, and eventually honeycombing develops. When honeycombing is present, the inflammatory infiltrate is significantly reduced. The prognosis for the patients with DIP is significantly better than that for patients with UIP.

Finally, it should be mentioned that some experts believe that DIP and UIP are two distinctly different interstitial lung disease entities. Others, however, believe that DIP and UIP are different stages of the same disease process. This disorder is most commonly seen in males between 40 and 70 years of age. Diagnosis is generally confirmed by an open lung biopsy. Most patients diagnosed with IPF have a more chronic progressive course, and death usually occurs in 4 to 10 years. Death is usually the result of progressive acute ventilatory failure, complicated by pulmonary infection.

Drug-induced Interstitial Lung Disease

As the list of pharmacologic agents continues to grow, so does the list of possible side effects. Unfortunately, the lungs are a major target organ affected by these side effects. While it is impossible to discuss in detail the various lung-related side effects of every drug, it is possible to describe some of the general concerns related to drug-induced lung disease and to list some of the pharmacological agents that may be responsible.

The chemotherapeutic or cytotoxic agents (anticancer agents) are by far the largest group of agents associated with interstitial lung disease. Bleomycin, mitomycin, busulfan, cyclophosphamide, methotrexate, and carmustine (BCNU) are the major offenders. Nitrofurantoin (an antibacterial drug used in the treatment of urinary tract infections) is also associated with interstitial lung disease. Gold and penicillamine for the treatment of rheumatoid arthritis has been shown to cause interstitial lung disease. The diagnosis may be difficult in these cases, since the underlying disease (rheumatoid arthritis) is also a possible cause of diffuse parenchymal disease.

The excessive administration of oxygen (oxygen toxicity) is also known to cause diffuse pulmonary injury and fibrosis (see Chapter 23). As a general rule, the risk of these drugs causing an interstitial lung disorder is directly related to the dosage. Drug-induced interstitial disease may be seen as early as one month to as late as several years after exposure to these agents.

The precise etiology of drug-induced interstitial lung disease is not known. Diagnosis is confirmed by an open lung biopsy. When interstitial fibrosis is found with no infectious organisms, a drug-induced interstitial process must be suspected.

Radiation-Induced Interstitial Lung Disease

Radiation therapy for tumors of the breast, lung, or thorax is a potential cause of interstitial lung disease. Radiation-induced lung disease is commonly divided into the following two major phases: the *acute,* or *early, pneumonitic phase* and the *late fibrotic phase.* Acute pneumonitis is rarely seen in patients who receive a total radiation dose of less than 3,500 rads. Doses in excess of 6,000 rads over six weeks almost always cause diffuse interstitial lung disease.

The acute pneumonitic phase develops approximately two to three months after exposure. Chronic radiation fibrosis is seen in all patients who develop acute pneumonitis. The late phase of fibrosis may develop (1) immediately after the development of acute pneumonitis, (2) without an acute pneumonitic period, or (3) after a symptom-free latent period. When fibrosis does develop, it generally does so between 6 to 12 months after radiation exposure. Pleural effusion is often associated with the late fibrotic phase.

The precise cause of radiation-induced lung disease is not known. Diagnosis is similar to that for drug-induced interstitial disease, i.e., by obtaining a history of recent radiation therapy and confirming the diagnosis with an open lung biopsy.

Irritant Gases

The inhalation of irritant gases may cause an acute chemical pneumonitis and, in severe cases, interstitial lung disease. Most exposures occur in an industrial setting. Table 25-4 lists some of the more common irritant gases and the industrial settings where they may be found.

Collagen Vascular Diseases

The collagen vascular diseases (also called connective tissue disorders) include rheumatoid arthritis, systemic lupus erythematosus, progressive systemic sclerosis (scleroderma), polymositis-dermatomyositis, and Sjögren's syndrome. All of these disorders are multisystem inflammatory diseases that are immunologically mediated. The organ systems that may be involved vary with each disease, but all may affect the lungs.

Rheumatoid arthritis.—Rheumatoid arthritis is primarily an inflammatory joint disease. It may, however, involve the lungs in the form of (1) pleurisy, with or without effusion, (2) interstitial pneumonitis, (3) necrobiotic nodules, with or without cavities, (4) Caplan's syndrome, and (5) pulmonary hypertension, secondary to pulmonary vasculitis.

Pleurisy with or without effusion is the most common pulmonary complication associated with rheumatoid arthritis. When present, the effusion is generally unilateral (often on the right side). Males appear to develop rheumatoid pleural complications more often than females. *Rheumatoid interstitial pneumonitis* is characterized by alveolar wall fibrosis, interstitial and intra-alveolar mononuclear cell infiltration, and lymphoid nodules. In severe cases,

Table 25-4 Common Irritant Gases Associated with Interstitial Lung Disease	
Gas	**Industrial Setting**
Chlorine	Chemical and plastic industries; Also used to disinfect water
Ammonia	Commercial refrigeration
Sulfur dioxide	Paper manufacture Smelting of sulfide ores
Ozone	Welding Manufacture of bleaches and peroxides
Nitrogen dioxide	May be liberated after exposure of nitric acid to air
Phosgene	Used in the production of aniline dyes

extensive fibrosing alveolitis and honeycombing may develop. Rheumatoid interstitial pneumonitis is more common in males. *Necrobiotic nodules* are characterized by the gradual degeneration and swelling of lung tissue. The pulmonary nodules generally appear as well-circumscribed masses that often progress to cavitation. The nodules usually develop in the periphery of the lungs and are more common in men. Histologically, the pulmonary nodules are identical to the subcutaneous nodules that develop in rheumatoid arthritis. *Caplan's syndrome* (also called rheumatoid pneumoconiosis) is a progressive pulmonary fibrosis of the lung commonly seen in coal miners. Caplan's syndrome is characterized by rounded densities in the lung periphery that often undergo cavity formation and, in some cases, calcification. *Pulmonary hypertension* is a common secondary complication caused by the progression of fibrosing alveolitis and pulmonary vasculitis.

Systemic lupus erythematosus.—Systemic lupus erythematosus (SLE) is a multisystem disorder that mainly involves the joints and skin. It may also cause serious problems in numerous other organs, including the kidneys, lungs, nervous system, and heart. Involvement of the lungs appears in about 50% to 70% of the cases. Pulmonary manifestations are characterized by (1) pleurisy with or without effusion, (2) atelectasis, (3) diffuse infiltrates and pneumonitis, (4) diffuse interstitial lung disease, (5) uremic pulmonary edema, (6) diaphragmatic dysfunction, and (7) infections.

Pleurisy with or without effusion is the most common pulmonary complication of SLE. The effusions are usually exudates with high protein concentration and are frequently bilateral. Atelectasis commonly develops in response to the pleurisy, effusion, and diaphragmatic elevation associated with SLE. Diffuse noninfectious pulmonary infiltrates and pneumonitis are common. In severe cases, chronic interstitial pneumonitis may develop. Because SLE frequently impairs the renal system, uremic pulmonary edema may occur. Recently, SLE has been found to be associated with diaphragmatic dysfunction and reduced lung volume. It is suggested that a diffuse myopathy affecting the diaphragm is the source of this problem. Approximately 50% of the cases have a complicating pulmonary infection.

Polymyositis-dermatomyositis.—*Polymyositis* is a diffuse inflammatory disorder of the striated muscles that primarily weakens the limbs, neck, and pharynx. *Dermatomyositis* is the term used when an erythematous skin rash accompanies the muscle weakness. Pulmonary involvement develops in response to (1) recurrent episodes of aspiration pneumonia caused by esophageal weakness and atrophy, (2) hypostatic pneumonia secondary to a weakened diaphragm, and (3) drug-induced interstitial pneumonitis.

Polymyositis-dermatomyositis is seen more often in females than males, at about a 2:1 ratio. The disease occurs primarily in two age groups: before the age of 10 and between 40 and 50 years of age. In about 40% of the patients, the pulmonary manifestations are seen 1 to 24 months before the striated muscle or skin signs of symptoms.

Progressive systemic sclerosis.—Progressive systemic sclerosis (also called scleroderma) is a disorder that primarily involves the skin and the small blood vessels. Involvement of other organ systems includes the esophagus, gastrointestinal tract, heart, lungs, and kidneys. The esophagus is the organ most often affected. Progressive systemic sclerosis of the lung appears in the form of interstitial lung disease and fibrosis. Of all the collagen vascular disorders, progressive systemic sclerosis is the one in which pulmonary involvement is most severe and most likely to cause significant scarring of the lung parenchyma.

The pulmonary complications include diffuse interstitial fibrosis, pulmonary vascular involvement, pleural disease, and aspiration pneumonitis (secondary to esophageal involvement). Progressive systemic sclerosis may also involve the small pulmonary blood vessels and appears to be independent of the fibrotic process involving the alveolar walls. The disease is most commonly seen in females between 30 and 50 years of age.

Sjögren's syndrome.—Sjögren's syndrome is a lymphocytic infiltration that primarily involves the salivary and lacrimal glands and is manifested by dry mucous membranes, usually of the mouth and eyes. Pulmonary involvement also frequently occurs in Sjögren's syndrome and includes (1) pleurisy with or without effusion, (2) interstitial fibrosis that is indistinguishable from that of other collagen vascular disorders, and (3) infiltration of lymphocytes of the tracheobronchial three mucus glands, which in turn causes atrophy of the mucous glands, mucus plugging, atelectasis, and secondary infections. Sjögren's syndrome occurs most often in women (90%) and is commonly associated with rheumatoid arthritis (50% of patients with Sjögren's syndrome).

Miscellaneous Diffuse Interstitial Lung Diseases
Goodpasture's Syndrome

Goodpasture's syndrome is a disease of unknown etiology that involves two organ systems—the lungs and the kidneys. In the lungs, there are recurrent episodes of pulmonary hemorrhage and, in some cases, pulmonary fibrosis—presumably as a consequence of the bleeding episodes. In the kidneys, there is a glomerulonephritis characterized by the infiltration of antibodies within the glomerular basement membrane. It is now known that these circulating antibodies function against the patient's own glomerular basement membrane. They are commonly abbreviated anti-GBM antibodies. It is believed that the anti-GBM antibodies cross-react with the basement membrane of the alveolar wall and that their deposition in the kidneys and lungs is responsible for producing the pathophysiologic processes of the disease.

Goodpasture's syndrome is usually seen in young adults. The average survival period after diagnosis is about 15 weeks. About 50% of the patients die from massive pulmonary hemorrhage, and about 50% die from chronic renal failure. An interesting feature of Goodpasture's syndrome is that the patient frequently demonstrates an increased D_{LCO}, which is in direct contrast to most interstitial lung disorders. The increased carbon monoxide uptake commonly seen in this disorder is thought to be due to the increased amount of retained blood in the alveolar spaces.

Idiopathic Pulmonary Hemosiderosis

Idiopathic pulmonary hemosiderosis is a disease entity of unknown etiology that is characterized by recurrent episodes of pulmonary hemorrhage similar to that seen in Goodpasture's syndrome. Histologic examination reveals an alveolar hemorrhage with hemosiderin-laden macrophages and hyperplasia of the alveolar epithelium. Unlike Goodpasture's syndrome, however, there is no evidence of circulating anti-GBM antibodies attacking the alveolar or glomerular basement membranes, and this disorder is not associated with renal disease.

Idiopathic pulmonary hemosiderosis is most often seen in children. As in Goodpasture's syndrome, patients commonly demonstrate an increased D_{LCO}, which is in direct contrast to most interstitial lung disorders. Again, the increased uptake of carbon monoxide is thought to be due to the increased amount of blood retained in the alveolar spaces.

Chronic Eosinophilic Pneumonia

Chronic eosinophilic pneumonia is characterized by infiltration of eosinophils and, to a lesser extent, macrophages into the alveolar and interstitial spaces. Clinically, a unique feature of this disorder is often seen on the chest radiograph, consisting of a peripheral distribution of pulmonary infiltrates. This radiographic pattern is commonly referred to as a *photographic negative of pulmonary edema.* This is because of the dense peripheral infiltration, with the sparing of the perihilar areas, seen in chronic eosinophilic pneumonia as compared to the central pulmonary infiltration, with the sparing of the lung periphery, seen in pulmonary edema. An increased number of eosinophils is also commonly seen in the peripheral blood. Histologic diagnosis is made by means of an open lung biopsy.

Bronchiolitis Obliterans with Organizing Pneumonia

Bronchiolitis obliterans with organizing pneumonia, more commonly known by the acronym BOOP, is characterized by connective tissue plugs in the small airways (hence the term bronchiolitis obliterans) and mononuclear cell infiltration of the surrounding parenchyma (hence the term organizing pneumonia). Although the majority of the BOOP cases have no identifiable cause and are therefore considered idiopathic, it has been associated with connective tissue disease, toxic gas inhalation, and infection. The chest radiograph commonly shows patchy infiltrates of alveolar rather than interstitial involvement.

Lymphangioleiomyomatosis

Lymphangioleiomyomatosis (LAM) is a rare disease of the smooth muscles of the lungs affecting women of childbearing age. It is characterized by the proliferation of nodules composed of atypical smooth muscles along the lymphatics of the lung, thorax, and abdomen. Common clinical features associated with LAM are recurrent pneumothorax, hemoptysis, and chylothorax. The diagnosis of LAM is confirmed with an open lung biopsy. The prognosis of LAM is poor; the disease slowly progresses over 2 to 10 years with death secondary to ventilatory failure.

Alveolar Proteinosis

Alveolar proteinosis is a disorder of unknown etiology. It is characterized by the filling of the alveoli with an amorphous proteinaceous material. The material is a lipoprotein similar to the pulmonary surfactant produced by the Type II cells. In addition, the alveolar macrophages are generally dysfunctional in this disorder. The disease is most commonly seen in adults between 20 and 50 years of age. Males are affected twice as often as females. The chest radiograph typically reveals bilateral infiltrates that are most prominent in the perihilar regions (butterfly pattern). It is often indistinguishable from pulmonary edema, but without cardiac enlargement. Air bronchograms are commonly seen. The diagnosis of alveolar proteinosis is confirmed by transbronchial or open lung biopsy.

OVERVIEW

OF THE CARDIOPULMONARY CLINICAL MANIFESTATIONS ASSOCIATED WITH
CHRONIC INTERSTITIAL LUNG DISEASES

❑ **INCREASED RESPIRATORY RATE**
Several pathophysiologic mechanisms operating simultaneously may lead to an increased ventilatory rate (see page 17):

- Stimulation of peripheral chemoreceptors
- Decreased lung compliance
- Stimulation of the J receptors
- Pain/anxiety

❏ **PULMONARY FUNCTION STUDY FINDINGS**

Expiratory Maneuver Findings (see page 39)

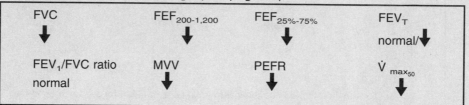

Lung Volume and Capacity Findings (see page 39)

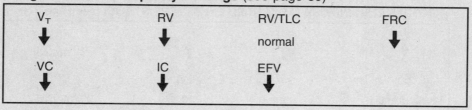

❏ **DECREASED DIFFUSION CAPACITY** (see page 48)

There is an exception to this finding in Goodpasture's syndrome and idiopathic pulmonary hemosiderosis. The D_{LCO} is commonly elevated in response to the increased amount of blood retained in the alveolar spaces that is associated with these two disorders.

❏ **INCREASED HEART RATE (PULSE), CARDIAC OUTPUT, AND BLOOD PRESSURE** (see page 86)

❏ **ARTERIAL BLOOD GASES**

Moderate Chronic Interstitial Lung Disease

Acute Alveolar Hyperventilation with Hypoxemia (see page 57)

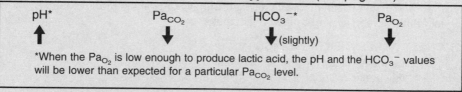

*When the Pa_{O_2} is low enough to produce lactic acid, the pH and the HCO_3^- values will be lower than expected for a particular Pa_{CO_2} level.

Severe Chronic Interstitial Lung Disease

Acute Ventilatory Failure with Hypoxemia (see page 59)

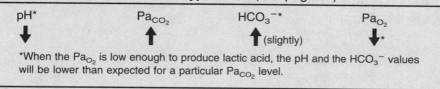

*When the Pa_{O_2} is low enough to produce lactic acid, the pH and the HCO_3^- values will be lower than expected for a particular Pa_{CO_2} level.

❑ **CYANOSIS** (see page 68)
❑ **OXYGENATION INDICES** (see page 69)

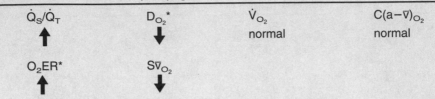

$$\dot{Q}_S/\dot{Q}_T \uparrow \qquad D_{O_2}{}^* \downarrow \qquad \dot{V}_{O_2} \text{ normal} \qquad C(a-\bar{v})_{O_2} \text{ normal}$$

$$O_2ER^* \uparrow \qquad S\bar{v}_{O_2} \downarrow$$

*The D_{O_2} may be normal in patients who have compensated for the decreased oxygenation status with an increased cardiac output. When the D_{O_2} is normal, the O_2ER is usually normal.

❑ **HEMODYNAMIC INDICES (ADVANCED OR SEVERE STAGE)** (see page 87)

CVP ↑	RAP ↑	$\overline{PA}$ ↑	PCWP normal
CO normal	SV normal	SVI normal	CI normal
RVSWI ↑	LVSWI normal	PVR ↑	SVR normal

❑ **POLYCYTHEMIA/COR PULMONALE** (see page 92)
- Distended neck veins
- Enlarged and tender liver
- Peripheral edema
- Pitting edema

❑ **DIGITAL CLUBBING** (see page 93)
❑ **COUGH (NONPRODUCTIVE)** (see page 93)
❑ **PLEURAL EFFUSION** (see chapter 19)
Pleural effusion is commonly associated with lymphomatoid granulomatosis, rheumatoid arthritis, and systemic lupus erythematosus.

❑ **CHEST ASSESSMENT FINDINGS** (see page 6)
- Increased tactile and vocal fremitus
- Dull percussion notes
- Bronchial breath sounds
- Crackles/rhonchi/wheezes
- Pleural friction rub
- Whispered pectoriloquy

❑ **RADIOLOGIC FINDINGS**
Chest radiograph
- Bilateral infiltrates
- Granulomas
- Cavity formation
- Honeycombing
- Air bronchograms
- Pleural effusion

Bilateral diffuse interstitial infiltrates and nodular densities in the lower lung lobes are the general radiographic appearance. Cavity formation is commonly associated with Wegener's granulomatosis, lymphomatoid granulomatosis, and rheumatoid arthritis (Fig. 25-2). Pleural effusion is commonly seen in patients with lymphomatoid granulomatosis, rheumatoid arthritis, systemic lupus erythematosus, and progressive systemic sclerosis (Fig. 25-3). A honeycomb or reticulonodular pattern may also be seen in patients with chronic interstitial lung disease (Fig. 25-4).

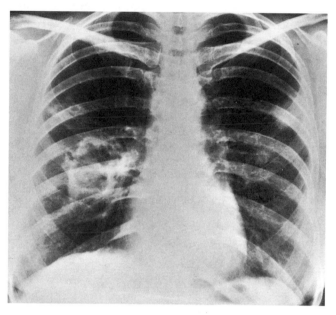

FIG 25-2

Wegener's granulomatosis. Multiple nodules with a large (6-cm) cavitary lesion adjacent to the right hilus. Its walls are thick and irregular. (Courtesy of Dr. G.J. Hunter, London.) (From Armstrong P, Wilson AG, Dee P: *Imaging of diseases of the chest,* St. Louis, 1990, Mosby-Year Book. Used by permission.)

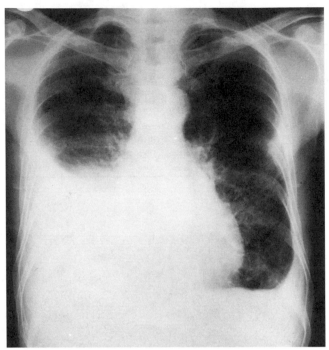

FIG 25-3
Pleural effusion in rheumatoid disease. Bilateral pleural effusions are present with mild changes of fibrosing alveolitis. The effusions were painless, and that on the right had been present, more or less unchanged, for 5 months. (From Armstrong P, Wilson AG, Dee P: *Imaging of diseases of the chest,* St. Louis, 1990, Mosby-Year Book. Used by permission.)

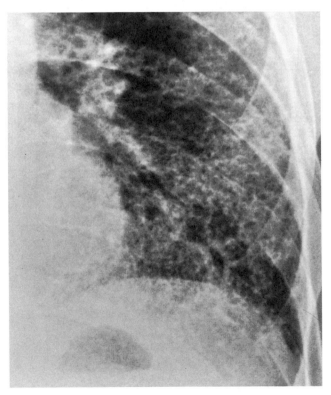

FIG 25-4
Reticulonodular pattern in a chest x-ray of a patient with interstitial pulmonary fibrosis due to scleroderma. (From Armstrong P, Wilson AG, Dee P: *Imaging of diseases of the chest,* St. Louis, 1990, Mosby-Year Book. Used by permission.)

GENERAL MANAGEMENT OF INTERSTITIAL LUNG DISEASES

The management of interstitial lung disorders is directed at the inflammation associated with the various disorders.

Medication

Corticosteroids.—Corticosteroids are commonly administered with reasonably good results, but the benefit varies remarkably from one patient to another (see Appendix V).

Sympathomimetics.—Sympathomimetic drugs may be helpful when smooth muscle constriction is present (see Appendix II).

Other agents.—In patients with Wegener's granulomatosis, the prognosis has dramatically improved since the development of cytotoxic agents (e.g., *cyclophosphamide*).

Supplemental Oxygen

Because of the hypoxemia associated with interstitial lung diseases, supplemental oxygen is often required. It should be noted, however, that the hypoxemia that develops in interstitial lung disorders is most commonly caused by the alveolar thickening, fibrosis, and capillary shunting associated with the disorder. Hypoxemia caused by capillary shunting is refractory to oxygen therapy.

Other

Plasmapheresis—Treatment of Goodpasture's syndrome is directed at reducing the circulating anti-GBM antibodies that attack the patient's glomerular basement membrane. Plasmapheresis, which directly removes the anti-GBM antibodies from the circulation, has been of some benefit.

• • • **INTERSTITIAL LUNG DISEASE CASE STUDY** • • •

ADMITTING HISTORY AND PHYSICAL EXAMINATION

This 57-year-old female had been well until seven years ago, when she noticed the onset of mild dyspnea and exertion. About the same time, a friend pointed out to her that her fingers were becoming clubbed; the patient had not been aware of this. Her past medical history revealed a 30 pack-year cigarette habit, and she had complained of a nonproductive "smoker's morning cough" for several years. Over the past four years, her dyspnea had increased gradually, until she had to resign from her job as a telephone operator. During this same period, she had occasional episodes of ankle swelling which were successfully treated with diuretics by her local physician. Six months prior to admission, she was given a course of corticosteroids, but this did not seem to improve her dyspnea to any appreciable degree.

Physical examination revealed a well-nourished, well-developed, middle-aged female in moderate respiratory distress while resting quietly in bed. There was marked clubbing of the fingers and toes, and there was obvious cyanosis of the lips and extremities. There was bilateral ankle and pretibial edema, described as +3. The neck veins were distended with the patient in a 30-degree head-up position, and the liver was tender. Blood pressure was 130/75 mm Hg, pulse 110/min, respirations 30/min. There were diffuse crackles at both bases.

A thoracoscopic lung biopsy was performed. A diagnosis of idiopathic pulmonary fibrosis was made. Laboratory examination revealed the following:

- Chest x-ray: diffuse interstitial fibrosis of lower 2/3 of both lungs
- ECG: right ventricular hypertrophy
- Lung scan: decreased ventilation and perfusion at both bases
- Pulmonary function studies

	Predicted normal	Patient	%
VC (cc)	2745	1350	49.2
RV (cc)	1945	750	38.6
TLC (cc)	4690	2050	43.7
D_{LCO}	25 ml/min/mm Hg	3.0 ml/min/mm Hg	12.0
FEF_{25-75}	2.36	2.05	80.0

- Blood Gases

	Rest Room Air	Rest O_2 3 l/min	Exercise O_2 5 l/min	Rest O_2 100%
pH	7.49	7.49	7.47	7.43
Pa_{CO_2}	29	28	29	35
Pa_{O_2}	27	52	33	96
Sa_{O_2}	62%	85%	66%	100%

RESPIRATORY ASSESSMENT AND PLAN

S: Complains of dyspnea and leg and ankle swelling.

O: Cyanotic on room air. BP 130/75; P 110; RR 30. +3 ankle and pretibial edema. Distended neck veins and tender liver. Crackles heard at both lung bases. CXR: fibrosis lower ⅔ of both lungs. Lung biopsy: idiopathic pulmonary fibrosis. ECG: cor pulmonale. PFTs: restrictive lung disease with severe diffusion blockade. ABG on room air and at rest: pH 7.49, Pa_{CO_2} 29, Pa_{O_2} 27.

A: • Idiopathic pulmonary fibrosis (biopsy)
  • Cor pulmonale (ECG)
  • Chronic alveolar hyperventilation with severe hypoxemia (ABG)

P: O_2 titration per oxygenation protocol. Deep breathing and coughing instruction. Smoking cessation protocol.

The possibility of lung transplantation was discussed with the patient. Although she was extremely concerned about the complexity and expense of such an operation, she agreed, with the full understanding that an appropriate donor would first have to be found. A modest diuresis followed aggressive oxygen titration. The physician prescribed home care oxygen therapy per protocol and discharged the patient the next day. A home care respiratory therapist visited her regularly and titrated her oxygen therapy as needed.

Over the next year the patient slowly but steadily deteriorated until she became almost totally incapacitated. Her ankle edema was +4. On continuous oxygen therapy, she could feed herself, but even this minimal activity exacerbated her already severe dyspnea. Sixteen months after she was discharged from the hospital, she was accepted as a lung transplant recipient candidate and, indeed, a double lung transplant was performed six weeks later. The patient did well and, at this writing, three months post-transplant, she is up and about. She remains on immunosuppressive therapy, but no longer requires supplemental oxygen.

DISCUSSION

In the past, the respiratory care of patients with interstitial lung disease was limited. Oxygen therapy was about all that was available to treat the uncomplicated disease. With the availability of lung transplantation, new vistas opened up. In this new setting, preoperative and postoperative evaluation of pulmonary function and exercise testing, diagnosis and treatment of infections associated with organ rejection, and intermittent bouts of reversible respiratory failure challenge the respiratory care practitioner.

Here, appropriately, we see that oxygen therapy is used for protocol. The hope obviously was that such therapy would improve not only the patient's symptoms, but her pulmonary arterial hypertension (cor pulmonale). Some centers are now studying the use of nitric acid aerosols in the treatment of both ARDS and the pulmonary hypertension seen in some lung transplant recipients.

SELF-ASSESSMENT QUESTIONS

Multiple Choice

1. Which of the following is another name for extrinsic allergic alveolitis?
    a. Sarcoidosis
    b. Hypersensitivity pneumonitis
    c. Alveolar proteinosis
    d. Idiopathic pulmonary hemosiderosis
    e. Chronic eosinophilic pneumonia
2. Which of the following allergic reactions appears to be the underlying cause for most of the pathologic changes associated with extrinsic allergic alveolitis?
    a. Type I: Anaphylaxis
    b. Type II: Cytotoxic
    c. Type III: Immune complex-mediated hypersensitivity
    d. Type IV: Cell-mediated reactions
    e. None of the above
3. Which of the following is/are associated with interstitial inflammation with granuloma formation?
    I. Rheumatoid arthritis
    II. Extrinsic allergic alveolitis
    III. Sarcoidosis
    IV. Churg-Strauss syndrome
    a. I only
    b. II only
    c. III and IV only
    d. II and III only
    e. II, III, and IV only
4. Eosinophilic granuloma is also called
    a. Histiocystosis X.
    b. Wegener's granulomatosis.
    c. Goodpasture's syndrome.
    d. Polymyositis-dermatomyositis.
    e. Alveolar proteinosis.
5. Which of the following is/are considered pulmonary vasculitides?
    I. Rheumatoid arthritis
    II. Wegener's granulomatosis
    III. Lymphomatoid granulomatosis
    IV. Churg-Strauss syndrome
    a. I only
    b. III only
    c. II, III, and IV only
    d. I, II, and III only
    e. I, II, III, and IV
6. Which of the following disorders is associated with desquamative interstitial pneumonia (DIP) and usual interstitial pneumonia (UIP)?
    a. Idiopathic pulmonary fibrosis
    b. Eosinophilic granuloma
    c. Rheumatoid arthritis
    d. Sarcoidosis
    e. Goodpasture's syndrome
7. Which of the following is/are collagen vascular diseases?
    I. Histiocystosis X
    II. Rheumatoid arthritis
    III. Sjögren's syndrome
    IV. Alveolar proteinosis
    a. I only
    b. III only
    c. II and IV only
    d. I and IV only
    e. II and III only

8. Which of the following pulmonary function study findings is/are associated with chronic interstitial lung diseases?
   I. Increased FRC
   II. Decreased FEV_T
   III. Increased RV
   IV. Decreased FVC
      a. I only
      b. III only
      c. II and IV only
      d. III and IV only
      e. II, III, and IV only

9. Which of the following hemodynamic indices is/are associated with advanced or severe interstitial lung disease?
   I. Increased CVP
   II. Decreased PCWP
   III. Increased $\overline{PA}$
   IV. Decreased RAP
      a. I only
      b. IV only
      c. I and III only
      d. II and IV only
      e. I, III, and IV only

10. A pleural effusion is commonly associated with which of the following chronic interstitial lung diseases?
    I. Systemic lupus erythematosus
    II. Rheumatoid arthritis
    III. Lymphomatoid granulomatosis
    IV. Goodpasture's syndrome
       a. I only
       b. III only
       c. II and IV only
       d. III and IV only
       e. I, II, and III only

Answers appear in Appendix XXI.

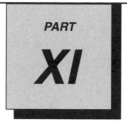

PART

XI

NEUROLOGIC DISORDERS AND SLEEP APNEA

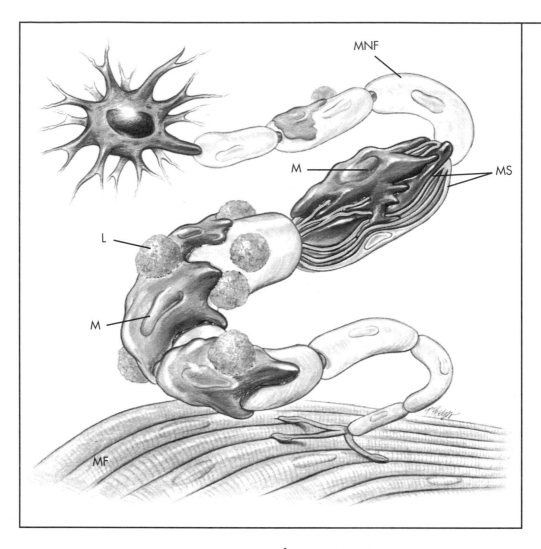

GUILLAIN-BARRÉ SYNDROME

FIG 26-1

Guillain-Barré syndrome. Lymphocytes and macrophages attacking and stripping away the myelin sheath of a peripheral nerve. *MNF* = myelinated nerve fiber; *L* = lymphocyte; *M* = macrophage; *MS* = myelin sheath (cross-sectional view; note the macrophage attacking the myelin sheath); *MF* = muscle fiber. (See also Plate 25.)

CHAPTER 26

Guillain-Barré Syndrome

ANATOMIC ALTERATIONS ASSOCIATED WITH THE GUILLAIN-BARRÉ SYNDROME

The Guillain-Barré syndrome is a relatively rare disorder of the peripheral nervous system in which flaccid paralysis of the skeletal muscles and loss of reflexes develop in a previously healthy patient. In severe cases, paralysis of the diaphragm and ventilatory failure can develop. Clinically, this is a medical emergency. If the ventilatory failure is not properly managed, mucus accumulation, airway obstruction, alveolar consolidation, and atelectasis can develop (see Fig 1-1).

Paralysis of the skeletal muscles develops in response to various pathologic changes in the peripheral nerves. Microscopically, the nerves show demyelination, inflammation, and edema. As the anatomic alterations of the peripheral nerves intensify, the ability of the neurons to properly transmit impulses to the muscles decreases, and eventually paralysis ensues (Fig 26-1).

Other names found in the literature for the Guillain-Barré syndrome are as follows:

- Postinfectious polyneuritis
- Acute idiopathic polyneuritis
- Landry-Guillain-Barré-Strohl syndrome
- Landry's paralysis
- Acute postinfections polyneuropathy
- Acute polyradiculitis
- Polyradiculoneuropathy

To summarize, the major pathologic or structural changes of the lungs associated with the ventilatory failure that may accompany Guillain-Barré syndrome are as follows:

- Mucus accumulation
- Airway obstruction
- Alveolar consolidation
- Atelectasis

ETIOLOGY

The precise cause of the Guillain-Barré syndrome is not known. It is probably an immune disorder (humoral factor) that causes inflammation and deterioration of the patient's peripheral nervous system. Studies of serial serum samples have shown high antibody titers during the early stages of the disorder. Elevated levels of specific antibodies include IgM and the presence of what are called the *complement-activating antibodies* against isolated human peripheral nerve myelin, or anti-PNM antibodies. Studies have shown that the serum antibody titers fall rapidly during the recovery period.

Lymphocytes and macrophages appear to attack and strip off the myelin sheath of the peripheral nerves and leave swelling and fragmentation of the neural axon (see Fig 26-1). It is believed that the myelin sheath covering the peripheral nerves (or the myelin-producing Schwann cell) is the actual target of the immune attack.

The onset of the Guillain-Barré syndrome frequently follows a febrile episode such as an upper respiratory or gastrointestinal illness within one to four weeks. Multiple viruses and some bacterial agents have been implicated as precursors to the Guillain-Barré syndrome. Infectious mononucleosis, for example, has been associated with as many as 25% of the cases. Other possible infective agents include parainfluenza 2, vaccinia, variola, measles, mumps, hepatitis A and B viruses, *Mycoplasma pneumoniae, Salmonella typhi,* and *Chlamydia psittaci.* Although the significance of the association is controversial, during the nationwide immunization campaign in the United States in 1976, more than 40 million adults were vaccinated with swine influenza vaccine, and more than 500 cases of the Guillain-Barré syndrome were reported among the vaccinated individuals, with 25 deaths.

The annual incidence of Guillain-Barré syndrome in the United States is about 1.7 cases per 100,000. Although uncommon in early childhood, the condition may occur in all age groups and in either sex. A greater incidence has been noted among people 45 years of age and older, among males, and among whites (50% to 60% greater in whites). There is no obvious seasonal clustering of cases.

If diagnosed early, patients with the Guillain-Barré syndrome have an excellent prognosis. The diagnosis is typically based on the history of the neurologic symptoms, the nature of the cerebrospinal fluid, and the electrodiagnostic studies. If the Guillain-Barré syndrome is present, the cerebrospinal fluid shows an increased protein concentration with a normal cell count. Serial electrodiagnostic studies in multiple nerves in both the upper and lower extremities provide important data in making the diagnosis as well as in determining the location and severity of the lesions. Functional, spontaneous recovery is expected in about 85% to 95% of the cases, although about 40% may have some minor residual symptoms.

COMMON NONCARDIOPULMONARY MANIFESTATIONS

- Progressive ascending skeletal muscle paralysis
- Tingling sensation and numbness (distal paresthesia)
- Loss of deep tendon reflexes
- Sensory nerve impairment
- Peripheral facial weakness
- Decreased gag reflex
- Decreased ability to swallow

The early symptoms of the Guillain-Barré syndrome include fever, malaise, nausea, and prostration, with a subsequent tingling sensation and numbness in the extremities (distal paresthesia). The feet and lower portions of the legs are usually affected first. The tingling and numbness are followed by skeletal muscle paralysis and the loss of deep tendon reflexes.

The muscle paralysis then moves upward (ascending paralysis) to the arms, neck, and pharyngeal and facial muscles (cranial nerves IX and X). The muscle weakness and paralysis commonly develop over a single day, although it may develop over a period of several days. Paralysis generally peaks in less than 10 days. Sensory nerve impairment may also be present. The patient's gag reflex is generally decreased or absent, and swallowing is usually difficult (dysphagia). Thus, the handling of oral secretions is usually a problem.

Although the Guillain-Barré syndrome is typically an ascending paralysis (i.e., moving from the lower portions of the legs upward), muscle paralysis may affect the facial and arm muscles first and then move downward. While it is more common for the weakness to be symmetrical, a single arm or leg may be involved before paralysis spreads. The paralysis may also affect all four limbs simultaneously. Progression of the paralysis may stop at any point. Once the paralysis reaches its maximum, it usually remains unchanged for a few days or weeks. Improvement generally begins spontaneously and continues for weeks or, in rare cases, months.

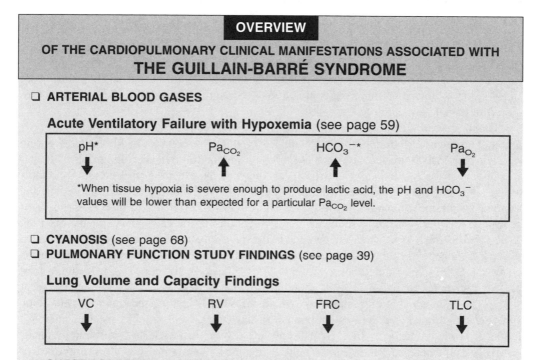

OVERVIEW

OF THE CARDIOPULMONARY CLINICAL MANIFESTATIONS ASSOCIATED WITH
THE GUILLAIN-BARRÉ SYNDROME

❏ **ARTERIAL BLOOD GASES**

Acute Ventilatory Failure with Hypoxemia (see page 59)

pH*	Pa_{CO_2}	HCO_3^-*	Pa_{O_2}
↓	↑	↑	↓

*When tissue hypoxia is severe enough to produce lactic acid, the pH and HCO_3^- values will be lower than expected for a particular Pa_{CO_2} level.

❏ **CYANOSIS** (see page 68)
❏ **PULMONARY FUNCTION STUDY FINDINGS** (see page 39)

Lung Volume and Capacity Findings

VC	RV	FRC	TLC
↓	↓	↓	↓

❏ **CHEST ASSESSMENT FINDINGS** (see page 6)
 • Diminished breath sounds
 • Crackles/rhonchi

❏ **RADIOLOGIC FINDINGS**
Chest radiograph
 • Normal
 • Increased opacity (when atelectasis is present)

If the ventilatory failure associated with Guillain-Barré syndrome is properly managed, the chest x-ray should be normal. If improperly managed, however, alveolar consolidation and atelectasis develop from excess secretion accumulation in the tracheobronchial tree. This increases the density of the lung segments affected.

❏ **AUTONOMIC NERVOUS SYSTEM DYSFUNCTIONS**
 • Heart rate and rhythm abnormalities
 • Blood pressure abnormalities

Autonomic nervous system dysfunction develops in about 50% of the cases. The autonomic dysfunction involves the overreaction or underreaction of the sympathetic or parasympathetic nervous system. Clinically the patient may manifest various cardiac arrhythmias such as sinus tachycardia (the most common), bradycardia, ventricular tachycardia, atrial flutter, atrial fibrillation, and asystole. Hypertension and hypotension may also be seen. Although the loss of bowel and bladder sphincter control is uncommon, transient sphincter paralysis may occur during the evolution of symptoms. The autonomic involvement may be transient or may persist throughout the duration of the disorder.

GENERAL MANAGEMENT OF THE GUILLAIN-BARRÉ SYNDROME

The Guillain-Barré syndrome is a potential medical emergency that must be monitored closely after the diagnosis has been made. The primary treatment should be directed at stabilization of vital signs and supportive care for the patient. Initially, such patients should be managed in an intensive care unit. Frequent measurements of the patient's vital capacity, blood pressure, oxygen saturation, and arterial blood gases should be performed. Mechanical ventilation should be administered when the clinical data demonstrate impending or acute ventilatory failure. Routine pulmonary toilet should be instituted to prevent mucus accumulation, airway obstruction, alveolar consolidation, and atelectasis.

As in any patient who is paralyzed, the risk of thromboembolic events increases. Because of this, the patient commonly receives subcutaneously administered heparin, elastic stockings, and passive range-of-motion exercises (every 3 to 4 hours) for all extremities.

To prevent skin breakdown and bedsores, the patient should be turned frequently from side to side. A rotary bed or Stryker frame may be required. Urinary catheterization is required in completely paralyzed patients.

Blood pressure disturbances and cardiac arrhythmias require immediate attention. For example, nitroprusside (Nipride) or phentolamine (Regitine) are commonly administered during severe hypertensive episodes. Episodes of bradycardia may be treated with atropine.

In severe cases, *plasmapheresis* has been shown to be effective in decreasing the morbidity and shortening the clinical course of Guillain-Barré syndrome. Plasmapheresis is the removal of plasma from withdrawn blood, with retransfusion of the formed elements. This procedure has been shown to reduce antibody titers during the early stages of the disorder. Type-specific fresh frozen plasma or albumin is generally used to replace the withdrawn plasma. As a general rule, a fairly conservative plasmapheresis regimen is performed: an exchange of 200 to 250 ml/kg over a period of 7 to 14 days. In the normal-sized adult, a total of five exchanges of 3 L each over a period of 8 to 10 days is usually adequate. Recent studies have shown that plasmapheresis within the first 7 days of the onset of neurologic symptoms significantly decreases the number of days the patient requires mechanical ventilation. It is recommended, however, that only the severely affected and worsening patients receive plasmapheresis. Patients with mild symptoms or symptoms that have improved or plateaued should not undergo plasmapheresis.

Because the Guillain-Barré syndrome is believed to be immunologically mediated, anti-inflammatory and immunosuppressive agents are commonly administered. Corticosteroids are frequently used, but their effectiveness is controversial.

Mobilization of Bronchial Secretions

Because of the mucus accumulation associated with Guillain-Barré syndrome, a number of respiratory therapy modalities may be used to enhance the mobilization of bronchial secretions (see Appendix XI).

Hyperinflation Techniques

Hyperinflation techniques may be ordered to offset the alveolar consolidation and atelectasis associated with Guillain-Barré syndrome (see Appendix XII).

Supplemental Oxygen

Because hypoxemia may develop in Guillain-Barré syndrome, supplemental oxygen may be required. It should be noted, however, that because of the alveolar consolidation and atelectasis associated with Guillain-Barré syndrome, capillary shunting may be present. Hypoxemia caused by capillary shunting and not alveolar hypoventilation is refractory to oxygen therapy.

• • • **GUILLAIN-BARRÉ SYNDROME CASE STUDY** • • •

ADMITTING HISTORY AND PHYSICAL EXAMINATION

A 46-year-old male lawyer was quite well until 10 days prior to admission when, after a polio and influenza vaccination, he developed generalized malaise. There was no evidence of an upper respiratory infection, and the malaise continued for four days. On awakening on the fifth day, he noticed some weakness of the pelvic girdle. This was followed by severe muscular and testicular pain, which responded poorly to aspirin. Two days prior to admission, he developed weakness in all four extremities. At this time, there was no difficulty in breathing and no change in the quality of his voice. His weakness progressed over the next 24 hours, and he was brought to the hospital by ambulance.

Physical examination revealed a well-nourished, well-developed male in obvious respiratory distress with rapid, shallow, abdominal breathing. Blood pressure was 186/116, pulse 84/min, and respirations 32/min. The cranial nerves, the sternocleidomastoids, and the trapezius were intact. There was decreased vibratory sense in the lower extremities, but otherwise the sensory exam results were negative. The remainder of the examination was negative, other than the obvious and profound weakness of all the affected muscles and diminished-to-absent deep tendon reflexes in all four extremities.

A chest x-ray was unremarkable. On room air, arterial blood gas values were pH 7.33, Pa_{CO_2} 47, HCO_3^- 24, Pa_{O_2} 71. A spinal tap revealed clear CSF. There were no cells, but the spinal fluid protein was 110 mg/dl. The respiratory therapist recorded the following:

RESPIRATORY ASSESSMENT AND PLAN

S: Complains of dyspnea and inability to take a deep breath.

O: Appears anxious; dyspneic. Voice is nasal. BP 186/116, P 84, RR 32 and shallow. Weak in all four extremities. Lungs clear. CXR: normal. On room air, pH 7.33, Pa_{CO_2} 47, HCO_3^- 24, Pa_{O_2} 71.

A: • Muscle weakness? Etiology? Physician ruling out Guillain-Barré syndrome.
  • Possible impending ventilatory failure (history, ABG trend)

P: Follow FVC and NIF every hour (qh). Continuous oximetry. Stand by to intubate and ventilate.

The physician made the diagnosis of Guillain-Barré syndrome and admitted the patient to the respiratory ICU to be monitored closely. His vital capacity was 3500 ml on admission but decreased to 700 ml during the subsequent 48 hours. During this time, he also developed mild difficulties in swallowing. Shortly after this development, the pulse oximeter alarm sounded and the physician was notified. Since it was anticipated that the patient would require respiratory assistance for several weeks, a tracheostomy was performed under local anesthesia, and the patient was connected to a ventilator with an $F_{I_{O_2}}$ 0.3, IMV rate 12/min, V_T 0.8 L, PSV mode. Twenty minutes later his blood gas values were pH 7.43, Pa_{CO_2} 38, HCO_3^- 23, Pa_{O_2} 104, Sa_{O_2} 97%. The following respiratory care assessment was then entered in the patient's chart:

RESPIRATORY ASSESSMENT AND PLAN

S: N/A (patient on ventilator)

O: Appears comfortable on present ventilator settings. Lungs clear. On present ventilatory setting, ABGs are pH 7.43, Pa_{CO_2} 38, HCO_3^- 23, Pa_{O_2} 104, Sa_{O_2} 97%.

A: • Stable on present ventilatory settings (ABG)
  • Slow recovery from Guillain-Barré syndrome (history)

P: Wean ventilator and O_2 therapy per ventilator weaning protocol as tolerated. Suction as needed.

Over the next three weeks, the patient remained almost totally paralyzed, with the exception of the extrinsic eye muscles, some muscles of facial expression, and the sternocleidomastoids. He also developed bilateral lower lobe pneumonia that required intensive antibiotic therapy. Tracheobronchial secretions were troublesome and required frequent suctioning.

One afternoon, there was a sudden onset of tachycardia, fever, and chest pain. At this point, this respiratory assessment was entered in the patient's chart:

RESPIRATORY ASSESSMENT AND PLAN

S: Indicates (by pointing) that he has left lower chest pain.

O: Anxious. P 170 regular, BP 160/90. T 39.6° C. Lungs clear. CXR: new left lower lobe infiltrate/atelectasis. Sa_{O_2} 78%.

A: Possible acute pulmonary embolism (chest pain & CXR)

P: Contact physician to discuss present condition and concerns. Increase $F_{I_{O_2}}$ per oxygenation protocol.

A ventilation-perfusion lung scan was ordered by the physician. It showed a small pulmonary embolism and infarction in the left lower lung lobe. The patient was heparinized, and the chest pain disappeared shortly. Plasmapheresis was performed on two occasions, but resulted in no appreciable improvement.

One month after admission, he started to regain muscle strength, and from that time on his recovery was dramatic. His vital capacity increased almost daily, and six weeks after admission the ventilator was discontinued. The tracheostomy tube was removed three days later, and the patient was discharged three days after this. Throughout his illness, he was given passive and then active physical therapy. One month after discharge, he was able to resume his practice, with only minimal residual weakness of the left leg.

DISCUSSION

The key to respiratory care in cases of Guillain-Barré syndrome is to have an attitude of "watchful expectancy." Serial NIF and FVC determinations are absolutely core to following the waxing and waning status of the muscular respiratory pump in this condition. Of course, alarming oximeters are also helpful, but frequent assessments of respiratory muscle strength are also necessary.

Although ventilatory care is usually straightforward in these individuals, since there is no basic intrinsic lung disease, the situation can always be complicated by pneumonia, excess secretions, or as in this case, pulmonary embolism. The latter condition almost certainly arose out of this patient's prolonged immobility. At any rate, the care of such patients is often prolonged, and the respiratory care practitioner has a good chance to become acquainted with his patient during this interval.

SELF-ASSESSMENT QUESTIONS

Multiple Choice

1. In Guillain-Barré syndrome, which of the following pathologic changes develop in the peripheral nerves?
   - I. Inflammation
   - II. Increased ability to transmit nerve impulses
   - III. Demyelination
   - IV. Edema
        - a. I and IV only
        - b. II and III only
        - c. III and IV only
        - d. II, III, and IV only
        - e. I, III, and IV only

2. Which of the following is associated with Guillain-Barré syndrome?
   - I. Alveolar consolidation
   - II. Mucus accumulation
   - III. Alveolar hyperinflation
   - IV. Atelectasis
        - a. I only
        - b. I and II only
        - c. III and IV only
        - d. I, II, and IV only
        - e. II, III, and IV only

3. The incidence of Guillain-Barré syndrome is greater in
   - I. People older than 45 years of age.
   - II. Blacks than in whites.
   - III. Males than in females.
   - IV. Early childhood.
        - a. I only
        - b. IV only
        - c. I and III only
        - d. III and IV only
        - e. II and III only

4. Which of the following is/are possible precursors to the Guillain-Barré syndrome?
   - I. Mumps
   - II. Swine influenza vaccine
   - III. Infectious mononucleosis
   - IV. Measles
        - a. I and III only
        - b. II and IV only
        - c. III and IV only
        - d. II, III, and IV only
        - e. I, II, III, and IV

5. Spontaneous recovery from Guillain-Barré syndrome is expected in about what percentage of cases?
        - a. 45 to 55
        - b. 55 to 65
        - c. 65 to 75
        - d. 75 to 85
        - e. 85 to 95

True or False

1. In Guillain-Barré syndrome a tingling sensation and numbness usually begins in the feet and lower portions of the legs.   True _____   False _____
2. Guillain-Barré syndrome is called a descending paralysis.   True _____   False _____

3. Paralysis in Guillain-Barré syndrome usually takes about 12 weeks to peak.   True _____   False _____

4. Hypertension and hypotension are associated with Guillain-Barré syndrome.   True _____   False _____

5. Plasmapheresis has been shown to reduce the antibody titers during the early stages of Guillain-Barré syndrome.   True _____   False _____

Answers appear in Appendix XXI.

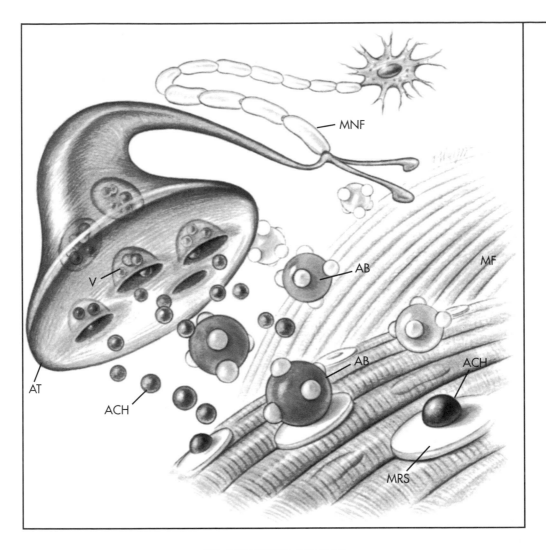

MYASTHENIA GRAVIS

FIG 27-1

Myasthenia gravis. Disorder of the neuromuscular junction that interferes with the chemical transmission of acetylcholine. *MNF* = myelinated nerve fiber; *AT* = axonal terminal; *V* = vesicle; *ACh* = acetylcholine; *MF* = muscle fiber; *MRS* = muscle receptor site; *AB* = antibody. Note that the antibodies have a similar physical structure to that of ACh, which in turn permits them to connect to (and block ACh from) the muscle receptor sites. (See also Plate 26.)

Myasthenia Gravis

ANATOMIC ALTERATIONS ASSOCIATED WITH MYASTHENIA GRAVIS

Myasthenia gravis is a chronic disorder of the neuromuscular junction that interferes with the chemical transmission of acetylcholine (ACh) between the axonal terminal and the receptor sites of voluntary muscles (Fig 27-1). It is characterized by periods of fatigue, with improvement following rest. Because the disorder affects only the myoneural junction, there is no loss of sensory function.

The abnormal fatigability may be confined to an isolated group of muscles (e.g., the drooping of one or both eyelids), or it may manifest as a generalized weakness that, in severe cases, includes the diaphragm. When the diaphragm is involved, ventilatory failure can develop. If the ventilatory failure is not properly managed, mucus accumulation, airway obstruction, alveolar consolidation, and atelectasis can develop (see Fig 1-1).

ETIOLOGY

The cause of myasthenia gravis appears to be related to circulating antibodies of the autoimmune system (anti-ACh receptor antibodies). It is believed that the antibodies disrupt the chemical transmission of ACh at the neuromuscular junction by (1) blocking the ACh from the receptor sites of the muscular cell, (2) accelerating the breakdown of ACh, and (3) destroying the receptor sites (see Fig 27-1). While it is not clear what events activate the formation of the antibodies, the thymus gland is almost always abnormal. Because of this fact, it is generally presumed that the antibodies arise within the thymus or in related tissue.

The incidence of myasthenia gravis ranges between 1 in 10,000 and 1 in 25,000 persons in the United States. It is at least twice as common in women as in men. The disease usually has a peak age of onset in females between 15 and 35 years as compared with 40 to 70 years of age in males. The clinical manifestations associated with myasthenia gravis are often provoked by emotional upset, physical stress, exposure to extreme temperature changes, febrile illness, or pregnancy. Death caused by myasthenia gravis is possible, especially during the first few years after onset. After the disease has been in progress for 10 years, however, death from myasthenia gravis is rare.

The diagnosis of myasthenia gravis is based on (1) the clinical history, (2) the clinical response to an intravenous injection of edrophonium chloride (Tensilon), (3) electrophysiological tests of neuromuscular transmission, and (4) the amount of circulating antibodies in the blood.

In regard to the clinical history, muscular weakness without sensory involvement, changes in consciousness, and autonomic dysfunction are early signs of myasthenia gravis. Because the disease is relatively uncommon and because the symptoms fluctuate from hour to hour, day to day, and week to week, the patient is often misdiagnosed or not diagnosed until the disorder has progressed to a more generalized and consistent weakness.

The diagnosis is usually confirmed with the *Tensilon test.* Tensilon (edrophonium chloride), which is a short-acting drug, blocks cholinesterase from breaking down ACh after is has been released from the terminal axon. This action increases the concentration of ACh, which in turn works to offset the influx of antibodies at the neuromuscular junction. When muscular weakness is caused by myasthenia gravis, a dramatic transitory improvement in muscle function (lasting about 10 minutes) is seen after the administration of Tensilon.

To further support the diagnosis of myasthenia gravis, *electromyography* is usually performed to confirm the diagnosis, identify specific muscles involved, and determine the degree of fatigability. Electromyography entails the repetitive stimulation of a nerve, such as the ulnar, with the simultaneous recording of the muscle response. Clinically, the degree of fatigability is often evaluated by having the patient use certain muscles for a sustained period of time. For example, the patient may be instructed to gaze upward for an extended period of time, to blink continuously, to hold both arms outstretched as long as possible, or to count aloud as long as possible in one breath (normal is about 50). A dynamometer is sometimes used to measure the force of repetitive muscle contractions.

Finally, measurement of the circulating anti-ACh receptor antibodies in the blood may also be helpful. Antibody titers are detectable in the serum of 50% to 85% of myasthenic patients. Special chest x-ray films can show an enlarged thymus gland, which may also support the diagnosis of myasthenia gravis.

COMMON NONCARDIOPULMONARY MANIFESTATIONS

Weakness of striated muscles

- Eye muscles (ptosis)
  - Drooping of the upper eyelids
- Extraocular muscles (diplopia)
  - Double vision
- Muscles of the lower portion of the face
  - Speech impairment
- Chewing and swallowing muscles (dysphagia)
- Muscles of the arms and legs

The onset of myasthenia gravis is usually gradual. The drooping of one or both upper eyelids (ptosis), followed by double vision (diplopia) due to weakness of the external ocular muscles, is usually the first symptom. Weakness of the external ocular muscles is usually asymmetrical and may progress to complete external paralysis in one or both eyes. For some patients, these may be the only symptoms. This condition is called *ocular myasthenia.*

In many patients, however, the disease progresses to a generalized skeletal muscle disorder. In such patients, the lower facial and neck muscles are almost always affected. The orbicularis oris is usually weak, which causes a vertical snarl when attempting to smile. Chewing and swallowing become difficult as the muscles of the jaw, soft palate, and pharynx weaken. The patient may also regurgitate food and fluid through the nose when swallowing. Muscle fatigue in the pharyngeal area represents a significant danger since food and fluids may be *aspirated.* During periods of muscle fatigue, the patient's ability to articulate frequently deteriorates, and the voice is usually high and nasal in quality. Weakness of the neck muscles commonly causes the patient's head to fall forward. Clinically, the patient is often seen to support the chin with one hand to either hold the head up or to assist in speaking.

As the disorder becomes more generalized, weakness develops in the arms and legs. The muscle weakness is usually more pronounced in the proximal parts of the extremities. The patient has difficulty in climbing stairs, lifting objects, maintaining balance, and walking. In severe cases, the weakness of the upper limbs may be such that the hand cannot be lifted to the mouth. Muscle atrophy or pain is rare. A notable characteristic of myasthenia gravis is that the tendon reflexes almost always remain intact.

Finally, it should be stressed that the clinical manifestations during the early stages of the disorder are often elusive. The patient may (1) demonstrate normal health for weeks or months at a time, (2) only show signs of weakness late in the day or evening, or (3) develop a sudden and transient generalized weakness that includes the diaphragm. *Ventilatory failure* is always a sinister possibility.

If the ventilatory failure associated with myasthenia gravis is properly managed, the chest x-ray findings should be normal. If improperly managed, however, alveolar consolidation and atelectasis develop from excess secretion accumulation in the tracheobronchial tree. Common cardiopulmonary clinical manifestations associated with these anatomic alterations are as follows:

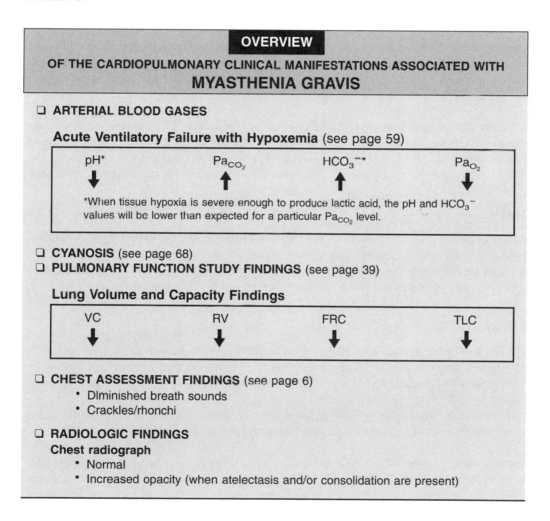

OVERVIEW
OF THE CARDIOPULMONARY CLINICAL MANIFESTATIONS ASSOCIATED WITH
MYASTHENIA GRAVIS

❏ **ARTERIAL BLOOD GASES**

Acute Ventilatory Failure with Hypoxemia (see page 59)

pH^*	Pa_{CO_2}	HCO_3^{-*}	Pa_{O_2}
↓	↑	↑	↓

*When tissue hypoxia is severe enough to produce lactic acid, the pH and HCO_3^- values will be lower than expected for a particular Pa_{CO_2} level.

❏ **CYANOSIS** (see page 68)
❏ **PULMONARY FUNCTION STUDY FINDINGS** (see page 39)

Lung Volume and Capacity Findings

VC	RV	FRC	TLC
↓	↓	↓	↓

❏ **CHEST ASSESSMENT FINDINGS** (see page 6)
- Diminished breath sounds
- Crackles/rhonchi

❏ **RADIOLOGIC FINDINGS**
Chest radiograph
- Normal
- Increased opacity (when atelectasis and/or consolidation are present)

GENERAL MANAGEMENT OF MYASTHENIA GRAVIS

Formerly many patients with myasthenia gravis died within the first few years of the disease. Today, there are a number of therapeutic measures that provide many patients with marked relief of symptoms and allow them to live a normal life span. Because there is the possibility of ventilatory failure in patients with myasthenia gravis, the patient should be monitored closely during critical periods. Frequent measurements of the patient's vital capacity, blood pressure, oxygen saturation, and arterial blood gases should be performed. Mechanical ventilation should be administered when the patient's clinical data demonstrate impending or acute ventilatory failure. The routine pulmonary hygiene protocol should be instituted to prevent mucus accumulation, airway obstruction, alveolar consolidation, and atelectasis.

During a myasthenic crisis, the following treatment modalities may also be used:

Drug Therapy

Drugs used to enhance the action of ACh are used to treat myasthenia gravis. The most popular agents are edrophonium chloride (Tensilon), neostigmine (Prostigmin), and pyridostigmine (Mestinon). These agents inhibit the function of cholinesterase. This action in effect increases the concentration of ACh to compete with the circulating anti-ACh antibodies, which interfere with the ability of ACh to stimulate the muscle receptors. Although the anticholinesterase drugs are very effective in mild cases of myasthenia gravis, they are not completely effective in severe cases.

Corticosteroid therapy.—The patient's strength often improves strikingly with steroids (e.g., prednisone). Patients receiving long-term steroid therapy, however, frequently develop various complications such as cataracts, gastrointestinal bleeding, infections, aseptic necrosis of the bone, osteoporosis, myopathies, and psychoses.

Adrenocorticotropic hormone therapy.—The administration of adrenocorticotropic hormone (ACTH) has proved useful in severely ill myasthenia gravis patients. A disadvantage to this therapy, however, is that patients tend to worsen before improving. Paradoxically, patients who demonstrate the greatest initial weakness often show the most improvement later.

Thymectomy

Although controversial, thymectomy has been helpful in many myasthenia gravis patients, especially young adult females. The thymus gland in the myasthenic patient frequently appears to be the source of anti-ACh receptor antibodies. In some patients, muscle strength improves soon after surgery, while in others it takes months or years.

Respiratory Care

Mobilization of bronchial secretions.—Because of the mucus accumulation associated with myasthenia gravis, a number of respiratory therapy modalities may be used to enhance the mobilization of bronchial secretions (see Appendix XI).

Hyperinflation techniques.—Hyperinflation techniques may be ordered to offset the alveolar consolidation and atelectasis associated with myasthenia gravis (see Appendix XII).

Supplemental oxygen.—Because hypoxemia may develop in myasthenia gravis, supplemental oxygen may be required. It should be noted, however, that because of the alveolar consolidation and atelectasis associated with myasthenia gravis, capillary shunting may be present. Hypoxemia caused by capillary shunting is refractory to oxygen therapy.

• • • • █ MYASTHENIA GRAVIS CASE STUDY █ • • • •

ADMITTING HISTORY AND PHYSICAL EXAMINATION

This was the second hospital admission for a 61-year-old male who was well until about eight months earlier when he noticed the development of diplopia, followed by the weakness of the neck muscles and the muscles of the shoulder girdle. On admission to the hospital at that time, a diagnosis of myasthenia gravis was made.

He was started on pyridostigmine bromide (Mestinon), 300 mg at 7 AM, 11 AM, and 2 PM; 240 mg at 5 PM; and 260 mg of Mestinon Timespan at 10 PM. He was also given ranitidine, ephedrine, and amytal. On this regime, he rapidly improved and was discharged from the hospital.

He did well for about six months, but then noticed that his voice tired quickly and that he could walk only about 100 feet. Four days prior to the current admission, he became nauseated and could not take all his medication. He felt progressively weaker until the morning of admission. He had not been taking any medication except ranitidine for the last 24 hours. In the emergency room, he was given edrophonium chloride (Tensilon), 2.5 mg IV, which improved the strength of his neck and arm muscles for a short while.

Physical examination revealed a chronically ill male in moderate distress. His blood pressure was 140/90, pulse was 110/min, and his respiratory rate was 12/min. His lungs were clear to auscultation, and he was afebrile. He had marked weakness of the extraocular muscles, with diplopia, and weakness of cranial nerves V and VII. All muscles of the extremities were weak, and the biceps and triceps reflexes were absent. All other reflexes were hypoactive. A chest x-ray was normal. His FEV_1 was 600 ml. On room air his ABG values were pH 7.28, Pa_{CO_2} 63, HCO_3^- 25, and Pa_{O_2} 59. The respiratory therapist recorded this SOAP note in the patient's chart:

RESPIRATORY ASSESSMENT AND PLAN

S: Complains of generalized weakness, anxiety, and mild shortness of breath.

O: Alert, afebrile. BP 140/90, P 110, RR 10. FEV_1 600 ml. Lungs clear. CXR unremarkable. On room air, pH 7.28 Pa_{CO_2} 63, HCO_3^- 25, Pa_{O_2} 59. Tensilon test results positive.

A: • Myasthenia gravis (clinical trends moving from stable to severe)
   • Acute ventilatory failure with moderate hypoxemia (ABG)

P: Contact physician and report clinical findings. Continuous oximetry, hourly FVC and FEV_1 measurements. Respiratory therapist to remain on standby to intubate and mechanically ventilate. O_2 per vent mask at 24% oxygen, then per oxygenation protocol.

Thirty minutes after the physician reviewed the above clinical findings, the patient was transferred to ICU. Initially, the patient was treated conservatively and monitored closely. In spite of increasing anticholinesterase medication, the patient's respiratory function and arterial blood gas status continued to decrease rapidly. Two hours after admission to ICU, the patient was intubated and ventilated. All medication was discontinued, and he remained on the ventilator for 14 days with no remarkable complications.

At the end of this period, the anticholinesterase regime was restarted and his strength began to return. He could breathe spontaneously for increasingly long periods of time. He was weaned from the respirator after 21 days. Over the next 10 days, his Mestinon dosage could be gradually reduced, and he was discharged from the hospital on less than his original daily dose of Mestinon.

DISCUSSION

As was the case with Guillain-Barré syndrome discussed in Chapter 26, again, we are here dealing with a neurologic disorder that impacts on skeletal muscle and, most importantly, on the function of the chest wall and diaphragm. The treatment here, as noted, is the use of anticholinesterase medications, which once adequately titered can usually control the situation.

Respiratory therapists should be aware that a condition called *pseudomyasthenia gravis* occurs in patients with pulmonary malignancy, and a careful look at the chest x-ray in this connection may be indicated. Otherwise, the care of these patients is much as is discussed in Chapter 26.

SELF-ASSESSMENT QUESTIONS

True or False

1. Alveolar hyperinflation is associated with myasthenia gravis.　　　　　True _____ False _____

2. The cause of myasthenia gravis appears to be related to circulating antibodies that disrupt the transmission of acetylcholine.　　　　　True _____ False _____

3. Myasthenia gravis is more common in men than women.　　　　　True _____ False _____

4. Tensilon is used to confirm the diagnosis of myasthenia gravis because of its ability to block cholinesterase.　　　　　True _____ False _____

5. The onset of myasthenia gravis is usually sudden.　　　　　True _____ False _____

6. In myasthenia gravis, the extremity muscles (arms and legs) are usually the first to weaken.　　　　　True _____ False _____

7. Neostigmine is used to treat patients with myasthenia gravis.　　　　　True _____ False _____

8. A thymectomy may be beneficial in young adult females with myasthenia gravis.　　　　　True _____ False _____

9. In males, the incidence of myasthenia gravis is greatest between 15 and 35 years of age.　　　　　True _____ False _____

10. After the disease has been in progress for 10 years, death from myasthenia gravis is rare.　　　　　True _____ False _____

Answers appear in Appendix XXI.

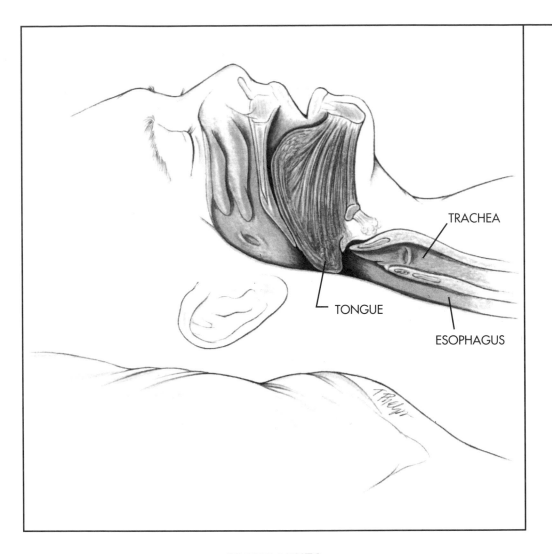

SLEEP APNEA

FIG 28-1

Obstructive sleep apnea. When the genioglossus muscle fails to oppose the collapsing force on the airway passage during inspiration, the tongue moves into the oropharyngeal area and obstructs the airway. (See also Plate 27.)

Sleep Apnea

Despite the fact that the clinical characteristics of sleep apnea have been described in the literature for centuries, it was not until the late 1970s or early 1980s that this disorder became generally acknowledged by the medical community. Prior to this time, it was assumed that individuals who breathed normally while awake also did so during sleep. It was also assumed that patients with lung disorders were not likely to develop more severe respiratory problems when asleep than when awake. Both of these assumptions are now recognized as being incorrect.

STAGES OF SLEEP AND CHARACTERISTIC CARDIOPULMONARY PATTERNS

During sleep, the normal individual slips in and out of two major stages: *nonrapid eye movement* (non-REM) sleep (also called quiet or slow-wave sleep) and *rapid eye movement* (REM) sleep (also called active or dreaming sleep). Each stage is associated with characteristic electroencephalographic (EEG), behavioral, and breathing patterns.

Non-REM Sleep

Non-REM sleep usually begins immediately after an individual dozes off. This stage consists of four separate phases, each progressing into a deeper sleep. During phases 1 and 2, the ventilatory rate and tidal volume continually increase and decrease, and brief periods of apnea may be seen. The EEG tracing shows an increased slow-wave activity (slow-wave sleep) and loss of alpha rhythm. The occurrence of apnea is greater in persons over 40 years of age. Cheyne-Stokes respiration is also commonly seen in older adult males during non-REM sleep, especially at high altitudes.

During phases 3 and 4, ventilation becomes slow and regular. The minute ventilation is commonly 1 to 2 L/min less than during the quiet wakeful state. Typically, the Pa_{CO_2} levels are higher (4 to 8 mm Hg), the Pa_{O_2} levels are lower (3 to 10 mm Hg), and the pH is lower (0.03 to 0.05 units).

Normally, non-REM sleep lasts for about 60 to 90 minutes. Although an individual typically moves in and out of all four phases during non-REM sleep, most of the time is spent in phase 2. An individual may move into REM sleep at any time and directly from any of the four non-REM sleep phases, although the lighter phases (1 and 2) are commonly the levels of sleep just prior to REM sleep.

REM Sleep

During REM sleep, there is a burst of fast alpha rhythms in the EEG tracing. During this period, the ventilatory rate becomes rapid and shallow. Sleep-related hypoventilation and apnea are frequently demonstrated during this period. Apnea in the normal adult lasts about 15 to 20 seconds; in the normal infant, apnea lasts about 10 seconds. There is a marked reduction in both the hypoxic ventilatory response and the hypercapnic ventilatory response during REM sleep. The heart rate also becomes irregular, and the eyes move rapidly. Dreaming occurs mainly during REM sleep, and there is a profound paralysis of movement. The skeletal muscle paralysis primarily affects the arms, legs, and intercostal and upper airway muscles. The activity of the diaphragm is maintained.

The muscle paralysis that occurs during REM sleep can affect an individual's ventilation in two major ways: *first,* since the muscle tone of the intercostal muscles is low during this period, the negative intrapleural pressure generated by the diaphragm often causes a paradoxical motion of the rib cage. That is, during inspiration the tissues between the ribs move inward, and during expiration the tissues bulge outward. This paradoxical motion of the rib cage causes the functional residual capacity to decrease. During the wakeful state, the intercostal muscle tone tends to stiffen the tissue between the ribs. *Second,* the loss of muscle tone in the upper airway involves muscles that normally contract during each inspiration and hold the upper airway open. These muscles include the posterior muscles of the pharynx, the genioglossus (which normally causes the tongue to protrude outward), and the posterior cricoarytenoid (the major abductor of the vocal cords). *The loss of muscle tone in the upper airway may result in airway obstruction.* The negative pressure produced when the diaphragm contracts during inspiration tends to bring the vocal cords together, collapse the pharyngeal wall, and suck the tongue back into the oral pharyngeal cavity.

REM sleep lasts about 5 to 40 minutes and recurs about every 60 to 90 minutes. The REM sleep period lengthens and becomes more frequent toward the end of a night's sleep. REM sleep constitutes about 20% to 25% of sleep time. Most studies show that it is more difficult to awaken a subject during REM sleep.

TYPES OF SLEEP APNEA

Apnea is defined as the cessation of breathing for a period of 10 seconds or longer. Sleep apnea is diagnosed in patients who have at least 30 episodes of apnea that occur in both non-REM and REM sleep over a 6-hour period. Generally, the episodes of apnea are more frequent and severe during REM sleep. They last about 20 to 30 seconds and occasionally may exceed 100 seconds. Some patients have as many as 500 periods of apnea per night. It may occur in all age groups; in infants, it may play an important role in sudden infant death syndrome (SIDS).

Sleep apnea is classified as *obstructive, central,* or *mixed apnea.* Patients often have more than one type and are classified according to the predominant type.

Obstructive Sleep Apnea

Obstructive sleep apnea is the sleep disorder most commonly encountered in the clinical setting. It is caused by an anatomic obstruction of the upper airway in the presence of continued ventilatory effort (Fig 28-1). During periods of obstruction patients commonly appear quiet and still, as if holding their breath, followed by increasingly desperate efforts to inhale. Often, the apneic episode ends only after an intense struggle. In severe cases, the patient may suddenly awaken, sit upright in bed, and gasp for air. Interestingly, however, patients with obstructive sleep apnea usually demonstrate perfectly normal and regular breathing patterns during the wakeful state.

Obstructive sleep apnea is seen more often in males than in females (8:1 ratio), and it is especially common in middle-aged men. It is estimated that 1% to 4% of the male population may be affected. It is commonly associated with obesity and with individuals who have a short neck, a combination that may significantly narrow the pharyngeal airway. In fact, a large number of patients with obstructive sleep apnea demonstrate the *pickwickian syndrome* (named after the fat boy in Charles Dickens' *The Posthumous Papers of the Pickwick Club,* published in 1837). Charles Dickens' description of Joe, the fat boy who snored and had excessive daytime sleepiness, included many of the classic features of what are now recognized as the sleep apnea syndrome. It should be emphasized, however, that many patients with sleep apnea are not obese and, therefore, clinical suspicion should not be limited to this group.

Some clinical disorders associated with the cause of obstructive sleep apnea are as follows:

- Obesity (hypoventilation syndrome)
- Anatomic narrowing of upper airway
  - Excessive pharyngeal tissue
  - Enlarged tonsils or adenoids
  - Deviated nasal septum
  - Laryngeal stenosis
  - Laryngeal web
  - Pharyngeal neoplasms
  - Micrognathia
  - Macroglossia
  - Goiter
- Hypothyroidism
- Testosterone administration
- Myotonic dystrophy
- Shy Drager syndrome
- Down syndrome

The general *noncardiopulmonary clinical manifestations of obstructive sleep apnea* can be summarized as follows:

- Loud snoring
- Morning headaches
- Nausea
- Excessive daytime sleepiness (hypersomnolence)
- Intellectual and personality changes
- Depression
- Sexual impotence
- Nocturnal enuresis

Central Sleep Apnea

Central sleep apnea occurs when the respiratory centers of the medulla fail to send signals to the respiratory muscles. It is characterized by cessation of airflow at the nose and mouth along with cessation of inspiratory efforts (absence of diaphragmatic excursions), as opposed to obstructive sleep apnea, which is characterized by the presence of inspiratory efforts during apneic periods. Central sleep apnea is associated with central nervous system disorders. As already mentioned, a small number of brief central apneas normally occur with the onset of sleep or the onset of REM sleep. Central sleep apnea, however, is diagnosed when the frequency of the apnea episodes is excessive (over 30 in a 6-hour period).

Clinical disorders associated with central sleep apnea include the following:

* Idiopathic (hypoventilation syndrome)
* Encephalitis
* Brain stem neoplasm
* Brain stem infarction
* Bulbar poliomyelitis
* Cervical cordotomy
* Spinal surgery
* Hypothyroidism

The general *noncardiopulmonary clinical manifestations of central sleep apnea* can be summarized as follows:

* Tendency for the patient to be of normal weight
* Mild snoring
* Insomnia
* Although not as great as in obstructive apnea, there may be some of the following:
  · Daytime fatigue
  · Depression
  · Sexual dysfunction

Mixed Sleep Apnea

Mixed sleep apnea is a combination of obstructive and central sleep apneas. It usually begins as central apnea followed by the onset of ventilatory effort without airflow (obstructive apnea). Clinically, patients with predominantly mixed apnea are classified as having obstructive sleep apnea.

Figure 28-2 summarizes the *patterns of airflow, respiratory effort* (reflected through the esophageal pressure), and *arterial oxygen saturation* in central, obstructive, and mixed apneas.

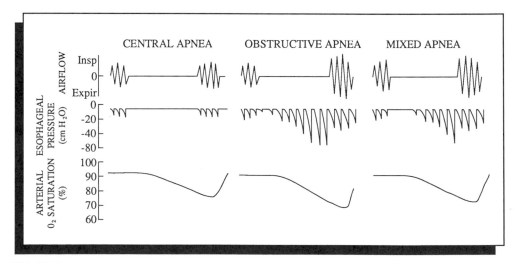

FIG 28-2

Patterns of airflow, respiratory efforts (reflected through the esophageal pressure), and arterial oxygen saturation produced by central, obstructive, and mixed apneas.

DIAGNOSIS

The diagnosis of sleep apnea begins with the history of the patient, especially the presence of snoring, sleep disturbance, and persistent daytime sleepiness. This is followed by a careful examination of the upper airway and by pulmonary function studies to determine whether there is an upper airway obstruction.

The patient's blood is evaluated for the presence of polycythemia and thyroid function. Arterial blood gas values are obtained to determine the oxygenation and acid-base status. A chest x-ray film and electrocardiogram (ECG) are helpful in evaluating the presence of pulmonary hypertension, the state of right and left ventricular compensation, and the presence of any other cardiopulmonary disease.

The diagnosis and type of sleep apnea is confirmed with polysomnographic sleep studies, which include (1) an EEG and an electro-oculogram to identify the sleep stages; (2) a monitoring device for airflow in and out of the patient's lungs; (3) an ECG to identify cardiac arrhythmias; (4) either impedance pneumography, intercostal electromyography, or esophageal manometry to monitor the patient's ventilatory rate and effort; and (5) ear oximetry or transcutaneous oxygen monitoring to detect changes in the patient's oxygen saturation.

Patients diagnosed as having predominantly central sleep apnea are evaluated carefully for lesions involving the brain stem. Patients diagnosed as having obstructive sleep apnea may undergo a computed tomographic evaluation or a cephalometric head x-ray of the upper airway to determine the site(s) and severity of the pharyngeal narrowing.

The steps typically involved in diagnosing sleep apnea can be summarized as follows:

* History
* Examination of the neck and upper airway
* Spirometry (flow-volume loops in the erect and supine positions)
* Arterial blood gases
* Hemoglobin
* Nocturnal recording oximetry
* Thyroid function
* Chest radiograph
* Electrocardiogram
* Polysomnographic (sleep) study
* Computed axial tomographic scan of the upper airway (obstructive apnea) or cephalometric head x-ray.

OVERVIEW

OF THE CARDIOPULMONARY CLINICAL MANIFESTATIONS ASSOCIATED WITH

SLEEP APNEA

❑ **ARTERIAL BLOOD GASES**

Severe Sleep Apnea

Chronic Ventilatory Failure with Hypoxemia (see page 59)

pH	Pa_{CO_2}	HCO_3^-	Pa_{O_2}
normal	↑	↑ (significantly)	↓

Acute Ventilatory Changes Superimposed on Chronic Ventilatory Failure (see page 65)

Because acute ventilatory changes are frequently seen in patients with chronic venti-latory failure, the respiratory care practitioner must be familiar with and be on alert for (1) *acute alveolar hyperventilation superimposed on chronic ventilatory failure,* and (2) *acute ventilatory failure superimposed on chronic ventilatory failure.*

❏ **CYANOSIS** (see page 68)
❏ **OXYGENATION INDICES** (see page 69)

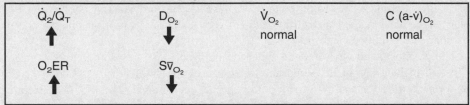

❏ **HEMODYNAMIC INDICES (SEVERE SLEEP APNEA)** (see page 87)

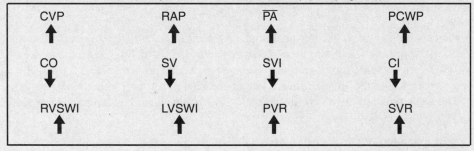

During periods of apnea, the heart rate decreases, followed by an increase after the termination of apnea. It is believed that the carotid body peripheral chemoreceptors are responsible for this response, i.e., when ventilation is kept constant or absent (e.g., apneic episode), it is known that hypoxic stimulation of the carotid body peripheral che-moreceptors *slows* the cardiac rate. Thus, it follows that when the lungs are unable to expand (e.g., periods of obstructive apnea), the depressive effect of the carotid bodies on the heart rate predominates. The increased heart rate noted when ventilation re-sumes is activated by the excitation of the pulmonary stretch receptors.

Although changes in cardiac output during periods of apnea have been difficult to study, several studies have reported a reduction in cardiac output (about 30%) during periods of apnea, followed by an increase (10% to 15% above controls) after the ter-mination of apnea.

Both pulmonary and systemic arterial blood pressures increase in response to the nocturnal oxygen desaturation that develops during periods of sleep apnea. The mag-nitude of the pulmonary hypertension is related to the severity of the alveolar hypoxia and hypercapnic acidosis. It is believed that repetition of these transient episodes of pulmonary hypertension, many times a night every night for years, may contribute to the development of the ventricular hypertrophy, cor pulmonale, and eventual decom-pensation seen in such patients. Systemic vasoconstriction secondary to sympathetic adrenergic neural activity is believed to be responsible for the elevation in systemic blood pressure that is seen during apneas.

❏ **CARDIAC ARRHYTHMIAS**
  • Sinus arrhythmia
  • Sinus bradycardia
  • Sinus pauses
  • Atrioventricular block (second degree)
  • Premature ventricular contraction
  • Ventricular tachycardia

In severe cases of sleep apnea, there is always a possibility of a sudden arrhythmia-related death. Periods of apnea are commonly associated with sinus arrhythmias, sinus bradycardia, and sinus pauses (greater than 2 seconds). The extent of sinus bradycardia is directly related to the severity of the oxygen desaturation. Obstructive apneas are usually associated with the greatest degrees of cardiac slowing. To a lesser extent, atrioventricular heart blocks (second degree), premature ventricular contractions, and ventricular tachycardia are seen. Identification of apnea-related ventricular tachycardia is viewed as a life-threatening event.

❑ **PULMONARY FUNCTION STUDY FINDINGS** (see page 39)

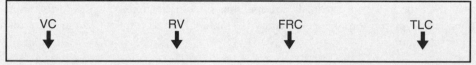

Patients with obstructive sleep apnea commonly demonstrate a sawtooth pattern on maximal inspiratory and expiratory flow-volume loops. Also characteristic of obstructive sleep apnea is a ratio of expiratory-to-inspiratory flow rates at 50% of the vital capacity ($FEF_{50\%}/FIF_{50\%}$) that exceeds 1.0 in the absence of obstructive airway disease.

In addition, because the muscle tone of the intercostal muscles is low during periods of REM apneas, the negative intrapleural pressure generated by the diaphragm often causes a paradoxical motion of the rib cage, that is, during inspiration the tissue between the ribs moves inward, and during expiration the tissue bulges outward. This paradoxical motion of the rib cage may cause the VC, RV, FRC, and TLC to decrease. This pathologic condition further contributes to the nocturnal hypoxemia seen in patients with sleep apnea syndrome.

❑ **RADIOLOGIC FINDINGS**
Chest radiograph
   • Right- or left-sided heart failure

Because of the pulmonary hypertension and polycythemia associated with persistent periods of apnea, right- and left-sided heart failure may develop. This condition is readily identified on a chest x-ray film and may help in diagnosis.

GENERAL MANAGEMENT OF SLEEP APNEA

Over the past few years, it has become apparent that many pathologic conditions are associated with sleep apnea, including hypoxemia, fragmented sleep, cardiac arrhythmias, and neurologic disorders. In general, the prognosis is more favorable for obstructive and mixed apneas than for central sleep apnea.

Weight Reduction

Many patients with obstructive sleep apnea are overweight, and although the weight alone is not the cause of the apnea, weight reduction clearly parallels the reduction in apnea severity. The precise reason is not known. Because weight reduction may take months and because it is often difficult to maintain a certain weight loss, weight reduction as a single form of therapy often fails.

Sleep Posture

It is generally believed that most obstructive apnea is more severe in the supine position and, in fact, may only be present in this position. Apnea and daytime hypersomnolence have significantly improved in some patients who have been instructed to sleep on their sides and avoid the supine posture. Others may benefit from sleeping in a head-up position—for example, in a lounge chair. The effect of this can be documented by recording oximetry in the supine and lateral decubitus positions.

Oxygen Therapy

Because of the hypoxemia-related cardiopulmonary complications of apnea (arrhythmias and pulmonary hypertension), oxygen therapy is commonly used to offset or minimize the oxygen desaturation.

Drug Therapy

There is one major type of drug used to treat sleep apnea: REM inhibitors.

REM Inhibitors

Protriptyline hydrochloride.—The most frequent and severe episodes of apnea occur during REM sleep in patients with obstructive sleep apnea. Protriptyline hydrochloride, which is a tricyclic antidepressant, causes a marked decrease in REM sleep. By decreasing the amount of REM sleep, the incidence of REM apneic episodes is also decreased. Some patients demonstrate improved upper airway muscle tone during REM and non-REM sleep when administered protriptyline hydrochloride. A reduction in daytime hypersomnolence may also be seen. Protriptyline hydrochloride is not therapeutic for central sleep apnea.

Surgery

Some non-obese patients with obstructive sleep apnea benefit from surgical correction or bypass of the anatomic defect or obstruction that is responsible for the apneic episodes. The following procedures are presently available:

Tracheostomy.—A tracheostomy is often the treatment of choice in emergency situations and in patients who do not respond satisfactorily to drug therapy or to other treatment interventions.

Palatopharyngoplasty.—A laser palatopharyngoplasty is a relatively new procedure in treating obstructive sleep apnea. In general, the soft palate is shortened by removing the posterior third, including the uvula. The pillars of the palatoglossal arch and the palatopharyngeal arch are sewn together, and the tonsils are removed if they are still present. As much excess lateral posterior wall tissue is removed as possible. Palatopharyngoplasty is effective in a small proportion of cases.

Mandibular advancement.—Approximately 6% of patients with obstructive sleep apnea have a mandibular malformation. For example, patients who have obstructive sleep apnea because of retrognathia or mandibular micrognathia may benefit from surgical mandibular advancement.

Mechanical Ventilation

Continuous positive airway pressure.—As mentioned earlier, the cause of many obstructive sleep apneas is related to (1) an anatomic configuration of the pharynx and (2) the decreased muscle tone that normally develops in the pharynx during REM sleep. When these patients inhale, the pharyngeal muscles and surrounding tissues are sucked inward in response to the negative airway pressure generated by the contracting diaphragm. Nocturnal continuous positive airway pressure (CPAP) is useful in preventing the collapse of the hypotonic airway and is the standard treatment for most cases of obstructive sleep apnea (Fig 28-3). CPAP is not indicated in pure central sleep apnea.

Continuous mechanical ventilation.—Intubation and continuous mechanical ventilation may be used for short-term therapy when acute ventilatory failure develops in central or obstructive sleep apnea.

Negative-pressure ventilation.—In patients with central sleep apnea, the noninvasive approach of negative-pressure ventilation without an endotracheal tube may be useful. For example, a negative-pressure cuirass, which is applied to the patient's chest and upper portion of the abdomen, may effectively control a patient's ventilation throughout the night. A negative-pressure cuirass is convenient for home use. Negative-pressure ventilation is contraindicated in obstructive sleep apnea.

Phrenic Nerve Pacemaker

The implantation of an external phrenic nerve pacemaker may be useful in patients with central sleep apnea since these patients experience apnea because of the absence of a signal sent from the central nervous system to the diaphragm by way of the phrenic nerve. This procedure, however, has not received wide application.

Medical Devices

Tongue-retaining device.—In some patients whose obstructive sleep apnea is caused by a large tongue, a tongue-retaining device may be helpful. A major problem with this therapy,

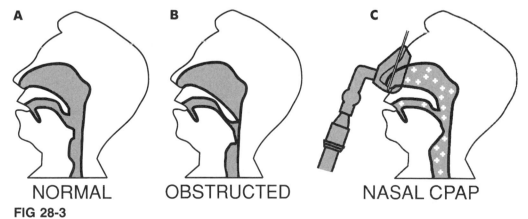

NORMAL   OBSTRUCTED   NASAL CPAP

FIG 28-3
A, Normal airway. **B,** Obstructed airway during sleep. **C,** Nasal CPAP generates a positive pressure and holds airway open during sleep.

Table 28-1 Therapy Modalities for Sleep Apnea

Therapy	Obstructive	Central
Oxygen therapy	Therapeutic	Therapeutic
Drugs		
REM inhibitor		
Protriptyline hydrochloride	Therapeutic	Not indicated
Surgical		
Tracheostomy	Therapeutic (100%)	Not indicated
Palatopharyngoplasty	Therapeutic	Not indicated
Mandibular advancement	Therapeutic	Not indicated
Mechanical ventilation		
Continuous positive airway pressure	Therapeutic	Not indicated
Mechanical ventilation	Short-term	Short-term
Negative-pressure ventilation	Contraindicated	Therapeutic
Endotracheal tube at night	Short-term	Not indicated
Phrenic nerve pacemaker	Not indicated	Experimental
Medical devices	Experimental	Not indicated

however, is that it is quite uncomfortable and, because of this fact, patient compliance is often low.

Neck collar.—It has been reported that a small number of patients have used a collar (similar to those used to stabilize cervical fractures) to increase the diameter of the airway and reduce the apnea. The therapeutic success of this procedure is questionable.

Other Therapeutic Approaches

Regardless of the type of sleep apnea, the patient should be advised to avoid drugs that depress the central nervous system. For example, alcohol and sedatives have been shown to increase the severity and frequency of sleep apnea. Weight loss should be encouraged in all obese apnea patients.

Table 28-1 summarizes the major therapy modalities for obstructive and central apnea and their effectiveness.

• • OBSTRUCTIVE SLEEP APNEA (OSA) CASE STUDY • •

ADMITTING HISTORY AND PHYSICAL EXAMINATION

A 42-year-old obese male sought medical advice because of excessive daytime sleepiness and impotence of increasing severity over a period of three months. History was not contributory except that the patient admitted moderate, but daily alcohol use. Discussion with the patient's wife revealed that the patient was snoring so consistently and so loudly that she was forced to sleep in a separate bedroom.

On physical examination he was found to be in no acute distress, and cooperative. He was 5'10" tall and weighed 147 kg. He had a blood pressure of 152/90 and pulse of 92 bpm. The remainder of the physical examination was within normal limits. The laboratory examination showed a Hct. of 46%. The remainder of the hemogram, urinalysis, and hepatic and renal functions were within normal limits.

The patient was referred to the sleep disorders laboratory of a nearby university hospital where monitoring during sleep revealed frequent (30/hr) apneic episodes (up to 60 seconds in duration), episodic oxygen desaturation to 70%, and cyclical bradycardia. A diagnosis of obstructive sleep apnea was made. An initial, conservative program of weight reduction was instituted, with advice to abstain from all alcoholic beverages and to sleep in the lateral decubitus position, with the head of the bed elevated.

On return visit two months later, it was found that the patient had gained 20 kg and had not abstained from alcohol. His daytime sleepiness was not improved. He snored just as much as before. There was 2+ leg edema. His lungs were clear to auscultation, and ECG revealed a sinus of tachycardia of 110 bpm. An S_3 heart sound was noticed, and P_2 was prominent. Chest x-ray showed right-sided cardiac enlargement without pulmonary infiltrates. In the sleep disorders laboratory, an awake room air ABG analysis showed pH 7.35, Pa_{CO_2} 55, HCO_3^- 30, and Pa_{O_2} 61. He was admitted to the hospital. At this time, the respiratory care practitioner entered the following:

RESPIRATORY ASSESSMENT AND PLAN

S: "I'm sleepy and my wife complains of my snoring."

O: Patient is somnolent. Obese (147 kg). 2+ pitting edema of legs. Heart enlarged in CXR. Lungs clear to auscultation. ABG: pH 7.35, Pa_{CO_2} 55, HCO_3^- 30, Pa_{O_2} 61. ECG: sinus rhythm, rate 110 ppm.

A: • Obstructive sleep apnea (diagnosis)
• Morbid obesity (physical exam)
• Cor pulmonale (x-ray & physical exam)
• Chronic ventilatory failure with mild hypoxemia (ABG)

P: Set up ECG and oximetric monitoring. Nasal oxygen at 1 lpm and titrate upward if Sa_{O_2} is less than 88%. Schedule nasal CPAP titration and trial.

The patient's apneic syndrome was found to be relieved by +10 cm H_2O CPAP delivered through a large CPAP mask. Despite use of a "ramping feature" and nasal pillows, he still could not tolerate the mask, and requested that it be discontinued after the third night. The possibility of a uvulopalatopharyngoplasty (UPPP) was discussed with him. He was informed that the chances of significant improvement with this procedure were less than 50%. The patient indicated that he understood this, but still wanted the procedure performed, since his present condition was increasingly burdensome.

Accordingly, a UPPP procedure was performed under general anesthesia. Following the procedure, the patient's condition was very much improved and the daytime somnolence was dramatically improved. He went on a strict weight reduction diet. Two months later, the patient agreed to a follow-up sleep study, which revealed only an occasional, mild apnea-related decrease in peripheral oxygen saturation and no bradyarrhythmia. The patient's wife reported that the snoring was very much decreased and that the couple had resumed normal sexual relations.

DISCUSSION

This patient with obstructive sleep apnea demonstrated the classic *pickwickian syndrome*. He was obese, snored, and had excessive daytime sleepiness. While asleep, he had frequent apneic and oxygen desaturation episodes. He was sexually impotent and had chronic ventilatory failure with hypoxemia, and cor pulmonale.

Nocturnal CPAP was initially administered to prevent the inward collapse of the oropharynx that develops during REM sleep. The low-flow oxygen was titrated to relieve the hypoxemia, but care was taken not to give too much oxygen and, possibly, knock out the patient's hypoxic drive. When this failed, a UPPP was performed to surgically widen the oral pharynx. Tracheostomy was the only other alternative. A strict weight reduction diet was ordered to supplement the benefit of the UPPP. Fortunately, this patient was in the group that responds favorably to this therapy.

The respiratory care practitioner will find himself caring for only the sickest of patients with obstructive sleep apnea, as the vast majority are diagnosed and treated as outpatients. When a preexisting cardiopulmonary disease such as chronic bronchitis is complicated by obesity and obstructive sleep apnea, the patient is clearly starting from a more vulnerable position, even when awake. In that situation, his resting awake hypoxemia is compounded by the nocturnal hypoventilation. Care of both the primary pulmonary disease and the coincidental respiratory pump disease is the key to success in this setting.

SELF-ASSESSMENT QUESTIONS

Multiple Choice

1. Nonrapid eye movement (non-REM) sleep is also called
   I. Slow-wave sleep.
   II. Active sleep.
   III. Dreaming sleep.
   IV. Quiet sleep.
      a. I only
      b. III only
      c. IV only
      d. I and IV only
      e. II and III only

2. During non-REM sleep, ventilation becomes slow and regular during which phase(s)?
   I. Phase 1
   II. Phase 2
   III. Phase 3
   IV. Phase 4
      a. II only
      b. III only
      c. I and II only
      d. II and III only
      e. III and IV only

3. The pickwickian syndrome is associated with which of the following?
   I. Central sleep apnea
   II. Obesity
   III. Loud snoring
   IV. Obstructive sleep apnea
   V. Absence of diaphragmatic excursion
      a. I only
      b. IV only
      c. I and V only
      d. IV and V only
      e. II, III, and IV only

4. During periods of apnea, the patient commonly demonstrates
   I. Systemic hypotension.
   II. Decreased cardiac output.
   III. Increased heart rate.
   IV. Pulmonary hypertension.
      a. I and III only
      b. II and IV only
      c. III and IV only
      d. I, II, and III only
      e. II, III, and IV only

5. Periods of severe sleep apnea are commonly associated with
   I. Ventricular tachycardia.
   II. Sinus bradycardia.
   III. Premature ventricular contraction.
   IV. Sinus arrhythmia.
      a. I and IV only
      b. II and III only
      c. III and IV only
      d. II, III, and IV only
      e. I, II, III, and IV

6. During REM sleep, there is paralysis of the
    I. Arm muscles.
    II. Upper airway muscles.
    III. Leg muscles.
    IV. Intercostal muscles.
    V. Diaphragm.
        a. IV only
        b. V only
        c. IV and V only
        d. I, II, III, and IV only
        e. I, II, III, IV, and V

7. Normally, REM sleep constitutes about what percentage of the total sleep time?
        a. 5 to 10
        b. 10 to 20
        c. 20 to 25
        d. 25 to 30
        e. 35 to 40

8. Which of the following therapy modalities are therapeutic for obstructive apnea?
    I. Phrenic pacemaker
    II. CPAP
    III. Theophylline
    IV. Negative-pressure ventilation
        a. I only
        b. II only
        c. III and IV only
        d. I and IV only
        e. I, II, III, and IV

9. Which of the following therapy modalities are therapeutic for central sleep apnea?
    I. Negative-pressure ventilation
    II. CPAP
    III. Tracheostomy
    IV. Endotracheal tube at night
        a. I only
        b. II only
        c. III only
        d. II and III only
        e. II, III, and IV only

10. Normal periods of apnea during REM sleep last about
        a. 0 to 5 seconds.
        b. 5 to 10 seconds.
        c. 10 to 15 seconds.
        d. 15 to 20 seconds.
        e. 30 to 40 seconds.

Answers appear in Appendix XXI.

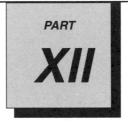

PART

XII

OTHER IMPORTANT
TOPICS

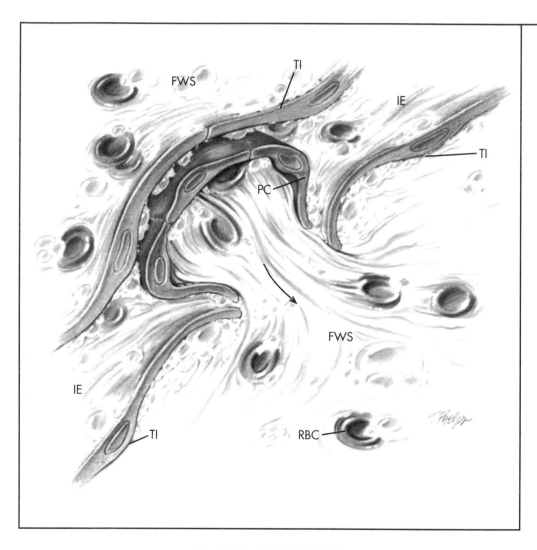

NEAR WET-DROWINING

FIG 29-1

Near wet-drowning. Cross-sectional, microscopic view of alveolar-capillary unit. Illustration shows fluid moving from a pulmonary capillary to an alveolus. *PC* = pulmonary capillary; *FWS* = frothy white secretions; *RBC* = red blood cell; *TI* = type I alveolar cell; *IE* = interstitial edema. (See also Plate 28.)

Near Drowning

ANATOMIC ALTERATIONS OF THE LUNGS

Drowning is defined as suffocation and death as a result of submersion in liquid. Drowning may further be defined as **near drowning, dry drowning,** and **wet drowning.** *Near drowning* refers to the situation in which a victim survives a liquid submersion, at least temporarily. In *dry drowning,* the glottis spasms and prevents water from passing into the lungs. The lungs of dry drowning victims are usually normal.

In *wet drowning,* the glottis relaxes and allows water to flood the tracheobronchial tree and the alveoli. Initially, when fluid is inhaled, the bronchi constrict in response to a parasympathetic-mediated reflex. As fluid enters the alveoli, the pathophysiologic processes responsible for *noncardiogenic pulmonary edema* begin. That is, fluid from the pulmonary capillaries moves into the perivascular spaces, peribronchial spaces, alveoli, bronchioles, and bronchi. As a consequence of this fluid movement, the alveolar walls and interstitial spaces swell, pulmonary surfactant concentration decreases, and the alveolar surface tension increases.

As this condition intensifies, the alveoli shrink and atelectasis develops. Excess fluid in the interstitial spaces causes the lymphatic vessels to dilate and the lymph flow to increase. In severe cases, the fluid that accumulates in the tracheobronchial tree is churned into a frothy, white (sometimes blood tinged) sputum as a result of air moving in and out of the lungs (generally by means of mechanical ventilation).

Finally, if the victim was submerged in unclean water (e.g., swamp, pond, sewage, or mud), a number of pathogens (e.g., *Pseudomonas*) and solid material may be aspirated. When this occurs, pneumonia may be seen and, in severe cases, ARDS may develop. Although it has been controversial in the past, it is now believed that the major pathologic changes of the lungs are essentially the same in *freshwater* and *seawater wet drownings;* both result in a reduction in pulmonary surfactant, alveolar injury, atelectasis, and pulmonary edema (Fig 29-1).

To summarize, the major pulmonary pathologic and structural changes associated with wet drowning are as follows:

* Laryngospasm and bronchial constriction
* Interstitial edema, including engorgement of the perivascular and peribronchial spaces, alveolar walls, and interstitial spaces
* Decreased pulmonary surfactant
* Increased surface tension
* Alveolar shrinkage and atelectasis
* Frothy, white secretions throughout the tracheobronchial tree

ETIOLOGY

It is estimated that worldwide about 150,000 people die each year as a result of drowning. The number of near drowning episodes each year is unknown. It is estimated that about 10% to 15% of drownings that occur each year are *dry drownings,* and that the remaining 85% to 90% are *wet drownings.*

Most drowning or near drowning victims are children and young adults. Males predominate in every age group, and black children are most at risk. Common factors associated with drowning victims include use of home swimming pools, alcohol, and trauma caused by such things as diving into shallow water, horseplay, and powerboats. Table 29-1 summarizes the general sequence of events that occur in drowning or near drowning victims. Victims submerged in cold water generally demonstrate a much higher survival rate than victims submerged in warm water. Table 29-2 lists favorable prognostic factors in cold-water near drowning.

Table 29-1 Drowning or Near Drowning Sequence

1. Panic and violent struggle to return to the surface
2. Period of calmness and apnea
3. Swallowing of large amounts of fluid, followed by vomiting
4. Gasping inspirations and aspiration
5. Convulsions
6. Coma
7. Death

Table 29-2 Favorable Prognostic Factors in Cold-Water Near Drowning

Age	The younger the better
Submersion times	The shorter the better (60 minutes appears to be the upper limit in cold-water submersions)
Water temperature	The colder the better (range, 27° F-70° F)
Water quality	The cleaner the better
Other injuries	None serious
Amount of struggle	The less struggle the better
CPR quality	Good CPR techniques increase the survival rate
Suicidal intent	Victims attempting suicide by drowning appear to have a smaller survival rate than victims of accidental submersion.

OVERVIEW
OF THE CARDIOPULMONARY CLINICAL MANIFESTATIONS ASSOCIATED WITH
NEAR WET-DROWNING VICTIMS

❑ **APNEA (**see page 17)
Apnea is directly related to the length of time the victim is submerged. The longer the submersion the more likely it is that the victim will not have spontaneous respiration. When spontaneous breathing is present, the respiratory rate is usually increased.

❑ **INCREASED RESPIRATORY RATE**

Several pathophysiologic mechanisms operating simultaneously may lead to an increased respiratory rate. These are (see page 17)

* Stimulation of peripheral chemoreceptors
* Decreased lung compliance/increased ventilatory relationship
* Stimulation of the J receptors
* Anxiety (conscious patient)

❑ **PULMONARY FUNCTION STUDIES (LATE STAGES OF NEAR WET DROWNING)**

Lung Volume and Capacity Findings (see page 39)

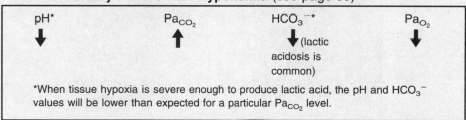

V_T	RV	RV/TLC	FRC
↓	↓	normal	↓
TLC	VC	IC	ERV
↓	↓	↓	↓

❑ **ARTERIAL BLOOD GASES**

Early and Advanced Stages of Near-Drowning Victims

Acute Ventilatory Failure with Hypoxemia (see page 59)

pH*	Pa_{CO_2}	HCO_3^-*	Pa_{O_2}
↓	↑	↓ (lactic acidosis is common)	↓

*When tissue hypoxia is severe enough to produce lactic acid, the pH and HCO_3^- values will be lower than expected for a particular Pa_{CO_2} level.

❑ **OXYGENATION INDICES** (see page 69)

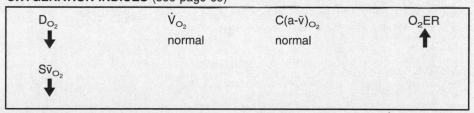

D_{O_2}	$\dot{V}_{O_2}$	$C(a-\bar{v})_{O_2}$	O_2ER
↓	normal	normal	↑
$S\bar{v}_{O_2}$			
↓			

❑ **CYANOSIS** (see page 68)
❑ **COUGH AND SPUTUM PRODUCTION (FROTHY, PINK STABLE BUBBLES)** (see page 93)
❑ **CHEST ASSESSMENT FINDINGS** (see page 6)
* Crackles/rhonchi

❑ **PNEUMOTHORAX** (see Chapter 19)

Pneumothorax and pneumomediastinum frequently occur in victims of near drowning who are being mechanically ventilated.

❑ **RADIOLOGIC FINDINGS**
Chest radiograph
* Fluffy infiltrates
* Pneumothorax/pneumomediastinum

The initial appearance of the radiograph may vary from complete normality through varying degrees of pulmonary edema (Fig 29-2). It should be emphasized, however, that an initially normal chest radiograph may still be associated with significant hypoxemia, hypercapnia, and acidosis. In any case, radiographic deterioration may occur in the first 48 to 72 hours. Because a pneumothorax or pneumomediastinum often occurs in near-drowning patients who are on ventilator support, the respiratory care practitioner must be on alert for this condition.

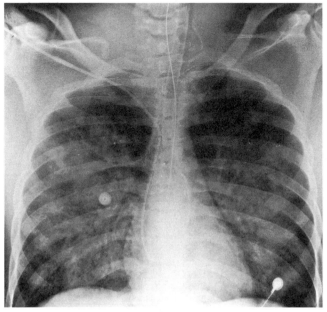

FIG 29-2
Radiograph of a young man just after an episode of near drowning shows a pulmonary edema pattern. (From Armstrong P, Wilson AG, Dee P: *Imaging of diseases of the chest,* St. Louis, 1990, Mosby-Year Book. Used by permission.)

GENERAL MANAGEMENT
The First Responder

The first objective in treating a drowning victim is to remove the person from the water and, if the patient has no spontaneous ventilations and pulse, to call for help and to immediately initiate *cardiopulmonary resuscitation* (CPR). When the patient has been submerged for less than 60 minutes in cold water, fixed and dilated pupils do not necessarily indicate a poor prognosis. Because water is an excellent conductor of body heat (cold water can cool the body 25 times faster than air at the same temperature) and because evaporation further reduces an individual's body heat, the victim's wet clothing should be removed immediately and replaced with warm, dry coverings.

Management During Transport

The primary goal in treating near-drowning victims during transport is good quality CPR, with 100% oxygen. Further conservation of the victim's body heat should be secured by removing any wet garments and covering the high heat-loss areas with warm, dry coverings.

High heat-loss areas of the body include the head and neck, axillae, and inguinal areas. The victim's vital signs, including rectal temperature, should be monitored closely while enroute to the hospital. It should be emphasized that the victim's body temperature frequently falls during transport and that any measures taken to conserve the patient's body heat are extremely important. Victims with spontaneous ventilation should be monitored with pulse oximetry during transport.

Management at the Hospital

Treatment at the hospital is an extension of the prehospital management. Virtually every near-drowning victim suffers from hypoxemia, hypercapnia, and acidosis (acute ventilatory failure). Hypoxemia generally persists after aspiration of fluids (wet drowning) because of alveolar capillary damage and continued intrapulmonary shunting. The degree of hypoxemia is directly related to the amount of alveolar-capillary damage. A chest radiograph should be obtained to help evaluate the magnitude of the alveolar-capillary injury. It should be noted, however, that a normal chest radiograph does not rule out the possibility of alveolar-capillary deterioration during the first 24 hours.

Intubation and mechanical ventilation should be administered immediately to any victim with no spontaneous ventilations, or to victims who are breathing spontaneously but unable to maintain a Pa_{O_2} of 60 mm Hg with an $F_{I_{O_2}}$ of 0.5 or lower. Because of the nature of the alveolar-capillary injury seen in near wet-drowning victims, mechanical ventilation with positive and end expiratory pressure (PEEP) or continuous positive airway pressure (CPAP) should be administered. It should be noted, however, that barotrauma is a common complication of ventilatory therapy in these patients. The patient may also benefit from inotropic agents and diuretics.

Finally, rewarming the victim should progress concomitantly with all the other treatment modalities. Nearly all near-drowning victims are hypothermic to some degree. Depending on the severity of the hypothermia and on the available resources, there are a number of rewarming techniques that may be employed. For example, the body temperature can be increased by the intravenous administration of heated solutions; by heated lavage of the gastric, intrathoracic, pericardial, and peritoneal spaces; or by the administration of heated lavage to the bladder and rectum. Additional external heat techniques include heating blankets, warm baths, and immersion in a heated Hubbard tank. In rare cases, extracorporeal circulation, with complete cardiopulmonary bypass, has been successful.

• • • • **NEAR DROWNING CASE STUDY** • • • •

ADMITTING HISTORY AND PHYSICAL EXAMINATION

This 12-year-old boy had a history of a seizure disorder, but had not taken his medication for almost a year. On the morning of admission, he participated in a regular swimming class in the junior high school pool. According to the coach on duty, there had been a "pool check" thirty seconds before the patient's partner reported that the patient seemed to stay under water "too long."

When taken from the water, he was unconscious and "blue." He was given mouth-to-mouth resuscitation and, by the time the EMT squad arrived about 20 minutes later, he was breathing at a rate of 10/min, but his lips and fingers were still cyanotic. He remained comatose and was taken to the nearest hospital.

An x-ray was reported as showing "symmetrical, diffuse, abnormal increase in density, involving both lungs. The appearance is most suggestive of pulmonary edema or, possibly, hemorrhage." Plans were made to transfer him to a nearby medical center. The respiratory therapist in the emergency department entered the following assessment:

RESPIRATORY ASSESSMENT AND PLAN

S: N/A (patient comatose). History of near drowning.

O: Comatose. Spontaneous breathing at 10/min, BP 100/60, P 140. Crackles bilaterally. Nasotracheal suctioning yields clear fluid. Cyanotic.

A: • Near drowning. R/O seizure disorder (history)
• Airway secretions (suctioning of clear fluid)
• Poor oxygenation (cyanosis)

P: Stat ABG on 4 lpm oxygen, then titrate per protocol. Have equipment to intubate on standby. Bag ventilate and suction. Continuous pulse oximetry. Continue nasotracheal suctioning. Seizure precautions. Will accompany on transfer.

On admission to the medical center, the patient was described as a well-developed, slightly obese adolescent in obvious respiratory distress. He was now alert, oriented, but extremely apprehensive, and his vitals were temperature (rectal) 100.8° F, blood pressure 112/70, pulse 140, and respirations 60. The lips and fingertips were cyanotic. The respirations were paradoxical. There was marked substernal retraction. Breath sounds were diminished bilaterally, and there were loud crackles heard over both lungs anteriorly.

Laboratory examination revealed a leukocytosis of 21,000/mm³ and 2+ albumin in the urine, but was otherwise within normal limits. There was no evidence of hemolysis. On an $F_{I_{O_2}}$ of 0.5, the arterial blood gases were pH 7.29, Pa_{CO_2} 52, HCO_3^- 25, and Pa_{O_2} 48. The patient's condition was rapidly deteriorating, and he developed even more severe crackles. He now had a spontaneous cough with frothy sputum production. The chest x-ray was described as pulmonary edema and showed nearly complete opacification of both lungs. The following was entered in the patient's chart:

RESPIRATORY ASSESSMENT AND PLAN

S: Anxious, dyspneic, crying. "I can't get my breath. Where am I? Am I going to die?"

O: Afebrile. BP 112/70. P 140/min, RR 60/min. Cyanotic. Paradoxical chest/abdomen movements, sternal retraction. Crackles in both lungs anteriorly. Spontaneous cough with frothy sputum production. WBC 21,000/mm³. On 50% oxygen: pH 7.29, Pa_{CO_2} 52, HCO_3^- 25, Pa_{O_2} 48. CXR: "white-out."

A: • Pulmonary edema secondary to near drowning (frothy sputum)
• Acute ventilatory failure with metabolic acidosis (lactic) with moderate/severe hypoxemia (ABG)

P: Place on 100% O_2. Page physician stat. Obtain intubation equipment and prepare to place on ventilator. Follow oximetry. Prepare to assist in placement of Swan-Ganz catheter.

He was intubated with thiopental sodium and succinylcholine. As soon as he was intubated, copious pink foam could be aspirated from the endotracheal tube. He was alternately suctioned and ventilated with an Ambu bag. He was given 7 mg of morphine for sedation and was mechanically ventilated at a rate of 10 breaths per minute. On an $F_{I_{O_2}}$ of 0.6 and PEEP of +10 cm H_2O, his blood gases were pH 7.44, Pa_{CO_2} 43, HCO_3^- 24, and Pa_{O_2} 109. Since he was still fighting the respirator, he was paralyzed. After several hours, the lungs were clear, the secretions were no longer present, and his blood gases remained within normal limits on an $F_{I_{O_2}}$ of 0.3 and PEEP of 10 cm H_2O. His hemodynamic status was normal. The following assessment was entered on the patient's ventilator chart:

RESPIRATORY ASSESSMENT AND PLAN

S: N/A (patient sedated, paralyzed)

O: Lungs clear. No secretions. On 30% O_2 and +10 PEEP: pH 7.42, Pa_{CO_2} 42, HCO_3^- 24, Pa_{O_2} 98. CXR: considerable improvement in bilateral infiltrates. No cardiomegaly. PWCP 10 mm Hg.

A: • Considerable improvement on CMV and PEEP (general improvement of clinical indicators)
  • Acceptable ventilatory and oxygenation status on present ventilatory settings (ABG)
  • Frothy airway secretions no longer present (clear lungs & no secretions)

P: Contact physician to wean from muscle relaxant. Wean from mechanically ventilated breaths, $F_{I_{O_2}}$, and PEEP per protocol. Change ventilator to SIMV.

The patient was weaned from the ventilator over a period of six hours, after which he was extubated. The following morning, arterial blood gases on a 28% HAFOE oxygen mask were pH 7.37, Pa_{CO_2} 35, HCO_3^- 23, and Pa_{O_2} 158. X-ray examination of the lungs showed no residual pathology. An oxygen titration protocol was performed. He was discharged two days later.

DISCUSSION

This case demonstrates initial worsening of the near-drowning victim despite intensive respiratory care. When suctioning, supplementary oxygen, and bag ventilation were no longer successful, the patient was intubated and mechanical ventilation with PEEP was begun.

Even on these modalities, the patient remained anxious and was ultimately paralyzed to allow better respiratory synchrony and to diminish the chance for barotrauma. Morphine was used for its sedative qualities and as an afterload reducer.

This case demonstrates again the necessity for frequent reassessment of the patient, and course adjustments to follow the findings so observed.

SELF-ASSESSMENT QUESTIONS

Fill In The Blanks

1. Near drowning refers to _____
   _____.

2. In dry drowning, the _____
   _____.

3. In wet drowning, the _____
   _____.

4. In wet drowning, as fluid enters the alveoli, the pathophysiologic processes responsible for
   _____begin.

5. Cold water can cool the body _____times faster than air at the same
   temperature.

Answers appear in Appendix XXI.

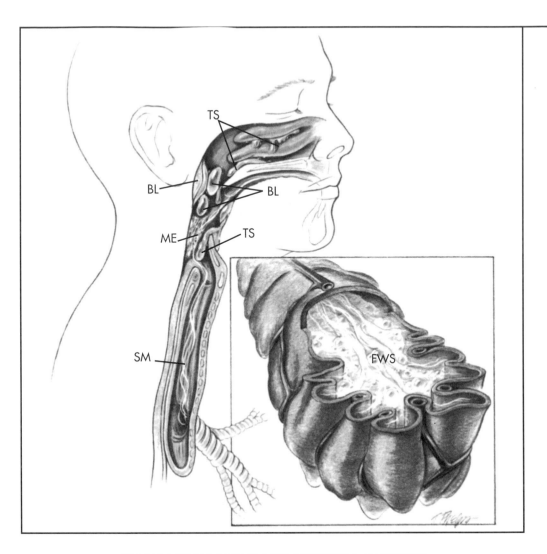

SMOKE INHALATION AND THERMAL INJURIES

FIG 30-1

Smoke inhalation and thermal injuries. *TS* = thick secretions; *BL* = blister; *ME* = mucosal edema; *SM* = smoke (toxic gas); *FWS* = frothy white secretions. (See also Plate 29.)

Smoke Inhalation
and Thermal Injuries

ANATOMIC ALTERATIONS OF THE LUNGS

The inhalation of *smoke* and *hot gases,* and *body surface burns*—in any combination—continue to be a major cause of morbidity and mortality among fire victims and fire fighters. In general, fire-related pulmonary injuries can be divided into *thermal* and *smoke* (toxic gases) injuries.

Thermal Injury

Thermal injury refers to the injuries caused by the inhalation of hot gases. Thermal injuries are usually confined to the upper airway—the nasal cavity, oral cavity, nasopharynx, oropharynx, and laryngopharynx. The airways distal to the larynx and the alveoli are usually spared serious injury because of the (1) remarkable ability of the upper airways to cool hot gases, (2) reflex laryngospasm, and (3) glottic closure. The upper airway is an extremely efficient "heat sink." In fact, in 1945, Moritz and associates demonstrated that the inhalation of hot gases alone did not produce significant damage to the lung. Anesthetized dogs were forced to breathe air heated to 500° C through an insulated endotracheal tube. Their results showed that the air temperature dropped to 50° C by the time it reached the level of the carina. No histologic damage was noticed in the lower trachea or lungs.

Even though thermal injury may occur with or without surface burns, the presence of facial burns is a "classic" predictor of thermal injury. Thermal injury to the upper airway results in blistering, mucosal edema, vascular congestion, epithelial sloughing, and accumulation of thick secretions. An acute upper airway obstruction (UAO) occurs in about 20% to 30% of hospitalized patients with thermal injury and is usually most marked in the supraglottic structures. When body surface burns require the rapid administration of resuscitative fluids, a UAO may develop rapidly (Fig 30-1).

Although rare, it should be noted that the inhalation of *steam* at 100 C° or greater usually results in severe damage at all levels of the respiratory tract. This is because steam has about 500 times the heat energy content than that of dry gas at the same temperature. Thermal injury to the distal airways results in mucosal edema, vascular congestion, epithelial sloughing, obliterative bronchiolitis, atelectasis, and pulmonary edema.

Thus, except for the rare instance of steam inhalation, direct thermal injuries do not usually occur below the level of the larynx. Damage to the distal airways is mostly caused by a variety of harmful products found in smoke.

Smoke Inhalation Injury

The pathologic changes in the distal airways and alveoli are mainly caused by the irritant and toxic gases, suspended soot particles, and vapors associated with incomplete combustion and smoke. Many of the substances found in smoke are extremely caustic to the tracheobronchial tree and poisonous to the body. The injuries that develop from smoke inhalation and burns are described as the *early stage, intermediate stage,* and *late stage.*

Early Stage (0-24 Hours Postinhalation)

The injuries associated with smoke inhalation do not always appear right away, even when there are extensive body surface burns. During the first 24 hours, however, the patient's pulmonary status often changes markedly. Initially, the tracheobronchial tree becomes more inflamed. This process causes (1) an overabundance of bronchial secretions to move into the airways and (2) bronchospasm. In addition, the toxic effects of smoke often slow the activity of the mucosal ciliary transport mechanism, causing further mucus retention.

   Smoke inhalation may also cause noncardiogenic, high-permeability pulmonary edema—commonly referred to in smoke inhalation cases as "leaky alveoli." Pulmonary edema is associated with overhydration due to fluid resuscitation for body surface burns (Fig 30-1). In severe cases, ARDS may also occur as an early problem.

Intermediate Stage (2-5 Days Postinhalation)

While the upper airway thermal injuries usually begin to improve during this period, the pathologic changes associated with smoke inhalation usually peak during this stage. Mucus production continues to increase while mucosal ciliary transport activity continues to decrease. The mucosa of the tracheobronchial tree frequently becomes necrotic and sloughs (usually between 3 and 4 days). The necrotic debris, excessive mucus production, and mucus retention lead to mucus plugging and atelectasis. In addition, the mucus accumulation often leads to bacterial colonization, bronchitis, and pneumonia. Organisms commonly cultured include gram-positive *Staphylococcus aureus* and gram-negative *Klebsiella, Enterobacter, Escherichia coli,* and *Pseudomonas.* If they are not already present, both noncardiogenic pulmonary edema and ARDS may develop at any time during this period.

   When chest burns are present, these pathologic conditions may be further aggravated by (1) the patient's inability to breathe deeply and cough as a result of pain, (2) the use of narcotics, (3) immobility, (4) increased airway resistance, and (5) decreased lung and chest compliance.

Late Stage (5 or More Days Postinhalation)

Body surface burn wound infections are the major concern during this period. Infected body surface burn wounds often lead to sepsis and multiorgan failure. Sepsis-induced multiorgan failure is the primary cause of death in seriously burned patients during this stage.

   Pneumonia also continues to be a major problem during this period. Pulmonary embolism may develop within two weeks after serious body surface burns. The pulmonary embolism ususally develops from a deep venous thrombosis secondary to a hypercoagulable state and prolonged immobility.

   Finally, the long-term effects of smoke inhalation can result in restrictive and obstructive lung disorders. In general, it is thought that a restrictive lung disorder develops from alveolar fibrosis and chronic lobar atelectasis. An obstructive lung disorder is believed to be caused by chronic bronchial secretions, bronchial stenosis, bronchial polyps, and bronchiectasis.

   To summarize, the major pathologic and structural changes of the respiratory system caused by thermal or smoke inhalation injuries are as follows:

Thermal injury (upper airway—nasal cavity, oral cavity, and pharynx)

* Blistering
* Mucosal edema
* Vascular congestion
* Epithelial sloughing
* Thick secretions
* Acute upper airway obstruction

Smoke inhalation injury (tracheobronchial tree and alveoli)

* Inflammation of the tracheobronchial tree
* Bronchospasm
* Excessive bronchial secretions and mucus plugging
* Decreased mucosal ciliary transport mechanism
* Atelectasis
* Alveolar edema and frothy secretions (pulmonary edema)
* ARDS (severe cases)
* Pulmonary embolism (severe cases)
* Alveolar fibrosis, bronchial stenosis, bronchial polyps, and bronchiectasis (severe cases)

ETIOLOGY

Fire-related death is the third most common cause of accidental death in the United States. The prognosis of fire victims is usually determined by the (1) extent and duration of smoke exposure, (2) chemical composition of the smoke, (3) size and depth of body surface burns, (4) temperature of gases inhaled, (5) age (the prognosis worsens in the very young or old), and (6) preexisting health. When smoke inhalation injury is accompanied by a full-thickness or third-degree burn, the mortality rate almost doubles.

Smoke can evolve from either *pyrolysis* (smoldering, in a low-oxygen environment) or *combustion* (burning, with visible flame, in an adequate-oxygen environment). Smoke is composed of a complex mixture of particulates, toxic gases, and vapors. The composition of smoke varies according to the chemical makeup of the material that is burning and the amount of oxygen that is being consumed by the fire. Table 30-1 lists some of the more common toxic

Table 30-1 Toxic Substances and Sources Commonly Associated with Fire and Smoke

Source	Substance
Wood, cotton, paper	Aldehydes (acrolein, acetaldehyde, formaldehyde)
	Organic acids (acetic and formic acids)
Polyvinylchloride (PVC)	Carbon monoxide, hydrogen chloride, phosgene
Polyurethanes	Hydrogen cyanide, isocyanate
Fluorinated resins	Hydrogen fluoride, hydrogen bromide
Melamine resins	Ammonia
Nitrocellulose film, fabrics	Oxides of nitrogen
Petroleum products	Benzene
Organic material	Carbon monoxide, carbon dioxide
Sulfur-containing compounds	Sulfur dioxide

substances produced by burning products frequently found in office, industrial, and residential buildings.

While in some instances the toxic components of the smoke may be obvious, in most cases the precise identification of the inhaled toxins is not feasible. In general, the inhalation of smoke with toxic agents that have high water solubility (e.g., ammonia, sulfur dioxide, and hydrogen flouride) affects the structures of the upper airway. In contrast, the inhalation of toxic agents that have a low water solubility (e.g., hydrogen chloride, chlorine, phosgene, and oxides of nitrogen) affects the distal airways and the alveoli. Many of the substances in smoke are caustic and can cause significant injury to the tracheobronchial tree, e.g., aldehydes (especially acrolein), hydrochloride, and oxides of sulfur.

BODY SURFACE BURNS

Because the amount and severity of body surface burns play a major role in the mortality and morbidity of the patient, an approximate estimate of the percentage of the body surface area burned is important. Table 30-2 lists the approximate percentage of surface area for various body regions of adults and infants. The severity and depth of burns are usually defined as follows:

First degree (minimal depth in skin): Superficial burn, damage limited to the outer layer of epidermis. Characterized by reddened skin, tenderness, and pain. Blisters are not present. Healing time is about 6 to 10 days. The end result of healing is normal skin.

Second degree (superficial to deep thickness of skin): Burns in which damage extends through the epidermis and into the dermis but not of sufficient extent to interfere with regeneration of epidermis. If secondary infection results, the damage from a second-degree burn may be equivalent to that of a third-degree burn. Blisters are usually present. Healing time is between 7 and 21 days. The end result of healing ranges from normal to a hairless and depigmented skin with a texture that is normal, pitted, or flat, and shiny.

Third degree (full thickness of skin including tissue beneath skin): Burns in which both epidermis and dermis are destroyed, with damage extending into underlying tissues. Tissue may be charred or coagulated. Healing may occur after 21 days or may never occur if the burned area is large. The end result is areas that heal with hypertrophic scars and chronic granulations.

Table 30-2 The Approximate Percentage of Body Surface Area (BSA) for Various Body Regions of Adults and Infants

Anatomic Region	Adult % BSA	Infant % BSA
Entire head and neck	9	18
Each arm	9	9
Anterior trunk	18	18
Posterior trunk	18	18
Genitalia	1	1
Each leg	18	13.5

Note: The *rule of nines* is used to estimate percentage of injury. This is because each of the above areas represents about 9% or 18% of the body surface area. This rule does not apply to the legs of infants.

OVERVIEW

OF THE CARDIOPULMONARY CLINICAL MANIFESTATIONS ASSOCIATED WITH

SMOKE INHALATION AND BURNS

❏ CARBON MONOXIDE POISONING

When a patient has been exposed to smoke, *carbon monoxide (CO) poisoning must be assumed!* Although CO has no direct injurious effect on the lungs, it can seriously reduce the patient's oxygen transport. This is because CO has an affinity for hemoglobin that is about 210 times greater than that of oxygen. CO attached to hemoglobin is called *carboxyhemoglobin* (HbCO). Breathing CO at a partial pressure of less than 2 mm Hg can result in an HbCO of 40% or more. In other words, 40% or more of the oxygen transport system is inactivated.

In addition, high concentrations of HbCO cause the oxyhemoglobin dissociation curve to move markedly to the left. This makes it more difficult for oxygen to leave the hemoglobin at the tissue sites. In essence, the tissue cells would be better oxygenated when 40% of the hemoglobin is absent (anemia) than when an HbCO of 40% is present. Table 30-3 lists the clinical manifestations associated with HbCO.

An HbCO in excess of 20% is usually considered CO poisoning, and an HbCO of 40% or greater is considered severe exposure. An HbCO level in excess of 50% may cause irreversible CNS damage. *It is important to note that pulse oximetry and Pa_{O_2} measurements are unreliable in the presence of HbCO!* Arterial blood gas measurements, however, do provide important information regarding the presence of hypoxemia, widened alveolar-arterial oxygen gradient, and acid-base status.

❏ CYANIDE POISONING

When smoke contains cyanide, oxygen utilization may be further impaired. Cyanide poisoning should be suspected in the comatose patient when plastic (polyurethane) or other synthetic materials are burned. Inhaled cyanide is easily transported in the blood to the tissue cells, where it bonds to the cytochrome oxidase enzymes of the mitochondria. This inhibits the metabolism of oxygen and causes the tissue cells to shift to an inefficient anaerobic form of metabolism. The end product of anaerobic metabolism is lactic acid. *It is interesting to note that cyanide poisoning may result in lactic acidemia, normally caused by an inadequate oxygen level, when the Pa_{O_2} is normal or above normal.* Clinically, cyanide concentrations are easily measured with commercially available kits. A cyanide blood level in excess of 1 mg/L is usually fatal.

❏ ACUTE UPPER AIRWAY OBSTRUCTION (THERMAL INJURY)

* Obvious pharyngeal edema and swelling
* Inspiratory stridor
* Hoarseness
* Altered voice
* Painful swallowing

Because the inhalation of hot gases often results in severe upper airway edema, the respiratory care practitioner should always be alert for any clinical manifestations of acute upper airway obstruction, even when the patient initially presents with no remarkable upper airway problems or upper body burns.

❏ INCREASED RESPIRATORY RATE

Several pathophysiologic mechanisms operating simultaneously may lead to an increased ventilatory rate. These are (see page 17)

* Stimulation of peripheral chemoreceptors
* Decreased lung compliance/increased ventilatory relationship
* Stimulation of the J receptors
* Pain/anxiety

❑ **PULMONARY FUNCTION STUDY FINDINGS**

Expiratory Maneuver Findings (see page 39)

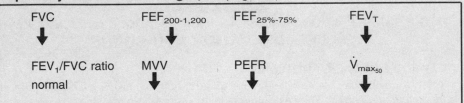

FVC	FEF$_{200-1,200}$	FEF$_{25\%-75\%}$	FEV$_T$
↓	↓	↓	↓
FEV$_1$/FVC ratio normal	MVV ↓	PEFR ↓	$\dot{V}_{max_{50}}$ ↓

Lung Volume and Capacity Findings (see page 39)

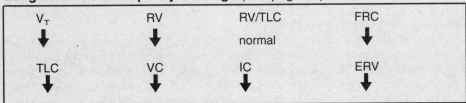

V$_T$	RV	RV/TLC	FRC
↓	↓	normal	↓
TLC ↓	VC ↓	IC ↓	ERV ↓

❑ **DECREASED DIFFUSION CAPACITY D$_{LCO}$** (see page 48)
❑ **INCREASED HEART RATE** (see page 86)
❑ **ARTERIAL BLOOD GASES**

Early Stages of Smoke Inhalation

Acute Alveolar Hyperventilation with Hypoxemia (see page 57)

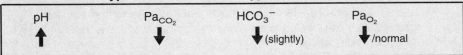

| pH | Pa$_{CO_2}$ | HCO$_3^-$ | Pa$_{O_2}$ |
| ↑ | ↓ | ↓ (slightly) | ↓ /normal |

Metabolic Acidosis (see page 67)

It should be noted that when carbon monoxide and/or cyanide poisoning are present, the pH may be decreased during the early stages of smoke inhalation. This is because patients with severe carbon monoxide and/or cyanide poisoning commonly have lactic acidemia (decreased pH) as a result of tissue hypoxia—even in the presence of a normal Pa$_{O_2}$. Thus, when carbon monoxide and/or cyanide poisoning are present, the patient may demonstrate the following arterial blood gas values:

| pH | Pa$_{CO_2}$ | HCO$_3^-$ | Pa$_{O_2}$ |
| ↓ (lactic acidemia) | ↓ | ↓ | normal (but patient has tissue hypoxia) |

Late Stages of Smoke Inhalation

Acute Ventilatory Failure with Hypoxemia (see page 59)

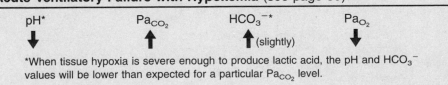

| pH* | Pa$_{CO_2}$ | HCO$_3^-$* | Pa$_{O_2}$ |
| ↓ | ↑ | ↑ (slightly) | ↓ |

*When tissue hypoxia is severe enough to produce lactic acid, the pH and HCO$_3^-$ values will be lower than expected for a particular Pa$_{CO_2}$ level.

❑ **CYANOSIS** (see page 68)

❑ **OXYGENATION INDICES (SMOKE INHALATION AND BURNS)** (see page 69)

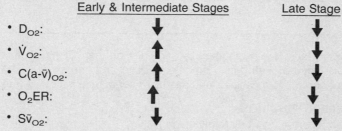

	Early & Intermediate Stages	Late Stage
• D_{O2}:	↓	↓
• $\dot{V}_{O2}$:	↑	↓
• $C(a\text{-}\bar{v})_{O2}$:	↑	↓
• O_2ER:	↑	↓
• $S\bar{v}_{O2}$:	↓	↓

It should be noted that when carbon monoxide and/or cyanide poisoning are present, the oxygenation indices are unreliable. This is because the Pa_{CO2} often appears normal in the presence of carbon monoxide poisoning and, when cyanide poisoning is present, the tissue cells are prevented from consuming oxygen. Both of these conditions cause false readings. For example, when CO is present, a normal D_{O2} value may be calculated when, in reality, the patient's oxygen transport status is extremely low. When cyanide poisoning is present, the patient's $\dot{V}_{O2}$ may appear normal or increased when, in actuality, the tissue cells are extremely hypoxic. Typically, these problems are not present during the intermediate and late stages with appropriate treatment.

❑ **HEMODYNAMIC INDICES IN THE PRESENCE OF BODY SURFACE BURNS** (see page 87)

	Early	Intermediate	Late
• CVP:	↓	normal	↓
• RAP:	↓	normal	↓
• $\overline{PA}$:	↓	normal	↓
• PCWP:	↓	normal	↓
• CO:	↓	normal	↓
• SV:	↓	normal	↓
• SVI:	↓	normal	↓
• CI:	↓	normal	↓
• RVSWI:	↓	normal	↓
• LVSWI:	↓	normal	↓
• PVR:	normal	normal	↑
• SVR:	↑	normal	↑

In general, the hemodynamic profile seen in patients with body surface burns relate to the amount of intravascular volume lost (hypovolemia) that occurs from third-space fluid shifts. For example, during the early stage, the decreased values shown for the CVP, RAP, $\overline{PA}$, PCWP, CO, SV, SVI, CI, RVSWI, and LVSWI all reflect the reduction in pulmonary intravascular and cardiac filling volumes. Hypovolemia causes a generalized peripheral vasoconstriction, which is reflected in an elevated SVR. When appropriate fluid resuscitation is administered, the patient's hemodynamic indices usually appear normal during the intermediate stage.

❑ **COUGH AND SPUTUM PRODUCTION** (see page 93)
When the patient has upper airway thermal injuries, an excessive amount of thick secretions are usually present. During the early stage of smoke inhalation, the patient generally expectorates a small amount of black, sooty sputum (carbonaceous sputum). During the intermediate stage, the patient may produce a moderate to large amount of frothy secretions. During the late stage, purulent mucus is frequently seen.

❑ **RADIOLOGIC FINDINGS**
Chest radiograph
- Usually normal (early stage)
- Pulmonary edema/ARDS (intermediate stage)
- Patchy or segmental infiltrate (late stage)

During the early stage, the radiograph is generally normal. Signs of pulmonary edema and ARDS may be seen during the intermediate and late stages. The chest x-ray film reveals dense, fluffy opacities, and patchy or segmental infiltrates (Fig 30-2).

❏ **CHEST ASSESSMENT FINDINGS**
  - Usually normal breath sounds (early stage)
  - Wheezing
  - Crackles
  - Rhonchi

Table 30-3 General HbCO Levels and Clinical Manifestations

HbCO%	Clinical Manifestations
0 to 10	Usually no symptoms
10 to 20	Mild headache, dilatation of cutaneous blood vessels
	Cherry red skin—but not always
20 to 30	Throbbing headache, nausea, vomiting, impaired judgment
30 to 50	Throbbing headache, possible syncope, increased respiratory and pulse rates
50 to 60	Syncope, increased respiratory and pulse rates, coma, convulsions, Cheyne-Stokes respiration
60 to 70	Coma, convulsions, cardiovascular and respiratory depression, and possible death
70 to 80	Cardiopulmonary failure and death

GENERAL MANAGEMENT OF HOT GAS AND SMOKE INHALATION
General Emergency Care

The principal goals in the initial care of patients with smoke inhalation and burns include the immediate assessment of the patient's airway and respiratory status, cardiovascular status and, if present, the percentage of body burned and the depth of burns. An IV line should be started immediately to administer medications and fluids. Easily separated clothing should be removed. Any remaining clothing should be soaked thoroughly. When present, burn wounds should be covered to prevent shock, fluid loss, heat loss, and pain. Infection control includes isolation, room pressurization, air filtration, and wound coverings.

Fluid resuscitation with Ringer's lactate solution is usually initiated according to the Parkland formula—4 ml/kg of body weight for each percent of body surface area burned over a 24-hour period. The patient's hemodynamic status usually remains stable, with an average urine output target of 30 to 50 ml and central venous target of 2 to 6 mm Hg. Because this process often leads to overhydration and acute upper airway obstruction and pulmonary edema, it is important to monitor the patient's fluid and electrolyte status (weight, input and output, and laboratory values).

Finally, the exposure characteristics of the fire-related accident may be helpful in assessing the potential clinical complications. For example, does the accident involve a closed-space setting or entrapment? The amount and concentration of smoke is usually much greater in these conditions. What type of material was burning in the fire? Are the inhaled toxins known? Was carbon monoxide or cyanide produced by the burning substances? Was the patient unconscious before entering the hospital?

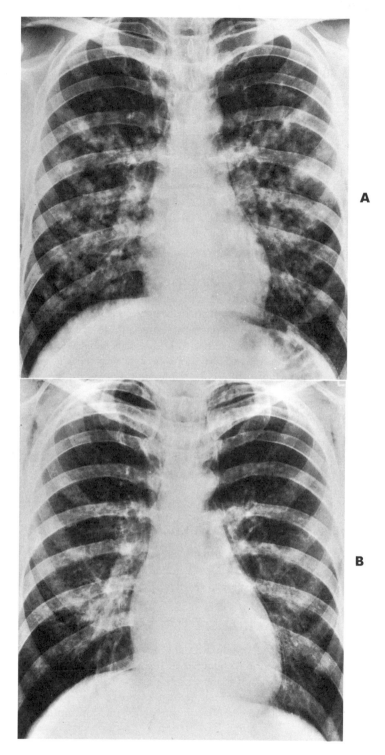

FIG 30-2
A, radiograph of a young man admitted after accidentally setting his kitchen on fire while intoxicated. **B,** prompt recovery after 72 hours. (Courtesy of Dr. K. Simpkins, Leeds, England.) (From Armstrong P, Wilson AG, Dee P: *Imaging of diseases of the chest,* St. Louis, 1990, Mosby-Year Book. Used by permission.)

Oxygen Therapy

Because of the hypoxemia, carbon monoxide, and cyanide poisoning associated with smoke inhalation, a high concentration of oxygen should always be administered immediately. The HbCO half-life when a patient is breathing room air at one atmosphere is approximately 5 hours. That is, a 40% HbCO will decrease to about 20% in 5 hours and to about 10% in another 5 hours. Breathing 100% oxygen at one atmosphere reduces the HbCO half-life to less than 1 hour.

Airway Management

Early elective endotracheal intubation should be performed on the patient who has inhaled hot gases and demonstrates any signs of impending upper airway obstruction (e.g., upper airway edema, blisters, inspiratory stridor, thick secretions). *This is a medical emergency!* Even though acute upper airway obstruction (UAO) is considered one of the most treatable complications of smoke inhalation, death still occurs from UAO (hence the well-supported clinical guideline that states "When in doubt, intubate").

It should be noted that securing an endotracheal tube is often difficult in the presence of facial burns (typically wet wounds). Adhesive tape may cause further trauma to the burn wounds. The ingenuity and creativity of the respiratory care practitioner may be required. The securing of the endotracheal tube without traumatizing the patient has been successful with umbilical tape and a variety of helmets, halo traction devices, and Velcro straps.

Because of the infections associated with body surface burns and smoke inhalation, a tracheostomy should be reserved for conditions in which an airway cannot be established otherwise or for the patient who will require prolonged mechanical ventilation.

Continuous Positive Airway Pressure (CPAP)

The administration of CPAP via an endotracheal tube or a mask (when there are no head or neck burns) may help to minimize the development of pulmonary edema. CPAP also provides support to edematous airways and maintains or increases the patient's functional residual capacity.

Mechanical Ventilation with Positive End-Expiratory Pressure (PEEP)

Mechanical ventilation with PEEP is usually required in patients who develop pulmonary edema, ARDS, and pneumonia. Mechanical ventilation should be established in the presence of acute ventilatory failure or impending ventilatory failure.

MOBILIZATION OF BRONCHIAL SECRETIONS

Because of the excessive mucus production and accumulation in the intermediate and late stages of smoke inhalation injuries, a number of respiratory therapy modalities may be used to enhance the mobilization of bronchial secretions (see Appendix XI). It should be noted, however, that even though chest physical therapy is an excellent treatment modality to mobilize secretions, patients with severe chest burns or recent skin grafts do not tolerate chest percussion and vibration.

Bronchoscopy

Bronchoscopy is often used to clear airways with mucus plugs. In addition, early bronchoscopy is often performed to inspect and evaluate the upper airways. Mucosal changes distal to the larynx serve as good indicators of subsequent respiratory problems.

Hyperbaric Oxygen

Although controversial, hyperbaric oxygenation may be useful in the rapid elimination of CO. While it is well established that a Pa_{O_2} greater than 1,500 mm Hg can be achieved with a hyperbaric chamber, it is generally not possible or practical to institute this therapy. The chamber may not be immediately available. Can the patient be transported safely? Will the interruption of the immediate therapy be detrimental?

Medications

Mucolytic agents.—Mucolytics may be used to break down the large amounts of thick tenacious mucus (see Appendix VI).

Sympathomimetics.—Sympathomimetic drugs are commonly administered to patients with smoke inhalation to offset bronchospasm (see Appendix II).

Antibiotic agents.—Antibiotics may be used to combat burn wounds and pulmonary infections (see Appendix VIII).

Expectorants.—Expectorants may be administered to facilitate expectoration (see Appendix VII).

Analgesic agents.—Analgesics are generally ordered when surface burns are present.

Prophylactic heparin therapy.—Heparin is often administered to patients with severe, long-term and immobile fire-related injuries to reduce the risk of pulmonary embolism.

Treatment for Cyanide Poisoning

The treatment for cyanide poisoning includes amyl nitrite inhalation and intravenous sodium thiosulfate.

• **SMOKE INHALATION AND THERMAL INJURY CASE STUDY** •

ADMITTING HISTORY AND PHYSICAL EXAMINATION

A 21-year-old male was in excellent health until a few hours prior to admission when, after smoking marijuana and falling asleep, his bed caught on fire and he suffered second- and third-degree burns on his face, chest, and abdomen. The total extent of second- and third-degree burns were only 6% to 8% of his total body surface and presented no significant problems.

It was noted shortly after admission that he was developing significant respiratory distress with evidence suggestive of pulmonary edema. His blood pressure was 110/60, pulse 100/min, and respiratory rate 30/min. Bilateral crackles and rhonchi were present. Spontaneous cough was productive of large amounts of thick whitish-grey sputum. The chest radiograph revealed bilateral patchy infiltrates and consolidation. On 4 L/min oxygen, his arterial blood gas values were pH 7.51, Pa_{CO_2} 28, HCO_3^- 21, and Pa_{O_2} 45.

He was treated conservatively, and the edema cleared in 36 hours, but the hypoxemia persisted, even on 50% oxygen by HAFOE mask. Fiberoptic bronchoscopy revealed extensive thermal damage to the trachea and large bronchi. At this time, the following respiratory assessment was entered in the patient's chart:

RESPIRATORY ASSESSMENT AND PLAN

S: Complains of productive cough, substernal chest pain when coughing, and moderate dyspnea.

O: Afebrile. BP 120/65, P 119 & regular, RR 35. On 50% O_2: pH 7.54, Pa_{CO_2} 25, HCO_3^- 20, Pa_{O_2} 38. CXR bilateral patchy infiltrates & consolidation. No cardiomegaly. Bronchoscopy—blackish eschar in oropharynx; reddened and inflamed larynx, trachea, and large airways. Thick, whitish-grey secretions noted.

A: • Smoke inhalation with thermal burns of oropharynx, larynx, and large airways (history & bronchoscopy)
  • Alveolar infiltrates and consolidation (CXR)
  • Acute alveolar hyperventilation with severe hypoxemia (ABG)
    • Impending ventilatory failure (general history & clinical trends)
  • Excessive and thick airway secretions (sputum)

P: Confer with attending physician to intubate and initiate ventilator care per protocol. Oxygen therapy protocol. Bronchial hygiene therapy per protocol. In-line USN, aerosolized steroids.

He was intubated and started on intravenously administered steroids. He was ventilated with an F_{I_O} of 0.50, rate of 12, and PEEP of +10 cm H_2O. Because of the upper body burns, chest physical therapy and postural drainage were prohibited. The bronchial secretions, however, were loosened and mobilized adequately with an in-line ultrasonic nebulizer and frequent endotracheal suctioning. In-line aerosolized steroids were also administered to the patient at this time.

On this regime, the patient's vital signs and blood gases were within normal limits. After 12 days of respiratory care, he was weaned to room air and extubated.

Three days after extubation, on room air, his pH was 7.46, Pa_{CO_2} 38, HCO_3^- 24, and Pa_{O_2} 59. On exercise, the Pa_{O_2} decreased to 47 mm Hg. His PEFR was 40% of predicted. At this time, the following respiratory assessment was written in the patient's chart:

RESPIRATORY ASSESSMENT AND PLAN

S: Complains of shortness of breath with any activity

O: Vital signs stable. Crackles heard over both lung bases. Some expiratory prolongation. Room air: pH 7.46, Pa_{CO_2} 38, HCO_3^- 24, and Pa_{O_2} 59. Room air Pa_{O_2} 59 decreased to 47 mm Hg with exercise. PEFR 40% of predicted. CXR: improvement in patchy lung infiltrates.

A: • Moderate hypoxemia secondary to thermal injury to lung (ABG & history)
  • Moderate obstructive pulmonary disease (PEFR)

P: Complete PFTs ordered. Oxygen per oxygen therapy protocol. If obstructive pulmonary disease confirmed, start bronchial hygiene and aerosolized medication protocols.

Pulmonary function studies showed severely reduced expiratory flows and a sharply decreased diffusion capacity. Chest x-rays, taken at regular intervals, began to show emphysematous changes. The diaphragms were flattened, and there were bilateral coarse reticular infiltrates. In spite of vigorous therapy over the next six weeks, the patient's cardiopulmonary status continued to worsen. The patient died on the 56th day, two months after his original thermal and inhalational injury. The antemortem diagnosis, confirmed by autopsy, was bronchiolitis fibrosa obliterans.

DISCUSSION

This interesting case is instructive for several reasons. The first is that all patients with burns of the upper chest, neck, or face should have a careful oropharyngeal examination to determine whether burns have indeed occurred in the upper airway. The presence of soot or eschar in the oropharynx is diagnostic of this problem and, predictably, respiratory distress will almost certainly ensue if such is found, although not immediately. There is often a 24- to 72-hour lag between the burn itself and clinical obstruction of the airway.

Second, a dreaded complication of smoke and heat inhalation is bronchiolitis fibrosa obliterans, which developed in this patient and ultimately was responsible for his demise.

These days, if such developed, consideration of the patient for lung transplantation might be given. A message for the therapist from this case is that STAT intubation over the diagnostic bronchoscope may be necessary in such patients, and that he/she should be prepared accordingly.

SELF-ASSESSMENT QUESTIONS

Multiple Choice

1. About what percentage of hospitalized patients with thermal injury have an acute upper airway obstruction?
    a. 0% to 10%
    b. 10% to 20%
    c. 20% to 30%
    d. 30% to 40%
    e. 40% to 50%

2. Except for the rare instance of steam inhalation, direct thermal injuries do not usually occur below the level of the
    a. Oral pharynx.
    b. Larynx.
    c. Carina.
    d. Bronchi.
    e. Bronchioles.

3. When chest burns are present, the patient's pulmonary condition may be further aggravated by
    I. Decreased lung and chest compliance.
    II. Increased airway resistance.
    III. The use of narcotics.
    IV. Immobility.
    a. I and III only
    b. II and III only
    c. I, II, and III only
    d. II, III, and IV only
    e. I, II, III, and IV

4. Which of the following is/are the pulmonary-related pathologic changes associated with smoke inhalation?
    I. Alveolar hyperinflation
    II. Bronchospasm
    III. Pulmonary edema
    IV. Pulmonary embolism
    a. I only
    b. II only
    c. III and IV only
    d. II, III, and IV only
    e. I, II, III, and IV

5. Which of the following produce carbon monoxide when burned?
    I. Polyurethanes
    II. Wood, cotton, paper
    III. Organic material
    IV. Polyvinylchloride (PVC)
    a. I only
    b. II only
    c. III and IV only
    d. I, II, and III only
    e. I, II, III, and IV

6. Which of the following oxygenation indices is/are associated with smoke inhalation and burns during the early and intermediate stages?
    I. Increased $\dot{V}_{O_2}$
    II. Decreased $C(a-\bar{v})_{O_2}$
    III. Increased D_{O_2}
    IV. Decreased $S\bar{v}_{O_2}$
    a. II only
    b. IV only
    c. II and III only
    d. I and IV only
    e. II, III, and IV only

7. Which of the following hemodynamic indices is/are associated with body surface burns during the early stage?
   I. Decreased CO
   II. Increased SVR
   III. Decreased $\overline{PA}$
   IV. Increased PCWP
       a. I only
       b. III only
       c. II and IV only
       d. I, II, and III only
       e. I, II, III, and IV

8. If an adult's entire right arm, right leg, and anterior trunk has been burned, approximately what percentage of the patient's body surface area is burned?
       a. 15%
       b. 25%
       c. 35%
       d. 45%
       e. 55%

9. Healing time for a second-degree burn is between
       a. 1 and 7 days.
       b. 7 and 21 days.
       c. 21 and 31 days.
       d. 1 and 2 months.
       e. 2 and 3 months.

10. Breathing 100% oxygen at one atmosphere reduces the HbCO half-life to less than
       a. 1 hour.
       b. 2 hours.
       c. 3 hours.
       d. 4 hours.
       e. 5 hours.

Answers appear in Appendix XXI.

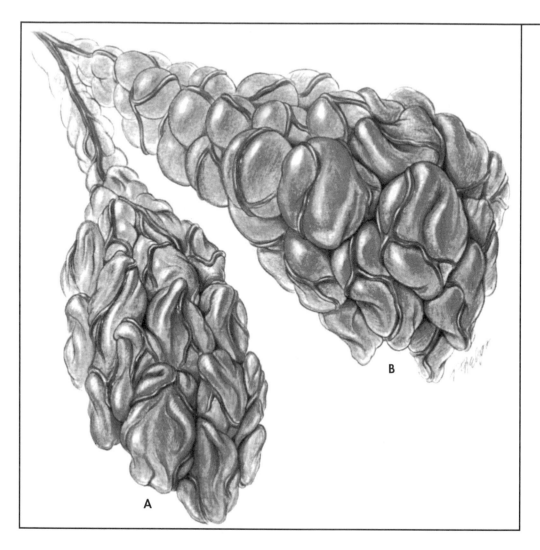

POSTOPERATIVE ATELECTASIS

FIG 31-1

Alveoli in postoperative atelectasis. A total or partial collapse of a previously expanded lung region. **A,** total alveolar collapse. **B,** partial alveolar collapse. (See also Plate 30.)

Postoperative Atelectasis

ANATOMIC ALTERATIONS OF THE LUNGS

Postoperative atelectasis is commonly seen after upper abdominal and thoracic surgical procedures. The term *atelectasis,* in the strict sense of the word, is defined as the condition in which the lungs of the newborn remain unexpanded (airless) at birth. In the clinical setting, however, the meaning of atelectasis is generally broadened to include partial or total collapse of previously expanded lung regions. Atelectasis may be limited to the smallest lung unit (i.e., alveoli or primary lobule*) or involve an entire lung segment, lobe, or lung (Fig 31-1).

To summarize, the major pathologic and anatomic alterations associated with postoperative atelectasis include partial or total collapse of the following:

- Alveoli or primary lobule
- Lung segment
- Lung lobe
- Entire lung

ETIOLOGY

Postoperative atelectasis is most commonly associated with (1) conditions that decrease lung expansion and (2) airway secretions and mucus plugs.

Decreased Lung Expansion

Good lung expansion is dependent on both the patient's ability to generate an appropriate intrapleural pressure and an intact chest cage. Thoracic, upper abdominal, and lower abdominal surgical procedures often result in a reduction in the patient's ability to generate good lung expansion and, therefore, are all considered high-risk factors for postoperative atelectasis. Upper abdominal surgery presents the greatest risk for atelectasis.

Other precipitating factors that decrease the patient's ability to generate a negative intrapleural pressure include (1) anesthesia, (2) postoperative pain, (3) reclining position, (4) obesity, (5) advanced age, (6) inadequate tidal volumes during mechanical ventilation, (7)

---

*A primary lobule is a cluster of alveoli that originates from a single terminal bronchiole. Each primary lobule is about 3.5 mm in diameter and contains about 2,000 alveoli. There are about 150,000 primary lobules in the lung. A primary lobule is also called acinus, terminal respiratory unit, lung parenchyma, and functional unit.

malnutrition, (8) ascites, (9) diaphragmatic apraxia (e.g., topical cooling of the left phrenic nerve often occurs during cardiac surgery and may lead to an inadequate diaphragmatic movement and left lower lobe atelectasis), and (10) restrictive lung disorders (e.g., pleural effusion, pneumothorax, ARDS, pulmonary edema, chronic interstitial lung disease, and pleural mass).

Airway Secretions and Mucus Plugs (Airway Obstruction)

Postoperative atelectasis is also associated with retained airway secretions and mucus plugs. Precipitating factors for retained secretions include (1) decreased mucociliary transport mechanism, (2) excessive secretions, (3) inadequate hydration, (3) weak or absent cough, (4) general anesthesia, (5) smoking history, and (6) certain pathologic conditions (e.g., bronchiectasis, chronic bronchitis, cystic fibrosis, and asthma). When mucus plugs develop, distal gases are absorbed into the pulmonary circulation and atelectasis ensues. The breathing of high oxygen concentrations enhances this pathologic process.

OVERVIEW

OF THE CARDIOPULMONARY CLINICAL MANIFESTATIONS ASSOCIATED WITH
POSTOPERATIVE ATELECTASIS

❑ **INCREASED RESPIRATORY RATE**

Several pathophysiologic mechanisms operating simultaneously may lead to an increased ventilatory rate. These are (see page 17)

- Stimulation of the peripheral chemoreceptors
- Decreased lung compliance/increased ventilatory rate relationship
- Stimulating of J receptors
- Pain/anxiety/fever

❑ **PULMONARY FUNCTION STUDY FINDINGS**

Expiratory Maneuver Findings (see page 39)

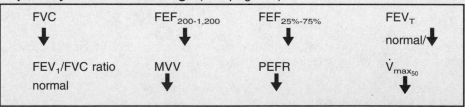

| FVC ↓ | FEF$_{200-1,200}$ ↓ | FEF$_{25\%-75\%}$ ↓ | FEV$_T$ normal/↓ |
| FEV$_1$/FVC ratio normal | MVV ↓ | PEFR ↓ | $\dot{V}_{max_{50}}$ ↓ |

Lung Volume and Capacity Findings (see page 39)

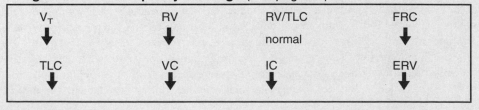

| V$_T$ ↓ | RV ↓ | RV/TLC normal | FRC ↓ |
| TLC ↓ | VC ↓ | IC ↓ | ERV ↓ |

❑ **INCREASED HEART RATE (PULSE), CARDIAC OUTPUT, AND BLOOD PRESSURE** (see page 86)

❑ **ARTERIAL BLOOD GASES**

Small or Localized Postoperative Atelectasis

Acute Alveolar Hyperventilation with Hypoxemia (see page 57)

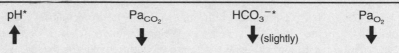

pH*	Pa_{CO_2}	HCO_3^-*	Pa_{O_2}
↑	↓	↓(slightly)	↓

*When tissue hypoxia is severe enough to produce lactic acid, the pH and HCO_3^- values will be lower than expected for a particular Pa_{CO_2} level.

Large or Widespread Postoperative Atelectasis

Acute Ventilatory Failure with Hypoxemia (see page 59)

pH*	Pa_{CO_2}	HCO_3^-*	Pa_{O_2}
↓	↑	↑(slightly)	↓

*When tissue hypoxia is severe enough to produce lactic acid, the pH and HCO_3^- values will be lower than expected for a particular Pa_{CO_2} level.

❑ **OXYGENATION INDICES** (see page 69)

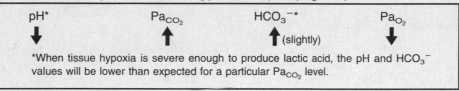

$\dot{Q}_S/\dot{Q}_T$	D_{O_2}*	$\dot{V}_{O_2}$	$C(a-\bar{v})_{O_2}$
↑	↓	normal	normal

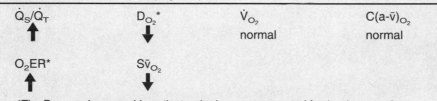

O_2ER*	$S\bar{v}_{O_2}$
↑	↓

*The D_{O_2} may be normal in patients who have compensated for the decreased oxygenation status with an increased cardiac output. When the D_{O_2} is normal, the O_2ER is usually normal.

❑ **CYANOSIS (see page 68)**
❑ **CHEST ASSESSMENT FINDINGS (see page 6)**
   • Increased tactile and vocal fremitus
   • Dull percussion note
   • Bronchial breath sounds
   • Diminished breath sounds (common when atelectasis is caused by mucus plugs
   • Crackles (usually heard initially in the dependent lung regions and during late inspiration)
   • Whispered pectoriloquy

❑ **RADIOLOGIC FINDINGS**
   Chest radiograph
   • Increased density in areas of atelectasis
   • Air bronchograms
   • Elevation of the hemidiaphragm on affected side
   • Mediastinal shift toward affected side

   Areas of increased density generally appear initially in the dependent lung regions. Air bronchograms can be seen when large areas of atelectasis are present. An elevation of the hemidiaphragm and/or mediastinal shift toward the affected side is often seen when large area of atelectasis exist.

GENERAL MANAGEMENT OF POSTOPERATIVE ATELECTASIS

Precipitating factors for postoperative atelectasis should be identified during the postoperative assessment (see etiology). High-risk patients should be monitored closely. For example, bedside spirometry (vital capacity and inspiratory capacity) is useful in the early detection of atelectasis. Preventive measures are also prescribed for high-risk patients. For example, incentive spirometry is frequently prescribed to encourage good lung expansion, or chest physical therapy may be given to the patient with mild to moderate bronchial secretions to offset the development of mucus plugs and atelectasis. When the diagnosis of postoperative atelectasis has been made, the following respiratory care procedures may be prescribed:

General Considerations

Whenever possible, treatment of the underlying cause of the postoperative atelectasis should be prescribed immediately (e.g., medication for pain, correction of inadequate tidal volumes during mechanical ventilation, or withdrawal of air or fluid from the pleural cavity).

Hyperinflation Techniques

Hyperinflation techniques are prescribed to reinflate the collapsed lung areas (see Appendix XII).

Mobilization of Bronchial Secretions

When postoperative atelectasis is caused by mucus accumulation and mucus plugs, a number of respiratory therapy modalities may be used to enhance the mobilization of bronchial secretions (see Appendix XI).

Supplemental Oxygen

Because hypoxemia is associated with postoperative atelectasis, supplemental oxygen may be required. It should be noted, however, that the hypoxemia that develops in postoperative atelectasis is caused by capillary shunting. Hypoxemia caused by capillary shunting is refractory to oxygen therapy.

Mechanical Ventilation

Mechanical ventilation is often prescribed after major surgery, especially if the patient demonstrates one or more high-risk factors for postoperative atelectasis. For example, in cardiac surgery patients, mechanical ventilation is generally maintained until all the cardiopulmonary parameters are stable.

• • • **POSTOPERATIVE ATELECTASIS CASE STUDY** • • •

ADMITTING HISTORY AND PHYSICAL EXAMINATION

This 62-year-old male with a 35-pack-year smoking history had the left upper lobe resected for small cell carcinoma. Anesthesia had been performed, using a right-sided double-lumen endotracheal tube. At the end of the procedure, the patient was breathing well and the tube was removed.

In the recovery room, 30 minutes after arrival, it was noted that his respiratory rate increased from 22 to 34/min. His pulse increased from 70 to 130 beats/min and regular, and his blood pressure increased from 115/85 to 160/95 mm Hg. His peripheral oxygen saturation dropped from 97% to 92% while on an $F_{I_{O_2}}$ of 0.30. A chest x-ray showed atelectasis of the right upper lobe. Arterial blood gas values were pH 7.29, Pa_{CO_2} 63, HCO_3^- 25, Pa_{O_2} 55. At this time, the respiratory therapist recorded the following:

RESPIRATORY ASSESSMENT AND PLAN

S: N/A. Patient still sedated from anesthesia.

O: RR 34, P 130 regular, BP 160/95. BS decreased in right upper chest anteriorly. CXR: right upper lobe atelectasis. On room air: pH 7.29, Pa_{CO_2} 63, HCO_3^- 25, Pa_{O_2} 55.

A: • Right upper lobe atelectasis. Rule out mucus plug. (CXR & decreased breath sounds)
 • Acute ventilatory failure with moderate hypoxemia (ABG)

P: Contact physician: reintubation and ventilation. Follow pulse oximetry. Institute bronchial hygiene & volume expansion protocols.

The patient was reintubated, ventilated, and oxygenated according to protocol. A mucolytic (acetylcysteine) was aerosolized and instilled into the patient's endotracheal tube. Aggressive tracheobronchial suctioning was performed. This was productive of small amounts of secretions with little or no benefit to the patient.

In view of this, a fiberoptic bronchoscope was inserted through the endotracheal tube, and a large mucus plug was identified in the orifice of the right upper lobe bronchus. This was removed under direct vision. Following the bronchoscopy, the patient improved rapidly and could be extubated after about 30 minutes. A chest x-ray taken at this time showed full expansion of the right upper lobe.

DISCUSSION

Postoperative atelectasis is one of the bread-and-butter responsibilities of the respiratory care practitioner. Accordingly, he must be extremely facile in the diagnosis and management of such patients. The development of immediate postoperative atelectasis is almost always related to airway obstruction, in this case due to a large mucus plug obstructing the right upper lobe. Since such patients (in the immediate postoperative period) often cannot cough vigorously, particularly after thoracotomy, the decision to immediately initiate bronchoscopy, rather than to rely on physical therapy and mucolytics, was certainly in order.

In patients with abdominal surgery, and/or those in whom atelectasis develops later, the simpler approaches should certainly be tried first. Atelectasis has a tendency to recur, and these patients need to be followed at least 72 hours postoperatively to be sure that has not happened. Thus, the therapist's suggestion to follow pulse oximetry is entirely appropriate.

As important as treatment is, prevention is better, and in this connection, the bronchial hygiene and volume expansion protocols ordered are very important. Indeed, institution of these simple protocols often prevents the late development of atelectasis in postoperative patients.

SELF ASSESSMENT QUESTIONS

Fill In The Blanks

1. List the three types of surgery that are considered high-risk for postoperative atelectasis.

    a. _____

    b. _____

    c. _____

2. List five precipitating factors that decrease the patient's ability to generate a negative intrapleural pressure.

    a. _____

    b. _____

    c. _____

    d. _____

    e. _____

3. List five precipitating factors associated with airway secretions and mucus plugs.

    a. _____

    b. _____

    c. _____

    d. _____

    e. _____

Answers appear in Appendix XXI.

APPENDIXES

APPENDIX I: SYMBOLS AND ABBREVIATIONS COMMONLY USED IN RESPIRATORY PHYSIOLOGY

PRIMARY SYMBOLS		
Gas Symbols		**Blood Symbols**
P	Pressure	Q Blood volume
V	Gas volume	$\dot{Q}$ Blood flow
$\dot{V}$	Gas volume per unit of time, or flow	C Content in blood
F	Fractional concentration of gas	S Saturation

SECONDARY SYMBOLS		
Gas Symbols		**Blood Symbols**
I	Inspired	a Arterial
E	Expired	c Capillary
A	Alveolar	v Venous
T	Tidal	$\bar{v}$ Mixed venous
D	Deadspace	

ABBREVIATIONS	
Lung Volume	
VC	Vital capacity
IC	Inspiratory capacity
IRV	Inspiratory reserve volume
ERV	Expiratory reserve volume
FRC	Functional residual capacity
RV	Residual volume
TLC	Total lung capacity
RV/TLC (%)	Residual volume-to-total lung capacity ratio, expressed as a percentage
V_T	Tidal volume
V_A	Alveolar ventilation
V_D	Dead-space ventilation
V_L	Actual lung volume

Spirometry	
FVC	Forced vital capacity with maximally forced expiratory effort
FEV_T	Forced expiratory volume, timed
$FEF_{200\text{-}1,200}$	Average rate of airflow between 200 and 1,200 mL of the FVC
$FEF_{25\%\text{-}75\%}$	Forced expiratory flow during the middle half of the FVC (formerly called the maximal midexpiratory flow [MMF])
PEFR	Maximum flow rate that can be achieved
$\dot{V}_{max_x}$	Forced expiratory flow related to the actual volume of the lungs as denoted by the subscript x, which refers to the amount of lung volume remaining when measurement is made
MVV	Maximal voluntary ventilation as the volume of air expired in a specified interval

Mechanics	
C_L	Lung compliance, volume change per unit of pressure change
R_{aw}	Airway resistance, pressure per unit of flow

Diffusion	
D_{LCO}	Diffusing capacity of carbon monoxide

Blood Gases	
$P_{A_{O_2}}$	Alveolar oxygen tension
$P_{c_{O_2}}$	Pulmonary capillary oxygen tension
Pa_{O_2}	Arterial oxygen tension
$P\bar{v}_{O_2}$	Mixed venous oxygen tension
$P_{A_{CO_2}}$	Alveolar carbon dioxide tension
$P_{c_{CO_2}}$	Pulmonary capillary carbon dioxide tension
Pa_{CO_2}	Arterial carbon dioxide tension
Sa_{O_2}	Arterial oxygen saturation
$S\bar{v}_{O_2}$	Mixed venous oxygen saturation
pH	Negative logarithm of the H^+ concentration used as a positive number
HCO_3^-	Plasma bicarbonate concentration
mEq/L	The number of grams of solute dissolved in a normal solution
Ca_{O_2}	Oxygen content of arterial blood
Cc_{O_2}	Oxygen content of capillary blood
$C\bar{v}_{O_2}$	Oxygen content of mixed venous blood
$\dot{V}/\dot{Q}$	Ventilation-perfusion ratio
$\dot{Q}_s/\dot{Q}_T$	Shunt
Q_T	Total cardiac output

APPENDIX II: SYMPATHOMIMETIC BRONCHODILATORS

Sympathomimetic agents are used to offset bronchial smooth muscle constriction.

Generic Name	Trade Name
Epinephrine	Adrenalin
Racemic epinephrine	MicroNefrin VapoNefrin AsthmaNefrin
Isoproterenol	Isuprel Mistometer Isuprel
Isoetharine	Brokosol Bronkometer
Metaproterenol	Alupent Metaprel
Terbutaline	Brethine Brethaire
Albuterol	Proventil Ventolin
Bitolterol (Colterol)	Tornalate
Pirbuterol	Maxair
Salmeterol	Serevent

APPENDIX III: PARASYMPATHOLYTIC (ANTICHOLINERGIC) BRONCHODILATORS

Parasympatholytic agents are used to offset bronchial smooth muscle constriction.

Generic Name	Trade Name
Atropine sulfate Ipratropium bromide Glycopyrrolate	Dey-Dose Atropine Sulfate Atrovent Robinul*

*Available in injectable solution; used experimentally as aerosol.

APPENDIX IV: XANTHINE BRONCHODILATORS

Xanthine bronchodilators are used to enhance bronchial smooth muscle relaxation.

Generic Name	Trade Name
Theophylline	Bronkodyl
	Elixophyllin
	Somophyllin-T
	Slo-Phyllin
	Theolair
	Theo-Dur
	Theo-Dur Sprinkle
	Constant-T
	Quibron-T/SR
	Respbid
Theophylline sodium glycinate	Synophylate
Oxtriphylline (choline theophyllinate)	Choledyl
Aminophylline (theophylline ethylenediamine)	Aminophyllin
	Phyllocontin
Dyphylline	Lufyllin

APPENDIX V: CORTICOSTEROIDS

Aerosolized corticosteroids are used to suppress bronchial inflammation and bronchial edema. They are also used for their ability to enhance the responsiveness of β_2 receptor sites to sympathomimetic agents.

Generic Name	Trade Name
Dexamethasone sodium phosphate	Decadron Respihaler
Beclomethasone dipropionate	Vanceril
	Beclovent
Triamcinolone acetonide	Azmacort
Flunisolide	AeroBid

APPENDIX VI: MUCOLYTIC AGENTS

The following agents are used to enhance the mobilization of bronchial secretions:

Generic Name	Trade Name
Acetylcysteine	Mucomyst
Recombinant human DNase (rhDNase)	Pulmozyme
Sodium bicarbonate	2% solution

APPENDIX VII: EXPECTORANTS

Expectorants are agents used to increase bronchial gland secretion, which in turn decreases mucus viscosity. This facilitates the mobilization and expectoration of bronchial secretions.

Generic Name	Trade Name
Guaifenesin	Robitussin, Naldecon Senior EX, Humibid L.A.
Terpin hydrate	(Various)
Iodinated glycerol	Organidin
Potassium iodide (SSKI)	(Various)

APPENDIX VIII: ANTIBIOTIC AGENTS

Agent	Therapeutic Uses

Penicillins
  Penicillin G
  Penicillin V
  Oxacillin (Prostaphilin)
  Cloxacillin (Tegopen)
  Methicillin (Staphcillin)
  Ampicillin (Omnipren)
  Amoxicillin (Polymox)
  Carbenicillin (Geopen)
  Ticarcillin (Ticar)
	Used in treating streptococcal species, staphylococcal species, *Haemophilus influenzae*. Also used in treating aspiration pneumonia

Cephalosporins
  First generation
    Cefaclor (Ceclor)
    Cephalexin (Keflex)
    Cefadroxil (Duricef)
    Cephalothin (Keflin)
  Second generation
    Cephamandole (Mandol)
    Cefoxitin (Mefoxin)
    Cefonicid (Monocid)
  Third generation
    Cefoperazone (Cefobid)
    Cefotaxime (Claforan)
    Ceftizoxime (Cefizox)
    Ceftazidime (Fortaz)
	Important for their broad-spectrum activity against common gram-positive cocci (primarily the first generation) and some gram-negative organisms (primarily the second and third generations). Also active against *Klebsiella* species, but lack efficacy against *Pseudomonas aeruginosa* and *Haemophilus influenzae*

Aminoglycosides
  Streptomycin
  Gentamicin (Garamycin)
  Netilmicin (Netromycin)
  Amikacin (Amikin)
  Kanamycin (Kantrex)
  Neomycin (Neosporin)
	Used for treating gram-negative organisms. Commonly used to treat *Pseudomonas* in cystic fibrosis. Streptomycin is also used in treating *M. tuberculosis*

Continued.

APPENDIX VIII: ANTIBIOTIC AGENTS—cont'd

Agent	Therapeutic Uses
Tetracyclines	
Tetracycline (Achromycin)	Used in treating mycoplasmal and other
Oxytetracycline (Terramycin)	atypical pneumonias and acute infections
Demeclocycline (Declomycin)	superimposed on chronic bronchitis
Methacycline (Rondomycin)	
Doxycycline (Vibramycin)	
Minocycline (Minocin)	
Other antibiotic agents	
Vancomycin (Vanocin)	Used in treating staphyloccal infections
Chloramphenicol (Chloromycetin)	Used in treating penicillinase-producing *Staphylococcus, Klebsiella, Haemophilus influenzae*
Erythromycin (Erythrocin, Ilotycin)	Used in treating penicillin-allergic patients with pneumococcal pneumonia
Polymyxins	Used in treating *Pseudomonas* and other gram-negative organisms
Polymyxin B	
Polymyxin E	
Clindamycin (Cleocin) and Lincomycin (Linococin)	Used in treating aspiration pneumonia
Metronidazole (Flagyl, Metizol)	Active against anaerobic infections
Quinolones	Used in treating *H. influenzae, Legionella pneumophila, M. pneumoniae, P. aeruginosa*
Pentamidine, isethionate (Pentam)	Used in treating the protozoan *Pneumocystis carinii* in AIDS patients

APPENDIX IX: POSITIVE INOTROPIC AGENTS

The following positive inotropic agents are used to increase cardiac output:

Generic Name	Trade Name
Digitalis	(Various)
Deslanoside	Cedilanid-D
Digoxin	Lanoxin
Digitoxin	Crystodigin
Amrinone	Inocor
Dobutamine	Dobutrex
Dopamine	Intropin
Epinephrine	(Various)
Isoproterenol	Isuprel

APPENDIX X: DIURETICS

Diuretics are drugs used to increase urine output.

Generic Name	Trade Name
Furosemide	Lasix
Ethacrynic acid	Edecrin
Bumetanide	Bumex
Hydrochlorothiazide	Esidrix, HydroDIURIL
Spironolactone	Aldactone

APPENDIX XI: TECHNIQUES USED TO MOBILIZE BRONCHIAL SECRETIONS

The following respiratory therapy modalities are used to enhance the mobilization of bronchial secretions:

- Ultrasonic nebulization
- Increased fluid intake (6 to 10 glasses of water daily)
- Chest physical therapy (CPT)
- Postural drainage (PD)
- Percussion and vibration with postural drainage
- Deep breathing and coughing
- Intermittent positive-pressure breathing (IPPB)
- Incentive spirometry
- Positive expiratory pressure (PEP) therapy
- Suctioning
- Bronchoscopy

Therapeutic bronchoscopy includes (1) suctioning of excessive secretions/retained secretions/mucus plugs, (2) removal of foreign bodies, (3) selective lavage (with normal saline or mucolytic agents), (4) management of life-threatening hemoptysis, and (5) endotracheal intubation. While the merits of therapeutic fiberoptic bronchoscopy are well documented, routine respiratory therapy modalities at the patient's bedside (e.g., chest physical therapy, postural drainage, deep breathing and coughing techniques, and positive expiratory pressure [PEP] therapy) are considered the first line of defense in the treatment of atelectasis from pooled secretions. Therapeutic bronchoscopy is commonly used in the management of bronchiectasis, lung abscess, smoke inhalation and thermal injuries, and lung cancer.

APPENDIX XII: HYPERINFLATION TECHNIQUES

Hyperinflation techniques are often used to offset alveolar consolidation and atelectasis. Common techniques include the following:

- Cough and deep breathing
- Incentive spirometry
- Intermittent positive-pressure breathing (IPPB)
- Continuous positive airway pressure (CPAP)
- Positive end-expiratory pressure (PEEP)

APPENDIX XIII: THE IDEAL ALVEOLAR GAS EQUATION

Clinically, the alveolar oxygen tension can be computed from the ideal alveolar gas equation. A useful clinical approximation of the ideal alveolar gas equation is as follows:

$$Pa_{O_2} = [PB - P_{H_2O}] \, FI_{O_2} - Pa_{CO_2} \, (1.25)$$

where PB is barometric pressure, Pa_{O_2} is the partial pressure of oxygen within the alveoli, P_{H_2O} is the partial pressure of water vapor in the alveoli (at body temperature and at sea level P_{H_2O} in the alveoli is 47 mm Hg), FI_{O_2} is the fractional concentration of inspired oxygen, and Pa_{CO_2} is the partial pressure of arterial carbon dioxide. The number 1.25 is a factor that adjusts for alterations in oxygen tension due to variations in the respiratory exchange ratio. The respiratory exchange ratio indicates that less carbon dioxide is transferred into the alveoli (about 200 cc/min) than the amount of oxygen that moves into the pulmonary capillary blood (about 250 mL/min). This ratio is normally about 0.8.

Therefore, if a patient is receiving an FI_{O_2} of 40% on a day when the barometric pressure is 755 mm Hg and the Pa_{CO_2} is 55 mm Hg, the patient's alveolar oxygen tension (Pa_{O_2}) can be calculated as follows:

$$
\begin{aligned}
P_{A_{O_2}} &= (PB - P_{H_2O}) \, FI_{O_2} - Pa_{CO_2} \, (1.25) \\
&= (755 - 47) \, .40 - 55 \, (1.25) \\
&= (708) \, .40 - 68.75 \\
&= (283.2) - 68.75 \\
&= 214.45
\end{aligned}
$$

The ideal alveolar gas equation is part of the clinical information needed to calculate the degree of pulmonary shunting.

APPENDIX XIV: PHYSIOLOGIC DEAD-SPACE CALCULATION

The amount of physiologic dead space (V_D) in the tidal volume (V_T) can be estimated by using the dead space-to-tidal volume ratio (V_D/V_T) equation. The equation is arranged as follows:

$$V_D/V_T = \frac{Pa_{CO_2} - P\bar{E}_{CO_2}}{Pa_{CO_2}}$$

For example, in a patient whose Pa_{CO_2} is 40 mm Hg and whose $P\bar{E}_{CO_2}$ is 28 mm Hg:

$$
\begin{aligned}
V_D/V_T &= \frac{40 - 28}{40} \\
&= \frac{12}{40} \\
&= .3
\end{aligned}
$$

In this case, approximately 30% of the patient's ventilation is dead-space ventilation. This is within the normal range.

APPENDIX XV: UNITS OF MEASUREMENT

Metric Weight

Grams	Centigrams	Milligrams	Micrograms	Nanograms
1	100	1000	1,000,000	1,000,000,000
.01	1	10	10,000	10,000,000
.001	.1	1	1000	1,000,000
.000001	.0001	.001	1	1000
.000000001	.0000001	.000001	.001	1

Weight

Metric	Approximate Apothecary Equivalents
Grams	*Grains*
.0002	$1/300$
.0003	$1/200$
.0004	$1/150$
.0005	$1/120$
.0006	$1/100$
.001	$1/60$
.002	$1/30$
.005	$1/12$
.010	$1/6$
.015	$1/4$
.025	$3/8$
.030	$1/2$
.050	$3/4$
.060	1
.100	$1\frac{1}{2}$
.120	2
.200	3
.300	5
.500	$7\frac{1}{2}$
.600	10
1	15
2	30
4	60

Liquid Measure

Metric	Approximate Apothecary Equivalents
Milliliters	
1,000	1 quart
750	1½ pints
500	1 pint
250	8 fluid ounces
200	7 fluid ounces
100	3½ fluid ounces
50	1¾ fluid ounces
30	1 fluid ounce
15	4 fluid drams
10	2½ fluid drams
8	2 fluid drams
5	1¼ fluid drams
4	1 fluid dram
3	45 minims
2	30 minims
1	15 minims
0.75	12 minims
0.6	10 minims
0.5	8 minims
0.3	5 minims
0.25	4 minims
0.2	3 minims
0.1	1½ minims
0.06	1 minim
0.05	¾ minim
0.03	½ minim

Metric Liquid

Liter	Centiliter	Milliliter	Microliter	Nanoliter
1	100	1000	1,000,000	1,000,000,000
.01	1	10	10,000	10,000,000
.001	.1	1	1000	1,000,000
.000001	.0001	.001	1	1000
.000000001	.0000001	.000001	.001	1

Metric Length

Meter	Centimeter	Millimeter	Micrometer	Nanometer
1	100	1000	1,000,000	1,000,000,000
.01	1	10	10,000	10,000,000
.001	.1	1	1000	1,000,000
.000001	.0001	.001	1	1000
.000000001	.0000001	.000001	.001	1

Weight Conversions (Metric and Avoirdupois)

Grams	Kilograms	Ounces	Pounds
1	.001	.0353	.0022
1000	1	35.3	2.2
28.35	.02835	1	$\frac{1}{16}$
454.5	.4545	16	1

Weight Conversions (Metric and Apothecary)

Grams	Milligrams	Grains	Drams	Ounces	Pounds
1	1000	15.4	.2577	.0322	.00268
.001	1	.0154	.00026	.0000322	.00000268
.0648	64.8	1	$\frac{1}{60}$	$\frac{1}{480}$	$\frac{1}{5760}$
3.888	3888	60	1	$\frac{1}{8}$	$\frac{1}{96}$
31.1	31104	480	8	1	$\frac{1}{12}$
363.25	373248	5760	96	12	1

Approximate Household Measurement Equivalents (volume)

```
                                        1 tsp =      5 ml
                             1 tbsp =  3 tsp =     15 ml
                  1 fl oz =  2 tbsp =  6 tsp =     30 ml
         1 cup =     8 fl oz                 =    240 ml
1 pt =   2 cups =  16 fl oz                  =    480 ml
1 qt =  2 pt =  4 cups =  32 fl oz           =    960 ml
1 gal = 4 qt = 8 pt = 16 cups = 128 fl oz    =   3840 ml
```

Volume Conversions (Metric and Apothecary)

Milliliters	Minims	Fluid Drams	Fluid Ounces	Pints	Liters	Gallons	Quarts	Fluid Ounces	Pints
1	16.2	.27	.0333	.0021	1	.2642	1.057	33.824	2.114
.0616	1	1/60	1/480	1/7680	3.785	1	4	128	8
3.697	60	1	1/8	1/128	.946	1/4	1	32	2
29.58	480	8	1	1/16	.473	1/8	1/2	16	1
473.2	7680	128	16	1	.0296	1/128	1/32	1	1/16

Length Conversions (Metric and English System)

	Millimeters	Centimeters	Inches	Feet	Yards	Meters
1 A =	$\dfrac{1}{10{,}000{,}000}$	$\dfrac{1}{100{,}000{,}000}$	$\dfrac{1}{254{,}000{,}000}$	$\dfrac{1}{3{,}050{,}000{,}000}$	$\dfrac{1}{9{,}140{,}000{,}000}$	$\dfrac{1}{10{,}000{,}000{,}000}$
1 nm =	$\dfrac{1}{1{,}000{,}000}$	$\dfrac{1}{10{,}000{,}000}$	$\dfrac{1}{25{,}400{,}000}$	$\dfrac{1}{305{,}000{,}000}$	$\dfrac{1}{914{,}000{,}000}$	$\dfrac{1}{1{,}000{,}000{,}000}$
1 μm =	$\dfrac{1}{1{,}000}$	$\dfrac{1}{10{,}000}$	$\dfrac{1}{25{,}400}$	$\dfrac{1}{305{,}000}$	$\dfrac{1}{914{,}000}$	$\dfrac{1}{1{,}000{,}000}$
1 mm =	1.0	0.1	0.03937	0.00328	0.0011	0.001
1 cm =	10.0	1.0	0.3937	0.03281	0.0109	0.01
1 in =	25.4	2.54	1.0	0.0833	0.0278	0.0254
1 ft =	304.8	30.48	12.0	1.0	0.333	0.3048
1 yd =	914.40	91.44	36.0	3.0	1.0	0.9144
1 m =	1000.0	100.0	39.37	3.2808	1.0936	1.0

APPENDIX XVI: POISEUILLE'S LAW
Poiseuille's Law for Flow Rearranged to a Simple Proportionality

$$\dot{V} \simeq \Delta P r^4, \text{ or rewritten as } \frac{\dot{V}}{r^4} \simeq \Delta P.$$

When ΔP remains constant, then

$$\frac{\dot{V}_1}{r_1^{\,4}} \simeq \frac{\dot{V}_2}{r_2^{\,4}}$$

Example 1.—If the radius (r_1) is decreased to half its previous radius ($r_2 = \frac{1}{2} r_1$), then

$$\frac{\dot{V}_1}{r_1^{\,4}} \simeq \frac{\dot{V}_2}{(\frac{1}{2} r_1)^4}$$

$$\frac{\dot{V}_1}{r_1^{\,4}} \simeq \frac{\dot{V}_2}{(\frac{1}{16})r_1^{\,4}}$$

$$(\cancel{r_1^{\,4}})\frac{\dot{V}_1}{\cancel{r_1^{\,4}}} \simeq (\cancel{r_1^{\,4}})\frac{\dot{V}_2}{(\frac{1}{16})\cancel{r_1^{\,4}}}$$

$$\dot{V}_1 \simeq \frac{\dot{V}_2}{\frac{1}{16}}$$

$$(\tfrac{1}{16})\dot{V}_1 \simeq (\tfrac{1}{16}) \frac{\dot{V}_2}{\tfrac{1}{16}}$$

$$(\tfrac{1}{16})\dot{V}_1 \simeq \dot{V}_2$$

The gas flow ($\dot{V}_1$) is reduced to $\tfrac{1}{16}$ its original flow rate [$\dot{V}_2 \simeq (\tfrac{1}{16})\,\dot{V}_1$].

Example 2.—If the radius (r_1) is decreased by 16% ($r_2 = r_1 - 0.16\,r_1 = 0.84r_1$), then

$$\frac{\dot{V}_1}{r_1^{\,4}} \simeq \frac{\dot{V}_2}{r_2^{\,4}}$$

$$\frac{\dot{V}_1}{r_1^{\,4}} \simeq \frac{\dot{V}_2}{(0.84r_1)^4}$$

$$\dot{V}_2 \simeq \frac{(0.84r_1^{\,4}\,\dot{V}_1}{r_1^{\,4}}$$

$$\dot{V}_2 \simeq \frac{0.4979\,r_1^{\,4}\,\dot{V}_1}{r_1^{\,4}}$$

$$\dot{V}_2 \simeq \tfrac{1}{2}\,\dot{V}_1$$

The flow rate ($\dot{V}_1$) would decrease to half the original flow rate ($\dot{V}_2 \simeq \tfrac{1}{2}\,\dot{V}_1$).

Poiseuille's Law for Pressure Rearranged to a Simple Proportionality

$$P \simeq \frac{\dot{V}}{r^4}, \text{ or rewritten as } P \cdot r^4 \simeq \dot{V}$$

When $\dot{V}$ remains constant, then

$$P_1 \cdot r_1^{\,4} \simeq P_2 \cdot r_2^{\,4}$$

Example 1.—If the radius (r_1) is reduced to half its original radius [$r_2 = (\tfrac{1}{2})\,r_1$], then

$$P_1 \cdot r_1^{\,4} \simeq P_2 \cdot r_2^{\,4}$$

$$P_1 \cdot r_1^{\,4} \simeq P_2[(\tfrac{1}{2})\,r_1]^4$$

$$P_1 \cdot r_1^{\,4} \simeq P_2 \cdot (\tfrac{1}{16})\,r_1^{\,4}$$

$$\frac{P_1 \cdot r_1^{\,4}}{r_1^{\,4}} \simeq \frac{P_2 \cdot (\tfrac{1}{16})\,r_1^{\,4}}{r_1^{\,4}}$$

$$P_1 \simeq P_2 \cdot (\tfrac{1}{16})$$

$$16\,P_1 \simeq 16 \cdot P_2 \cdot (\tfrac{1}{16})$$

$$16\,P_1 \simeq P_2$$

The pressure (P_1) will increase to 16 times its original level ($P_2 \simeq 16 \cdot P_1$).

Example 2.—If the radius (r_1) is decreased by 16% ($r_2 = r_1 - 0.16\,r_1 = 0.84\,r_1$), then

$$P_1 \cdot r_1^{\,4} \simeq P_2 \cdot r_2^{\,4}$$

$$P_1 \cdot r_1^{\,4} \simeq P_2\,(0.4979)r_1^{\,4}$$

$$\frac{P_1\,r_1^{\,4}}{(0.4979r_1)^4} = P_2$$

$$2\,P_1 = P_2$$

The pressure (P_1) would increase to twice its original pressure ($P_2 \simeq 2 \cdot P_1$).

APPENDIX XVII: P$_{CO_2}$/HCO$_3^-$/pH NOMOGRAM

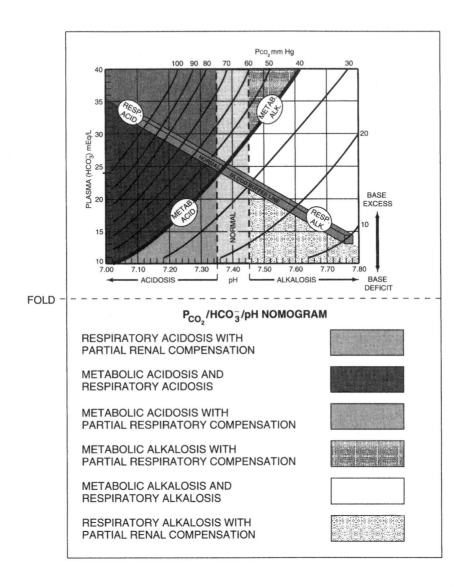

Copy the above P$_{CO_2}$/HCO$_3^-$/pH nomogram, color it in if you like, and have it laminated for use as a handy, pocket-size reference tool.

(From Des Jardins T: Cardiopulmonary Anatomy and Physiology: Essentials for Respiratory Care, 2nd Ed., Albany, NY, Delmar Publishers Inc, 1993. Used by permission.)

APPENDIX XVIII: CALCULATED HEMODYNAMIC MEASUREMENTS

The following are the major hemodynamic values that can be calculated from the direct hemodynamic measurements listed in Table 1-16. The calculated hemodynamic values are easily obtained from a programmed calculator or by using the specific hemodynamic formula and a handheld calculator. Because the calculated hemodynamic measurements vary with the size of an individual, some hemodynamic values are "indexed" by body surface area (BSA). Clinically, the BSA is obtained from a height-weight nomogram (see Appendix XVIX). In the normal adult, the BSA is 1.5 to 2 m^2.

Stroke Volume

The stroke volume (SV) is the volume of blood ejected by the ventricles with each contraction. The preload, afterload, and myocardial contractility are the major determinants of stroke volume. Stroke volume is derived by dividing the cardiac output (CO) by the heart rate (HR).

$$SV = \frac{CO}{HR}$$

For example, if an individual has a cardiac output of 4 L/min (4000 mL/min) and a heart rate of 80 beats/min, the stroke volume would be calculated as follows:

$$SV = \frac{CO}{HR}$$

$$= \frac{4000 \text{ mL/min}}{80 \text{ beats/min}}$$

$$= 50 \text{ mL/beat}$$

Stroke Volume Index

The stroke volume index (SVI), also known as stroke index, is calculated by dividing the stroke volume (SV) by the body surface area (BSA).

$$SVI = \frac{SV}{BSA}$$

For example, if a patient has a stroke volume of 50 mL and a body surface area of 2 m^2, the stroke volume index would be determined as follows:

$$SVI = \frac{SV}{BSA}$$

$$= \frac{50 \text{ mL/beat}}{2 \text{ m}^2}$$

$$= 25 \text{ mL/beat/m}^2$$

Assuming that the heart rate remains the same, as the stroke volume index increases or decreases, the cardiac index also increases or decreases. The stroke volume index reflects the (1) contractility of the heart, (2) overall blood volume status, and (3) amount of venous return.

Cardiac Index

The cardiac index (CI) is calculated by dividing the cardiac output (CO) by the body surface area (BSA).

$$CI = \frac{CO}{BSA}$$

For example, if a patient has a cardiac output of 6 L/min and a body surface area of 2 m^2, the cardiac index is computed as follows:

$$CI = \frac{CO}{BSA}$$

$$= \frac{6 \text{ L/min}}{2 \text{ m}^2}$$

$$= 3 \text{ L/min/m}^2$$

Right Ventricular Stroke Work Index

The right ventricular stroke work index (RVSWI) measures the amount of work required by the right ventricle to pump blood. The RVSWI is a reflection of the contractility of the right ventricle. In the presence of normal right ventricular contractility, increases in afterload (e.g., caused by pulmonary vascular constriction) cause the RVSWI to increase until a plateau is reached. When the contractility of the right ventricle is diminished by disease states, however, the RVSWI does not appropriately increase. The RVSWI is derived from the following formula:

$$RVSWI = SVI \times (\overline{PA} - CVP) \times 0.0136 \text{ g/mL}$$

where SVI is stroke volume index, $\overline{PA}$ is mean pulmonary artery pressure, and CVP is central venous pressure. The density of mercury factor 0.0136 g/mL is needed to convert the equation to the proper units of measurement—i.e., gram meters/m^2 (g m/m^2).

For example, if a patient has an SVI of 40 mL, a $\overline{PA}$ of 20 mm Hg, and a CVP of 5 mm Hg, the patient's RVSWI is calculated as follows:

$$RVSWI = SVI \times (\overline{PA} - CVP) \times 0.0136 \text{ g/mL}$$

$$= 40 \text{ mL/beat/m}^2 \times (15 \text{ mm Hg} - 5 \text{ mm Hg}) \times 0.0136 \text{ g/mL}$$

$$= 40 \text{ mL/beat/m}^2 \times 10 \text{ mm Hg} \times 0.0136 \text{ g/mL}$$

$$= 5.44 \text{ g m/m}^2$$

Left Ventricular Stroke Work Index

The left ventricular stroke work index (LVSWI) measures the amount of work required by the left ventricle to pump blood. The LVSWI is a reflection of the contractility of the left ventricle. In the presence of normal left ventricular contractility, increases in afterload (e.g., caused by systemic vascular constriction) cause the LVSWI to increase until a plateau is reached. When the contractility of the left ventricle is diminished by disease states, however, the LVSWI does not increase appropriately. The following formula is used for determining this hemodynamic variable:

$$LVSWI = SVI \times (MAP - PCWP) \times 0.0136 \text{ g/mL}$$

where SVI is stroke volume index, MAP is mean arterial pressure, and PCWP is pulmonary capillary wedge pressure. The density of mercury factor 0.0136 g/mL is needed to convert the equation to the proper units of measurements—i.e., gram meters/m^2 (g m/m^2).

For example, if a patient has an SVI of 40 mL, an MAP of 110 mm Hg, and a PCWP of 5 mm Hg, the patient's LVSWI is calculated as follows:

$$LVSWI = SVI \times (MAP - PCWP) \times 0.0136 \text{ g/mL}$$

$$= 40 \text{ mL/beat/m}^2 \times (110 \text{ mm Hg} - 5 \text{ mm Hg}) \times 0.0136 \text{ g/mL}$$

$$= 40 \text{ mL/beat/m}^2 \times (105 \text{ mm Hg}) \times 0.0136 \text{ g/mL}$$

$$= 59.84 \text{ g m/m}^2$$

Vascular Resistance

As blood flows through the pulmonary and the systemic vascular systems, there is resistance to flow. The pulmonary system is a *low-resistance* system. The systemic vascular system is a *high-resistance* system.

Pulmonary vascular resistance (PVR).—The PVR measurement reflects the afterload of the right ventricle. It is calculated by the following formula:

$$PVR = \frac{\overline{PA} - PCWP}{CO} \times 80$$

where $\overline{PA}$ is the mean pulmonary artery pressure, PCWP is the capillary wedge pressure, CO is the cardiac output, and 80 is a conversion factor for adjusting to the correct units of measurement (dyne $\times$ sec $\times$ cm^{-5}).

For example, if a patient has a $\overline{PA}$ of 20 mm Hg, a PCWP of 5 mm Hg, and a CO of 6 L/min, the patient's PVR is calculated as follows:

$$PVR = \frac{\overline{PA} - PCWP}{CO} \times 80$$

$$= \frac{20 \text{ mm Hg} - 5 \text{ mm Hg}}{6 \text{ L/min}} \times 80$$

$$= \frac{15 \text{ mm Hg}}{6 \text{ L/min}} \times 80$$

$$= 200 \text{ dynes} \times \sec \times \text{cm}^{-5}$$

Systemic or peripheral vascular resistance (SVR).—The SVR measurement reflects the afterload of the left ventricle. It is calculated by the following formula:

$$SVR = \frac{MAP - CVP}{CO} \times 80$$

where MAP is the mean arterial pressure, CVP is the central venous pressure, CO is the cardiac output, and 80 is a conversion factor for adjusting to the correct units of measurement (dyne $\times$ sec $\times$ cm^{-5}). (Note: The right atrial pressure [RAP] can be used in place of the CVP value.)

For example, if a patient has an MAP of 90 mm Hg, a CVP of 5 mm Hg, and a CO of 4 L/min, the patient's SVR is calculated as follows:

$$SVR = \frac{MAP - CVP}{CO} \times 80$$

$$= \frac{90 \text{ mm Hg} - 5 \text{ mm Hg}}{4 \text{ L/min}} \times 80$$

$$= \frac{85 \text{ mm Hg} \times 80}{4 \text{ L/min}}$$

$$= 1700 \text{ dynes} \times \sec \times \text{cm}^{-5}$$

APPENDIX XIX: DUBOIS BODY SURFACE AREA CHART

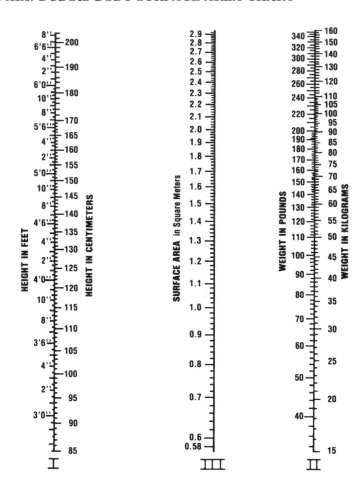

DIRECTIONS

To find the body surface area of a patient, locate the height in inches (or centimeters) on Scale I and the weight in pounds (or kilograms) on Scale II and place a straightedge (ruler) between these two points, which will intersect Scale III at the patient's surface area.

APPENDIX XX: CARDIOPULMONARY PROFILE

A representative example of a cardiopulmonary profile sheet used to monitor the critically ill patient.

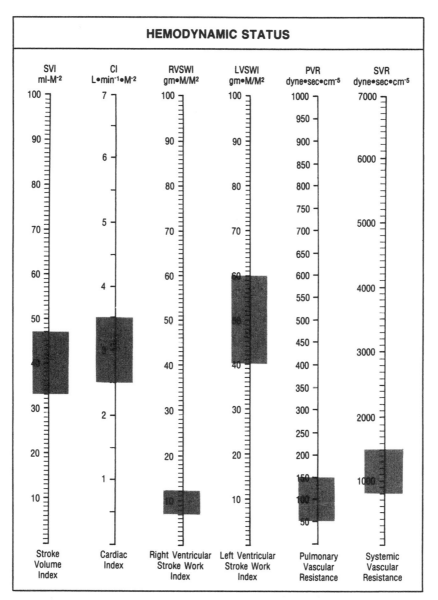

Shaded areas represent normal range.

(From Des Jardins T: Cardiopulmonary Anatomy and Physiology: Essentials for Respiratory Care, 2nd ed, Albany, NY, Delmar Publishers, 1993. Used by permission.)

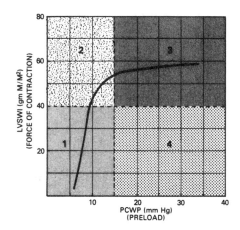

Quadrant 1: Hypovolemia
Quadrant 2: Optimal Function
Quadrant 3: Hypervolemia
Quadrant 4: Cardiac Failure

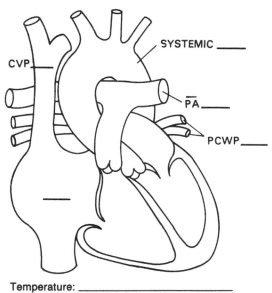

Temperature: _____

Heart Rate: _____

Cardiac Output: _____

Medications: _____

_____

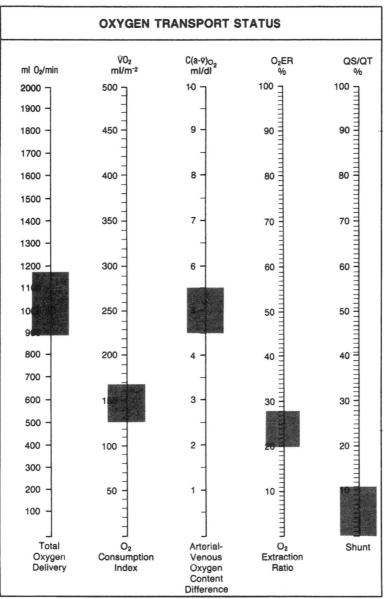

OXYGEN TRANSPORT STATUS

ml O₂/min	$\dot{V}O_2$ ml/m⁻²	$C(a-\bar{v})O_2$ ml/dl	O₂ER %	QS/QT %
Total Oxygen Delivery	O₂ Consumption Index	Arterial-Venous Oxygen Content Difference	O₂ Extraction Ratio	Shunt

Blood Gas Values

pH _____

Pa$_{CO_2}$ _____

HCO₃⁻ _____

Pa$_{O_2}$ _____   P$\bar{v}_{O_2}$ _____

Sa$_{O_2}$ _____ %   S$\bar{v}_{O_2}$ _____ %

F$_{IO_2}$ _____   Hb _____

Mode(s) of Ventilatory

Support: _____

_____

_____

_____

_____

Patient's Name _____

Date _____

Time _____

APPENDIX XXI: SELF-ASSESSMENT ANSWERS

Chapter 1

1. e	26. d
2. d	27. e
3. d	28. a
4. e	29. d
5. c	30. e
6. d	31. c
7. b	32. b
8. c	33. b
9. b	34. e
10. b	35. a
11. d	36. b
12. b	37. e
13. d	38. a
14. e	39. b
15. a	40. d
16. a	41. a
17. d	42. c
18. c	43. e
19. e	44. b
20. b	45. c
21. b	46. e
22. d	47. b
23. b	48. c
24. b	49. d
25. c	

50. a. $PA_{O_2} = (PB - (P_{H_2O})) FI_{O_2} - Pa_{CO_2} (1.25)$

$= (745 - 47) .70 - 46 (1.25)$

$= (698) .70 - 57.5$

$= (488.6) - 57.5$

$= 431.1$

Answer: 431.1

b. $Cc_{O_2} = (Hb \times 1.34) + (Pa_{O_2} \times 0.003)$

$= (11 \times 1.34) + (431.1 \times 0.003)$

$= (14.74) + (1.293)$

$= 16.033$

Answer: 16.033

c. $Ca_{O_2} = (Hb \times 1.34 \times Sa_{O_2}) + (Pa_{O_2} \times 0.003)$

$= (11 \times 1.34 \times .90) + (60 \times 0.003)$

$= (13.266) + (.18)$

$= 13.446$

Answer: 13.446

d. $C\bar{v}_{O_2} = (Hb \times 1.34 \times S\bar{v}_{O_2}) + (P\bar{v}_{O_2} \times 0.003)$

$= (11 \times 1.34 \times .75) + (38 \times 0.003)$

$= (11.055) + (.114)$

$= 11.169$

Answer: 11.169

e. $\dfrac{\dot{Q}_S}{\dot{Q}_T} = \dfrac{Cc_{O_2} - Ca_{O_2}}{Cc_{O_2} - C\overline{v}_{O_2}}$

$\qquad = \dfrac{16.033 - 13.446}{16.033 - 11.169}$

$\qquad = \dfrac{2.587}{4.864}$

$\qquad = .531$

Answer: 53%

51. e
52. e
53. c
54. e
55. c
56. e
57. a
58. e

59. e
60. e
61. c
62. c
63. b
64. d
65. e

Chapter 2

1. c
2. e
3. c
4. a
5. d

6. d
7. e
8. d
9. b
10. e

Chapter 3

1. d
2. a. Summarize pertinent clinical data.
   b. Analyze and assess it.
   c. Record the formulation of an appropriate treatment plan.
   d. Document the adjustments of the treatment plan.
3. e
4. b
5. a. Subjective and objective information
   b. An assessment
   c. The treatment plan (which has measurable outcomes)
   d. An evaluation of the patient's response to the treatment plan
   e. A section to record any adjustments made to the original treatment plan
6. S: Subjective information refers to information about the patient's feelings, concerns, or sensations presented by the patient.

   Example(s): • "I coughed hard all night!"
   • "My chest feels very tight."

   O: Objective information refers to the data that the respiratory care practitioner can measure, factually describe, or obtain from other professional reports or test results.

   Example(s): • Heart rate
   • Respiratory rate
   • Blood pressure

A: Assessment refers to the practitioner's professional conclusion about what is the cause of the subjective and objective data presented by the patient.

Example(s): • Bronchospasm
• Atelectasis
• Acute alveolar hyperventilation
• Mild hypoxemia

P: Plan is the therapeutic procedure(s) selected to remedy the cause (identified in the assessment) that is responsible for the subjective and objective data demonstrated by the patient.

Example(s): • Bronchodilator to offset bronchial smooth muscle constriction
• Continuous positive airway pressure to offset atelectasis

7. e
8. a. Impending ventilatory failure
   b. Ventilatory failure
   c. Apnea
9. Impending ventilatory failure
10. S: "It feels like there is a rope around my neck."
    O: Heart rate, 136; blood pressure, 165/120; respiratory rate, 32; breath sounds—wheezing & rhonchi bilaterally; arterial blood gases: pH 7.56, Pa_{CO_2} 28, HCO_3^- 21, Pa_{O_2} 47; strong cough effect; moderate amount of thin white secretions; peak expiratory flow rate, 185 L/min; x-ray: depressed diaphragm and hyperinflated alveoli.

    A: • Acute alveolar hyperventilation with moderate hypoxemia (ABG)
    • Bronchospasm (wheezing and low peak flow)
    • Accumulation of bronchial secretions (rhonchi and sputum production)
    • Good ability to mobilize secretions (strong cough effort)
    • Hyperinflated alveoli (x-ray)

    P: • Bronchodilator therapy (to offset bronchospasm, air trapping, and acute alveolar hyperventilation and hypoxemia)
    • Oxygen therapy (to offset hypoxemia and acute alveolar hyperventilation)
    • Encourage cough and deep breathing (to enhance secretion mobilization)
    • Reassess patient's response to therapy.

Chapter 4

1. b		6. c	
2. e		7. d	
3. d		8. b	
4. a		9. c	
5. b		10. e	

Chapter 5

1. e		6. e	
2. b		7. c	
3. b		8. d	
4. d		9. e	
5. c		10. b	

Chapter 6

1. e	6. d
2. b	7. c
3. b	8. d
4. e	9. b
5. a	10. c

Chapter 7

Multiple Choice

1. b	6. c
2. c	7. c
3. d	8. e
4. c	9. e
5. e	10. c

True or False

1. True	4. True
2. False	5. True
3. True	6. True

Matching

1. e	6. e
2. c	7. a
3. b	8. c
4. i	9. g
5. g	10. j

Chapter 8

1. e	6. d
2. c	7. b
3. c	8. e
4. e	9. b
5. d	10. d

Chapter 9

1. False	6. False
2. True	7. True
3. False	8. False
4. True	9. False
5. True	10. False

Chapter 10

1. d	6. c
2. b	7. a
3. b	8. b
4. d	9. b
5. e	10. b

Chapter 11
Multiple Choice
   1. d
   2. b
   3. b

   4. e
   5. e

Fill in the Blanks
   1. Western blot assay
   2. Reverse transcriptase
   3. Pentamidine

   4. Kaposi's sarcoma
   5. Integration

Chapter 12
Multiple Choice
   1. b
   2. e
   3. d

   4. c
   5. e

True or False
   1. True
   2. False
   3. True

   4. True
   5. False

Chapter 13
Multiple Choice
   1. e
   2. d
   3. e

   4. d
   5. c

True or False
   1. True
   2. False
   3. True

   4. True
   5. False

Chapter 14
Multiple Choice
   1. b
   2. a
   3. c

   4. d
   5. b

True or False
   1. True
   2. False
   3. False

   4. True
   5. True

Chapter 15
Multiple Choice
   1. e
   2. b
   3. e

   4. e
   5. a

True or False
   1. True
   2. True
   3. False

   4. True
   5. False

Fill in the Blank
    1. Albumin

Chapter 16

    1. c   6. b
    2. d   7. d
    3. c   8. d
    4. e   9. b
    5. a   10. a

Chapter 17
Multiple Choice
    1. c   4. c
    2. d   5. a
    3. b
True or False
    1. True   4. True
    2. True   5. True
    3. False

Chapter 18
    1. e   6. d
    2. c   7. e
    3. e   8. b
    4. d   9. b
    5. a   10. b

Chapter 19
Multiple Choice
    1. e   4. c
    2. b   5. d
    3. d
True or False
    1. True   4. True
    2. False   5. True
    3. True

Chapter 20
Multiple Choice
    1. a   4. a
    2. c   5. e
    3. c
True or False
    1. True   4. False
    2. False   5. False
    3. True

Chapter 21

Multiple Choice

1. e
2. d
3. c

4. b
5. e

Fill in the Blanks

1. the size of the dust particle
2. its chemical nature
3. its concentration
4. the time of exposure
5. the individual's susceptibility to specific inorganic dusts

Chapter 22

Multiple Choice

1. a
2. b
3. c

4. b
5. e

True or False

1. True
2. True
3. True

4. False
5. True

Chapter 23

Multiple Choice

1. d
2. b
3. a

4. b
5. b

True or False

1. True
2. False
3. True

4. False
5. False

Chapter 24

Multiple Choice

1. e
2. b
3. b

4. e
5. e

True or False

1. True
2. True
3. False

4. False
5. False

Fill in the Blank

1. 2.5 kg

Chapter 25

1. b
2. c
3. e
4. a
5. c

6. a
7. e
8. c
9. c
10. e

Chapter 26
Multiple Choice
1. e
2. d
3. c

4. e
5. e

True or False
1. True
2. False
3. False

4. True
5. True

Chapter 27
True or False
1. False
2. True
3. False
4. True
5. False

6. False
7. True
8. True
9. False
10. True

Chapter 28

1. d
2. c
3. e
4. b
5. e

6. d
7. c
8. b
9. a
10. d

Chapter 29
Fill in the Blanks
1. the situation in which a victim survives a liquid submersion, at least temporarily.
2. glottis spasms and prevents water from passing into the lungs.
3. glottis relaxes and allows water to flood the tracheobronchial tree and alveoli.
4. noncardiogenic pulmonary edema
5. 25

Chapter 30

1. c
2. b
3. e
4. d
5. c

6. d
7. d
8. d
9. b
10. a

Chapter 31

1. a. thoracic surgery
   b. upper abdominal surgery
   c. lower abdominal surgery

2. See text.
3. See text.

GLOSSARY

Abscess Localized collection of pus that results from disintegration or displacement of tissue in any part of the body.

Acetylcholine A neurotransmitter substance widely distributed in body tissue with a primary function of mediating synaptic activity of the nervous system.

Acidemia Decreased pH or an increased hydrogen ion concentration of the blood.

Acidosis Pathologic condition resulting from accumulation of acid or loss of base from the body.

Acinus Smallest division of a gland; a group of secretory cells surrounding a cavity; the functional part of an organ. (The respiratory acinus includes respiratory bronchioles, alveolar ducts, alveoli, and all other structures therein.)

Acute Sharp, severe; of rapid onset and characterized by severe symptoms and a short course; not chronic.

Adhesion Fibrous band that holds together parts that are normally separated.

Adrenergic Term applied to nerve fibers that, when stimulated, release epinephrine at their endings. Includes nearly all sympathetic postganglionic fibers except those innervating sweat glands.

Adrenocorticotropic hormone (ACTH) A hormone secreted by the anterior pituitary. It is regulated by the corticotropin-releasing factor (CRF) from the hypothalamus and is essential to growth, development, and continued function of the adrenal cortex.

Aerosol Gaseous suspension of fine solid or liquid particles.

Afebrile Without fever.

Afferent Carrying impulses toward a center.

Afferent nerves Nerves that transmit impulses from the peripheral to the central nervous system.

Air trapping Trapping of alveolar gas during exhalation.

Albumin One of a group of simple proteins widely distributed in plant and animal tissues. It is found in the blood as serum albumin, in milk as lactalbumin, and in the white of an egg as ovalbumin.

Alkalemia Increased pH or decreased hydrogen ion concentration of the blood.

Allele One of two or more different genes containing specific inheritable characteristics that occupy corresponding positions on paired chromosomes.

Allergen Any substance that causes manifestations of allergy. It may or may not be a protein.

Allergy Acquired hypersensitivity to a substance (allergen) that normally does not cause a reaction. An allergic reaction is essentially an antibody-antigen reaction, but in some cases the antibody cannot be demonstrated. The reaction is caused by the release of histamine-like or histamine-like substances from injured cells.

α_1-Antitrypsin Inhibitor of trypsin that may be deficient in persons with emphysema.

α-Receptor Site in the autonomic nerve pathways where excitatory responses occur when adrenergic agents such as norepinephrine and epinephrine are released.

Anaerobic Metabolic pathway that does not require oxygen; such processes usually produce lactic acid.

Anaphylaxis Allergic hypersensitivity reaction of the body to a foreign protein or drug.

Anemia Condition in which there is a reduction in the number of circulating red blood cells per cubic millimeter, the amount of hemoglobin per 100 ml, or the volume of packed red cells per 100 ml of blood.

Aneurysm Localized dilation of a blood vessel, usually an artery.

Angiogram Serial roentgenograms of a blood vessel taken in rapid sequence following injection of a radiopaque substance into the vessel.

Angiography Roentgenography of blood vessels after injection of a radiopaque substance.

Anoxia Deficiency of oxygen.

Anterolateral In front and to one side.

Antibody Protein substance that develops in response to and interacts with an antigen. The antigen-antibody reaction forms the basis of immunity. Antibodies are produced by plasma cells in lymphoid tissue. Antibodies may be present due to previous infection, vaccination, or transfer from the mother to the fetus in utero or may occur without known antigenic stimulus, usually as a result of unknown, accidental exposure.

Antigen Substance that induces the formation of antibodies that interact specifically with it. An antigen may be introduced into the body or may be formed within the body.

Aortic valve Valve between the left ventricle and the ascending aorta that prevents regurgitation of blood into the left ventricle.

Aperture Opening or orifice.

Apex Top, end, or tip of a structure.

Apnea Complete absence of spontaneous ventilation.

Aponeurosis Flat, fibrous sheet of connective tissue that attaches muscle to bone or other tissues. May sometimes serve as a fascia.

Arrhythmia Irregularity or loss of rhythm.

Arteriole Minute artery that, at its distal end, leads into a capillary.

Arthralgia Any pain that affects a joint.

Arthropod Any member of a large group of animals that possess a hard external skeleton and jointed legs and other appendages. Many arthropods are of medical importance (e.g., mites, ticks, and insects).

Asepsis The absence of germs; sterile.

Asphyxia Condition caused by an insufficient uptake of oxygen.

Aspiration Inhalation of pharyngeal contents into the pulmonary tree.

Asymmetric Unequal correspondence in shape, size, and relative position of parts on opposite sides of the midline.

Asystole Absence of contractions of the heart.

Atelectasis Collapsed or airless lung. May be caused by obstruction by foreign bodies, mucus plugs, or excessive secretions or by compression from without, as by tumors, aneurysms, or enlarged lymph nodes.

Atmospheric pressure Pressure of the air on the earth at mean sea level. Approximately 14.7 pounds to the square inch (760 mm Hg).

Atopic Of or pertaining to a hereditary tendency to develop immediate allergic reactions because of the presence of an antibody in the skin and sometimes the bloodstream.

Atrial fibrillation Irregular and rapid randomized contractions of the atria working independently of the ventricles.

Atrial flutter Extremely rapid (200 to 400/min) contractions of the atrium. In pure flutter, a regular rhythm is maintained; in impure flutter, the rhythm is irregular.

Atrophy A wasting or decrease in size of an organ or tissue.

Atropine An alkaloid obtained from belladonna. It is a parasympatholytic agent.

Autosomal recessive trait Pattern of inheritance in which the transmission of a recessive gene results in a carrier state if the person is heterozygous for the trait and in an affected state if the person is homozygous for the trait. Males and females are affected with equal frequency.

Bacillus Any rod-shaped bacterium.

Bacteria Unicellular, ovoid, or rod-shaped organisms existing in free-living or parasitic forms. They display a wide range of biochemical and pathogenic properties.

Bedsonia Former genus name for *Chlamydia,* now used as a common term denoting species of *Chlamydia* (e.g., bedsonias, *Bedsonia* organisms, bedsonial agents).

Benign Noncancerous and therefore not an immediate threat, even though treatment eventually may be required for health or cosmetic reasons.

β-Receptor Site in autonomic nerve pathways wherein inhibitory responses occur when adrenergic agents such as norepinephrine and epinephrine are released.

Bicarbonate Any salt containing the HCO_3^- anion.

Bifurcation A separation into two branches; the point of forking.

Biopsy Excision of a small piece of living tissue for microscopic examination; usually performed to establish a diagnosis.

Bleb Blister or bulla. Blebs may vary in size from that of a bean to that of a goose egg and may contain serous, seropurulent, or bloody fluid.

Blood-brain barrier Membrane between circulating blood and the brain that prevents certain substances from reaching brain tissue and cerebrospinal fluid.

Bradykinin Kinin composed of a chain of nine amino acids liberated by the action of trypsin or of certain snake venoms on a globulin of blood plasma

Bronchoconstriction Constriction of the bronchial tubes.

Bronchodilation Dilation of a bronchus.

Bronchograms Film of the airways after a radiopaque substance has been injected into them.

Bronchoscopy A visual examination of the tracheobronchial tree with the bronchoscope.

Bronchospasm Involuntary sudden movement or convulsive contraction of the muscular layer of the bronchus.

Bulla Blister, cavity, or vesicle filled with air or fluid; a bleb.

Cachexia General ill health and malnutrition marked by weakness and emaciation, usually associated with serious disease (e.g., tuberculosis, cancer).

Calcification Process in which organic tissue becomes hardened by the deposition of calcium salts in tissue.

Cannulation Placement of a tube or sheath enclosing a trocar to allow the escape of fluid after the trocar is withdrawn from the body.

Capillary stasis Stagnation of the normal flow of fluids or blood in capillaries.

Carbon dioxide (CO_2) Colorless, odorless, incombustible gas formed during respiration and combustion; normally constitutes only 0.03% of the atmosphere. Concentrations above 5% in inspired air stimulate respiration.

Carcinoma Malignant tumor that occurs in epithelial tissue. These neoplasms tend to infiltrate and give rise to metastases.

Cardiogenic Originating in the heart.

Cardiotonic drugs Drugs that increase the tonicity of the heart.

Carotid sinus baroreceptors Sensory nerve endings located in the carotid sinus. Changes in pressure stimulate the nerve endings.

Cartilage Dense, firm, compact connective tissue capable of withstanding considerable pressure and tension; located in all true joints, the outer ear, bronchi, and movable sections of the ribs.

Catecholamines Biologically active amines that behave as epinephrine and norepinephrine. Catecholamines have marked effects on the nervous and cardiovascular systems, metabolic rate, temperature, and smooth muscle.

Cavitation The formation of cavities or hollow spaces within the body, e.g., formed in the lung by tuberculosis.

Central venous pressure (CVP) Pressure within the superior vena cava. The pressure under which the blood is returned to the right atrium.

Cerebrospinal fluid (CSF) Water cushion protecting the brain and spinal cord from shock.

Chemoreceptor Sense organ or sensory nerve ending that is stimulated by and reacts to chemical stimuli and that is located outside the central nervous system. Chemoreceptors are found in the large arteries of the thorax and neck (carotid and aortic bodies), the taste buds, and the olfactory cells of the nose.

Chemotactic Attraction and repulsion of living protoplasm to a chemical stimulus.

Chlamydia Genus of viruslike microorganisms that cause disease in humans and birds. Some *Chlamydia* infections of birds can be transmitted to humans (ornithosis, parrot disease). The organisms resemble bacteria but are of similar size to viruses and are obligate parasites.

Chronic Denoting a process that shows little change and slow progression and is of long duration.

Cilia Small hairlike projections on the surface of epithelial cells. In the bronchi, they propel mucus and foreign particles in a whiplike movement toward the throat.

Clinical manifestations Symptoms or signs demonstrated by a patient; may be subjective or objective in nature.

Coagulation Process of clotting. Coagulation requires the presence of several substances, the most important of which are prothrombin, thrombin, thromboplastin, calcium in ionic form, and fibrinogen.

Coalesce To fuse, run, or grow together.

Coccobacillus Short, thick bacterial rod in the shape of an oval or slightly elongated coccus.

Coccus Bacterium with a spherical shape.

Collagen Fibrous insoluble protein found in connective tissue, including skin, bone, ligaments, and cartilage. Collagen represents about 30% of the total body protein.

Colloid Type of solution; a gluelike substance such as protein or starch whose particles (molecules or aggregates of molecules), when dispersed in a solvent to the greatest degree, remain uniformly distributed and fail to form a true solution.

Compromise A blending of the qualities of two different things; an unfavorable change.

Congenital Existing at and usually before birth; referring to conditions that are present at birth, regardless of their cause.

Congestion Excessive amount of blood or tissue fluid in an organ or in tissue.

Consolidation The process of becoming solid; a mass that has solidified.

Contusion Injury in which the skin is not broken; a bruise. Symptoms are pain, swelling, and discoloration.

Convex Having a rounded, somewhat elevated surface resembling a segment of the external surface of a sphere.

Cor pulmonale Hypertrophy or failure of the right ventricle resulting from disorders of the lungs, pulmonary vessels, or chest wall.

Corticosteroids Any of a number of hormonal steroid substances obtained from the cortex of the adrenal gland.

Costophrenic angle The junction of the rib cage and the diaphragm.

Cuirass A chest covering; breastplate.

Cyclic adenosine monophosphate (cAMP) Cyclic nucleotide participating in the activities of many hormones, including catecholamines, adrenocorticotropin, and vasopressin. It is synthesized from adenosine triphosphate and is stimulated by the enzyme adenylate cyclase.

Cyst Closed pouch or sac with a definite wall that contains fluid, semifluid, or solid material.

Cytoplasm Protoplasm of a cell exclusive of the nucleus.

Demarcate To set or mark boundaries or limits.

Demyelination The destruction or removal of the myelin sheath from a nerve or nerve fiber.

Density Mass of a substance per unit of volume; the relative weight of a substance compared with a reference standard.

Deoxyribonucleic acid (DNA) Type of nucleic acid containing deoxyribose as the sugar component and found principally in the nuclei of animal and vegetable cells, usually loosely bound to protein (hence termed deoxyribonucleoprotein).

Depolarize To reduce to a nonpolarized condition. To reduce the amount of electrical charge between oppositely charged particles.

Desensitization Prevention of anaphylaxis.

Diabetes mellitus Chronic disease of pancreatic origin that is characterized by insulin deficiency and a subsequent inability to utilize carbohydrates. This condition results in excess sugar in the blood and urine; excessive thirst, hunger, urination, weakness, and emaciation; and imperfect combustion of fats. If untreated, diabetes mellitus leads to acidosis, coma, and death.

Diagnostic Pertaining to the use of scientific and skillful methods to establish the cause and nature of a sick person's disease.

Diastole Period in the heart cycle during which the muscle fibers lengthen, the heart dilates, and the cavities fill with blood.

Dilation Expansion of an organ, orifice, or vessel.

Dimorphic fungus A condition where the organism has two distinct types of fungus.

Dimorphism The quality of existing in two distinct forms.

Disseminate Scatter or distribute over a considerable area; when applied to disease organisms, scattered throughout an organ or the body.

Distal Farthest from the center, from a medial line, or from the trunk.

Driving pressure Pressure difference between two areas.

Ductus arteriosus Vessel between the pulmonary artery and the aorta. It bypasses the lungs in the fetus.

Dynamometer An instrument for measuring the force of muscular contractions. For example, a squeeze dynamometer is one by which the grip of the hand is measured.

Dysplasia Abnormal development of organ tissues or cells.

Dyspnea Air hunger resulting in labored or difficult breathing, sometimes accompanied by pain. Symptoms include audible labored breathing, distressed anxious expression, dilated nostrils, protrusion of the abdomen with an expanded chest, and gasping.

Edema A local or generalized condition in which the body tissues contain an excessive amount of tissue fluid.

Efferent Carrying away from a central organ or section. Efferent nerves conduct impulses from the brain or spinal cord to the periphery.

Efferent nerves Nerves that carry impulses having the following effects: motor, causing contraction of the muscles; secretory, causing glands to secrete; and inhibitory, causing some organs to become quiescent.

Effusion Seeping of serous, purulent, or bloody fluid into a cavity; the result of such a seeping.

Elastase Enzyme that dissolves elastin.

Electrocardiogram (ECG) Record of the electrical activity of the heart.

Electrodiagnostic Use of electric and electronic devices for diagnostic purposes.

Electrolyte Substance that, in solution, conducts an electrical current and is decomposed by the passage of an electrical current. Acids, bases, and salts are electrolytes.

Electromyogram A graphic record of the contraction of a muscle as a result of electrical stimulation.

Electrophoresis Movement of charged colloidal particles through the medium in which they are dispersed as a result of changes in electrical potential.

Embolus Mass of undissolved matter present in blood or lymphatic vessels to which it has been brought by the blood or lymph current. Emboli may be solid, liquid, or gaseous.

Empyema Pus in a body cavity, especially in the pleural cavity; usually the result of a primary infection in the lungs.

Encapsulated Enclosed in a fibrous or membranous sheath.

Encephalitis Inflammation of the brain.

Endemic A disease that occurs continuously in a particular population but has low mortality, such as measles.

Endocarditis Inflammation of the endocardium. It may involve only the membrane covering the valves or it may involve the general lining of the chambers of the heart.

Endothelium The layer of epithelial cells that lines the cavities of the heart, blood and lymph vessels, and the serous cavities of the body; originating from the mesoderm.

Enuresis Involuntary discharge of urine, usually referring to involuntary discharge of urine during sleep at night; bed-wetting beyond the age when bladder control should have been achieved.

Enzyme Complex protein capable of inducing chemical changes in other substances without being changed itself. Enzymes speed chemical reactions.

Eosinophil Cell or cellular structure that stains readily with the acid stain eosin. Specifically refers to a granular leukocyte.

Epidemiology Science concerned with defining and explaining the interrelationships of factors that determine disease frequency and distribution.

Epinephrine Hormone secreted by the adrenal medulla in response to splanchnic stimulation.

Epithelium Covering of the internal and the external organs of the body, including the lining of vessels. It consists of cells bound together by connective material and varies in the number of layers and the kinds of cells.

Erythema multiforme A hypersensitivity syndrome characterized by polymorphous eruptions of the skin and mucous membranes.

Erythropoiesis Formation of red blood cells.

Etiology Cause of disease.

Exocrine gland Gland whose secretion reaches an epithelial surface either directly or through a duct.

Expectoration To clear out the chest and lungs by coughing up and spitting out matter.

Extravascular Outside a vessel.

Exudate Accumulation of a fluid in a cavity; matter that penetrates through vessel walls into adjoining tissue.

Fascia Fibrous membrane covering, supporting, and separating muscles.

Febrile Pertaining to a fever.

Fibrin Whitish, filamentous protein formed by the action of prothrombin on fibrinogen. The conversion of fibrinogen into fibrin is the basis for blood clotting. Fibrin is deposited as fine interlacing filaments in which are entangled red and white blood cells and platelets, the whole forming a coagulum or clot.

Fibrinolytic Pertaining to the splitting of fibrin.

Fibroelastic Composed of fibrous and elastic tissue.

Fibrosis Formation of scar tissue in the connective tissue framework of the lungs.

Fissure Cleft or groove on the surface of an organ, often marking division of the organ into parts, as the lobes of the lung.

Fistula Abnormal passage or communication, usually between two internal organs or leading from an internal organ to the surface of the body; designated according to the organs or parts with which it communicates.

Flaccid paralysis Paralysis in which there is loss of muscle tone, loss or reduction of tendon reflexes, atrophy and degeneration of muscles.

Flare Flush or spreading area of redness that surrounds a line made by drawing a pointed instrument across the skin. It is the second reaction in the triple response of skin to injury and is due to dilation of the arterioles.

Fluorescent antibody microscopy Microscopic examination of antibodies tagged with fluorescent material for the diagnosis of infections.

Foramen ovale Opening between the atria of the heart in the fetus. This opening normally closes shortly after birth.

Fossa Hollow or depression, especially on the surface of the end of a bone.

Galactosemia Presence of galactose in the blood.

Gastric juice Juice of the gastric glands of the stomach. It contains pepsin, hydrochloric acid, mucin, small quantities of inorganic salts, and the intrinsic antianemic principle. Gastric juice is strongly acid, having a pH of 0.9 to 1.5.

Genus In natural history classification, the division between the family or tribe and the species; a group of species alike in the broad features of their organization but different in detail.

Globulin One of a group of simple proteins insoluble in pure water but soluble in neutral solutions of salts of strong acids; the fraction of the blood serum with which antibodies are associated.

Glossopharyngeal nerve Ninth cranial nerve. Function: special sensory (taste), visceral sensory, and motor. Distribution: pharynx, ear, meninges, posterior third of the tongue, and parotid gland.

Glycolysis Breakdown of sugar by enzymes in the body. This occurs without oxygen.

Glycoprotein Any of a class of conjugated proteins consisting of a compound of protein with a carbohydrate group.

Hematocrit Volume of erythrocytes packed by centrifugation in a given volume of blood. Hematocrit is expressed as a percentage of the total blood volume that consists of erythrocytes or as the volume in cubic centimeters of erythrocytes packed by centrifugation of the blood.

Hematopoietic Pertaining to the production and development of blood cells.

Hemoptysis Expectoration of blood.

Hemorrhage Abnormal internal or external discharge of blood; may be venous, arterial, or capillary.

Heparin Polysaccharide that has been isolated from the liver, lung, and other tissues. It is produced by the mast cells of the liver and by basophil leukocytes. It inhibits coagulation by preventing conversion of prothrombin to thrombin and the liberation of thromboplastin from blood platelets.

Hepatosplenomegaly Enlargement of both the liver and spleen.

Heterozygote Individual with different alleles for a given characteristic.

Hilus Root of the lungs at the level of the fourth and fifth dorsal vertebrae.

Histamine Substance normally present in the body; it exerts a pharmacologic action when released from injured cells. The red flush of a burn is due to the local production of histamine. It is produced from the amino acid histidine.

Homozygote Individual developing from gametes with similar alleles and thus possessing like pairs of genes for a given hereditary characteristic.

Hormone Substance originating in an organ or gland that is conveyed through the blood to another part of the body where by chemical action, it stimulates increased functional activity and increased secretion.

Humoral Pertaining to body fluids or substances contained in them.

Hydrostatic Pertaining to the pressure of liquids in equilibrium and that exerted on liquids.

Hydrous Containing water, usually chemically combined.

Hypercarbia, hypercapnea Excess carbon dioxide in the blood; indicated by an elevated P_{CO_2}.

Hypercoagulation Greater-than-normal clotting.

Hyperinflation Distention of a part by air, gas, or liquid.

Hyperplasia Excessive proliferation of normal cells in the normal tissue arrangement of an organ.

Hyperpnea Increased depth (volume) of breathing with or without an increased frequency.

Hypersecretions Substance or fluid separated and elaborated by cells of glands in an excessive amount or more than normal.

Hypersensitivity Abnormal sensitivity to a stimulus of any kind.

Hypertension Higher-than-normal blood pressure; greater-than-normal tension or tonus.

Hypertrophy Increase in size of an organ or structure that does not involve tumor formation.

Hyperventilation Increased rate and depth of breathing.

Hypoperfusion Deficiency of blood coursing through the vessels of the circulatory system.

Hypoproteinemia Decrease in the amount of protein in the blood.

Hypoventilation Reduced rate and depth of breathing.

Hypoxemia Below-normal oxygen content in blood.

Hypoxia Tissue oxygen deficiency.

Iatrogenic Any adverse mental or physical condition induced in a patient by the effects of treatment by a physician or by the patient himself.

Idiopathic Disease or condition without a recognizable cause.

Ileocecal valve Valve between the ileum of the small intestine and the cecum of the large intestine. It consists of two flaps that project into the lumen of the large intestine just above the vermiform appendix.

Immunoglobulin One of a family of closely related but not identical proteins that are capable of acting as antibodies. Five major types of immunoglobulins are normally present in the human adult: IgG, IgA, IgM, IgD, and IgE.

Immunoglobulin α E (IgE) An α-globulin produced by cells of the lining of the respiratory and intestinal tract. IgE is important in forming reagin antibodies.

Immunologic mechanism Reaction of the body to substances that are foreign or are interpreted as foreign.

Immunotherapy Production or enhancement of immunity.

Incubation period Development of an infection from the time of entry into an organism up to the time of the first appearance of signs or symptoms.

Infarction Necrosis of tissue following cessation of blood supply.

Inferior vena cava (IVC) Venous trunk draining the lower extremities, the pelvis, and abdominal viscera.

Inflammation Localized heat, redness, swelling, and pain as a result of irritation, injury, or infection.

Inotropic (positive) Increasing myocardial contractibility.

Insertion Manner or place of attachment of a muscle to the bone.

Intercostal retraction Also known as retraction of the chest. Visible sinking-in of the soft tissues of the chest between and around the cartilaginous and bony ribs.

Interstitial Placed or lying between; pertaining to interstices or spaces within an organ or tissue.

Intrapleural pressure Pressure within the pleural cavity.

Iodine Nonmetallic element belonging to the halogen group.

Ion Atom, group of atoms, or molecule that has acquired a net electrical charge by gaining or losing electrons.

Ischemia Local and temporary deficiency of blood supply due to obstruction of the circulation to a part.

Isotope One of a series of chemical elements that have nearly identical chemical properties but differ in their atomic weights and electrical charges. Many isotopes are radioactive.

Kerley's lines Thickening of the interlobular septa as seen in chest roentgenography; may be due to cellular infiltration or edema associated with pulmonary venous hypertension.

Kinetic Pertaining to or consisting of motion.

Kulchitsky's cell A cell containing serotonin-secreting granules that stain readily with silver and chromium, also known as an argentaffin cell.

Lactic acid Acid formed in muscles during activity by the breakdown of sugar without oxygen.

Latency State of being concealed, hidden, inactive, or inapparent.

Lesion A wound, injury, or pathologic change in body tissue.

Lethargy The state or quality of being indifferent, apathetic, or sluggish; stupor.

Leukocytes White blood corpuscles, including cells both with and without granules within their cytoplasm.

Leukopenia An abnormal decrease in the number of white blood cells to fewer than 5,000 cells/mm^3.

Ligamentum nuchae Upward continuation of the supraspinous ligament, extending from the seventh cervical vertebra to the occipital bone.

Linea alba White line of connective tissue in the middle of the abdomen from sternum to pubis.

Lipid Any of numerous fats generally insoluble in water that constitute one of the principal structural materials of cells.

Longitudinal Parallel to the long axis of the body or part.

Lubricant Agent, usually a liquid oil, that reduces friction between parts that brush against each other as they move. Joints are lubricated by synovial fluid.

Lumen Inner open space of a tubular organ such as a blood vessel or intestine.

Lymphangitis carcinomatosa The condition of having widespread dissemination of carcinoma in lymphatic channels or vessels.

Lymphatic vessels Thin-walled vessels conveying lymph from the tissues. Like veins, they possess valves ensuring one-way flow and eventually empty into the venous system at the junction of the internal jugular and subclavian veins.

Lymph node Rounded body consisting of accumulations of lymphatic tissue found at intervals in the course of lymphatic vessels.

Macrophage Cell whose major function is phagocytosis of foreign matter.

Malaise A vague feeling of body weakness or discomfort that often marks the onset of disease.

Malleolus The protuberance on both sides of the ankle joint, the lower extremity of the fibula being known as the lateral malleolus and lower end of the tibia as the medial malleolus.

Mast cell Connective tissue cells that contain heparin and histamine in their granules; important in cellular defense mechanisms, including blood coagulation; needed during injury or infection.

Mechanoreceptor Receptor that receives mechanical stimuli such as pressure from sound or touch.

Meconium ileus Obstruction of the small intestine in the newborn by impaction of thick, dry, tenacious meconium, usually at or near the ileocecal valve. The condition results from a deficiency in pancreatic enzymes and is the earliest manifestation of cystic fibrosis.

Meningitis Any infection or inflammation of the membrane covering the brain and spinal cord.

Mesotheliomas A rare, malignant tumor of the mesothelium of the pleura or peritoneum; associated with earlier exposure to asbestos.

Metabolism Sum of all physical and chemical changes that take place with an organism, all energy and material transformations that occur within living cells.

Metaplasia Conversion of one kind of tissue into a form that is not normal for that tissue.

Methylxanthine Methylated xanthine. A nitrogenous extraction contained in muscle tissue, liver, spleen, pancreas, other organs, and urine; formed during the metabolism of nucleoproteins. The three methylated xanthines are caffeine, theophylline, and theobromine.

Microvilli Minute cylindrical processes on the free surface of a cell, especially cells of the proximal convoluted renal tubule and of the intestinal epithelium; they increase the surface area of the cell.

Mitosis A type of cell division of somatic cells where each daughter cell contains the same number of chromosomes as the parent cell.

Mitral valve Bicuspid valve between the left atrium and left ventricle.

Mononucleosis Presence of an abnormally high number of mononuclear leukocytes in the blood.

Motile Having the power to move spontaneously.

Mucociliary clearing action In the large airways a continuous blanket of mucus covering the tracheobronchial tree epithelium is mobilized by the forward motion of cilia. The ciliary action causes the mucus blanket to be mobilized in a continuous motion toward the hilus of the lung, eventually moving to the larynx where the mucus is moved into the pharynx and swallowed or expectorated.

Mucous Pertaining to or resembling mucus; also secreting mucus.

Mucus The free slime of the mucous membranes. It is composed of secretions of the glands along with various inorganic salts, desquamated cells, and leukocytes.

Myelin Insulating material covering the axons of many neurons; increases the velocity of the nerve impulse along the axon.

Myeloma Tumor originating in cells of the hematopoietic portion of bone marrow.

Myocardial infarction Development of an infarct in the myocardium, the result of myocardial ischemia following occlusion of a coronary artery.

Myocarditis Inflammation of the myocardium.

Myocardium Middle layer of the walls of the heart, composed of cardiac muscle.

Myopathy An abnormal condition of skeletal muscle characterized by muscle weakness, wasting, and histologic changes within muscle tissue.

Necrosis Death of areas of tissue.

Neoplasm New and abnormal formation of tissue, such as a tumor or growth. It serves no useful function but grows at the expense of the healthy organism.

Nephritis Inflammation of the kidney. The glomeruli, tubules, and interstitial tissue may be affected.

Neuroendocrine Pertaining to the nervous and endocrine systems as an integrated functioning mechanism.

Neuromuscular junction The area of contact between the ends of a large myelinated nerve fiber and a fiber of skeletal muscle.

Nitrogen oxides Automotive air pollutant. Depending on concentration, these gases cause respiratory irritation, bronchitis, and pneumonitis. Concentrations over 100 ppm usually cause pulmonary edema and result in death.

Nocturnal Pertaining to or occurring in the night.

Nodule A small aggregation of cells; a small node.

Nomogram Graph consisting of three lines or curves (usually parallel) graduated for different variables in such a way that a straight line cutting the three lines gives the related values of the three variables.

Norepinephrine Hormone produced by the adrenal medulla, similar in chemical and pharmacologic properties to epinephrine.

Normal flora Naturally occurring bacteria found in specific bodily areas. Normal flora has no detrimental effect.

Occlude To close, obstruct, or join together.

Olfactory Pertaining to the sense of smell.

Oncotic pressure Osmotic pressure due to the presence of colloids in a solution.

Opacity Opaque spot or area; the condition of being opaque.

Opaque Impervious to light rays or, by extension, to roentgen rays or other electromagnetic vibrations; neither transparent nor translucent.

Orbicularis oculi The muscular body of the eyelid composed of the palpebral, orbital, and lacrimal parts.

Orifice Mouth, entrance, or outlet to any aperture.

Origin The more fixed attachment (usually proximal or central) part of a muscle.

Orthopnea Respiratory complaint of discomfort in any but an erect sitting or standing position.

Osmotic pressure Pressure that develops when two unequally osmolar solutions are separated by a semipermeable membrane.

Osteoporosis Increased brittleness of bone seen most often in the elderly.

Oxygen content Total oxygen in blood.

Ozone Formed by the action of sunlight on oxygen in which three atoms form the molecule O_3. It is an irritant to the respiratory tract.

Palatine arches Vault-shaped muscular structures forming the soft palate between the mouth and the nasopharynx.

Pancreas Fish-shaped, grayish pink gland that stretches transversely across the posterior abdominal wall in the epigastric region of the body. It secretes various substances such as digestive enzymes, insulin, and glucagon.

Pancreatic juice Clear alkaline pancreatic secretion that contains at least three different enzymes (trypsin, amylopsin, and lipase). It is poured into the duodenum where, mixed with bile and intestinal juices, it furthers the digestion of foodstuffs.

Paracentesis A procedure in which fluid is withdrawn from the abdominal cavity.

Paradoxical Occurring at variance with the normal rule.

Paramyxovirus Subgroup of viruses including parainfluenza, measles, mumps, German measles, and respiratory syncytial viruses.

Parasite Any organism that grows, feeds, and is sheltered on or in a different organism while contributing nothing to the survival of the host.

Parenchyma Essential parts of an organ that are concerned with its function.

Paroxysmal Concerning the sudden, periodic attack or recurrence of symptoms of a disease.

Particulate Made up of particles.

Patent ductus Open, narrow, tubular channel.

Pathogen Any agent causing disease, especially a microorganism.

Pendelluft Shunting of air from one lung to another.

Perforation Hole made through a substance or part.

Peribronchial Located around the bronchi.

Peripheral airways Small bronchi on the outer portion of the lung where most gas transfer takes place.

Peritoneal dialysis Removal of toxic substances from the body by perfusing specific warm sterile chemical solutions through the peritoneal cavity.

Perivascular Located around a vessel, especially a blood vessel.

Permeability The quality of being permeable.

Permeable Capable of allowing the passage of fluids or substances in solution.

pH Symbol for the logarithm of the reciprocal of the hydrogen ion concentration.

Phagocytosis Envelopment and digestion of bacteria or other foreign bodies by cells.

Phalanges Bones of the fingers or toes.

Phenotype Physical makeup of an individual. Some phenotypes, such as the blood groups, are completely determined by heredity, while others such as stature are readily altered by environmental agents.

Phenylketonuria Abnormal presence of phenylketone in the urine.

Phlegmasia alba dolens Acute edema, especially of the leg, from venous obstruction, usually a thrombosis.

Phosgene Carbonyl chloride ($COCl_2$), a poisonous gas causing nausea and suffocation.

Phosphodiesterase Enzyme that catalyzes the breakdown of the second messenger cyclic adenosine monophosphate to adenosine monophosphate.

Plaque Patch on the skin or on a mucous surface.

Pleomorphic Multiform; occurring in more than one form.

Pleurisy Inflammation of the pleura.

Pleuritis Inflammation of the pleura.

Polyarteritis nodosa Necrosis and inflammation of small and medium-sized arteries and subsequent involvement of tissue supplied by these arteries.

Polycythemia Excess of red blood cells.

Polymorphonuclear leukocyte Subclass of white blood cells, including neutrophils, eosinophils, and basophils.

Polyneuritis Inflammation of two or more nerves at once.

Polyneuropathy Term applied to any disorder of peripheral nerves, but preferably to those of a noninflammatory nature.

Polyradiculitis Inflammation of nerve roots, especially those of spinal nerves as found in Guillain-Barré syndrome.

Polyradiculoneuropathy Guillain-Barré syndrome.

Postpartum Occurring after childbirth.

Postural drainage Drainage of secretions from the bronchi or a cavity in the lung by positioning the patient so that gravity will allow drainage of the particular lobe or lobes of the lung involved.

Pressure The quotient obtained by dividing a force by the area of the surface on which it acts.

Primigravida A woman pregnant for the first time.

Prognostic Related to prediction of the outcome of a disease.

Proliferation Increasing or spreading at a rapid rate; the process or results of rapid reproduction.

Prophylactic Any agent or regimen that contributes to the prevention of infection and disease.

Propranolol Beta-adrenergic blocker drug used in treating cardiac arrhythmias, particularly supraventricular tachycardia.

Prostaglandin F One of a group of fatty acid derivatives present in many tissues, including the prostate gland, menstrual fluid, brain, lung, kidney, thymus, seminal fluid, and pancreas. Prostaglandin F is believed to cause bronchoconstriction and vasoconstriction.

Prostration A condition of extreme exhaustion.

Proteolytic An enzyme producing proteolysis.

Proximal Nearest the point of attachment, center of the body, or point of reference.

Pulmonary Concerning or involving the lungs.

Pulmonary blood vessels Vessels that transport blood from the heart to the lungs and then back to the heart.

Pulmonary circulation Passage of blood from the heart to the lungs and back again for gas exchange. The blood flows from the right ventricle to the lungs, where it is oxygenated, and carbon dioxide is removed. The blood then flows back to the left atrium.

Pulsus paradoxus An exaggeration of the normal variation in the pulse volume with respiration. The pulse becomes weaker with inspiration and stronger with expiration. Pulsus paradoxus is characteristic of constrictive pericarditis and pericardial effusion. The changes are independent of changes in pulse rate.

Purulent Containing or forming pus.

Radiopaque Impenetrable to x-irradiation or other forms of radiation.

Recumbent Lying down or leaning backward.

Refractory Resistant to ordinary treatment; obstinate, stubborn.

Remission Lessening of severity or abatement of symptoms; the period during which symptoms abate.

Reticular formation Located in the brain stem, it acts as a filter from sense organs to the conscious brain. It analyzes incoming information for importance and influences alertness, waking, sleeping, and some reflexes.

Ribonucleic acid (RNA) Nucleic acid occurring in the nucleus and cytoplasm of cells that is involved in the synthesis of proteins. The RNA molecule is a single strand made up of nucleotides.

Roentgenogram Film produced by roentgenography.

Roentgenography Process of obtaining pictures by the use of roentgen rays.

Scintillation camera Camera used to photograph the emissions that come from radioactive substances injected into the body.

Semilunar valves Valves separating the left ventricle and aorta and right ventricle and pulmonary artery.

Semipermeable Permitting diffusion or flow of some liquids or particles but preventing the transmission of others, usually in reference to a membrane.

Septicemia Systemic disease caused by pathogenic organisms or toxins in the blood; may be a late development of any purulent infections.

Septum Wall dividing two cavities.

Serotonin Chemical present in platelets, gastrointestinal mucosa, mast cells, and carcinoid tumors; a potent vasoconstrictor.

Serum (1) Clear, watery fluid, especially that moistening surfaces of serous membranes, (2) exuded in inflammation of any of those membranes, (3) the fluid portion of the blood obtained after removal of the fibrin clot and blood cells, (4) sometimes used as a synonym for antiserum.

Sibilant Hissing or whistling; applied to sounds heard in a certain crackle (or rhonchus).

Sign Any objective evidence or manifestation of an illness or disordered function of the body. Signs are more or less definitive, obvious, and, apart from the patient's impressions, in contrast to symptoms, which are subjective.

Silicate Salt of silicic acid.

Sinus tachycardia Uncomplicated tachycardia when sinus rhythm is faster than 100 beats per minute.

Smooth muscle Muscle tissue that lacks cross-striations on its fibers; involuntary in action and found principally in visceral organs.

Somatic nerve Nerve that innervates somatic structures, i.e., those constituting the body wall and extremities.

Spasm Involuntary sudden movement or convulsive muscular contraction. Spasms may be clonic or tonic.

Sphygomomanometer Instrument for determining arterial blood pressure indirectly.

Sputum Substance expelled by coughing or clearing the throat. It may contain cellular debris, mucus, blood, pus, caseous material, and microorganisms.

Stasis Stagnation of the normal flow of fluids, as of the blood, urine, or intestinal mechanism.

Status asthmaticus Persistent and intractable asthma.

Streptokinase Enzyme produced by certain strains of streptococci, capable of converting plasminogen to plasmin.

Stroke volume Amount of blood ejected by the ventricle at each beat.

Subarachnoid space Space occupied by cerebrospinal fluid beneath the arachnoid membrane surrounding the brain and spinal cord.

Subcutaneous Beneath the skin.

Sulfur dioxide Common industrial air pollutant; causes bronchospasms and cell destruction.

Superficial Confined to the surface.

Superior vena cava Venous trunk draining blood from the head, neck, upper extremities, and chest. It begins by union of the two brachiocephalic veins, passes directly downward, and empties into the right atrium of the heart.

Surface tension Condition at the surface of a liquid in contact with a gas or another liquid. It is the result of the mutual attraction of molecules to produce a cohesive state, which causes liquids to assume a shape presenting the smallest surface area to the surrounding medium. It accounts for the spherical shape assumed by fluids such as drops of oil or water.

Surfactant Phospholipoid substance important in controlling the surface tension of the air-liquid emulsion in the lungs; an agent that lowers the surface tension.

Symmetric Equal correspondence in shape, size, and relative position of parts on opposite sides of the body.

Sympathomimetic Producing effects resembling those resulting from stimulation of the sympathetic nervous system, such as the effects following the injection of epinephrine.

Symptom Any perceptible change in the body or its functions that indicates disease or the kind of phases of a disease. Symptoms may be classified as objective, subjective, cardinal, and sometimes constitutional. However, another classification considers all symptoms as being subjective, with objective indications being called signs.

Syncope Transient loss of consciousness due to inadequate blood flow to the brain.

Syncytial Group of cells in which the protoplasm of one cell is continuous with that of adjoining cells.

Systemic Pertaining to the whole body rather than to one of its parts.

Systemic reaction Whole-body response to a stimulus.

Systole Part of the heart cycle in which the heart is in contraction.

Systolic pressure Maximum blood pressure; occurs during contraction of the ventricle.

Tachycardia Abnormal rapidity of heart action, usually defined as a heart rate over 100 beats per minute.

Tachypnea A rapid breathing rate.

Technetium 99m Radioisotope of technetium that emits α-rays; used in determining blood flow to certain organs by use of a scanning technique. It has a half-life of 6 hours.

Tenacious Adhering to; adhesive; retentive.

Tension of gas Gas pressure measured in millimeters of mercury (mm Hg).

Thoracentesis Puncture of the chest wall for removal of fluid.

Thrombocytopenia Abnormal decrease in the number of blood platelets.

Thromboembolism Blood clot caused by an embolus obstructing a vessel.

Thrombophlebitis Inflammation of a vein in conjunction with the formation of a thrombus; usually occurs in an extremity, most frequently a leg.

Thrombus Blood clot that obstructs a blood vessel or a cavity of the heart.

Thymectomy Surgical removal of the thymus gland.

Thymus Ductless, gland situated in the anterior mediastinal cavity that reaches maximum development during early childhood and then undergoes involution. It usually has two longitudinal lobes. An endocrine gland, the thymus is now thought to be a lymphoid body. It is a site of lymphopoiesis and plays a role in immunologic competence.

Titer A measurement of the concentration of a substance in a solution.

Tone That state of a body or any of its organs or parts in which the functions are healthy and normal. In a more restricted sense, the resistance of muscles to passive elongation or stretch; normal tension or responsiveness to stimuli.

Toxemia The condition resulting from the spread of bacterial products via the bloodstream; toxemic condition resulting from metabolic disturbances.

Toxin Poisonous substance of animal or plant origin.

Trachea Largest airway; a fibroelastic tube found at the level of the sixth cervical vertebra to the fifth thoracic vertebra; carries air to and from the lungs. At the carina it divides into two bronchi, one leading to each lung. The trachea is lined with mucous membrane, and its inner surface is lined with ciliated epithelium.

Tracheobronchial clearance Mechanism by which the airways are cleared of foreign substances; the act of clearing the airways by mucociliary action, coughing, macrophages, etc.

Tracheostomy Operation entailing cutting into the trachea through the neck, usually for insertion of a tube to overcome upper airway obstruction.

Tracheotomy Incision of the skin, muscles, and trachea.

Transfusion Injection of blood or a blood component into the bloodstream; transfer of the blood of one person into the blood vessels of another.

Translucent Transmitting light, but diffusing it so that objects beyond are not clearly distinguishable.

Transmission Transference of disease or infection.

Transpulmonary pressure The pressure difference between the mouth and intrapleural pressure.

Transverse Describing the state of something that is lying across or at right angles to something else; lying at right angles to the long axis of the body.

Trauma Physical injury or wound caused by external forces.

Tricuspid valve Right atrioventricular valve separating the right atrium from the right ventricle.

Trypsin Proteolytic enzyme of the pancreas.

Tuberculosis Infectious disease caused by the tubercle bacillus *Mycobacterium tuberculosis* and characterized by inflammatory infiltrations, formations of tubercles, caseation, necrosis, abscesses, fibrosis, and calcification. It most commonly affects the respiratory system.

Ulcerate To produce or become affected with an open sore or lesion of the skin.

Underventilation Reduced rate and depth of breathing.

Uremia Toxic condition associated with renal insufficiency that is produced by retention in the blood of nitrogenous substances normally excreted by the kidney.

Urokinase Enzyme obtained from human urine and used for dissolving intravascular clots. It is administered intravenously.

Vaccinia A contagious disease of cattle that is produced in humans by inoculation with cowpox virus to confer immunity against smallpox.

Vagus Pneumogastric or tenth cranial nerve. It is a mixed nerve, having motor and sensory functions and a wider distribution than any of the other cranial nerves.

Varicella Chickenpox.

Variola An acute contagious febrile disease with skin eruptions. It is also known as smallpox.

Vasoconstriction Constriction of the blood vessels.

Venous stasis Stagnation of the normal flow of blood, caused by venous congestion.

Ventilation Mechanical movement of air into and out of the lungs in a cyclic fashion. The activity is autonomic and voluntary and has two components—an in ward flow of air, called inhalation or inspiration, and an outward flow, called exhalation or expiration.

Ventricle Either of the two lower chambers of the heart. The right ventricle forces blood into the pulmonary artery; the left into the aorta.

Vernix Protective fatty deposit covering the fetus.

Visceral pleura Pleura that invests the lungs and enters into and lines the interlobar fissures.

Viscosity Stickiness or gumminess; resistance offered by a fluid to change of form or relative position of its particles due to the attraction of molecules to each other.

Viscous Sticky, gummy, gelatinous.

Viscus Any internal organ enclosed within a cavity such as the thorax or abdomen.

Volume percent (vol%) The number of cubic centimeters (millimeters) of a substance contained in 100 cc (or ml) of another substance.

Wheal More or less round and evanescent elevation of the skin, white in the center, with a red periphery. It is accompanied by itching and is seen in urticaria, insect bites, anaphylaxis, and angioneurotic edema.

Xenon 133 Radioactive isotope of xenon used in photoscanning studies of the lung.

REFERENCES

General Respiratory Care

Fundamentals of Respiratory Care

Barnes TA: *Core textbook of respiratory care practice,* ed 2, St. Louis, 1994, Mosby-Year Book.
Burton GG et al: *Respiratory care: a guide to clinical practice,* ed 3, Philadelphia, 1991, JB Lippincott.
Kacmarek RM et al: *Essentials of respiratory care,* ed 3, St. Louis, 1990, Mosby-Year Book.
Kacmarek RM, Stoller JK: *Current respiratory care,* St. Louis, 1988, Mosby-Year Book.
Scanlan CL et al: *Egan's fundamentals of respiratory care,* ed 5, St. Louis, 1990, Mosby-Year Book.
Shapiro BA et al: *Clinical application of respiratory care,* ed 4, St. Louis, 1991, Mosby-Year Book.

General Respiratory Care Equipment

McPherson SP: *Respiratory therapy equipment,* ed 4, St. Louis, 1990, Mosby-Year Book.
White GC: *Equipment theory for respiratory care,* Albany, NY, 1992, Delmar Publishers.

Mechanical Ventilation

Dupuis YG: *Ventilators: theory and clinical applications,* ed 2, St. Louis, 1992, Mosby-Year Book.
Pilbeam SP: *Mechanical ventilation,* ed 2, St. Louis, 1992, Mosby-Year Book.

Respiratory Care Monitoring

General

Kacmarek RM et al: *Monitoring in respiratory care,* St. Louis, 1993, Mosby-Year Book.

Hemodynamic Monitoring

Daily EK, Schroeder JS: *Technique in bedside hemodynamic monitoring,* ed 4, St. Louis, 1989, Mosby-Year Book.

Oblouk Darovic G: *Hemodynamic monitoring: invasive and noninvasive clinical application,* Philadelphia, 1987, WB Saunders.

General Pulmonary Function

Madama VC: *Pulmonary function testing and cardiopulmonary stress testing,* Albany, NY, 1993, Delmar Publishers.

Ruppel G: *Manual of pulmonary function testing,* ed 6, St. Louis, 1991, Mosby-Year Book.

Selected Pulmonary Function

Lal S, Ferguson AD, Campbell EJM: Forced expiratory time: a simple test for airways obstruction, *Br Med J* 28:814-817, 1964.

Kern DG, Patel SR: Auscultated forced expiratory time as a clinical and epidemiologic test of airway obstruction, *Chest* 100:636-639, 1991.

Rosenblatt G, Stein M: Clinical value of the forced expiratory time measured during auscultation, *N Engl J Med* 267:432-435, 1962.

Schapira RM et al: The value of the forced expiratory time in the physical diagnosis of obstructive airways disease, *JAMA* 270:731-736, 1993.

Arterial Blood Gases

Malley WJ: *Clinical blood gases: application and noninvasive alternatives,* Philadelphia, 1990, WB Saunders.

Shapiro BA et al: *Clinical application of blood gases,* ed 5, St. Louis, 1994, Mosby-Year Book.

Oxygenation

Cane RD et al: Unreliability of oxygen tension-bases indices in reflecting intrapulmonary shunting in critically ill patients, *Crit Care Med* 16:1243-1245, 1988.

Hess D, Kacmarek RM: Techniques and devices for monitoring oxygenation, *Respir Care* 38:646-671, 1993.

Kandel G, Aberman A: Mixed venous oxygen saturation: its role in the assessment of the critically ill patient, *Arch Intern Med* 143:1400-1402, 1993.

Nelson LD: Assessment of oxygenation: oxygenation indices, *Respir Care* 38:631-640, 1993.

Nelson LD: Monitoring lung injury, in: *Critical care: state of the art,* Fullerton, Calif, 1987 Society of Critical Care Medicine.

Nelson LD, Rutherford EJ: Monitoring mixed venous oxygen, *Respir Care* 37:154-164, 1992.

Rasanen J et al: Oxygen tension and oxyhemoglobin saturations in the assessment of pulmonary gas exchange, *Crit Care Med* 15:1058-1062, 1987.

Respiratory Pharmacology

Bills GW, Soderberg RC: *Principles of pharmacology for respiratory care,* Albany, NY, 1994, Delmar Publishers.

Howder CL: *Cardiopulmonary pharmacology: a handbook for respiratory practitioners and other allied health personnel,* Baltimore, 1992, Williams & Wilkins.

Witek TJ, Schachter EN: *Pharmacology and therapeutics in respiratory care,* Philadelphia, 1993, WB Saunders.

Rau JL: *Respiratory care pharmacology,* ed 4, St. Louis, 1994, Mosby-Year Book.

Assessment

General

Bates B: *A guide to physical examination and history taking,* ed 5, Philadelphia, 1991, JB Lippincott.

Christensen BL, Kockrow EO: *Foundations of nursing,* St. Louis, 1991, Mosby-Year Book.

Craven RR, Hirnle CJ: *Fundamentals of nursing: human health and function,* Philadelphia, 1992, JB Lippincott.

Harkness-Hood G, Dincher JR: *Total patient care: foundations and practice of adult health nursing,* St. Louis, 1992, Mosby-Year Book.

Jarvis C: *Physical examination and health assessment,* Philadelphia, 1992, WB Saunders.

Lewis L, Timby B: *Fundamental skills and concepts in patient care,* ed 4, Philadelphia, 1988, JB Lippincott.

Assessment in Respiratory Care

Op't Holt TB: *Assessment based respiratory care,* New York, 1986, John Wiley & Sons.
Wilkins RL et al: *Clinical assessment in respiratory care,* ed 2, St. Louis, 1990, Mosby-Year Book.
Witkowski AS: *Pulmonary assessment: a clinical guide,* Philadelphia, 1985, JB Lippincott.

Selected References on Assessment

Bergerson S: More about charting with a jury in mind, *Nurs 88* 18:51, 1988.
Frisch N, Coscarelli W: Systematic instructional strategies in clinical teachings: outcomes in student charting, *Nurse Educator* 11:29-32, 1986.
Kilpack V, Dobson-Brassard S: Intershift report: oral communication using the nursing process, *J Neurosci Nurs* 19:266-270, 1987.
Meredith RL, Pilbeam S: Assessing respiratory care practitioners assessment skills by performance on case studies: students vs. therapist vs. instructors, *Respir Care* 38:1219, 1993.
McPhee A: Teaching students how to chart, *Nurse Educator* 12:33, 1987.
Philpott M: 20 Rules for good charting, *Nurs 86* 16:63, 1986.
Rutkowski B: How D.R.G.'s Are Changing Your Charting, *Nurs 85* 15:49, 1985.
Stoller JK: Misallocation of respiratory care services, *Respir Care* 38:1219, 1993.
Thornton L: We teach nurses to chart defensively, *RN 57* 1986.
Weed LL: *Medical record, medical education, and patient care: the problem-oriented record as a basic tool,* Cleveland, Ohio, 1971, Case Western Reserve University Press.
Weed LL: *Medical record, medical education, and patient care,* St. Louis, 1969, Mosby-Year Book.

AARC Clinical Practice Guidelines

(In Chronological Order of Publication)

Hess D: The AARC clinical practice guidelines, *Respir Care* 36:1398-1401, 1991.
American Association for Respiratory Care: Clinical practice guidelines, *Respir Care* 36:1402-1405, 1991.
Hess D: More clinical practice guidelines: now what?, *Respir Care* 37:855-856, 1992.
American Association for Respiratory Care: Clinical practice guidelines, *Respir Care* 37:855-856, 882-922, 1992.
American Association for Respiratory Care: Clinical practice guidelines, *Respir Care* 38:495-521, 1993.
American Association for Respiratory Care: Clinical practice guidelines, *Respir Care* 38:1173-1200, 1993.
American Association for Respiratory Care: Clinical practice guidelines, *Respir Care* 39:797-836, 1994.

Radiography

General

Armstrong P, et al: *Imaging of diseases of the chest,* St. Louis, 1990, Mosby-Year Book.

Ballinger PW: *Merrill's atlas of radiographic positions and radiologic procedures,* ed 7, St. Louis, 1991, Mosby-Year Book.

Bontrager K: *Textbook of radiographic positioning and related anatomy,* ed 3, St. Louis, 1993, Mosby-Year Book.

Bushong SC: *Magnetic resonance imaging: physical and biological principles,* St. Louis, 1988, Mosby-Year Book.

Gurley LT: *Introduction to radiologic technology,* ed 3, St. Louis, 1992, Mosby-Year Book.

Malott JC, Fodor J III: *The art and science of medical radiography,* St. Louis, 1993, Mosby-Year Book.

Computed Tomography

Brown LR, Muhm JR: Computed tomography of the thorax: current perspectives, *Chest* 83:806-813, 1983.

Zerhouni E: Computed tomography of the pulmonary parenchyma: an overview, *Chest* 95:901-907, 1989.

Magnetic Resonance Imaging

Fisher MR: Magnetic resonance for evaluation of the thorax, *Chest* 95:166-173, 1989.

Lung Scanning

Spies WG et al: Radionuclide imaging in diseases of the chest, *Chest* 83:122-127, 250-255, 1983.

Pulmonary Angiography

Fedullo PF, Shure D: Pulmonary vascular imaging, *Clin Chest Med* 8:53-64, 1987.

General Anatomy and Physiology

Anthony CP, Thibodeau GA: *Anthony's textbook of anatomy and physiology,* ed 13, St. Louis, 1990, Mosby-Year Book.

Gray H: *Anatomy of the human body,* ed 30, Philadelphia, 1985, Lea & Febiger.

Guyton AC: *Anatomy and physiology,* Philadelphia, 1985, WB Saunders.

Guyton AC: *Physiology of the human body,* ed 6, Philadelphia, 1984, WB Saunders.

Hole JW: *Essentials of human anatomy and physiology,* ed 4, Dubuque, Iowa, 1992, Wm. C. Brown.

Thibodeau GA, Patton K: *Anatomy and physiology,* ed 2, St. Louis, 1992, Mosby-Year Book.

Thibodeau GA: *Structure and function of the body,* ed 9, St. Louis, 1992, Mosby-Year Book.

Tortora GJ, Anagnostakos NP: *Principles of anatomy and physiology,* ed 6, New York, 1990, Harper Collins.

Tortora GJ, Ronald EL: *Principles of human physiology,* ed 2, New York, 1986, Harper & Row.

VanDeGraaff KM: *Human anatomy,* ed 3, Dubuque, Iowa, Wm. C. Brown.

Vander AJ, Sherman JH, Luciano DS: *Human physiology: the mechanisms of body function,* ed 5, New York, 1990, McGraw-Hill.

Woodburne RT: *Essentials of human anatomy,* ed 8, Oxford, 1988, Oxford University Press.

Cardiopulmonary Anatomy and Physiology

Berne RM, Levy MN: *Cardiovascular physiology,* ed 6, St. Louis, 1992, Mosby-Year Book.

Cherniack RM, Cherniack LC: *Respiration in health and disease,* ed 3, Philadelphia, 1983, WB Saunders.

Conover MH, Zalis EG: *Understanding electrocardiography: physiological and interpretive concepts,* ed 6, St. Louis, 1992, Mosby-Year Book.

Comroe JH: *Physiology of respiration,* ed 2, St. Louis, 1974, Mosby-Year Book.

Des Jardins TD: *Cardiopulmonary anatomy and physiology: essentials for respiratory care,* ed 2, Albany, NY, 1993, Delmar Publishers.

Green JF: *Fundamental cardiovascular and pulmonary physiology,* ed 2, Philadelphia, 1987, Lea & Febiger.

Honig CR: *Modern cardiovascular physiology,* ed 2, Boston, 1988, Little, Brown & Co.

Hurst JW, Logue RB, eds: *The heart,* ed 7, New York, 1987, McGraw-Hill.

Leff AR, Schumacker PT: *Respiratory physiology: basics and applications,* Philadelphia, 1993, WB Saunders.

Levitzky MG: *Pulmonary physiology,* ed 3, New York, 1991, McGraw-Hill.

Mines AH: *Respiratory physiology,* ed 2, New York, 1986, Raven Press.

Mohrman DE, Heller LJ: *Cardiovascular physiology,* ed 3, New York, 1993, McGraw-Hill.

Murray JF: *The normal lung,* ed 2, Philadelphia, 1986, WB Saunders.

Slonim NB, Hamilton LH: *Respiratory physiology,* ed 5, St. Louis, 1987, Mosby-Year Book.

Smith JJ, Kampine JP: *Circulatory physiology: the essentials,* ed 3, Baltimore, 1990, Williams & Wilkins.

West JB: *Respiratory physiology: the essentials,* ed 4, Baltimore, 1990, Williams & Wilkins.

Microbiology

Alcamo IE: *Fundamentals of microbiology,* ed 3, Redwood City, Calif, 1991, Benjamin/Cummings Publishing.

Creager JG et al: *Microbiology; principles & applications,* Englewood Cliffs, NJ, 1990, Prentice Hall.

Pelczar MJ, Jr et al: *Microbiology,* ed 5, New York, 1986, McGraw-Hill.

Talaro K, Talaro A: *Foundations in microbiology,* Dubuque, Iowa, 1993, Wm. C. Brown.

General Pathophysiology

Cawson RA et al: *Pathology: the mechanisms of disease,* ed 2, St. Louis, 1987, Mosby-Year Book.

Porth CM: *Pathophysiology: concepts of altered health states,* ed 3, Philadelphia, 1990, JB Lippincott.

Sheldon H: *Boyd's introduction to the study of disease,* ed 11, Philadelphia, 1992, Lea & Febiger.

Walter JB: *An introduction to the principles of disease,* ed 3, Philadelphia, 1992, WB Saunders.

General Pulmonary Disorders

Bates DV et al: *Respiratory function in disease,* ed 3, Philadelphia, 1989, WB Saunders.

Braun SR: *Concise textbook of pulmonary medicine,* New York, 1989, Elsevier.

Cherniak NS (ed): *Chronic obstructive pulmonary disease,* Philadelphia, 1991, WB Saunders.

Farzan S: *A concise handbook of respiratory disease,* ed 3, Norwalk, Connecticut, 1992, Appleton & Lange.

Fishman AP (ed): *Pulmonary diseases and disorders,* ed 2, New York, 1994, McGraw-Hill.

Glauser FL (ed): *Signs and symptoms in pulmonary medicine,* Philadelphia, 1983, JB Lippincott.

Mackay AD, Cole RB: *Essentials of respiratory disease,* ed 3, New York, 1990, Churchill Livingstone.

Mitchell RS, Petty TL: *Synopsis of clinical pulmonary disease,* ed 4, St. Louis, 1989, Mosby-Year Book.

Murray JF, Nadel JA (eds): *Textbook of respiratory medicine,* ed 2, Philadelphia, 1988, WB Saunders.

Weinberger SE: *Principles of pulmonary medicine,* Philadelphia, 1992, WB Saunders.

West JB: *Pulmonary pathophysiology: the essentials,* Baltimore, 1991, Williams & Wilkins.

Wilkins RL, Dexter JR: *Respiratory disease: principles of patient care,* Philadelphia, 1993, FA Davis.

General Neonatal/Pediatric Pulmonary Disorders

Aloan CA: *Respiratory care of the newborn: a clinical manual,* Philadelphia, 1987, JB Lippincott.

Avery ME et al: *The lung and its disorders in the newborn,* ed 4, Philadelphia, 1981, WB Saunders.

Gerbeaux JJ, Tournier G (eds): *Pediatric respiratory disease,* ed 2, New York, 1982, John Wiley & Sons.

Koff PB et al: *Neonatal and pediatric respiratory care,* St Louis, 1993, Mosby-Year Book.

Whitaker K: *Comprehensive perinatal and pediatric respiratory care,* Albany, NY, 1992, Delmar Publishers.

Yeh TF: *Neonatal therapeutics,* ed 2, St. Louis, 1991, Mosby-Year Book.

Selected Pulmonary Disorder References

Chronic Bronchitis and Emphysema

American Thoracic Society, Statement by Committee on Diagnostic Standards for Non-Tuberculous Respiratory Diseases: Definitions and classifications of chronic bronchitis, asthma, and pulmonary emphysema, *Am Rev Respir Dis* 85:762-768, 1962.

Make B: *Clinics in chest medicine: pulmonary rehabilitation,* Philadelphia, 1986, WB Saunders.

Mamilli AE et al: Longitudinal changes in forced expiratory volume in one second in adults, *Am Rev Respir Dis* 135:794, 1987.

Ploysongsang Y et al: Lung sounds in patients with emphysema, *Am Rev Respir Dis* 124:45, 1981.

Robins AG: Pathophysiology of emphysema. *Clin Chest Med* 4:413-420, 1983.

Snider GL: Chronic bronchitis and emphysema, in Murray JF, Nadel JA (eds): *Textbook of respiratory medicine,* Philadelphia, 1988, WB Saunders.

Snider GL: The pathogenesis of emphysema—20 years of progress, *Am Rev Respir Dis* 124:321-324, 1981.

Snider GL et al: The definition of emphysema (Report of National Heart, Lung and Blood Institute, Division of Lung Diseases Workshop), *Am Rev Respir Dis* 132:182, 1985.

Weingberger SE: Chronic obstructive pulmonary diseases, in Weinberger SE (ed): *Principles of pulmonary medicine,* Philadelphia, 1992, WB Saunders.

Wewers MD et al: Replacement therapy for alpha$_1$-antitrypsin deficiency associated with emphysema, *N Engl J Med* 316:1055, 1987.

Bronchiectasis

Barker AF, Bardana EJ, Jr.: Bronchiectasis: update of an orphan disease, *Am Rev Respir Dis* 137:969-978, 1988.

George RB et al: *Bronchiectasis, chest Medicine,* New York, 1983, Churchill Livingstone.

Hodgkin JE: Bronchiectasis, in Conn RB (ed): *Current diagnosis,* Philadelphia, 1985, WB Saunders.

Mazzocco M, Owens GR: Chest percussion and postural drainage on patients with bronchiectasis, *Chest* 88:360-363, 1985.

Smith C: *Bronchiectasis in core pathology—fundamental concepts and principles,* Oradell, NJ, 1981, Medical Economics.

Asthma

Blumenthal MN et al: A multicenter evaluation of the clinical benefits of cromolyn sodium aerosol by metered-dose inhaler in the treatment of asthma, *J Allergy Clin Immunol* 81:681, 1988.

Cardan DL et al: Vital signs including pulsus paradoxus in the assessment of acute bronchial asthma, *Ann Emerg* 12:80, 1983.

Henkind SJ et al: The paradox of pulsus paradoxus, *Am Heart J* 114:198, 1987.

Konig P: Conflicting viewpoints about the treatment of asthma with cromolyn: a review of the literature, *Ann Allergy* 43:293, 1979.

Martin AJ: The natural history of childhood asthma to adult life, *Br Med J* 1:1397, 1980.

Moler FW et al: Improvement in clinical asthma score and Pa_{CO_2} in children with severe asthma treated with continuously nebulized terbutaline, *J Allergy Clin Immunol* 81:1101, 1988.

Portnow J, Aggarwal J: Continuous terbutaline nebulization for the treatment of severe exacerbations of asthma in children, *Ann Allergy* 60:368, 1988.

Williams MH: The nature of asthma: definition and natural history, *Semin Respir Med* 1:283, 1980.

Cystic Fibrosis

Aitken ML et al: Recombinant human DNase inhalation in normal subjects and patients with cystic fibrosis, *JAMA* 267:1947, 1992.

App EM et al: Acute and long term amiloride inhalation in cystic fibrosis lung disease: a rationale approach to cystic fibrosis therapy, *Am Rev Respir Dis* 141:605, 1990.

Davis PB, diSant'Agnese PA: A review: cystic fibrosis at forty—quo vadis?, *Pediatr Res* 14:83-87, 1980.

Desmond KJ et al: Immediate and long term effects of chest physiotherapy in patients with cystic fibrosis, *J Pediatr* 103:538, 1983.

Fink RJ et al: Pulmonary function and morbidity in 40 adult patients with cystic fibrosis, *Chest* 74:643, 1978.

Fowler RS et al: Cor pulmonale in cystic fibrosis, *J Electrocardiol* 14:319-324, 1981.

Hilman BC: Cystic fibrosis: not just a pediatric disease, *J Respir Dis* 2:83-97, 1981.

Hen J et al: Meconium plug syndrome associated with cystic fibrosis and Hirschsprung's disease, *Pediatrics* 66:466-468, 1980.

Hodson ME et al: Aerosolized carbenicillin and gentamicin treatment of *Pseudomonas aeruginosa* infection in patients with cystic fibrosis, *Lancet* 2:1137, 1981.

Holsclaw DS: Cystic fibrosis: overview and pulmonary aspects in young adults, *Clin Chest Med* 1:407, 1980.

Huang NN et al: Clinical features, survival rate, and prognostic factors in young adults with cystic fibrosis, *Am J Med* 82:871-879, 1987.

Hubbard RC et al: A preliminary study of aerosolized recombinant deoxyribonuclease I in the treatment of cystic fibrosis, *N Engl J Med* 326:812, 1992.

Kerem E et al: The relation between genotype and phenotype in cystic fibrosis of the most common mutation (delta F_{508}), *N Engl J Med* 323:1517, 1990.

Knowles MR et al: A pilot study of aerosolized amiloride for treatment of lung disease in cystic fibrosis, *N Engl J Med* 322:1189, 1990.

Larter N: Cystic fibrosis, *Am J Nurs* 81:527-532, 1981

Ledger S: Nursing care study: a young patient with cystic fibrosis, *Nurs Times* 77:1291-1294, 1981.

Lester LA: Complications of cystic fibrosis pulmonary disease, *Semin Respir Med* 6:285-298, 1985.

Marks MI: The pathogenesis and treatment of pulmonary infections in patients with cystic fibrosis, *J Pediatr* 98:173-179, 1981.

Maxwell M: Review of literature of physiotherapy in cystic fibrosis, *Physiotherapy* 66:245-246, 1980.

Mischler EH: Treatment of pulmonary disease in cystic fibrosis, *Semin Respir Med* 6:271-284, 1985.

Quinton PM, Bujman J: Higher bioelectric potentials due to decreased chloride absorption in the sweat glands of patients with cystic fibrosis, *N Engl J Med* 308:1185, 1983.

Riordan JR et al: Identification of the cystic fibrosis gene: cloning and characterization of the complementary DNA, *Science* 245:1066, 1989.

Rommens JM et al: Identification of the cystic fibrosis gene: chromosome walking and jumping, *Science* 245:1059, 1989.

Russell NJ et al: Lung function in young adults with cystic fibrosis, *Br J Dis Chest* 76:35-43, 1982.

Statement from the National Institutes of Health workshop in population screening for the cystic fibrosis gene, *N Engl J Med* 323:70, 1990.

Steen JH et al: Evaluation of the PEP mask in cystic fibrosis, *Acta Paediatr Scand* 80:51, 1991.

Taussig LM: *Cystic fibrosis,* New York, 1984, Thieme-Stratton.

Croup and Epiglottis

Ashcrage CK, Russell WS: Epiglottis: a pediatric emergency, *J Respir Dis* 7:40-60, 1988.

Barker GA: Current management of croup and epiglottis, *Pediatr Clin North Am* 26:565, 1979.

Bass JW, Wehrie PF: Croup and epiglottis, in Nussbaum E, Galant SP (eds): *Pediatric respiratory disorders,* Orlando, Fla, 1984, Grune & Stratton.

Butt W et al: Acute epiglottis: a different approach to management, *Crit Care Med* 16:43, 1988.

Cherry JD: The treatment of croup: continued controversy due to failure of recognition of historic, ecologic, etiological, and clinical perspectives, *J Pediatr* 94:352, 1979.

Denny FW: Croup: an 11-year study in a pediatric practice, *Pediatrics* 71:871, 1983.

Eigen H: Croup or epiglottis: differential diagnosis and treatment, *Respir Care* 20:1158-1163, 1975.

Kimmons HC, Peterson BM: Management of acute epiglottis in pediatric patients, *Crit Care Med* 14:278, 1986.

Letourneau MA: Respiratory disorders, in Berkin RM et al (eds): *Pediatric emergency medicine,* St. Louis, 1992, Mosby-Year Book.

Mayo-Smith MF et al: Acute epiglottitis in adults, an eight-year experience in the state of Rhode Island, *N Engl J Med* 314:1133-1139, 1986.

Robotham, JL: Obstructive airways disease in infants and children, in Kirby RR, Taylor RW (eds): *Respiratory failure,* St. Louis, 1986, Mosby-Year Book.

Simkins R: Croup and epiglottis, *Am J Nurs* 81:519-520, 1981.

Thomas DO: Are you sure it's only croup? *RN* 47:40-43, 1984.

Vernon DD, Ashok PS: Acute epiglottis in children: a conservative approach to diagnosis and management, *Crit Care Med* 14:1, 1986.

Pneumonia

General Reviews

Alcamo IE: *Study guide to accompany fundamentals of microbiology,* Reading, Mass, 1983, Addison-Wesley Publishing.

Fang G-D et al: New and emerging etiologies for community-acquired pneumonia with implications for therapy: a prospective multicenter study of 359 cases, *Medicine* 69:307, 1990.

Nester EW et al: *Microbiology,* Philadelphia, 1983, WB Saunders.

Pennington JE (ed): *Respiratory infections: diagnosis and management,* ed 2, New York, 1988, Raven Press.

Ross FC: *Introductory microbiology,* Columbus, Ohio, 1983, Charles E. Merrill Publishing.

Bacterial Pneumonia

Davis GS, Winn WC, Jr.: Legionnaires' disease: respiratory infections caused by *legionella bacteria, Clin Chest Med* 8:419-439, 1987.

Edelstein PH, Meyer RD: Legionnaires' disease: a review, *Chest* 85:114-120, 1984.

George WL, Finegold SM: Bacterial infections of the lung, *Chest* 81:502-507, 1982.

Grayston JT: Chlamydia pneumoniae, strain TWAR, *Chest* 95:664-669, 1989.

Marrie TJ et al: Pneumonia associated with the TWAR strain of Chlamydia, *Ann Intern Med* 106:507-511, 1987.

Rytel MW: Pneumococcal pneumonia: still a serious problem, *J Respir Dis* 11:83-95, 1990.

Viral Pneumonia

Anderson LJ et al: Viral respiratory illness, *Med Clin North Am* 67:1009-1030, 1983.

McIntosh K: Respiratory syncytial virus infection infants and children: diagnosis and treatment, *Pediatr Rev* 9:191-196, 1987.

Reichman RC, Dolin R: Viral pneumonia, *Med Clin North Am* 64:491-506, 1980.

Rose RM et al: Viral infection of the lower respiratory tract, *Clin Chest Med* 8:405-418, 1987.

Miscellaneous Pneumonia

Bartlett JG, Gorbach SL: The triple threat of aspiration pneumonia, *Chest* 68:560-566, 1975.

Mansel JK et al: Mycoplasma pneumoniae pneumonia, *Chest* 95:639-646, 1989.

Acquired Immunodeficiency Syndrome

Baskin MI et al: Regional deposition of aerosolized pentamidine: effects of body position and breathing pattern, *Ann Intern Med* 113:677-683, 1990.

Braun MM et al: Acquired immunodeficiency syndrome and extrapulmonary tuberculosis in the United States, *Arch Intern Med* 150:1913-1916, 1990.

Centers for Disease Control: Guidelines for prophylaxis against *Pneumocystis carinii* pneumonia for persons infected with human immunodeficiency virus, *MMWR* 38:1-9, 1989.

Chaisson RE, Slutkin G: Tuberculosis and human immunodeficiency virus infection, *J Infect Dis* 159:96-100, 1989.

Conte JE, Jr. et al: Intravenous or inhaled pentamidine for treating *Pneumocystis carinii* pneumonia in AIDS, *Ann Intern Med* 113:203-209, 1990.

DeVita VT et al: *AIDS,* ed 3, Philadelphia, 1992, JB Lippincott.

Luce JM: HIV, AIDS, and the Respiratory Care Practitioner, *Respir Care* 38:189-196, 1993.

Murray JF, Mills J: Pulmonary infectious complications of human immunodeficiency virus infection, *Am Rev Respir Dis* 141:1356-1372, 1582-1598, 1990.

Rankin JA et al: Acquired immune deficiency syndrome and the lung, *Chest* 94:155-164, 1988.

Wallace JM, Hannah J: Cytomegalovirus pneumonitis in patients with AIDS, *Chest* 92:198-203, 1987.

White DA, Stover DE (ed): Pulmonary effects of AIDS, *Clin Chest Med* 9:363-533, 1988.

Lung Abscess

Bartlett JG: Anaerobic bacterial infections of the lung, *Chest* 91:901-909, 1987.

Bartlett JG: Lung abscess, *Johns Hopkins Med J* 15:141-147, 1982.

Estrera AS et al: Primary lung abscess, *J Thorac Cardiovasc Surg* 79:275-282, 1980.

Pohlson EC et al: Lung abscess: a changing pattern of the disease, *Am J Surg* 150:97-101, 1985.

Spencer H: Lung abscesses, in *Pathology of the lung,* vol 1, New York, 1985, Pergamon Press.

Fungal Disorders of the Lungs

General

American Thoracic Society: Laboratory diagnosis of mycotic and specific fungal infections, *Am Rev Respir Dis* 132:1373-1379, 1985.

Davies SF: An overview of pulmonary fungal infections, *Clin Chest Med* 8:495-512, 1987.

Histoplasmosis

Goodwin RA, Jr., Des Prez RM: Histoplasmosis, state of the art, *Am Rev Respir Dis* 117:929-956, 1978.

Goodwin RA, Jr. et al: Histoplasmosis in normal hosts, *Medicine* 60:231-266, 1981.

Sagg MS, Dismukes WE: Treatment of histoplasmosis and blastomycosis, *Chest* 93:848-851, 1988.

Wheat LJ et al: Cavitary histoplasmosis occurring during two large urban outbreaks, *Medicine* 63:201-209, 1984.

Coccidioidomycosis

Bayer AS: Fungal pneumonias: pulmonary coccidioidal syndromes, Parts 1 and 2, *Chest* 79:686-691, 1981.

Einstein HE: Coccidioidomycosis, *Respir Care* 26:563-568, 1981.

Ross JB et al: Ketoconazole for treatment of chronic pulmonary coccidioidomycosis, *Ann Intern Med* 86:440-443, 1982.

Blastomycosis

Bradsher RW et al: Ketoconazole therapy for endemic blastomycosis, *Ann Intern Med* 103:872-879, 1983.

Gabr-Habte E, Smith IM: North American blastomycosis in Iowa: review of 34 cases, *J Chron Dis* 26:1-10, 1973.

Cryptococcosis

Kerkening TM et al: The evaluation of pulmonary cryptococcosis, *Ann Intern Med* 94:611-616, 1981.

Aspergillosis

Binder RE et al: Chronic necrotizing pulmonary aspergillosis: a discrete clinical entity, *Medicine* 61:109-124, 1982.

Ricketti AJ et al: Allergic bronchopulmonary aspergillosis, *Chest* 86:773-778, 1984.

Candidiasis

Masur H et al: Pulmonary disease caused by candida species, *Am J Med* 63:914-926, 1977.

Tuberculosis

American Thoracic Society: Control of tuberculosis in the United States (ATS statement), *Am Rev Respir Dis* 146:1623-1633, 1992.

American Thoracic Society: Diagnostic standards and classification of tuberculosis, *Am Rev Respir Dis* 142:725-735, 1990.

American Thoracic Society: Treatment of tuberculosis and tuberculosis infection in adults and children, *Am Rev Respir Dis* 134:355, 1986.

Bailey WC et al: Preventive treatment of tuberculosis, *Chest* 85:1285-1325, 1984.

Barnes PF et al: Tuberculosis in patients with human immunodeficiency virus infection, *N Engl J Med* 324:1644-1650, 1991.

Brudney K, Dobkin J: Resurgent tuberculosis in New York City: human immunodeficiency virus, homelessness, and the decline of tuberculosis control programs, *Am Rev Respir Dis* 144:745-749, 1991.

Gracey DR: Tuberculosis in the world today, *Mayo Clin Proc* 63:1251-1255, 1988.

Perez-Stable EJ, Hopewell P: Chemotherapy of tuberculosis, *Semin Respir Med* 9:459-469, 1988.

Raleigh JW: Disease due to *mycobacterium kansasii, Semin Respir Med* 9:498-504, 1988.

Rieder HL et al: Tuberculosis in the United States, *JAMA* 262:385-389, 1989.

Rook GA: The role of vitamin D in tuberculosis, *Respir Dis* 138:768-770, 1988.

Smith MJ, Citron KM: Clinical review of pulmonary disease caused by *Mycobacterium, Thorax* 28:197, 1983.

Snider DE et al: Standard therapy for tuberculosis, *Chest* 87:1175-1235, 1985.

Snider DE: Current and future priorities in tuberculosis, *Semin Respir Med* 9:514-520, 1988.

Spires R: Tuberculosis today: the siege isn't over yet, *RN* 43:43-46, 1980.

Pulmonary Edema

Ayres SM: Mechanisms and consequences of pulmonary edema: cardiac lung, shock lung, and principles of ventilatory therapy in adult respiratory distress syndrome, *Am Heart J* 103:97-112, 1982.

Braunwald E: Clinical manifestations of heart failure, in Braunwald E (ed): *Heart disease: a textbook of cardiovascular medicine,* Philadelphia, 1984, WB Saunders.

Branson RD et al: Mask CPAP: state of the art, *Respir Care* 30:846, 1985.

Chesebro JH, Burnett JC: Cardiac failure: characteristics and clinical manifestations, in Brandenburg RO et al (eds): *Cardiology: fundamentals and practice,* St. Louis, 1987, Mosby-Year Book.

Chesebro JH: Cardiac failure: medical management, in Brandenburg RO et al (eds): *Clinical assessment in respiratory care,* St. Louis, 1990, Mosby-Year Book.

Fuster V et al: The natural history of idiopathic dilated cardiomyopathy, *Am J Cardiol* 47:525, 1981.

Krider SJ: Invasively monitored hemodynamic pressures, in Wilkins RL et al (eds): *Clinical assessment in respiratory care,* St. Louis, 1990, Mosby-Year Book.

Marland AM, Glauser FL: Hemodynamic and pulmonary edema protein measurements in a case of re-expansion pulmonary edema, *Chest* 81:250-251, 1982.

Pastore JO: Cardiac disease in respiratory patients in the intensive care unit, in MacDonnell KF et al (eds): *Respiratory intensive care,* Boston, 1987, Little, Brown & Co.

Perel A et al: Effectiveness of CPAP via face mask for pulmonary edema associated with hypercarbia, *Intensive Care Med* 9:17, 1983.

Rasanen J et al: Continuous positive pressure by face mask in acute cardiogenic pulmonary edema. A randomized study, *Crit Care Med* 12:A325, 1983.

Pulmonary Embolism and Infarction

Dalen JE: Clinical diagnosis of acute pulmonary embolism. When should a V̇/Q̇ scan be ordered?, *Chest* 100:1185, 1991.

Dossey B, Passons JM: Pulmonary embolism: preventing it, treating it, *Nursing 81* 11:26-33, 1981.

Moser KM: Pulmonary embolism, in Murray JF, Nadel JA (eds): *Textbook of respiratory medicine,* Philadelphia, 1988, WB Saunders.

Moser KM: Pulmonary embolism, *Am Rev Respir Dis* 115:829, 1977.

Moser KM, Fedullo PF: Venous thromboembolism: three simple decisions, *Chest* 83:117, 256, 1983.

Moser KM: Venous thromboembolism, *Am Rev Respir Dis* 141:235-249, 1990.

Stein PD et al: Clinical, laboratory, roentgenographic, and electrocardiographic findings in patients with acute pulmonary embolism and no pre-existing cardiac or pulmonary disease, *Chest* 100:598, 1991.

Wenger NK: Pulmonary embolism: recognition and management, *Consultant* 6:85-98, 1980.

West JW: Pulmonary embolism, in Wu K (ed): *Pathophysiology and management of thromboembolic disorders,* Littleton, Mass, 1984, PGS Publishing.

Flail Chest

Bollinger CT, Van Eeden SF: Treatment of multiple rib fractures: randomized controlled trial comparing ventilatory with nonventilatory management, *Chest* 97:943-948, 1990.

Carpintero JL et al: Methods of management of flail chest, *Intensive Care Med* 6:217-221, 1980.

Christensson P et al: Early and late results of controlled ventilation in flail chest, *Chest* 75:456-460, 1979.

Craven KD et al: Effects of contusion and flail chest on pulmonary perfusion and oxygen exchange, *J Appl Physiol* 47:729-737, 1979.

Cullen P: Treatment of patients with flail chest by intermittent mandatory ventilation and PEEP, *Crit Care Med* 3:45, 1975.

Hankins JR et al: Management of flail chest: an analysis of 99 cases, *Am Surg* 45:176, 1979.

Hood RM: Trauma to the chest, in Sabiston DC, Jr., Spencer FC (eds): *Gibbon's surgery of the chest,* ed 4, Philadelphia, 1983, WB Saunders.

Jackson H: Nursing care of patients with chest injuries, *Nursing* 11:303-309, 1979.

Jette NT, Barash PG: Treatment of a flail injury of the chest: a case report with consideration of the evolution of therapy, *Anaesthesia* 32:475-479, 1977.

Maloney JV et al: Paradoxical respiration and "pendelluft," *J Thorac Cardiovasc Surg* 41:291-298, 1961.

Miller HAB et al: Management of flail chest, *Can Med Assoc J* 129:1104-1107, 1983.

Richardson JD et al: Selective management of flail chest and pulmonary contusion, *Ann Surg* 196:481-487, 1982.

Relihan M, Litwin MS: Morbidity and mortality associated with flail chest injury: a review of 85 cases, *J Trauma* 13:663, 1973.

Pneumothorax

Gustman P et al: Immediate cardiovascular effects of tension pneumothorax, *Am Rev Respir Dis* 127:171-174, 1983.

Harvery JE, Jeyasingham K: The difficult pneumothorax, *Br J Dis Chest* 81:209-216, 1987.

Jerkinson SG: Pneumothorax, *Clin Chest Med* 6:153-161, 1985.

O'Rourke JP, Yee ES: Clivilian spontaneous pneumothorax: treatment options and long-term results, *Chest* 96:1302-1306, 1989.

Yamazaki S et al: Pulmonary blood flow to rapidly reexpanded lung in spontaneous pneumothorax, *Chest* 81:118-120, 1982.

Pleural Diseases

Ali I, Unruh H: Management of empyema thoracis, *Ann Thorac Surg* 50:355-359, 1990.

Bynum LJ, Wilson JE III: Radiographic features of pleural effusion in pulmonary embolism, *Am Rev Respir Dis* 117:829-852, 1978.

Collins TR, Sahn SA: Thoracocentesis: clinical value, complications, technical problems, and patient experience, *Chest* 91:817-822, 1987.

Hughes RL et al: The management of chylothorax, *Chest* 76:212-218, 1979.

Light RW: *Pleural diseases,* ed 2, Philadelphia, 1990, Lea & Febiger.

Nielsen PH et al: Postoperative pleural effusion following upper abdominal surgery, *Chest* 96:1133-1135, 1989.

Sahn SA: The pathophysiology of pleural effusion, *Annu Rev Med* 41:7-13, 1990.

Sahn SA: The pleura, *Am Rev Respir Dis* 138:184-234, 1988.

Smyrnios NS et al: Pleural effusion in an asymptomatic patient, *Chest* 97:192-196, 1990.

Kyphoscoliosis

Bergofsky EH: Respiratory failure in disorders of the thoracic cage, *Am Rev Respir Dis* 119:643-669, 1979.

Fulkerson WJ et al: Life threatening hypoventilation in kyphoscoliosis: successful treatment with a molded body brace-ventilator, *Am Rev Respir Dis* 129:185-187, 1984.

Guilleminault C et al: Severe kyphoscoliosis, breathing and sleep, *Chest* 79:626-630, 1981.

Keim HA, Hensinger RN: Spinal deformities: scoliosis and kyphosis, *Clin Symp* 41:3-32, 1989.

Pneumoconioses

Albelda SM et al: Pleural thickening: its significance and relationship to asbestos dust and exposure, *Am Rev Respir Dis* 126:621-624, 1982.

Arzt GH: Review of lung function data in 195 patients with asbestosis of the lung, *Int Arch Occup Environ Health* 45:63-79, 1980.

Becklake MR: Pneumoconiosis, in Murray JF, Nadel JA (eds): *Textbook of respiratory medicine,* Philadelphia, 1988, WB Saunders.

Churg A: Asbestos fibers in the general population, *Am Rev Respir Dis* 122:660-678, 1980.

Craishead JE et al: The pathology of asbestos-associated diseases of the lungs and pleural cavities: diagnostic criteria and proposed grading schema. Report of the pneumonoconiosis Committee of the College of American Pathologists and the National Institute for Occupational Safety and Health, *Arch Pathol Lab Med* 106:544-596, 1982.

deShazo RD: Current concepts about the pathogenesis of silicosis and asbestosis, *J Allergy Clin Immunol* 70:41-49, 1982.

Epler GR: Asbestos-related disease from household exposure, *Respiration* 39:229-240, 1980.

Finkelstein MM: Asbestosis in long-term employees of an Ontario asbestos-cement factory, *Am Rev Respir Dis* 125:496-501, 1982.

Gee JB: Cellular mechanisms in occupational lung disease, *Chest* 78:384-387, 1980.

Goodman LR: Radiology of asbestos disease, *JAMA* 249:644-646, 1983.

Morgan WHC, Seaton A: *Occupational lung diseases,* ed 2, Philadelphia, 1984, WB Saunders.

Motley RL: Asbestos and lung cancer: evaluation of legal requirements of medical causation, *N Y State J Med* 80:1143-1147, 1980.

Pearle J: Exercise performance and functional impairment in asbestos-exposed workers, *Chest* 80:1701-1705, 1981.

Roggli VL: Comparison of sputum and lung asbestos body counts in former asbestos workers, *Am Rev Respir Dis* 122:941, 1980.

Sargent EN et al: Calcified interlobar pleural plaques: visceral pleural involvement due to asbestos, *Radiology* 140:634, 1981.

Victor LD, Talamonti WJ: Asbestos lung disease, *Hosp Pract* 21:257-268, 1986.

Weill H: Asbestos-associated diseases: science, public policy, and litigation, *Chest* 84:601-608, 1983.

Cancer of the Lung

Bone RC, Balk RB: Staging of bronchogenic carcinoma, *Chest* 82:473-480, 1982.

Carr DT: Malignant lung disease, *Hosp Pract* 16:97-115, 1981.

Doyle LA, Aisner J: Clinical presentation of lung cancer, in Roth JA et al (eds): *Thoracic oncology,* Philadelphia, 1989, WB Saunders.

Engelking C: Lung cancer: the language of staging, *Am J Nurs* 87:1434-1437, 1987.

Faber LP: Lung cancer, in Holleb AI et al (eds): *American Cancer Society textbook of clinical oncology,* Atlanta, 1991, American Cancer Society.

Filderman AE, Matthay RA: Update on lung cancer, *Respir Ther* 15:21-31, 1985.

Ginsberg RJ, Joss RA, Feld R: Fifth world conference on lung cancer, *Chest* 96:1S-107S, 1989.

Hande KR, Des Prez RM: Current perspectives in small cell lung cancer, *Chest* 85:669-677, 1984.

Khouri NF et al: The solitary pulmonary nodule: assessment, diagnosis and management, *Chest* 91:128, 1987.

Tisi GM et al: *Clinical staging of primary lung cancer,* New York, 1981, American Thoracic Society.

Adult Respiratory Distress Syndrome

Ashbaugh DG et al: Acute respiratory distress in adults, *Lancet* 2:319-323, 1967.

Bone RC (ed): Adult respiratory distress syndrome, *Clin Chest Med* 3:1-213, 1982.

Hudson LD: Ventilatory management of patients with adult respiratory distress syndrome, *Semin Respir Med* 2:128-139, 1981.

Hyers TM: Pathogenesis of adult respiratory distress syndrome: current concepts, *Semin Respir Med* 2:104-108, 1981.

Petty TL, Ashbaugh DG: The adult respiratory distress syndrome: clinical features, factors influencing prognosis and principles of management, *Chest* 60:233, 1971.

Petty TL: Adult respiratory distress syndrome: historical perspective and definition, *Semin Respir Med* 2:99-103, 1981.

Petty TL et al: Characteristics of pulmonary surfactant in adult respiratory distress syndrome associated with trauma and shock, *Am Rev Respir Dis* 115:531, 1977.

Rinalds JE, Rogers RM: Adult respiratory distress syndrome: changing concepts of lung injury and repair, *N Engl J Med* 306:900-909, 1982.

Shapiro BA et al: Changes in intrapulmonary shunting with administration of 100 percent oxygen, *Chest* 77:138-141, 1980.

Shapiro DL: Respiratory distress syndrome, *N Y State Med J* 80:257-259, 1980.

Stoller JK, Kacmarek RM: Ventilatory strategies in the management of the adult respiratory distress syndrome, *Clin Chest Med* 11:755, 1990.

Tomashefski JF: Pulmonary pathology of the adult respiratory distress syndrome, *Clin Chest Med* 11:593, 1990.

Idiopathic Respiratory Distress Syndrome

Barrie H: Simple method of applying continuous positive airway pressure in respiratory distress syndrome, *Lancet* 1:776, 1972.

Belani KG et al: Respiratory failure in newborns, infants, and children, *Indian J Pediatr* 48:21-36, 1981.

Bryan H et al: Perinatal factors associated with the respiratory distress syndrome, *Am J Obstet Gynecol* 162:476, 1990.

Carlo WA et al: The effect of respiratory distress syndrome on chest wall movements and respiratory pauses in preterm infants, *Am Rev Respir Dis* 126:103-107, 1982.

Chatburn R: Similarities and differences in the management of acute lung injury in neonates (IRDS) and in adults (ARDS), *Respir Care* 33:539, 1988.

Gregory G et al: Treatment of the idiopathic respiratory-distress syndrome with continuous positive airway pressure, *N Engl J Med* 284:1333, 1971.

Hallman M, Gluck L: Respiratory distress syndrome—update 1982, *Pediatr Clin North Am* 29:1057, 1982.

Lapido M: Respiratory distress revisited, *Neonatal Network* 8:9, 1989.

Chronic Interstitial Lung Diseases

Becklake MR: Pneumoconiosis, in Murray JF, Nadel JA (eds): *Textbook of respiratory medicine,* Philadelphia, 1988, WB Saunders.

Flint A: Pathologic features of interstitial lung disease, in Schwarz MI, King TE (eds): *Interstitial lung disease,* Toronto, 1988, BC Decker.

Fulmer JD: The interstitial lung diseases, *Chest* 82:172-178, 1982.

Fulmer JD: An introduction to the interstitial lung diseases, *Clin Chest Med* 3:457, 1982.

Morgan WKC, Seaton A: *Occupational lung diseases,* ed 2, Philadelphia, 1984, WB Saunders.

Rosenow EC, Martin WJ: Drug induced interstitial lung disease, in Schwarz MI, King TE (eds): *Interstitial lung disease,* Toronto, 1988, BC Decker.

Guillain-Barré Syndrome

Asbury AK: Diagnostic considerations in Guillain-Barré syndrome, *Ann Neurol* 9:1-5, 1981.

England JD: Guillain-Barre syndrome, *Ann Rev Med* 41:1-6, 1990.

Guillain-Barré Syndrome Study Group: Plasmapheresis and acute Guillain-Barré syndrome, *Neurology* 35:1096-1104, 1985.

Koski CL et al: Guillain-Barré syndrome, *Am Fam Physician* 34:190-210, 1986.

Schonberger LB et al: Guillain-Barré syndrome following vaccination in the National Influenza Immunization Program, United States, 1976-1977, *Am J Epidemiol* 100:105-123, 1979.

Myasthenia Gravis

Barry L: The patient with myasthenia gravis really needs you, *Nursing* 12:50-53, 1982.

Gracey D et al: Mechanical ventilation for respiratory failure in myasthenia gravis, *Mayo Clin Proc* 58:597-602, 1983.

Gracey DR et al: Postoperative respiratory care after transsternal thymectomy in myasthenia gravis, *Chest* 86:67-71, 1984.

Lisak R: Myasthenia gravis: mechanisms and management, *Hosp Pract* 18:101-109, 1983.

Mulder DG et al: Thymectomy for myasthenia gravis: recent observation and comparison with past experience, *Ann Thorac Surg* 48:551-555, 1989.

Sleep Apnea

Becker K, Cummiskey J: Managing sleep apnea: what are today's options?, *J Respir Dis*, 50-71, 1985.

Cherniack NS: Breathing disorders during sleep, *Hosp Pract* 21:81-104, 1986.

Douglas NJ: Breathing during sleep in patients with respiratory disease, *Semin Respir Med* 9:586-593, 1988.

George C, Kryger M: Management of sleep apnea, *Semin Respir Med* 9:569-576, 1988.

Guilleminault C et al: Determinants of daytime sleepiness in obstructive sleep apnea, *Chest* 94:32-37, 1988.

Jiang H et al: Mortality and apnea index in obstructive sleep apena, *Chest* 94:9-14, 1988.

Kales A et al: Sleep disorders: sleep apnea and narcolepsy, *Ann Intern Med* 106:434-443, 1987.

Kryger MH (ed): Symposium on sleep disorders, *Clin Chest Med* 6(4)-Dec, 1985.

Lugaresi E et al: Snoring: pathophysiology and clinical consequences, *Semin Respir Med* 9:577-585, 1988.

Mishoe SC: The diagnosis and treatment of sleep apnea syndrome, *Respir Care* 32:183-201, 1987.

Oesting HH, Manza RJ: Sleep apnea, *Geriatr Nurs* 9:232-233, 1988.

Onal E: Central sleep apnea, *Semin Respir Med* 9:547-553, 1988.

Patrinen M et al: Long-term outcome for obstructive sleep apnea syndrome patients: mortality, *Chest* 94:1200-1204, 1988.

Roth T et al: Behavioral morbidity of apnea, *Semin Respir Med* 9:554-559, 1988.

Shepard JW, Jr.: Pathophysiology and medical therapy of sleep apnea, *Ear Nose Throat J* 63:24-48, 1984.

Shepard JR, Jr.: Physiologic and clinical consequences of sleep apnea, *Semin Respir Med* 9:560-568, 1988.

Smith PL: Evaluation of patients with sleep disorders, *Semin Respir Med* 9:534-539, 1988.

Stauffer JL et al: Pharyngeal size and resistance in obstructive sleep apnea, *Am J Respir Dis* 136:623-627, 1987.

Stradling JR, Phillipson EA: Breathing disorders during sleep, *Q J Med* 58:3-18, 1986.

Strohl KP et al: Physiologic basis of therapy for sleep apnea (state of the art), *Am Rev Respir Dis* 134:791-802, 1986.

Tobin MJ et al: Breathing abnormalities during sleep, *Arch Intern Med* 143:1221-1228, 1983.

White DP: Disorders of breathing during sleep: introduction, epidemiology, and incidence, *Semin Respir Med* 1988; 9:529-533.

Wiegand L et al: Pathogenesis of obstructive sleep apnea: role of the pharynx, *Semin Respir Med* 9:540-546, 1988.

Near Drowning

Conn A, Barker G: Fresh water drowning and near-drowning: an update, *Can Anaesth Soc J* 31:S38, 1984.

Gilbert J et al: Near drowning: current concepts of management, *Respir Care* 30:108, 1985.

Gonzalez-Rothi R: Near drowning: consensus and controversies in pulmonary and cerebral resuscitation, *Heart Lung* 16:474, 1987.

Karch SB: Pathophysiology of the lung in near drowning, *Am J Emerg Med* 4:4-7, 1986.

Nemiroff MJ: Near-drowning, *Respir Care* 37:600-608, 1992.

Orlowski J: Drowning, near-drowning, and ice-water submersions, *Pediatr Clin North Am* 34:75, 1987.

Ornato J: The resuscitation of near-drowning victims, *JAMA* 256:75, 1986.

Pearn J: Pathophysiology of drowning, *Med J Aust* 142:586-588, 1985.

Shaw K: Management of near drowning patient, *Respir Mgmt* 21:32-38, 1991.

Siebke H et al: Survival after 40 minutes' submersion without cerebral sequelae, *Lancet* 1:1275, 1975.

Smoke Inhalation

Baud FJ et al: Elevated blood cyanide concentrations in victims of smoke inhalation, *N Engl J Med* 325:1761-1766, 1991.

Cahalane M, Demling RF: Early respiratory abnormalities from smoke inhalation, *JAMA* 251:771, 1984.

Chu C: Early and late pathological changes in severe chemical burns to the respiratory tract complicated with acute respiratory failure, *Burns* 8:387, 1982.

Clark CJ et al: Blood carboxyhaemoglobin and cyanide levels in fire survivors, *Lancet* 1:1332-1335, 1981.

Clark WR, Nieman GF: Smoke inhalation, *Burns* 14:473, 1988.

Demling RH: Management of the burn patient, in Shoemaker WC et al (eds): *Textbook of critical care,* ed 2, Philadelphia, 1989, WB Saunders.

Haponik EF: Smoke inhalation injury: some priorities for respiratory care professionals, *Respir Care* 37:609-627, 1992.

Haponik EF et al: Smoke inhalation, *Am Rev Respir Dis* 138:1060-1063, 1988.

Haponik EF, Lykens MG: Acute upper obstruction in burned patients, *Crit Care Report* 2:28-49, 1990.

Haponik EF, Summer WR: Respiratory complications in burned patients: diagnosis and management of inhalation injury, *J Crit Care* 2:121-143, 1987.

Herndon DN et al: Incidence, mortality, pathogenesis, and treatment of pulmonary injury, *J Burn Care Rehabil* 7:184, 1986.

Kinsella J: Smoke inhalation, *Burns* 14:269-279, 1988.

Moritz AR et al: The effects of inhaled heat on the air passages and lungs: an experimental investigation, *Am J Pathol* 21:311-331, 1945.

Myers RAM et al: Subacute sequelae of carbon monoxide poisoning, *Ann Emerg Med* 14:1163, 1985.

Nishimura N, Hiranuman N: Respiratory changes after major burn injury, *Crit Care Med* 10:25, 1982.

Traber DL et al: The pathophysiology of inhalation injury—a review, *Burns* 14:357-364, 1988.

Postoperative Atelectasis

Luce JM: Clinical risk factors for postoperative pulmonary complications, *Respir Care* 29:484, 1984.

Johnson NT, Pierson DJ: The spectrum of pulmonary atelectasis: pathophysiology, diagnosis, and therapy, *Respir Care* 31:1107, 1986.

Marini JJ: Postoperative atelectasis: pathophysiology, clinical importance, and principles of management, *Respir Care* 29:516, 1984.

Hodgkin JE: Preoperative assessment of respiratory function, *Respir Care* 29:496, 1984.

Matthay MA, Wiener-Kronish JP: Respiratory management after surgery, *Chest* 95:424, 1989.

Ricksten SE et al: Effects of periodic positive pressure breathing by mask on postoperative pulmonary function, *Chest* 89:774, 1986.

Medical Dictionaries

Anderson KN, Anderson LE: *Mosby's medical, nursing, and allied health dictionary,* ed 4, St. Louis, 1994, Mosby-Year Book.

McDonough JT: *Stedman's concise medical dictionary,* ed 2, Baltimore, 1994, Williams & Wilkins.

Thomas CL (ed): *Taber's cyclopedic medical dictionary,* ed 17, Philadelphia, 1993, FA Davis.

Index

A